Elsevier's Integrated
Pathology

Elsevier's Integrated
Pathology

Thomas C. King MD, PhD

Associate Professor of Pathology and Laboratory Medicine
Boston University School of Medicine
Boston, Massachusetts

Adjunct Associate Professor of Pathology and
Laboratory Medicine
Brown University School of Medicine
Providence, Rhode Island

Member, Board of Directors
Medpace Inc.
Cincinnati, Ohio

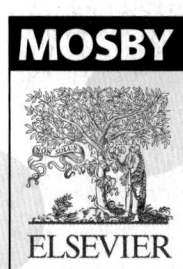

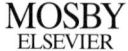

MOSBY
ELSEVIER

1600 John F. Kennedy Blvd
Suite 1800
Philadelphia, PA 19103-2899

ELSEVIER'S INTEGRATED PATHOLOGY

ISBN-13: 978-0-323-04328-1
ISBN-10: 0-323-04328-3

Notice

Knowledge and best practice in this field are constantly changing. As new research and experience broaden our knowledge, changes in practice, treatment and drug therapy may become necessary or appropriate. Readers are advised to check the most current information provided (i) on procedures featured or (ii) by the manufacturer of each product to be administered, to verify the recommended dose or formula, the method and duration of administration, and contraindications. It is the responsibility of the practitioner, relying on their own experience and knowledge of the patient, to make diagnoses, to determine dosages and the best treatment for each individual patient, and to take all appropriate safety precautions. To the fullest extent of the law, neither the Publisher nor the Author assumes any liability for any injury and/or damage to persons or property arising out or related to any use of the material contained in this book.

The Publisher

Library of Congress Cataloging-in-Publication Data

King, Thomas Charles.
  Elsevier's integrated pathology / Thomas C. King.
    p.; cm. — (Elsevier's integrated series)
  ISBN 0-323-04328-3
    1. Pathology. I. Title. II. Title: Integrated pathology. III. Series.
    [DNLM: 1. Pathology. QZ 4 K54e 2007]
  RB118.K562 2007
  616.07—dc22

                              2006046660

Acquisitions Editor: Alex Stibbe
Developmental Editor: Andrew Hall

Working together to grow
libraries in developing countries

www.elsevier.com | www.bookaid.org | www.sabre.org

ELSEVIER | BOOK AID International | Sabre Foundation

Printed in China

Last digit is the print number: 9 8 7 6 5 4 3 2 1

This book is dedicated to the memory of my parents,
Ernest and Violet King

Preface

Pathology involves the investigation of the pathophysiology at the cellular and molecular levels as well as the study and characterization of diseases through the morphologic and biochemical examination of organs, tissues, and body fluids. This focus juxtaposes pathology between clinical medicine and the basic sciences. Much of the detailed features of the pathology of different organ systems can be understood in the context of basic pathophysiologic principles that apply to all cell types. This text is organized first to provide a relatively detailed introduction to these basic pathophysiologic principles (Chapters 1–5), followed by a consideration of important pathologic processes in specific organ systems (Chapters 5–14). This book should provide a comprehensive overview of important pathophysiologic mechanisms as they are understood today, but the short length of this text precludes the complete description of all diseases of each organ system. Emphasis has been placed on common diseases and diseases in which the underlying pathophysiology is becoming clearly understood or which serve as useful examples of important pathophysiologic principles. This text also emphasizes the interactions between different organ systems in disease and the necessity to consider these relationships when diagnosing and treating individual patients.

Thomas C. King, MD, PhD

Editorial Review Board

Contents

Series Preface

How to Use This Book

The idea for Elsevier's Integrated Series came about at a seminar on the USMLE Step 1 exam at an American Medical Student Association (AMSA) meeting. We noticed that the discussion between faculty and students focused on how the exams were becoming increasingly integrated—with case scenarios and questions often combining two or three science disciplines. The students were clearly concerned about how they could best integrate their basic science knowledge.

One faculty member gave some interesting advice: "read through your textbook in, say, biochemistry, and every time you come across a section that mentions a concept or piece of information relating to another basic science—for example, immunology—highlight that section in the book. Then go to your immunology textbook and look up this information, and make sure you have a good understanding of it. When you have, go back to your biochemistry textbook and carry on reading."

This was a great suggestion—if only students had the time, and all of the books necessary at hand, to do it! At Elsevier we thought long and hard about a way of simplifying this process, and eventually the idea for Elsevier's Integrated Series was born.

The series centers on the concept of the *integration box*. These boxes occur throughout the text whenever a link to another basic science is relevant. They're easy to spot in the text—with their color-coded headings and logos. Each box contains a title for the integration topic and then a brief summary of the topic. The information is complete in itself—you probably won't have to go to any other sources—and you have the basic knowledge to use as a foundation if you want to expand your knowledge of the topic.

You can use this book in two ways. First, as a review book . . . When you are using the book for review, the integration boxes will jog your memory on topics you have already covered. You'll be able to reassure yourself that you can identify the link, and you can quickly compare your knowledge of the topic with the summary in the box. The integration boxes might highlight gaps in your knowledge, and then you can use them to determine what topics you need to cover in more detail.

Second, the book can be used as a short text to have at hand while you are taking your course . . . You may come across an integration box that deals with a topic you haven't covered yet, and this will ensure that you're one step ahead in identifying the links to other subjects (especially useful if you're working on a PBL exercise). On a simpler level, the links in the boxes to other sciences and to clinical medicine will help you see clearly the relevance of the basic science topic you are studying. You may already be confident in the subject matter of many of the integration boxes, so they will serve as helpful reminders.

At the back of the book we have included case study questions relating to each chapter so that you can test yourself as you work your way through the book.

Online Version

An online version of the book is available on our Student Consult site. Use of this site is free to anyone who has bought the printed book. Please see the inside front cover for full details on the Student Consult and how to access the electronic version of this book.

In addition to containing USMLE test questions, fully searchable text, and an image bank, the Student Consult site offers additional integration links, both to the other books in Elsevier's Integrated Series and to other key Elsevier textbooks.

Books in Elsevier's Integrated Series

The nine books in the series cover all of the basic sciences. The more books you buy in the series, the more links that are made accessible across the series, both in print and online.

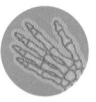 Anatomy and Embryology

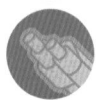 Histology

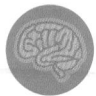 Neuroscience

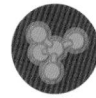 Biochemistry

 Physiology

 Pathology

 Immunology and Microbiology

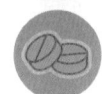 Pharmacology

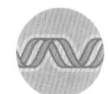 Genetics

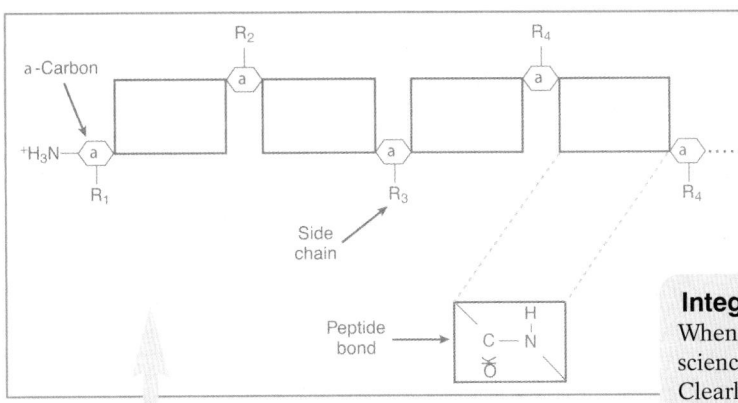

Figure 3-1. The peptide bond linking α-carbons and their side chains together into a polypeptide. The *trans* conformation is favored, producing a rigid structure that restricts freedom of movement except for rotation around bonds that join to the α-carbons.

Integration boxes:
Whenever the subject matter can be related to another science discipline, we've put in an Integration Box. Clearly labeled and color-coded, these boxes include nuggets of information on topics that require an integrated knowledge of the sciences to be fully understood. The material in these boxes is complete in itself, and you can use them as a way of reminding yourself of information you already know and reinforcing key links between the sciences. Or the boxes may contain information you have not come across before, in which case you can use them a springboard for further research or simply to appreciate the relevance of the subject matter of the book to the study of medicine.

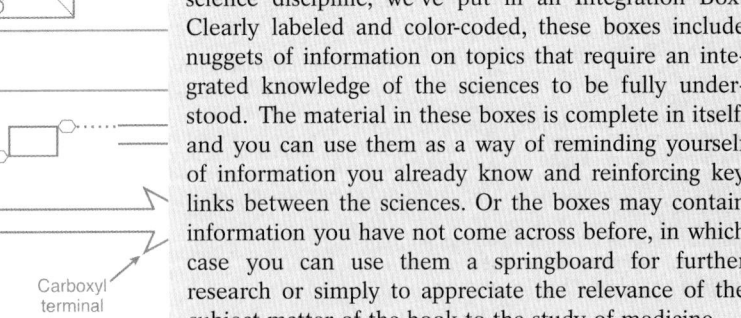

Artwork:
The books are packed with 4-color illustrations and photographs. When a concept can be better explained with a picture, we've drawn one. Where possible, the pictures tell a dynamic story that will help you remember the information far more effectively than a paragraph of text.

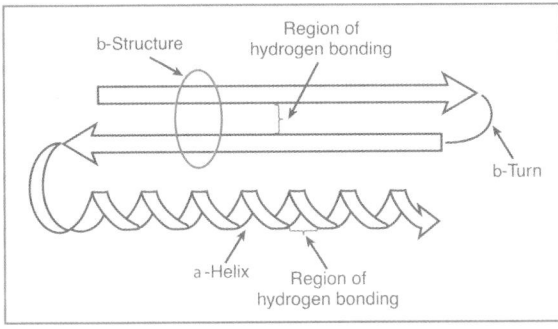

Figure 3-3. Secondary structure includes α-helix and β-pleated sheet (β-sheet).

MICROBIOLOGY

Prion Diseases

Prions (PrP^Sc) are formed from otherwise normal neurologic proteins (PrP) and are responsible for encephalopathies in humans (Creutzfeldt-Jakob disease, kuru), scrapie in sheep, and bovine spongiform encephalopathy. Contact between the normal PrP and PrP^Sc results in conversion of the secondary structure of PrP from predominantly α-helical to predominantly β-pleated sheet. The altered structure of the protein forms long, filamentous aggregates that gradually damage neuronal tissue. The harmful PrP^Sc form is highly resistant to heat, UV irradiation, and protease enzymes.

Since proline has no free hydrogen to contribute to helix stability, it is referred to as a "helix breaker." The α-helix is found in most globular proteins and in some fibrous proteins (e.g., α-keratin).

Text:
Succinct, clearly written text, focusing on the core information you need to know and no more. It's the same level as a carefully prepared course syllabus or lecture notes.

...rmation
...-structure) consists of
... tabilized by hydrogen
...f adjacent sequences.
...ains can be the same (parallel) or opposite (antiparallel) direction. β-Structures are found in 80% of all globular proteins and in silk fibroin.

Supersecondary Structure and Domains

Supersecondary structures, or *motifs*, are characteristic combinations of secondary structure 10–40 residues in length that recur in different proteins. They bridge the gap between the less specific regularity of secondary structure and the highly specific folding of tertiary structure. The same motif can perform similar functions in different proteins.

- The four-helix bundle motif provides a cavity for enzymes to bind prosthetic groups or cofactors.
- The β-barrel motif can bind hydrophobic molecules such as retinol in the interior of the barrel.
- Motifs may also be mixtures of both α and β conformations.

Cell Injury, Cellular Responses to Injury, and Cell Death

1

●●● MECHANISMS OF CELL INJURY

The variety and possible mechanisms of cell injury are almost infinite, but cellular responses to various types of injury are relatively stereotyped. Indeed, many responses to injury are common to almost all types of cells, although the degree of response evoked varies considerably between different cells. Different classes of injury tend to result in relatively similar responses in a single cell type although some tissues or organs can have unique and characteristic responses to some forms of injury. Acute injuries that rapidly cause the death of an organism may not allow sufficient time for typical cellular responses to develop, so characteristic pathologic changes may be minimal or absent. For example, an acute myocardial infarct can cause sudden death and will not show morphologic features of myocyte necrosis because death occurs before the body can respond to this injury.

Cell injury that is severe enough to cause cell death tends to evolve through a series of biochemical and morphologic changes that follow a relatively consistent time scale. Ischemic injury (see Ischemia section) resulting from the occlusion of a tissue's vascular supply is a useful example to illustrate the changes that develop as cells respond to severe injury (Fig. 1-1). Biochemical changes develop within seconds to minutes after injury with marked depletion of intracellular ATP.

Morphologic changes are not apparent by electron microscopy until at least 10 minutes after injury with swelling of the endoplasmic reticulum and dissociation of ribosomes from the rough endoplasmic reticulum. These changes develop directly as a consequence of ATP depletion. Loss of ATP also results in the degradation of ionic gradients across cell membranes because ion pumps are no longer supplied with energy. These changes may be reversed if blood supply is rapidly restored to the injured cells.

Rupture and fragmentation of plasma and organelle membranes (which can be observed by electron microscopy but not by light microscopy) are a signal that irreversible injury has occurred. Approximately 15 minutes after the onset of severe ischemic injury, there is a large influx of calcium into damaged cells through membrane tears. Calcium entry activates lipases and proteases that begin to autodigest the irreversibly injured cell (Fig. 1-2). Light microscopic evidence of cell injury appears well after ultrastructural changes are well developed (usually hours after ischemic injury). These light microscopic changes correspond to the evolution of coagulative necrosis (discussed in detail below). The time scale of these events depends critically on the metabolic activity of the injured cell. Very active cells deplete ATP more quickly (e.g., proximal tubular cells in the kidney) and can undergo irreversible injury within a few minutes, whereas quiescent cells (e.g., collecting duct epithelia in the kidney) may survive more prolonged episodes of ischemia.

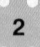

	Pathologic findings					
Time	Seconds	Minutes	15 to 60 minutes		4 to 8 hours	
Normal	No change	No change	ER swelling and ribosome dissociation	Membrane rupture, mitochondrial inclusions	Hypereosinophilia of cytoplasm; other features variable depending on the involved tissue	Karyolysis, coagulative necrosis, influx of neutrophils

Figure 1-1. Time scale of reversible and irreversible cell injury.

BIOCHEMISTRY

Oxidative Phosphorylation

Oxidative phosphorylation occurs in mitochondria and involves five protein complexes as well as electron carriers coenzyme Q and cytochrome c, all of which are embedded in the inner mitochondrial membrane.

These complexes catalyze reactions that sequentially liberate energy and result in the translocation of protons through the inner membrane to create a pH gradient.

This pH gradient is then used to synthesize ATP from ADP by the passage of H^+ protons out of the inner membrane.

- Complex I converts NADH to NAD^+ with the translocation of 2 H^+ protons.
- Complex II and III convert succinate to fumarate and translocate 4 H^+ protons.
- Complex IV converts $\frac{1}{2}$ oxygen molecule to water and translocates 2 H^+ protons.
- Complex V allows reverse passage of 3 H^+ protons down the concentration gradient with the synthesis of one ATP molecule in the mitochondrial matrix.

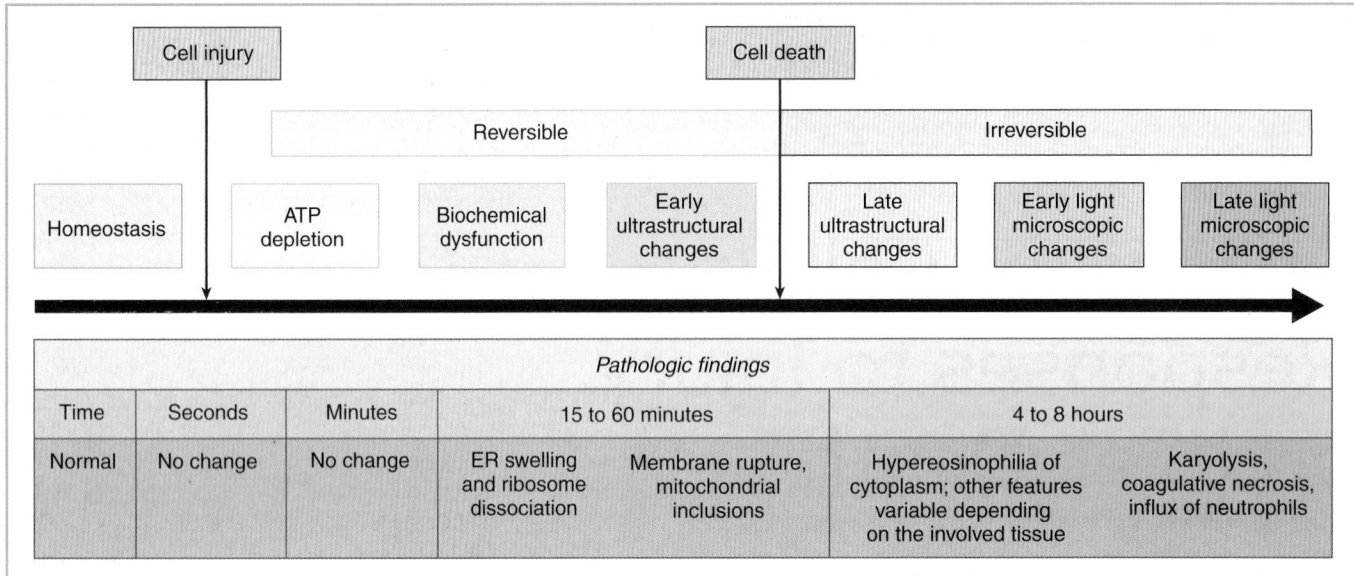

Figure 1-2. Biochemical alterations in ischemic injury.

Hypoxia

Hypoxic injury implies damage to cells resulting only from decreased oxygen tension. This is a relatively unusual pattern of injury in its pure form. Hypoxia can result from decreased atmospheric oxygen concentration, abnormal lung function, and decreased oxygen-carrying capacity in the blood (e.g., severe anemia). Acute hypoxia results in depletion of ATP in cells that triggers a switch to anaerobic glycolysis.

Since the energy yield from glycolysis is much less than from oxidative phosphorylation, energy demands are not met and the continuing decrease in ATP levels results in additional cellular dysfunction. Increased lactic acid produced by glycolysis also decreases intracellular pH, resulting in additional dysfunction.

As discussed above, different types of cells have markedly different metabolic rates and cells with high metabolic rates tend to be injured or killed very rapidly by hypoxia. For example, proximal tubular cells in the kidney may undergo necrosis (acute tubular necrosis, ATN) as a result of even transient hypoxia (Fig. 1-3). The light microscopic changes associated with necrosis include condensation and shrinking (pyknosis) or disappearance (karyolysis) of cell nuclei, which is evident in the necrotic renal tubular cells in Figure 1-3. These cells also show increased eosin staining (hypereosinophilia) of their cytoplasm as a result of the degradation of cellular proteins and loss of cytoplasmic RNA. Other cell types (e.g., neurons) may initiate apoptosis in response to hypoxic injury (see Apoptosis section). Chronic, sublethal hypoxia can activate transcription of genes that can initiate angiogenesis (new blood vessel formation), resulting in neovascularization of the affected tissue.

BIOCHEMISTRY

Glycolysis

Glycolysis metabolizes glucose and rapidly produces a small amount of ATP as well as acid, pyruvate, and NADH that can feed into the Krebs cycle. The overall reaction is

$$\text{Glucose} + 2\,\text{ADP} + 2\,P_i + 2\,\text{NAD}^+ \rightarrow$$
$$2\,\text{pyruvate} + 2\,\text{ATP} + 2\,\text{NADH} + 2\,\text{H}^+ + 2\,\text{H}_2\text{O}$$

Metabolism of glycolysis end products in the Krebs cycle produces much larger amounts of ATP than glycolysis does. In the absence of oxygen, the Krebs cycle is not active and acid and pyruvate can quickly accumulate. Since the amount of ATP produced from glucose by glycolysis is quite small relative to oxidative phosphorylation, energy charge declines rapidly in most hypoxic cells even if large glucose stores are available.

Ischemia

Ischemic injury is caused by diminished or absent blood flow. The main mechanism of injury in ischemia is hypoxia (as described above). Ischemic injury also results in more rapid and severe cellular acidosis than pure hypoxic injury because the absence of blood flow causes the localized accumulation of cellular metabolic by-products (e.g., lactic acid from anaerobic glycolysis). Ischemia may be relative or complete, in which case it usually results in coagulative necrosis. Relative ischemia can occur as a result of low blood pressure (hypotension), marked increases in cellular metabolism, and vascular stenosis. Relative ischemia typically results in cellular dysfunction but does not cause death in most cell types. Some cell types that are more sensitive to ischemic damage (e.g., neurons) may undergo apoptosis or necrosis while other cell types remain viable. Complete ischemia most often results from blockage of an arterial branch that causes infarction of the tissue supplied by that blood vessel. If an occluded blood vessel is reopened soon after ischemic injury, reversibly injured cells may recover. This situation is referred to as reperfusion and has become more common in the setting of myocardial infarction treated emergently by angioplasty and thrombolysis. Reperfusion may be too late to permit recovery of irreversibly injured cells and is often associated with hemorrhage owing to ischemic damage to endothelial cells in blood vessels that occurs prior to restoration of blood flow.

Free Radical–Induced Injury

Free radicals are active chemical compounds that can react directly with proteins, lipids, and DNA. Biologic free radicals

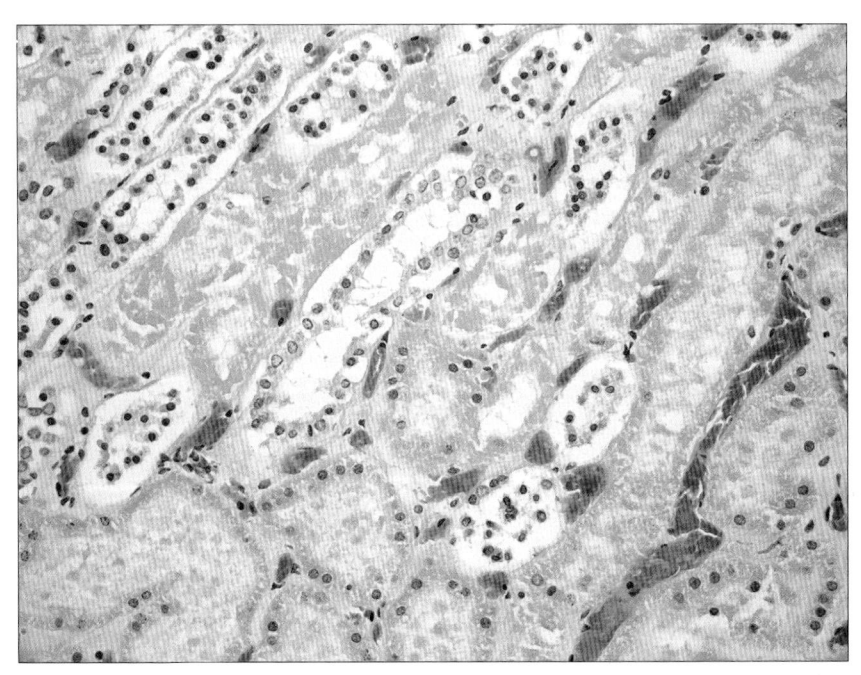

Figure 1-3. Acute tubular necrosis in the kidney. Note the eosinophilic staining of proximal tubular cells with loss of nuclear staining. The high metabolic rate of proximal tubular cells results in their rapid necrosis under ischemic or hypoxic conditions. Less active distal tubule and collecting duct epithelial cells appear morphologically normal in this photomicrograph.

are generated predominantly from oxygen metabolism. High oxygen tension and increased oxidative phosphorylation favor the formation of free radicals and can lead to severe cellular injury if protective mechanisms are not effective. Cellular macromolecules that react chemically with free radicals (phospholipids and proteins) often lose their normal function and cannot be repaired. These oxidized macromolecules are not effectively degraded by lysosomal enzymes, and oxidized protein and lipid fragments tend to accumulate in cells with free radical damage. These oxidized macromolecules tend to aggregate to form lipofuscin pigment that is retained in the damaged cell and provides an indication of the degree of oxidative stress a cell has experienced. Oxidative phosphorylation and β–fatty acid oxidation in mitochondria produce significant oxidative stress that may result in mitochondrial damage and trigger apoptosis by releasing mitochondrial proteins (e.g., cytochrome c) into the cytoplasm.

Specific enzyme systems are present in all cells to react with and detoxify free radicals. Superoxide dismutase (SOD) and catalase are important components of this system (Fig. 1-4). Cells that are frequently exposed to oxidative stress (high oxygen tension, very active oxidative phosphorylation, or β-oxidation of fatty acids) tend to express these enzyme systems at higher levels. Glutathione is another important protectant from free radical damage. Sulfhydryl groups on glutathione act as free radicals scavengers, and oxidation of glutathione can prevent damage to key cellular components. Hepatocytes contain relatively large amounts of glutathione to manage oxidative stress from the metabolism of various compounds and drugs by their cytochrome P-450 enzymes. Depletion of glutathione renders hepatocytes sensitive to free radical damage that can result in massive hepatic necrosis (e.g., acetaminophen poisoning). β-Carotene and other vitamins can act as free radical scavengers and may assist in detoxifying free radicals.

Inflammatory Injury

Inflammatory cells are very important in the response to injury in all tissues. Inflammation is the primary host response to infection, but it is also an essential component of the response to most other forms of injury. One consequence of the recruitment of inflammatory cells is the generation of large amounts of oxygen-derived free radicals by these cells. Cytokines, growth factors, and degradative enzymes also are produced and released into the extracellular environment by inflammatory cells. These molecules and proteins can damage parenchymal cells in inflamed tissues and may lead to cell death. Other forms of immune-mediated injury caused by antibodies and activated T cells may directly damage or kill parenchymal cells (e.g., viral infection and autoimmune disease; Fig. 1-5).

Infectious Injury

Infectious agents can damage cells and tissues directly by the production of toxins and/or degradative enzymes. Viruses directly infect host cells and may produce cell dysfunction or death. In addition to their direct effects, almost all infectious agents stimulate an immune and/or inflammatory response that can cause severe cellular damage.

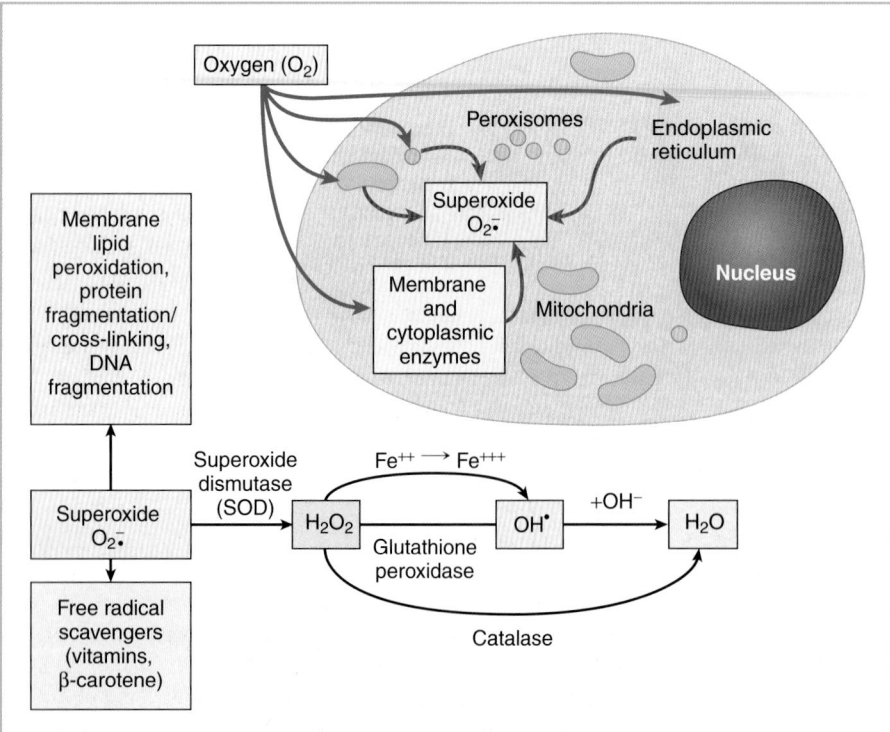

Figure 1-4. Generation, production, and detoxification of oxygen free radicals.

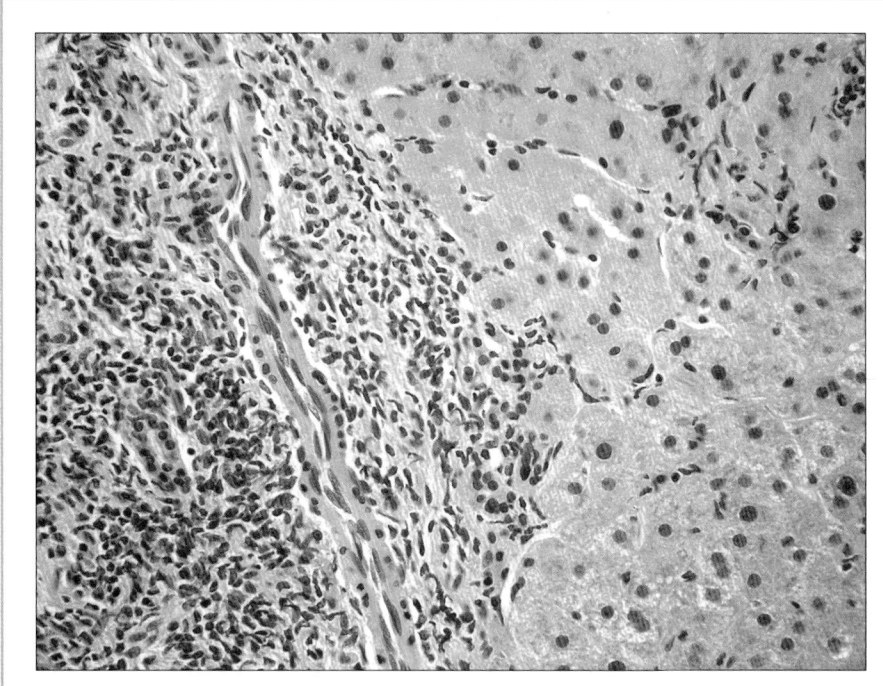

Figure 1-5. Immune-mediated injury in the liver. Microscopic section from a case of chronic hepatitis C virus infection showing piecemeal necrosis at the periphery of a portal tract. Individual hepatocytes are surrounded by T cells that trigger them to undergo apoptosis.

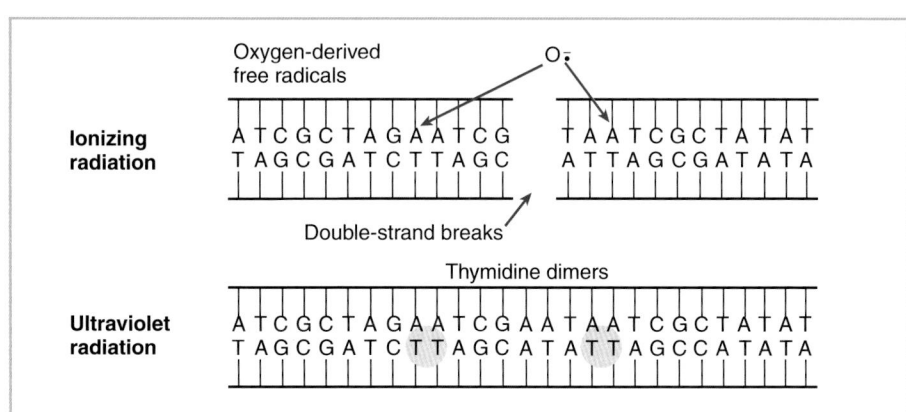

Figure 1-6. Radiation-induced injury.

Physical Injury

Physical injury typically refers to mechanical trauma but additionally includes injury secondary to solar and ionizing radiation. Mechanical injury can result from projectiles such as bullets, penetrating trauma, or blunt trauma. Trauma can initiate infection by directly introducing microorganisms (penetrating trauma) or by causing the breaks in host defenses (skin, mucosal surfaces, or intestinal tract perforation). Trauma can also damage tissues and organs by transmitting energy (e.g., deceleration of a bullet passing through tissue can transfer large amounts of kinetic energy resulting in damage to or destruction of a large tissue volume around the bullet track). In addition, trauma can result in vascular damage that causes hemorrhage.

Ultraviolet radiation can damage collagen to the extracellular matrix, but its main toxicity results from direct interaction with DNA to form thymidine dimers (Fig. 1-6).

Thymidine dimers may trigger apoptosis if they are not effectively repaired, or cell division may result in mutations in daughter cells. Damage from ultraviolet radiation is limited to exposed skin and mucous membranes, whereas ionizing radiation can penetrate deep within the body.

Ionizing radiation can produce free radicals by interaction with water molecules, or it may directly interact with DNA, resulting in single- and double-strand breaks that may not be repairable.

High levels of ionizing radiation can be acutely fatal because of severe free radical damage to neurons while somewhat lower doses can result in death subacutely because of extensive damage to replicating progenitor cells (e.g., gastrointestinal tract and bone marrow). The rapid cycling of progenitor cells means that a high percentage are undergoing replication at all times. After radiation injury, there is insufficient time for most progenitor cells to repair DNA damage before they enter the cell cycle. These cells then

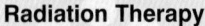
either trigger apoptosis or propagate mutations in their daughter cells. Loss of progenitor cells causes the breakdown of the mucosal layer after hours to days as well as marked myelosuppression with bone marrow failure over the course of days.

Chemical Injury

Chemical injury ranges from direct damage to cells and tissues by caustic agents (e.g., strong acid or bases) to damage due to toxins that may have very specific targets in a limited number of cell types (e.g., organophosphate compounds that simulate neurotransmitters in neurons, causing uncontrolled depolarization that can lead to cell death). Some chemicals result in the production of toxic substances (e.g., free radical production in hepatocytes) that are the ultimate mediators of injury. Many chemicals and drugs must be metabolized (usually by the liver's cytochrome P-450 system) before they are toxic to cells. Genetic polymorphisms in these drug-metabolizing enzymes in each individual can result in great differences in the effective doses of drugs and in the potential to generate toxic metabolites from various compounds.

Nutritional Injury

Nutritional injury corresponds to a lack of adequate intake of calories or protein that results in cellular or tissue dysfunction. Caloric malnutrition impairs a cell's ability to generate ATP and to maintain normal cellular functions. Protein malnutrition with adequate caloric intake can result in the inability to synthesize normal cellular proteins because of an inadequate amount of essential amino acids (i.e., amino acids that cannot be synthesized de novo). The consequences of nutritional injury differ greatly in children and adults. Growth retardation in children may be irreversible. The developing nervous system is particularly sensitive to both calorie and protein malnutrition. Deficiency of essential vitamins can lead to marked cellular dysfunction, which may cause irreversible damage to some specialized cells (e.g., severe vitamin A deficiency can cause blindness).

Genetic Injury

Genetic injury can result from the absence or abnormality of an essential enzymatic activity. Storage diseases result from the accumulation of metabolic products that normally would be digested and removed by normal degradative enzymes. Storage diseases tend to affect long-lived cells most severely. For example, Tay-Sachs disease results from the accumulation of sphingomyelin (a normal metabolic product) in neurons because the enzyme activity that would normally degrade sphingomyelin has been inactivated by homozygous mutation. More subtle forms of genetic injury may result from changes in cellular metabolism that predispose to, or accelerate, different types of disease (e.g., deficiency of the low-density lipoprotein receptor results in markedly increased cholesterol levels in blood that greatly accelerate atherosclerosis). Genetic polymorphisms can cause more subtle disease predispositions (see Chapter 4).

Aging and Senescence

Normal aging is not usually considered a pathologic condition although dysfunctional changes associated with cellular aging are not always distinct from disease processes. Aging almost always results in a decreased capacity of cells to proliferate and to respond to injury. Cells from older individuals have decreased replicative capacity because of age-dependent shortening of the length of telomeres at the ends of their chromosomes. Telomeres consist of numerous repeats of the sequence $TTAGGG_n$ and are on the order of 5 to 15 kilobases in length in normal cells in young individuals. DNA

Telomerase Enzymatic Structure

Chromosomal telomeres range from 5 to 15 kilobases in length in normal cells in younger individuals. As a consequence of the $3' \rightarrow 5'$ directionality of DNA polymerase, approximately 50 to 200 nucleotides of telomere sequence are lost from the lagging DNA strand during cell division. If these lost sequences are not replaced, cells become unable to initiate S phase after approximately 60 to 70 doublings (the so-called Hayflick limit). Telomerase can replace these sequences and restore telomeres to full length to prevent cellular senescence.

Telomerase is a ribonucleoprotein complex that consists of the TERT (telomerase reverse transcriptase) protein (130 kD) and the TERC (telomerase RNA component) in combination with several smaller accessory proteins including GAR1 and dyskerin that are all required for normal telomerase function. The TERC has a stem loop structure that provides the template sequence (CCCTAA) that codes for synthesis of telomere repeats.

Mutations or deletions in any of these proteins or in the TERC can cause loss of telomerase function and result in cellular senescence.

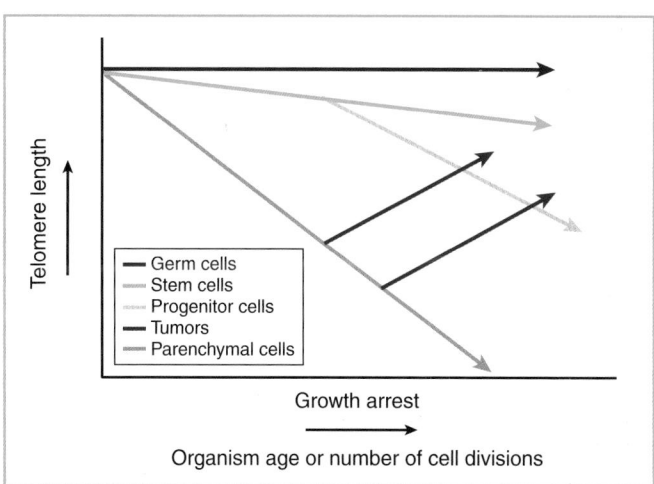

Figure 1-7. Maintenance of telomere length in different cell types.

syndromes (e.g., progeria) result in the rapid senescence of many tissues that resembles normal aging but results in death in childhood.

●●● CELLULAR RESPONSES TO INJURY

Analysis of cellular and tissue responses to injury is the core of the discipline of pathology. Because cells and organ systems respond to insults in a relatively stereotyped manner, these responses can be used to infer the cause or nature of injury in many cases. Cellular responses include dysfunctional changes in injured cells as well as inflammation in response to different insults. Many cells undergo (compensatory or adaptive) changes in response to injury or alterations in their environment. Tissues and organs can also undergo adaptive changes that are coordinated to manage internal or environmental stresses (e.g., alterations in heart rate and blood pressure). Coordination of these changes can occur at many levels including cell-cell interactions, localized signaling (paracrine signaling), and hormonal and neural signaling. The detailed repertoire of responses of different cells and tissues to different forms of injury occupies the bulk of later chapters in this text. Some basic mechanisms of response to injury are shared by most cell types and serve as a basis for understanding the more complicated responses of tissues and organs. These basic mechanisms include hyperplasia, hypertrophy, metaplasia, and atrophy (Fig. 1-8).

Hyperplasia

Hyperplasia is an increase in cell number (due to cell replication) in response to various stimuli. For some cell types (so-called "labile tissues"), replication is constantly required to replace lost cells (e.g., replication of basal cells in the skin provides a constant supply of new cells to replace those desquamated from the surface and is essential to maintain a steady state). Hyperplasia in a labile tissue can be accom-

polymerase synthesizes DNA only in a 5' to 3' direction, so the terminal ends of chromosomes cannot be fully copied during each cycle of replication. Telomeres normally prevent chromosomes from adhering to one another during mitosis, and their absence causes cells to trigger apoptosis (see below) and die. This process would eventually result in the disappearance of telomeres after many cycles of cell division. Cells that normally replicate many times (e.g., stem cells and progenitor cells) express an enzyme called telomerase, which replaces lost telomere sequences by adding new repetitive DNA sequences.

Telomerase activity declines in most cells with aging (Fig. 1-7), resulting in age-dependent telomere shortening that ultimately results in growth arrest (senescence). Normal stem cells continue to express telomerase and maintain telomere length. Genetic abnormalities in telomerase can cause stem cell failure resulting in some cases of aplastic anemia (see Chapter 11). Telomerase expression is frequently reactivated in malignant tumors, allowing them to escape from growth control by senescence.

Accumulated free radical stress in mitochondria can lead to dysfunction that may result in decreased energy production or trigger apoptosis. Apoptosis of permanent cells results in permanent loss of function, and this mechanism may also be important in aging. Higher caloric intake in lower animals is known to result in a shorter life span, and mitochondrial stress may explain these results.

Some of the changes observed in normal aging are accelerated in specific pathologic conditions (e.g., Alzheimer's disease), and this acceleration usually is considered pathologic (e.g., familial Alzheimer's disease). A few rare genetic

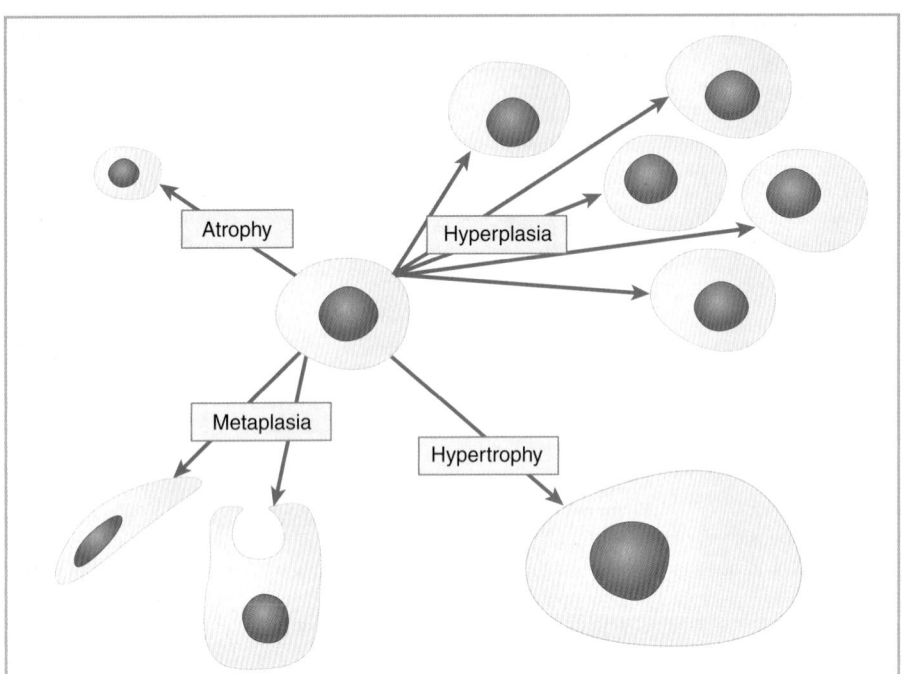

Figure 1-8. Mechanisms of cellular adaptation.

Labile (constant active self-renewal)	**Stable** (low level of renewal with capacity to replace cells)	**Permanent** (no capacity to replace cells)
Gastrointestinal mucosa	Liver	Adult neurons
Skin	Renal tubular cells	Renal glomeruli
Hematopoietic cells	Glial cells in the CNS	Retinal epithelial cells

Figure 1-9. Properties of labile, stable, and permanent tissues.

plished by increasing the replicative rate of precursor cells or by recruiting additional cells into the replicating pool. Increased proliferation may maintain steady state in the face of increased cell loss or may lead to a net increase in the number of mature cells present. "Stable tissues" have a much lower rate of cell turnover in steady state and so require a much lower rate of cell division to maintain homeostasis under normal conditions. Many stable tissues such as the liver retain a robust capacity for hyperplasia in response to injury or destruction of parenchymal cells (Fig. 1-9). These stable tissues have the capacity to greatly increase the number of replicating progenitor cells to replace cells destroyed by various forms of injury. When the injury has been repaired, the replicative rate usually diminishes to maintain a steady-state number of parenchymal cells. A third type of tissue often is called "permanent tissue" because its parenchymal cells have no capacity for hyperplasia or self-renewal in response to injury. The parenchymal cells in permanent tissues (e.g., neurons in the adult central nervous system and cardiac myocytes) are long-lived cells that can survive throughout a person's lifetime under normal conditions. If these cells are destroyed, however, there is no normal, effective way to

replace them (although there may be the potential to artificially manipulate stem cells to replace some types of "permanent" cell).

Sustained hyperplasia in response to chronic injury can strain the replicative capacity of a tissue. The progenitor pool may become inadequate to manage demand for new cells, or nutritional demands to support cell replication (vitamins, amino acids, calories) may not be met. Marked and prolonged hyperplasia may also predispose to the development of genetic abnormalities in cells that may eventually lead to unregulated cell growth (i.e., dysplasia and neoplasia; see below). Hyperplasia by itself may produce significant dysfunction (e.g., nodular hyperplasia of the prostate gland tends to block urine flow, leading to urinary retention and bladder infection, and metabolic syndromes can result from hyperplasia of endocrine organs).

Hypertrophy

Hypertrophy is an increase in the size of cells (or tissues) in response to various stimuli. A typical example is muscular hypertrophy in response to exercise. Exercise stimulates skeletal and cardiac muscle fibers to increase in diameter and to accumulate more structural contractile proteins. Hypertrophy may occur as a compensatory response to injury when parenchymal cells are damaged or lost. For instance, following myocardial infarction, cardiac myocytes cannot undergo hyperplasia to replace destroyed muscle fibers but residual myocytes enlarge (hypertrophy) in an attempt to replace some of the function of the lost myofibers (Fig. 1-10). Most forms of hypertrophy are actually far more complex than a simple increase in cell size (e.g., hypertrophy of cardiac myocytes is associated with changes in the pattern of gene expression that result in the reactivation of embryonic genes and alter the structure of contractile proteins and modify the density of hormone receptors). Physiologic hypertrophy is usually adaptive and improves function. Pathologic hypertrophy may be adaptive in some situations but often results in changes in gene expression that can exacerbate organ dysfunction.

Atrophy

Atrophy is essentially the opposite of hypertrophy and results in a decrease in cell size. Atrophic cells typically have diminished amounts of specialized organelles within their cytoplasm and are less functionally capable than normal cells. Atrophy of some cell types occurs as a consequence of normal aging and decreases in trophic hormone levels (e.g., endometrial and ovarian atrophy after menopause). Atrophy may also result from some forms of injury that diminish or block neural or hormonal stimulation of a tissue (e.g., marked skeletal muscle atrophy occurs if neural stimulation is inter-rupted for a prolonged period of time—so-called denervation atrophy). Indeed, inactivity (bed rest) or exposure to microgravity (in prolonged space flight) causes marked atrophy of the musculoskeletal system that can result in severe dysfunction.

Atrophy may also result from the accumulation of abnormal substances in a cell's cytoplasm that displaces organelles and cytoskeletal components (see Dystrophic Changes and Abnormal Accumulations section) (Figs. 1-11 and 1-12). Similarly, expansion of the extracellular matrix (e.g., accumulation of abnormal materials or fibrosis) can compress parenchymal cells and result in atrophy.

Metaplasia

Metaplasia is the conversion from one type of normal adult cell to another type of normal adult cell. The most common types of metaplasia observed by pathologists involve the conversion from squamous to glandular cells and vice versa. Glandular metaplasia can occur as a response to injury, as can occur in the distal esophagus with acid reflux from the stomach. This form of chronic injury may induce the conversion of the inflamed squamous mucosa to glandular mucosa that has many features of normal small intestinal mucosa. Metaplasia can also occur as a normal physiologic response. An example of physiologic metaplasia is the squamous metaplasia that occurs in the uterine cervix during the menstrual cycle as the squamocolumnar junction migrates across the transformation zone (Fig. 1-13). Although some forms of metaplasia are adaptive and may mitigate the effects of chronic injury, other types of metaplasia can result in

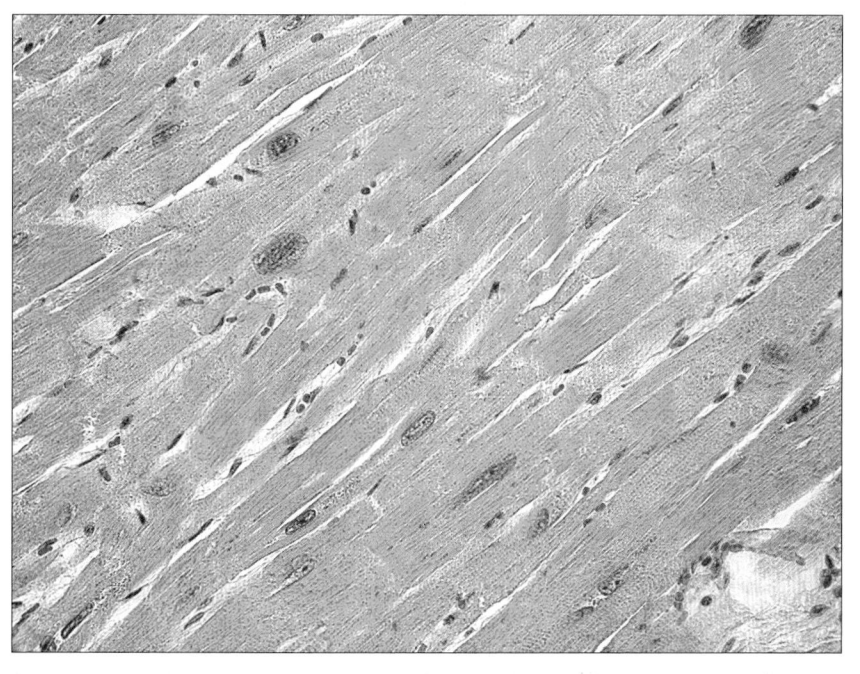

Figure 1-10. Hypertrophy of cardiac myocytes. Photomicrograph of cardiac myocytes showing increased fiber diameter and increased nuclear size. Hypertrophy of cardiac myocytes is accompanied by an increase in cellular DNA content (polyploidy) with corresponding nuclear enlargement and change from an oval to a rectangular configuration (so-called "boxcar" nuclei).

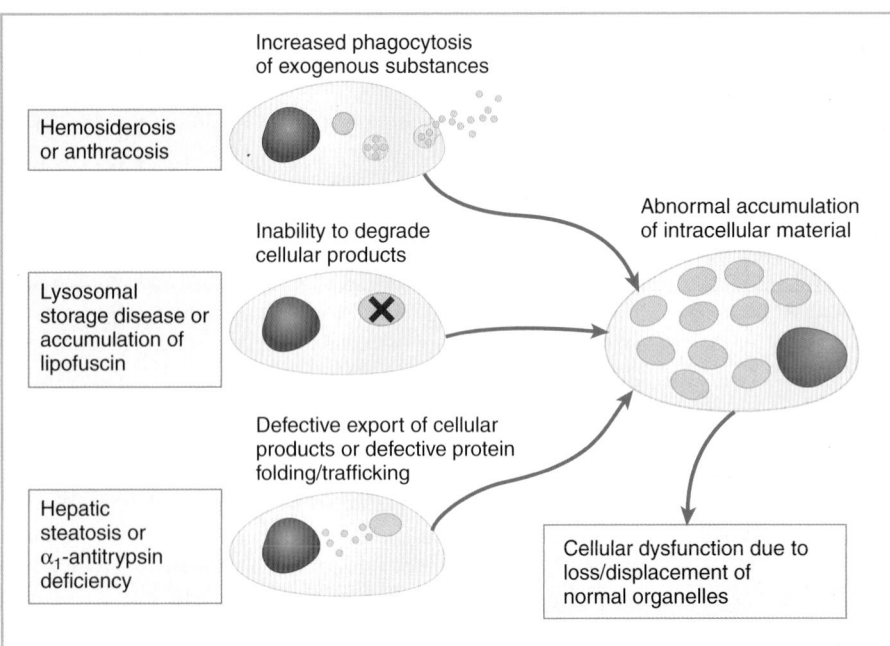

Figure 1-11. Intracellular accumulations.

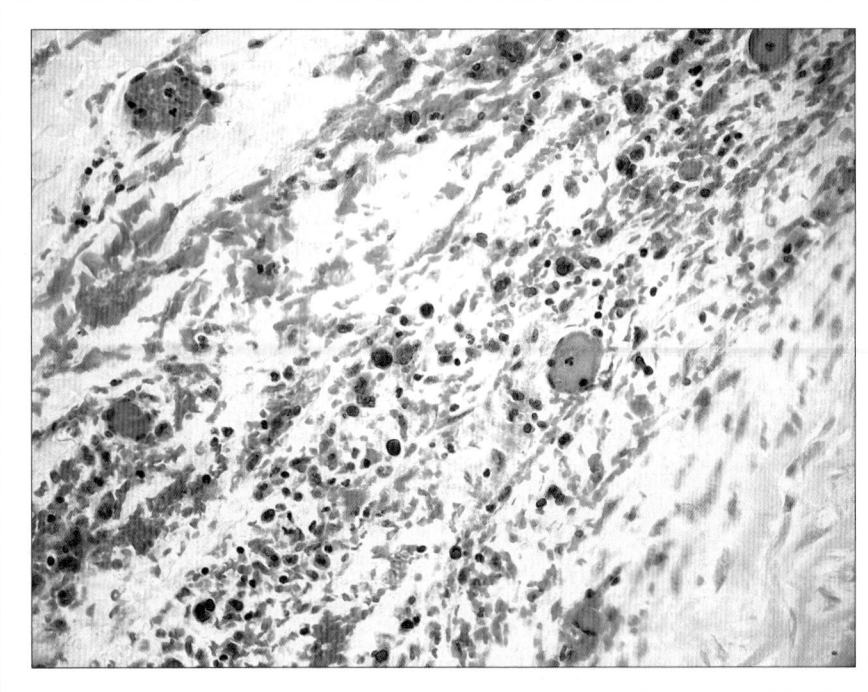

Figure 1-12. Intracellular accumulation of hemosiderin. Hemosiderin predominantly derives from the recycling of iron in senescent red blood cells. Hemosiderin accumulates in macrophages that phagocytize red blood cells and appears as golden brown, granular pigment forming slightly refractile globules in routine sections.

significant dysfunction. For example, squamous metaplasia of respiratory epithelium develops as a consequence of cigarette smoking and results in the loss of the normal mucociliary blanket, which is a major host barrier to infection and toxic substances in the environment. Most forms of metaplasia are reversible if the stimulus is removed, whereas a few (e.g., intestinal metaplasia of the esophagus in response to gastric acid reflux) tend to be permanent once they are established.

Dysplasia

Dysplasia implies that changes have taken place in affected cells that predispose them to develop into a malignant neoplasm. Dysplasia is not usually classified as a response to injury although many types of dysplasia can mimic cellular responses to injury and inflammation. Indeed, in some inflammatory processes, it may not be possible to reliably distinguish

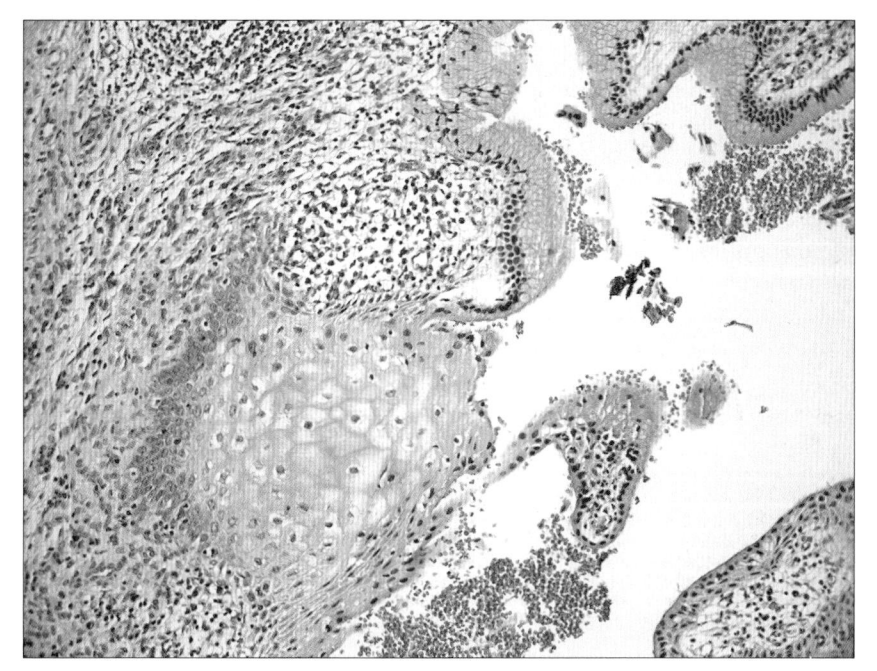

Figure 1-13. Squamous metaplasia at the transition zone of the uterine cervix. Metaplastic squamous epithelium is present in the central portion of the photomicrograph and is surrounded by glandular mucosa composed of columnar cells. This is a physiologic form of metaplasia.

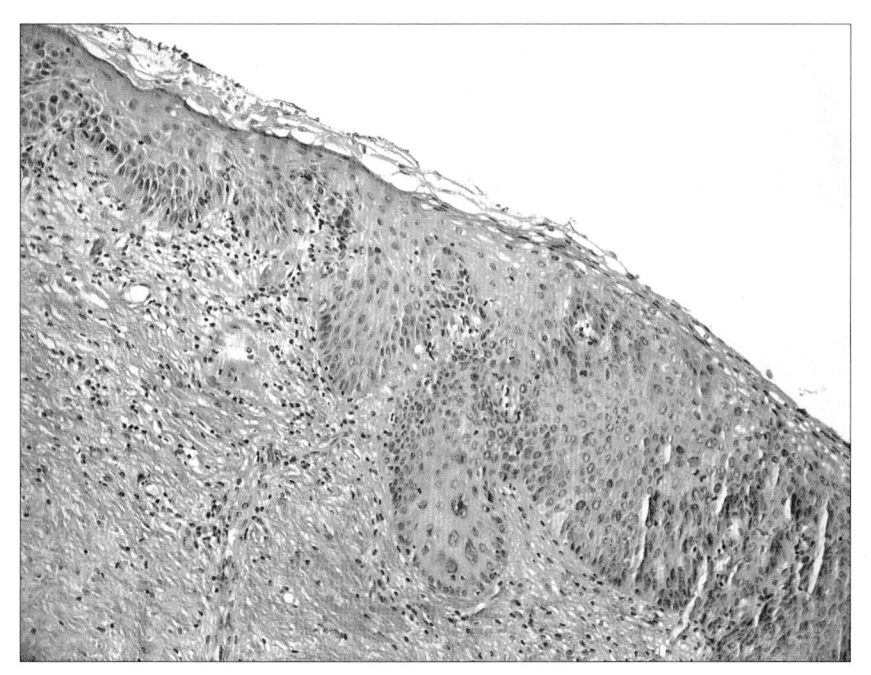

Figure 1-14. Squamous dysplasia of the uterine cervix. Dysplasia is a preneoplastic phenomenon that is always pathologic. There is increased nuclear size and disruption of normal, orderly maturation as squamous cells migrate upward from the basal layer toward the surface.

metaplasia from reactive cellular changes in response to inflammation that are not preneoplastic. Dysplasia is usually judged on the basis of changes in cell nuclei (irregularity of the nuclear envelope and of chromatin distribution), changes in the ratio of nuclear area to cytoplasmic area, and abnormalities in epithelial maturation. Dysplasia can be observed in mucosal surfaces in response to chronic injury (e.g., chemical injury in the bronchi of cigarette smokers or viral injury in the setting of dysplasia of the uterine cervix; Fig. 1-14). Dysplasia is almost always associated with somatic genetic changes in affected cells that can ultimately result in the formation of malignant tumors (see Chapter 5).

Dystrophic Changes and Abnormal Accumulations

Cells have complex mechanisms for sorting newly synthesized proteins to different subcellular compartments and for exporting them into the extracellular environment. These mechanisms involve chaperone proteins, which also assist in the proper folding of different proteins and help prevent their aggregation. Protein denaturation (formation of an abnormal tertiary structure) and aggregation (abnormal clumping of proteins to form macromolecular aggregates) can produce insoluble precipitates in the cell that may accumulate and

cause cellular dysfunction. Chaperone proteins associate with newly forming peptides to ensure that they achieve the appropriate tertiary structure and then help coordinate their movement to the appropriate cellular compartment (Fig. 1-15A). "Heat-shock proteins" are a form of chaperone protein that can actively refold denatured proteins and restore them to normal conformation (see Fig. 1-15B). Heat-shock proteins can be induced by many forms of cellular stress in addition to temperature changes (as their name implies). Genetic abnormalities of some proteins may cause them to be misdirected or misfolded by chaperones, resulting in their abnormal accumulation in various cellular or

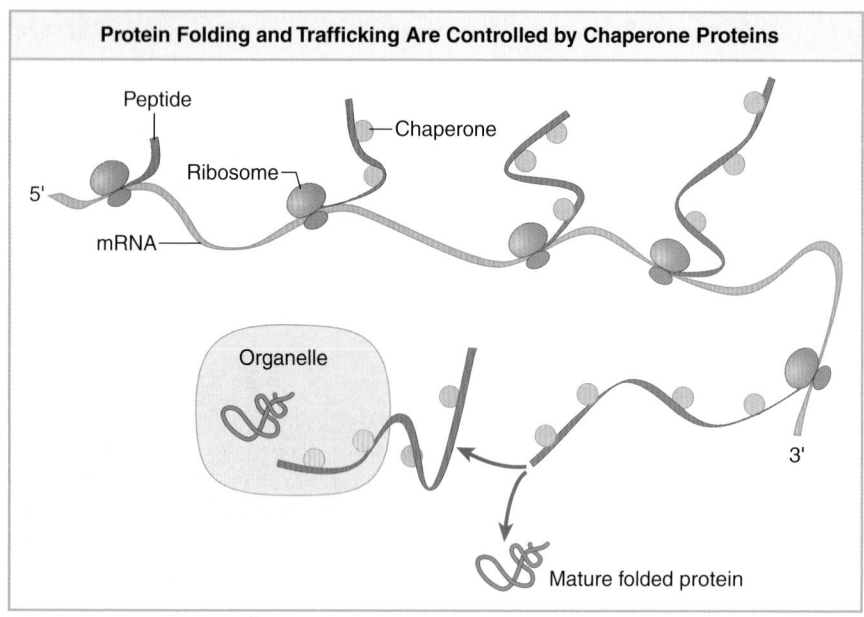

A

Figure 1-15. A, Nascent protein folding and intracellular trafficking. **B,** Refolding or destruction of denatured or abnormal cellular proteins.

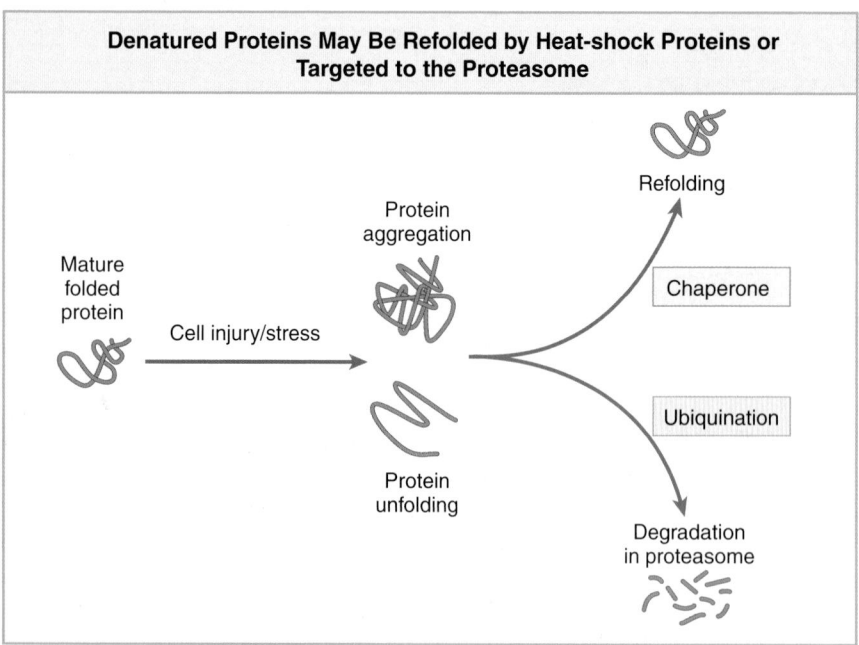

B

extracellular compartments. Proteins that cannot be refolded may be ubiquitinated (i.e., multiple ubiquitin moieties are added by ubiquitin ligase), which targets them to the proteosome for destruction.

Some proteins or fragments of proteins may be resistant to degradative enzymes because of their abnormal conformation or posttranslational modification, and they may accumulate over time. In long-lived cells (especially neurons), such accumulations can result in cellular dysfunction by displacement of normal organelles. Some abnormal materials may be directly toxic to cells. Genetic abnormalities and polymorphisms in chaperone proteins and proteases may also predispose to the mistargeting or accumulation of proteins or peptides with abnormal conformations that cause disease.

Cells and the extracellular matrix may also undergo dystrophic changes as a result of different types of damage (e.g., exposure of dermal collagen to ultraviolet light) or as a result of abnormal metabolic conditions in individuals (e.g., abnormally high concentrations of calcium and phosphorus in the blood can cause widespread calcification of normal tissues). Inadequate nutrition (oxygen and other nutrients) can cause cells to lose some of their differentiated functions and show morphologic evidence of dysfunction. For example, myocytolysis (Fig. 1-16A) occurs in subendocardial myocytes in ischemic heart disease. The affected myocytes are nutritionally deprived and develop vacuolization as a morphologic sign of their underlying cellular dysfunction.

Calcification

Abnormal cells, tissues, and extracellular matrix components often develop an increased affinity for calcium phosphate

---

BIOCHEMISTRY

Proteasome

The 26S proteasome (2.5 megadaltons) is a large multimeric structure composed of one 20S proteolytic complex (a large, barrel-shaped, multiprotein complex) and two 19S regulatory complexes. Proteasomes are present in both cytoplasm and nucleus.

Proteins that are targeted for destruction (e.g., proteins with abnormal folding, phosphorylation-dependent conformational changes, etc.) are ubiquitinated by ubiquitin ligase (E_{3S}). This ligase covalently links the C-terminal glycine of ubiquitin to specific lysine residues on target proteins. Additional ubiquitin molecules are added to lysine 48 on the attached ubiquitin to form a chain.

Polyubiquitinated proteins are directed to the proteasome, where they are recognized and unfolded by the 19S regulatory complex. They are fed into the 20S proteolytic complex and degraded in an energy-dependent process. The ubiquitin monomers are recycled by E_{1S} and E_{2S} (ubiquitin activating and carrier proteins).

Proteasome inhibitors can be used as antineoplastic agents and may function in part by inhibiting the destruction of IκB to block NFκB signaling.

---

binding, which can result in calcification. Calcification typically occurs in fat necrosis and results from the saponification of calcium salts (see Fig. 1-16B). Calcification in abnormal tissue is referred to as dystrophic calcification and may cause additional dysfunction of the affected tissue. High extracellular levels of calcium and phosphorus (e.g., in patients with chronic renal failure) can result in calcification of normal tissues, and this process is referred to as "metastatic" calcification.

Uric Acid

A diet that is high in protein content produces larger amounts of uric acid as a waste product. If the concentration of uric acid in the urine or in the extracellular matrix exceeds its solubility, uric acid crystals spontaneously form. These needle-shaped crystals tend to puncture the membranes of inflammatory cells that attempt to engulf them, releasing proteolytic enzymes and causing a marked inflammatory reaction. Over time, this can result in the formation of masses of extracellular uric acid (tophi) with associated fibrosis. Crystallization of uric acid in the kidney can block individual tubules and may form larger stones that cause obstruction of urine outflow, possibly damaging or destroying the kidney. Some individuals are prone to gout because their metabolism favors the formation of uric acid or its crystallization.

Lipofuscin

Lipofuscin (often referred to as "wear and tear" pigment) results from the oxidation of membrane lipids and proteins by free radicals. These abnormal molecules are not readily degraded by cellular enzymes and accumulate over time as gray-brown pigment aggregates in long-lived cells such as cardiac myocytes and hepatocytes (see Fig. 1-16C). The presence of large amounts of intracellular lipofuscin may be an indication of unusual oxidative stress or defective detoxification of free radicals in the affected cells. So called "brown atrophy" of the myocardium results from a combination of cellular atrophy and the accumulation of large amounts of lipofuscin pigment.

Amyloid

Amyloid is an abnormal protein composed of peptides or peptide fragments with a β-pleated sheet conformation at the molecular level. Amyloid tends to form fibrils that are 7 nm in diameter and can be visualized by electron microscopy. Multiple different proteins or protein fragments can give rise to amyloid, but some amino acid sequences are much more likely than others to assume a β-pleated sheet conformation. Polymorphisms in some proteins result in amino acid substitutions that greatly predispose to the formation of amyloid. Alternatively, abnormal cleavage of some proteins may release peptide fragments that tend to form amyloid.

Amyloid accumulates in the extracellular space (see Fig. 1-16D) and causes damage by compressing normal parenchymal cells and by altering the physical properties of the extracellular matrix (e.g., amyloid deposition in the heart results in both atrophy of cardiac myocytes and in a stiffer extracellular matrix that resists diastolic filling of the left

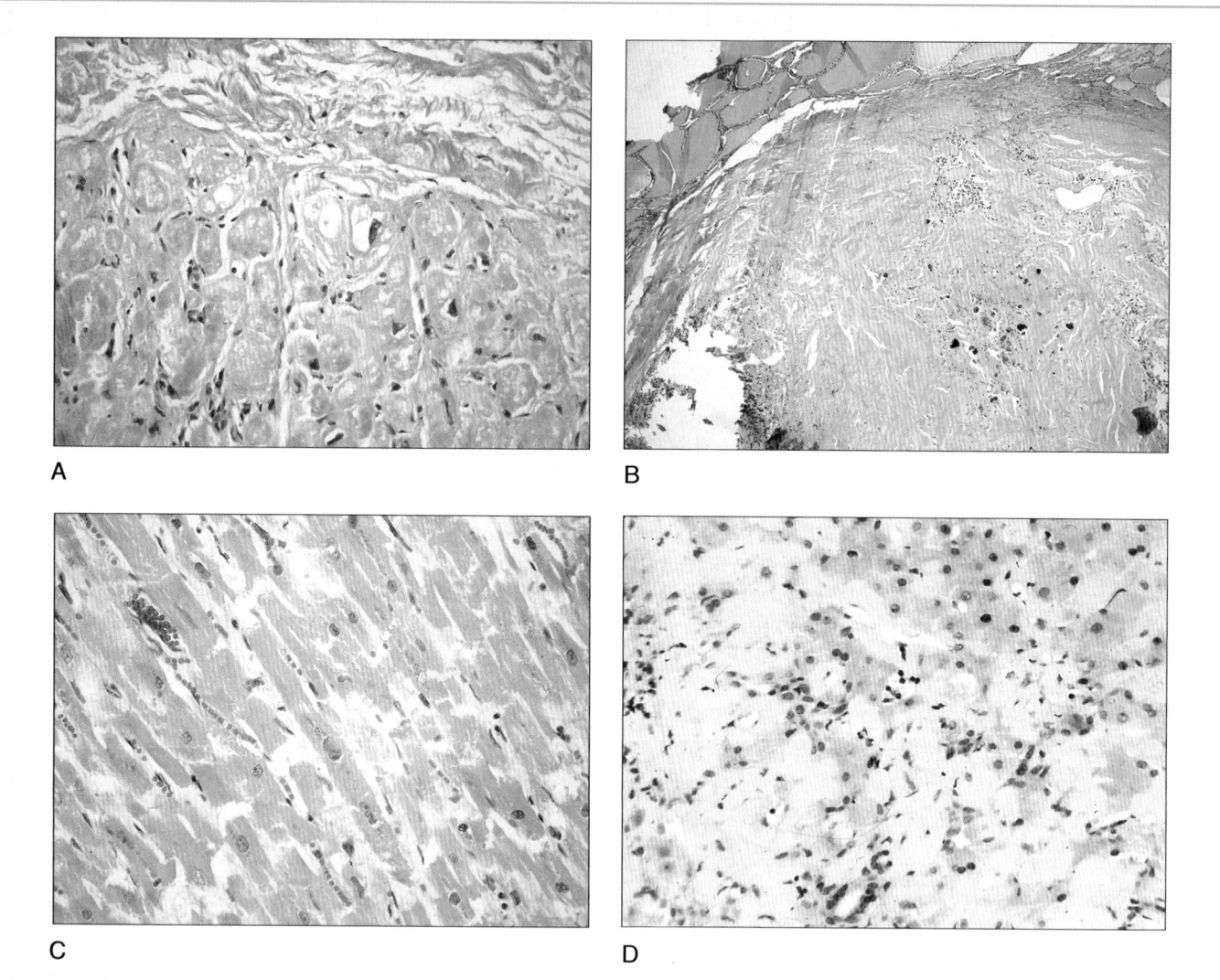

Figure 1-16. A, Myocytolysis of cardiac myocytes. Note the vacuoles present in the cytoplasm of cardiac myocytes in this photomicrograph of subendocardium from a patient with chronic ischemic heart disease. **B**, Dystrophic calcification in the thyroid gland. Calcium phosphate deposits in a fibrous nodule in a thyroid gland with nodular goiter are visible as punctuated bluish-purple crystals. **C**, Lipofuscin pigment in cardiac myocytes. The brown-gray, granular pigment within the perinuclear cytoplasm of cardiac myocytes (best seen in the central myofiber in this photomicrograph) is lipofuscin. **D**, Amyloid deposition in the liver. The pink amorphous material deposited in the interstitium (spaces between cells) is amyloid. There is pressure-induced atrophy of entrapped hepatocytes.

ventricle with blood, i.e., restrictive cardiomyopathy). Amyloid has a glassy, eosinophilic appearance in routine (hematoxylin and eosin–stained) sections and is described as having a hyaline appearance. A Congo red stain specifically stains amyloid fibers an orange-reddish color that is converted to "apple green" birefringence when the section is viewed under polarized light.

Cell Death

Severe or prolonged cell injury can result in cell death. Two different forms of cell death are distinguished: apoptosis and necrosis. Necrosis is always a pathologic process and usually corresponds to the abnormal death of a group of contiguous cells or of a whole tissue or organ, as depicted in Figure 1-17.

Necrosis can result from many different forms of injury, but a very common form of necrosis is ischemic necrosis due to arterial occlusion.

Apoptosis (often referred to as programmed cell death) is an energy-dependent process that usually results in the death of single, isolated cells within a tissue or an organ rather than of many contiguous cells. Apoptosis occurs as a physiologic process during normal embryogenesis as well as in some specialized tissues during postnatal life. Apoptosis also may be pathologic (e.g., death of hepatocytes due to viral hepatitis). While the distinction between apoptosis and necrosis is critical for understanding different pathologic processes, it is clear that some forms of injury result in cell death that shares some features of both apoptosis and necrosis.

BIOCHEMISTRY

Amyloid

Amyloid is formed from misfolded proteins or peptides (at least 21 proteins are known to form amyloid in humans) and tends to deposit in the extracellular space, where it causes tissue damage. Point mutations or abnormal proteolytic processing can predispose to amyloid formation. Increased concentrations of proteins susceptible to amyloid formation (e.g., lambda light chains in plasma cell myeloma) can greatly accelerate this process.

All forms of amyloid share a β-pleated sheet conformation (antiparallel arrangement in which the N and C termini of adjacent chains are in opposite orientations). This molecular organization produces polypeptide strands with a zigzag configuration. Amyloid forms fibers are nonbranching and range from 7.5 to 10 nm in diameter. All molecular forms of amyloid are morphologically indistinguishable from one another.

Congo red is a vital dye that intercalates in amyloid fibrils to stain them red under normal illumination and produces characteristic green birefringence under polarized light.

Precursor	Amyloid Protein	Disease	Organ Affected
Aβ protein precursor	Aβ	Alzheimer's disease	Brain
β₂-Microglogulin	Aβ2M	Complication of chronic hemodialysis	Systemic
Immunoglobulin light chain	AL	Myeloma-associated amyloidosis	Systemic
Serum amyloid A	AA	Secondary amyloidosis due to chronic inflammation	Systemic
Transthyretin	ATTR	Senile amyloidosis	Heart and blood vessels
Transthyretin	ATTR	Hereditary amyloidosis	Nerves
Lysozyme	ALys	Hereditary amyloidosis	Kidney, lever, spleen
Apolipoprotein A-1	AApoAl	Hereditary amyloidosis	Liver, kidney, heart

Apoptosis

Although apoptosis has been observed for many years by embryologists, it has only been recognized as a unique and critical form of cell death in adults during the last 30 years. In the developing embryo, the formation of different structures is accomplished by first forming scaffolding that is then removed to allow final morphogenesis. For example, the webs between individual digits in the limb buds of developing embryos are specifically signaled to initiate apoptosis to allow the formation of separate fingers and toes. Apoptosis causes

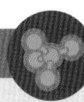

BIOCHEMISTRY

TUNEL Assay for Apoptosis

The TUNEL assay allows the in situ detection of apoptosis in tissue sections.

TUNEL is an acronym for terminal deoxynucleotidyl transferase biotin-dUTP nick end labeling. Terminal deoxynucleotidyl transferase (TdT) is a template-independent DNA polymerase that is normally active in primitive lymphoid cells to increase receptor diversity.

TdT can add random nucleotides to the ends of DNA fragments produced by endonucleases during apoptosis, since 3′ phosphate groups are the substrate for TdT (3′ phosphate groups are not produced during cell necrosis). Treating tissue sections with TdT and labeled nucleotides then provides a convenient assay for apoptosis. In practice, necrotic debris may nonspecifically trap either fluorescent or chromogenic signals and result in a false-positive assay.

Apoptosis can also be detected by means of assays for activated caspase-3, Fas ligand, and annexin V.

these cells to die and fall away without damaging adjacent cells that are fated to form final body parts.

Apoptosis is a stereotyped, energy-dependent process that results in nuclear fragmentation and cell death. Apoptosis can be induced in different types of cells by multiple internal and external triggers (Fig. 1-18A). These include Fas ligand binding, removal of trophic hormone or cytokine stimulation, and signaling by cytotoxic T lymphocytes. In sensitive cells, these signals can activate a cascade of enzymes that ultimately result in the activation of caspases, which trigger cell destruction. Nuclear destruction is accomplished by fragmentation of nuclear DNA by endonucleases that cleave between nucleosomes to produce DNA fragments of discrete length. Since the distance between nucleosomes is approximately 200 nucleotides, these DNA fragments tend to vary in length by multiples of 200 nucleotides. This specific pattern of DNA degradation can be detected by gel electrophoresis of DNA isolated from cells that have undergone apoptosis. As apoptosis proceeds, fragments of nuclear and cytoplasmic material are characteristically extruded from dying cells as apoptotic bodies (see Fig. 1-18B). This pattern of cell death can often be recognized in routine tissue sections by the presence of karyorrhectic debris (Fig. 1-19). The so-called TUNEL assay is a more specific slide-based assay for apoptosis.

Since apoptosis typically affects isolated cells, viable cells usually surround an apoptotic cell. Apoptosis induces a limited inflammatory response that is often restricted to a few histiocytes that engulf and remove the apoptotic cell, leaving a hole in the tissue. The lack of a marked inflammatory response in response to apoptosis is clearly important for its physiologic function in normal embryogenesis. In contrast, necrosis always induces an intense inflammatory response that usually results in additional cellular and tissue injury.

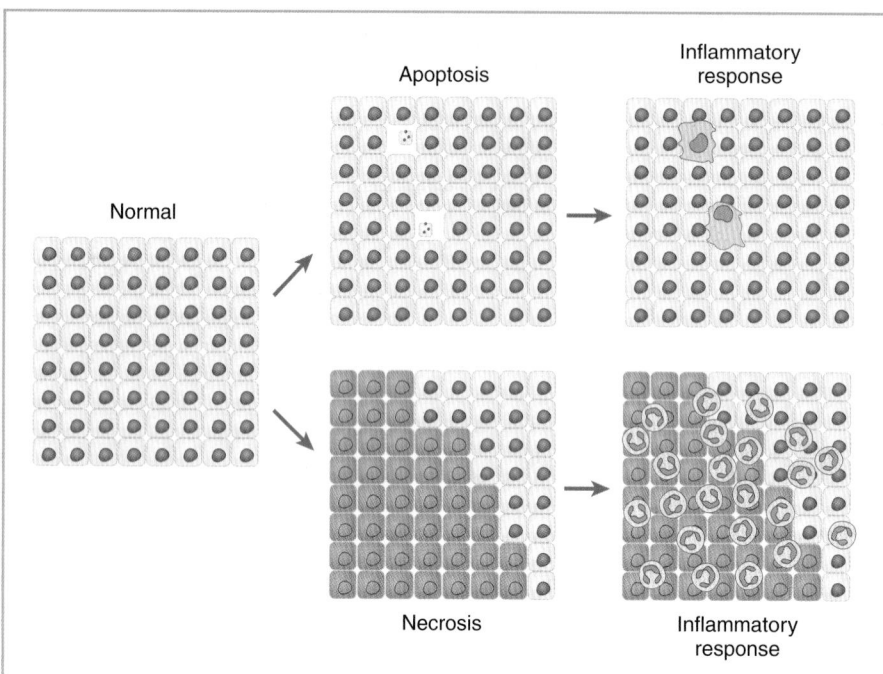

Figure 1-17. Apoptosis versus necrosis.

Cell Necrosis

Necrosis is a form of cell death that typically results in the destruction of many contiguous parenchymal cells and may involve an entire tissue or organ. Ischemic necrosis resulting from vascular occlusion is the most common form of necrosis encountered clinically. Ischemic necrosis usually produces the morphologic pattern of coagulation (coagulative) necrosis. In coagulative necrosis, cells do not undergo an energy-dependent, orchestrated process that results in cell fragmentation. Rather, energy depletion results in the breakdown of ionic gradients across cell membranes that initially causes influx of sodium and water (cell swelling) and ultimately results in the entry of calcium into the cell cytoplasm from the external environment and from mitochondria (in which oxidative phosphorylation has ceased because of hypoxia). These changes can rapidly lead to irreversible injury to cells with high metabolic requirements, whereas other cell types are more resistant to ischemic damage. Greater metabolic demands on a tissue (high replicative rate, essential contractile function) tend to hasten cell injury and promote necrosis.

Membrane rupture is a signal of irreversible injury in all cell types. Calcium activates cellular proteases and lipases that destroy essential macromolecules and organelles. Decreased pH (due to lactic acid produced by anaerobic glycolysis while cells are still living) inhibits or blocks many normal enzymatic activities and results in additional dysfunction.

These changes create an environment in which cellular proteins coagulate (i.e., become denatured and fall out of solution). Protein coagulation results in increased eosin staining of the cytoplasm of necrotic cells (hypereosinophilia), which is one of the typical morphologic features of coagulation necrosis (Fig. 1-20). Messenger RNA in the cytoplasm of necrotic cells is rapidly degraded, resulting in the loss of basophilic staining in the cytoplasm (nucleic acids show basophilic staining with hematoxylin) that further increases cytoplasmic eosinophilia. The nucleus of necrotic cells also loses its basophilic staining characteristics as endonucleases and exonucleases randomly degrade DNA. In contrast with apoptosis (in which endonucleases cleave between nucleosomes), the breakdown of chromatin structure in necrosis results in the nonspecific fragmentation of DNA that produces a smear of different-sized nucleic acid fragments on gel electrophoresis (Fig. 1-21).

In some necrotic cells, the nucleus may shrink (pyknosis) before disappearing (karyolysis). In some forms of necrosis, karyolysis occurs without pyknosis. Necrosis is always associated with marked acute inflammation (in contrast with apoptosis) and induces a predominantly neutrophilic infiltrate. Degradative enzymes from inflammatory cells digest necrotic tissue and prepare the site for healing or repair (Fig. 1-22). The presence of excess inflammatory cell enzymes can also lead to additional or exaggerated tissue destruction greater than the original insult.

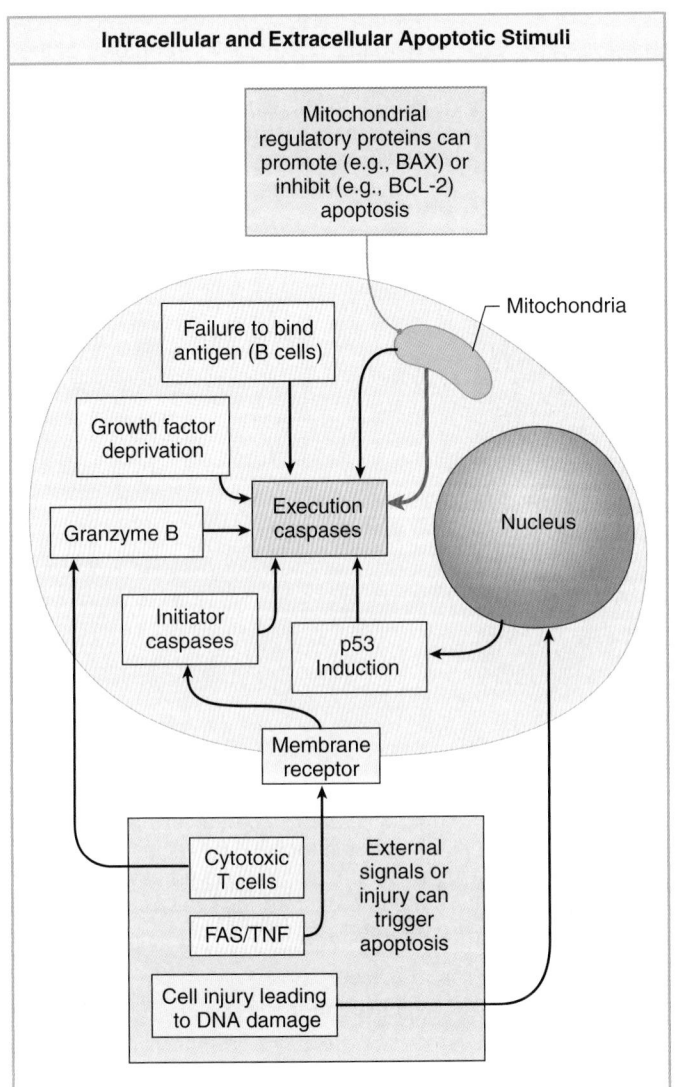

Intracellular and Extracellular Apoptotic Stimuli

A

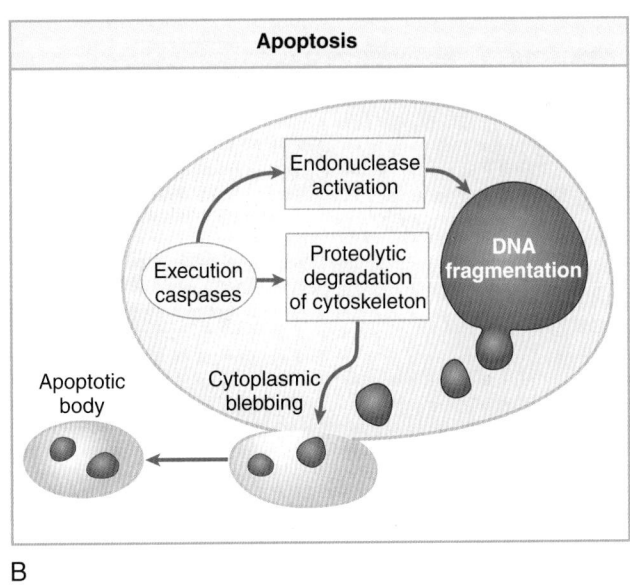

Apoptosis

B

Figure 1-18. **A**, Intrinsic and extrinsic apoptotic stimuli. **B**, Metabolic and morphologic changes during apoptosis.

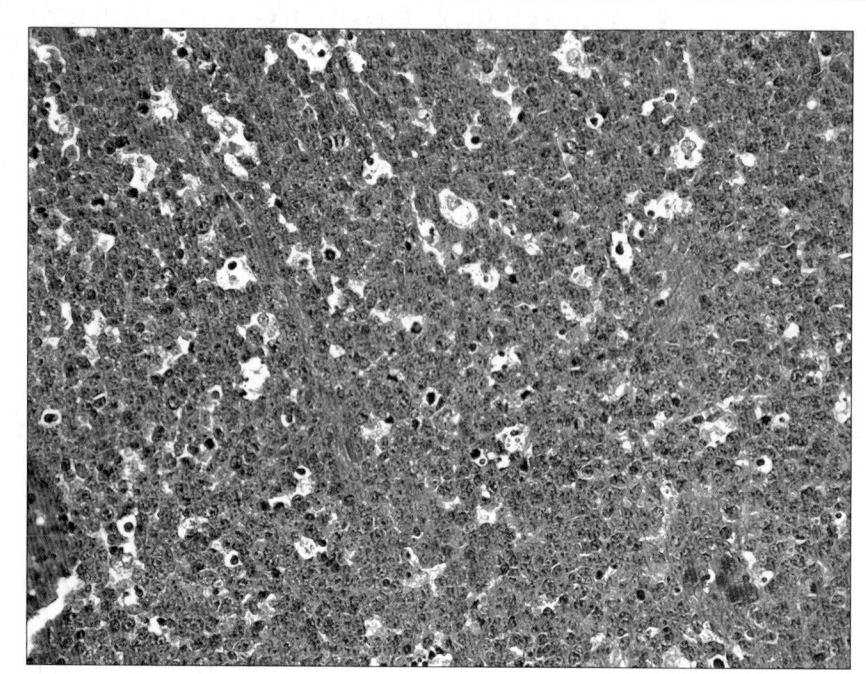

Figure 1-19. Apoptosis in lymph node germinal center cells. Apoptosis of the individual B cells undergoing antigen selection is seen as empty spaces containing fragments of apoptotic debris. Unlike necrosis, apoptosis does not provoke an acute inflammatory reaction.

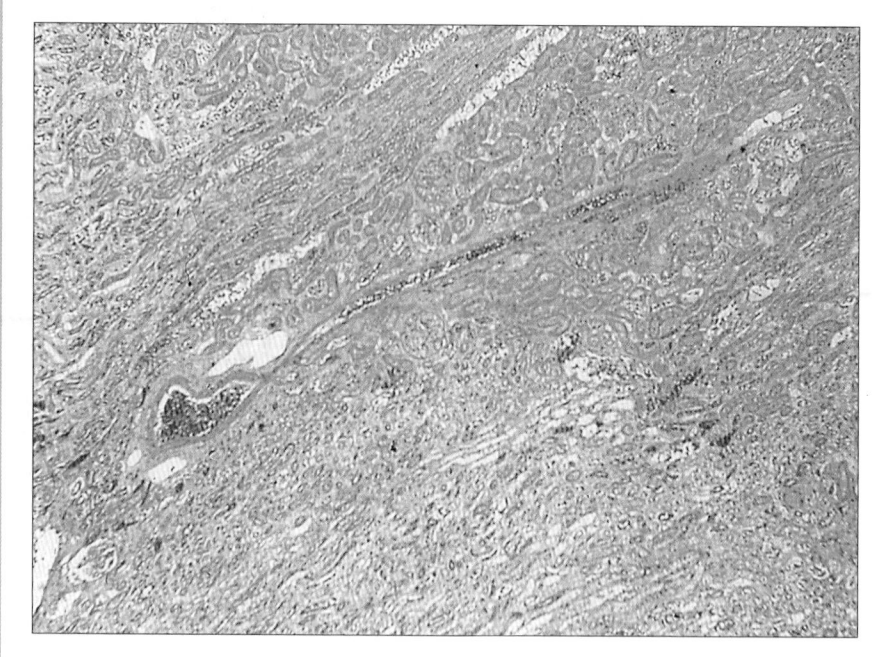

Figure 1-20. Coagulation necrosis in a renal infarct. Necrotic cells show hypereosinophilia as well as the loss of nuclear staining. Inflammatory cells have not yet reached the central portion of the infarct.

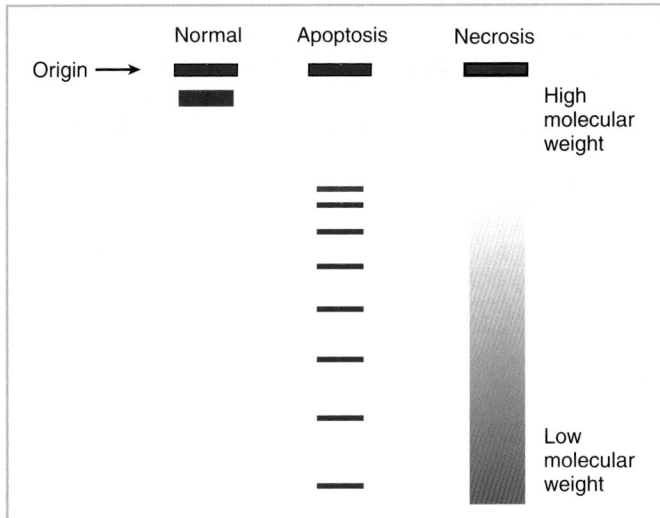

Figure 1-21. Gel electrophoresis pattern of DNA from normal, necrotic, and apoptotic cells.

PHYSIOLOGY

Gel Electrophoresis

Gel electrophoresis is an analytical technique that allows size separation of DNA as well as other macromolecules.

For gel electrophoresis, a DNA sample is loaded at one end of a gel matrix (usually agarose or acrylamide) that provides a uniform pore size through which the DNA molecules can move. Application of a constant electric field causes DNA fragments (all have a uniform, strong negative charge) to migrate toward the cathode. As they move through the gel, longer fragments are retarded more than shorter fragments and their migration rate is proportional to the logarithm of the length of the DNA fragment. This relationship holds over a range of DNA sizes, and useful separation can be achieved for DNA fragments from a few nucleotides in length up to 25,000 nucleotides using a range of gels of different concentration.

Molecular weight standards provide a means of calibrating the gel and estimating molecular weight.

Larger DNA molecules can be separated using pulsed-field electrophoresis, which employs different separation principles.

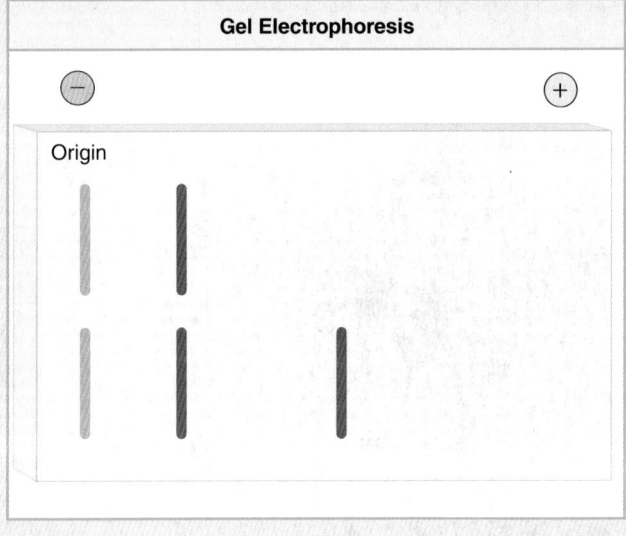

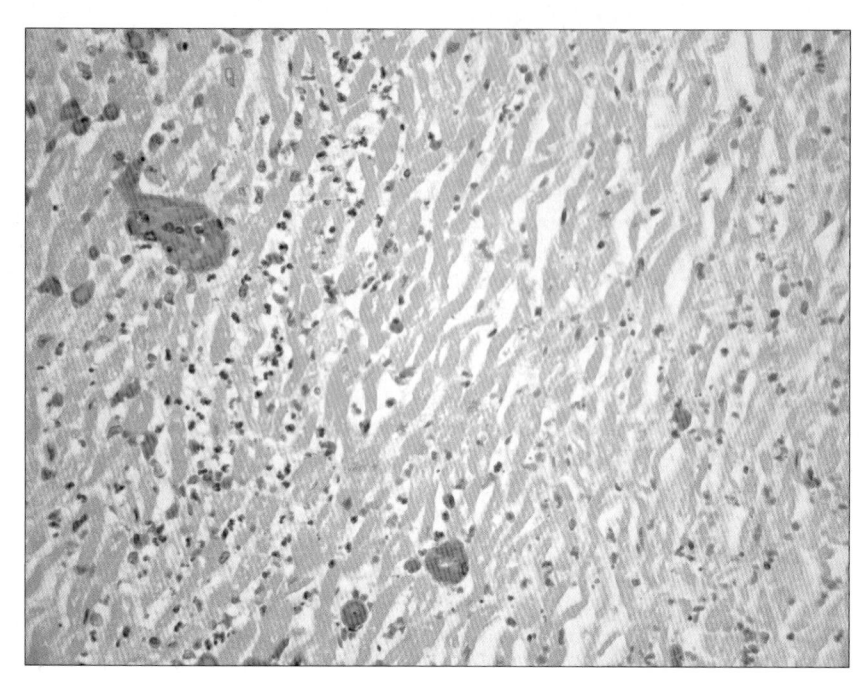

Figure 1-22. Ischemic necrosis of cardiac myocytes. Note the prominent, acute inflammatory infiltrate and features of coagulation necrosis (hypereosinophilia, karyolysis, etc.) in this case of acute myocardial infarction.

Inflammation, Inflammatory Mediators, and Immune-Mediated Disease

2

CONTENTS

Inflammation is an essential process that is critical to host defense against microorganisms and parasites. Inflammation is also the initial response to most types of physical injuries, providing a clean-up function that segues to tissue repair. Most inflammatory and immune-mediated reactions are primarily adaptive or reparative, but these processes can easily result in excessive tissue damage that may cause acute or chronic dysfunction of tissues, organs, or the entire organism. Networks of stimulatory and inhibitory factors that interact to initiate, modulate, and terminate these reactions control most inflammatory processes. Different types of inflammatory reactions occur over greatly differing time scales. Vascular changes can occur within seconds, while chronic inflammatory reactions may take days or weeks to fully develop. Genetic abnormalities in various components of the inflammation system or polymorphisms in some genes that control inflammatory processes can predispose to the development of abnormal inflammatory processes that can result in tissue damage or destruction.

Conventionally, inflammation is either acute or chronic. Acute inflammation involves predominantly alterations in blood vessels (that produce increased blood flow and edema) and the action of neutrophils. Some of these changes can be activated within seconds and the remainder over minutes to hours. Vascular changes are followed by a cellular response (predominantly neutrophils) over the course of hours. Many acute inflammatory reactions are innate immune responses that are not dependent on antigen-specific effector cells or antibodies. The presence of specific antibodies for a particular pathogen can usually accelerate the acute inflammatory reaction and may greatly enhance its effectiveness.

Chronic inflammation typically evolves over the course of days to weeks and is usually characterized by the presence of lymphocytes, macrophages, and plasma cells. Chronic inflammation usually coexists with and cooperates with tissue repair processes. Tissue repair is discussed in detail in Chapter 3. Specific types of infectious organisms and specific types of insults can incite specialized types of chronic inflammation such as granulomatous inflammation. Coexistence of acute and chronic inflammation is typical within the first few days after many types of insults. The character of an inflammatory infiltrate can be helpful in assessing the acuteness or chronicity of an insult and in identifying the causative agent.

●●● VASCULAR CHANGES

Vascular changes in acute inflammation underlie the classic findings of *rubor*, *tumor*, *dolor*, and *calor*. Changes in the vasculature enhance blood flow to the affected tissue causing hyperemia (rubor), which also results in increased delivery of heat to peripheral tissues (calor). Hyperemia is an active process whereby the blood volume and flow are increased by active dilatation of arterioles supplying the tissue (increased blood flow) as well as dilatation of venules to expand blood volume. Various soluble inflammatory mediators including histamine and nitric oxide (which will be discussed later in this chapter) can mediate vasodilatation. Vasodilation slows blood flow in the affected vessels and permits increased inter-action between endothelial cells and circulating inflammatory cells that facilitates their localization to sites of inflammation.

Congestion is a passive process in which blood accumulates in organ or tissue as the result of decreased venous return. Congestion usually results from increased central venous pressure or from blockage or obstruction of venous return from a particular vascular bed. Congestion is usually a patho-logic process, whereas hyperemia is an active, physiologic reaction to injury. Chronic congestion predisposes to hemor-rhage into tissue, resulting in inflammation that can ultimately cause fibrosis and organ dysfunction. A typical example is long-standing hepatic congestion secondary to increased central venous pressure in congestive heart failure. Increased pressure in central veins causes them to expand, putting pressure on adjacent hepatocytes that disrupts their normal function and, if severe enough, causes cell death (i.e., centrilobular necrosis; Fig. 2-1). Repeated cycles of injury lead to microhemorrhages and fibrosis around central veins that can cause permanent dysfunction. Similarly, chronic congestion in the lungs causes many microhemorrhages that result in the accumulation of hemosiderin-containing macrophages in alveoli and chronic inflammation and fibrosis in interstitial lung tissue that result in scarring, leading to decreased lung compliance and impaired gas exchange.

Edema

In homeostasis, opposing forces of hydrostatic and oncotic pressure in plasma and tissue maintain a balance between intravascular and extravascular fluid. Higher hydrostatic pressure in arterioles forces a net movement of water from blood into tissue while the lower hydrostatic pressure and increased oncotic pressure in venules result in a net move-ment of water back into vasculature (Fig. 2-2A). Changes in hydrostatic oncotic pressure in either blood vessels or tissue can disrupt this equilibrium and cause a net loss or gain of water in a tissue. Acute inflammatory mediators in an inflamed tissue result in the contraction of vascular endothelial cells with loosening of their tight junctions. These gaps permit movement of fluid with plasma proteins and electrolytes from plasma into the inflamed tissue. The increase in oncotic pressure in the interstitium shifts the equilibrium of oncotic and hydrostatic pressure, resulting in a net fluid accumulation in the interstitium (see Fig. 2-2B). This fluid movement occurs most prominently in postcapillary venules, in which endothe-lial cells are sensitive to several inflammatory mediators. The accumulation of extracellular fluid results in tissue swelling because of increased interstitial volume (tumor). Pain (dolor) results from the direct action of inflammatory mediators such as bradykinin and substance P on small nerves.

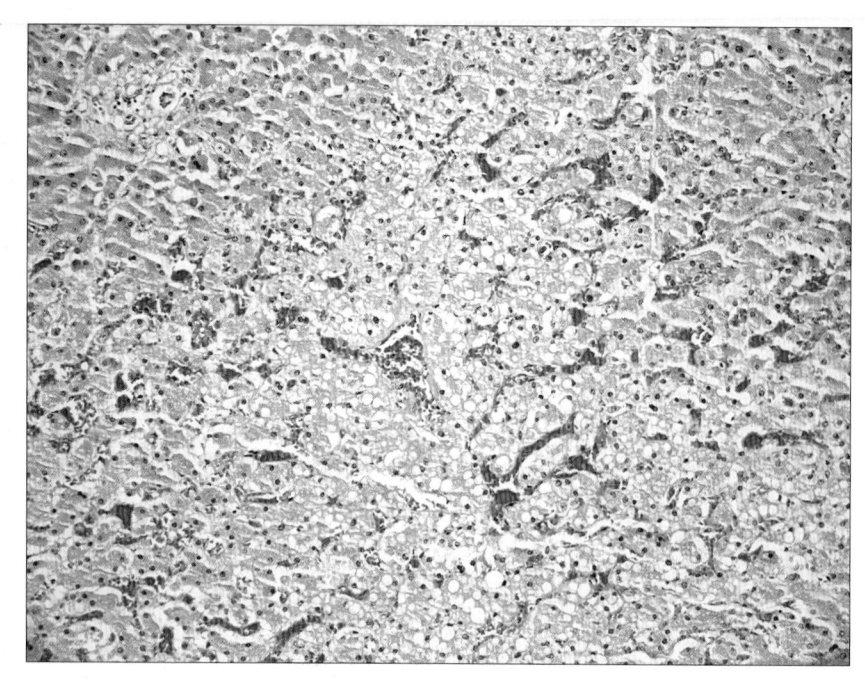

Figure 2-1. Hepatic congestion. Photomicrograph of liver showing marked centrilobular congestion with dilated vascular spaces filled with red blood cells. Cytoplasmic vacuolization of hepatocytes is indicative of cellular dysfunction resulting from abnormally increased central venous pressure.

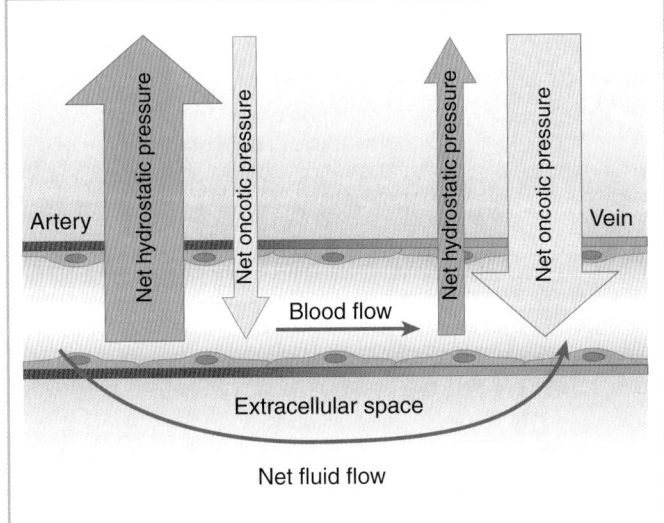

A

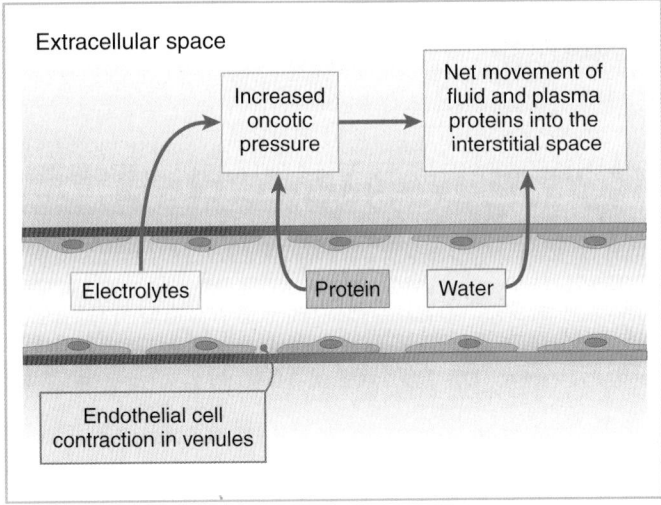

B

Figure 2-2. A, Forces controlling fluid flow across a vascular bed. **B**, Endothelial cell contraction in the venules causes edema.

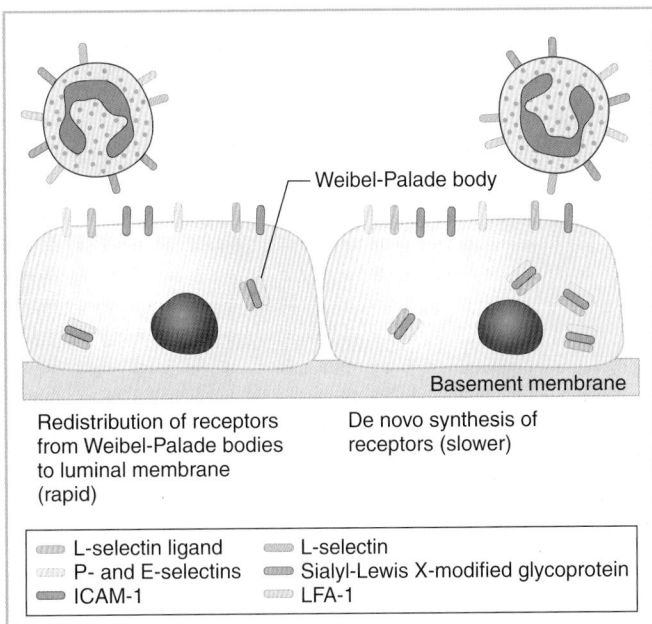

Figure 2-3. Endothelial cell activation.

Endothelial Cell Activation

Activation of endothelial cells results in the surface expression of selectin and integrin proteins through redistribution of preformed proteins (from intracellular Weibel-Palade bodies) and de novo synthesis (Fig. 2-3). Morphologically, activated endothelial cells become plump with easily visible cytoplasm (Fig. 2-4) in contrast with quiescent endothelial cells that are flat and barely visible in histologic sections. Integrins and selectins promote the binding of inflammatory cells to the endothelial surface and can trigger the initial activation of these inflammatory cells. These interactions are initially transient, with neutrophils "rolling" along the endothelial surface. Histologically, this corresponds to margination of neutrophils

at the periphery of blood vessels (Fig. 2-5A). After inflammatory cells have firmly adhered, they undergo further activation triggered by their interaction with endothelial cells, causing them to actively transmigrate between endothelial junctions into the interstitium (see Fig. 2-5B).

●●● INFLAMMATORY CELLS

Inflammatory cells are the main agents of most inflammatory processes (Fig. 2-6). They may kill microorganisms by ingesting and transporting them to phagolysosomes, where specialized enzyme systems produce hydrogen peroxide and hypochlorite, which are effective in killing most types of microorganisms. Activated inflammatory cells also release mediators and chemotactic factors that recruit and activate additional inflammatory cells, resulting in the amplification of the inflammatory response. Neutrophils are the most important agents of response to pyogenic bacterial infections and are the initial responders to most types of mechanical or physical injury. Neutrophils have surface Fc receptors for immunoglobulin constant regions as well as receptors for complement components that allow them to phagocytose cells and other materials that have been coated (opsonized) with these proinflammatory molecules.

Neutrophils have selectins and integrins on their surfaces, which allow them to interact with activated endothelial cells. This interaction is facilitated by vasodilatation, which typically occurs early in the inflammatory response. Dilatation of small blood vessels results in decreased flow rates that promote the margination of inflammatory cells, which then have an opportunity to interact with receptors on activated endothelial cells. These interactions first result in the so-called rolling of neutrophils along the endothelial surface (Fig. 2-7A). Cross-

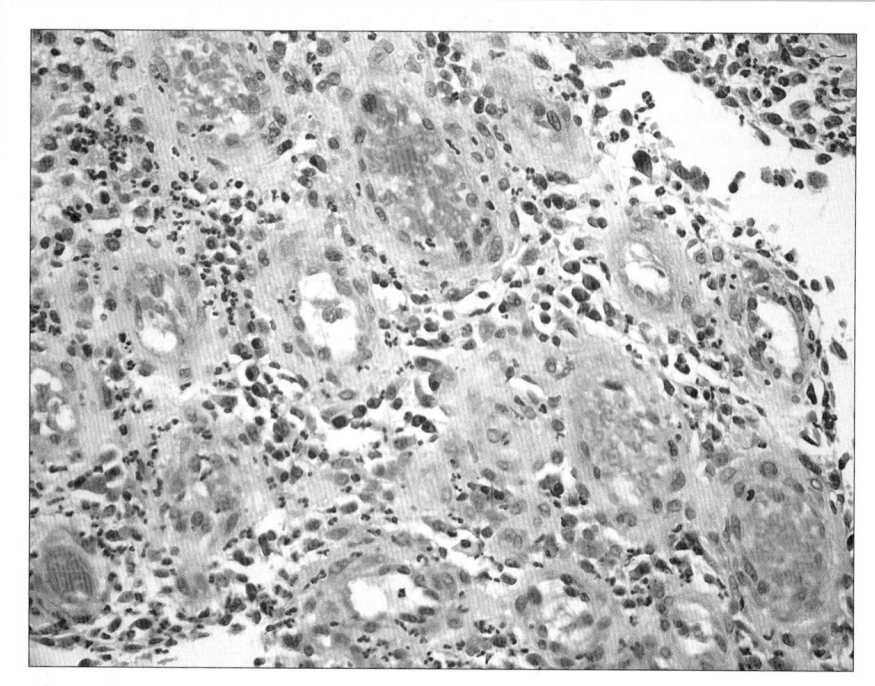

Figure 2-4. Inflamed granulation tissue. Acute inflammatory cells are present among newly formed blood vessels. Endothelial cells are activated and have prominent nuclei and easily recognizable cytoplasm (quiescent endothelial cells would be inconspicuous at this magnification).

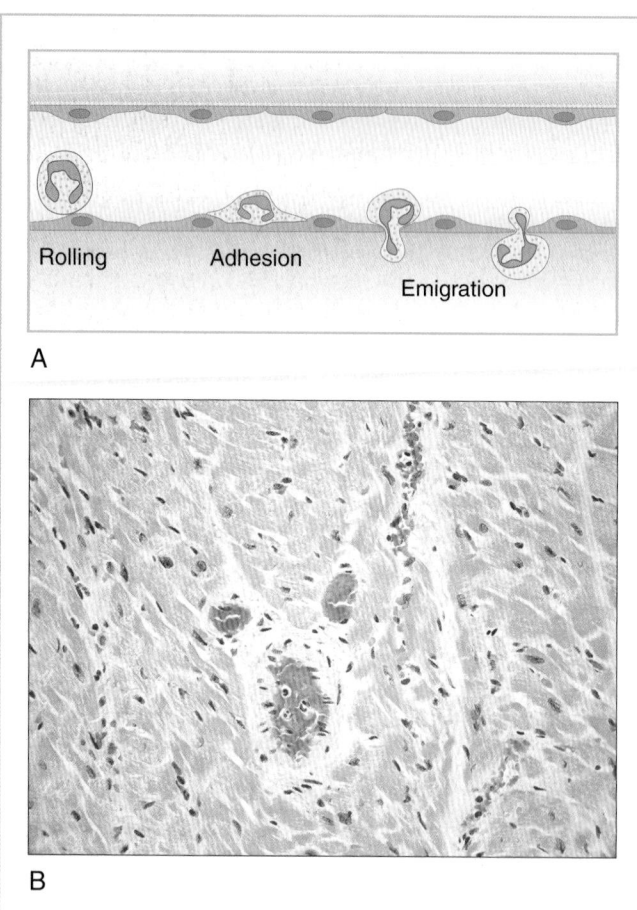

Figure 2-5. A, Leukocyte transmigration in venules. **B,** Margination of granulocytes in an early acute myocardial infarct. The peripheral location of acute inflammatory cells within the vasculature is the initial step in recruitment of inflammatory cells to a site of inflammation.

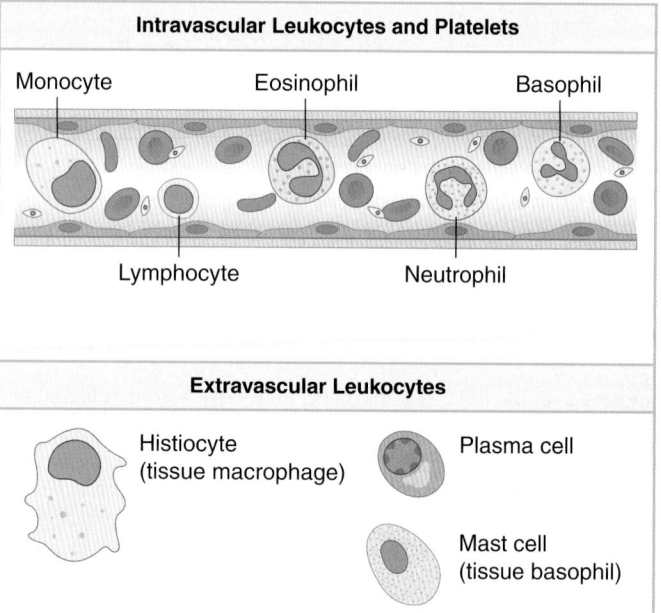

Figure 2-6. Intravascular and extravascular inflammatory cells.

talk between neutrophil and endothelial cell receptors results in further activation, causing the neutrophils to flatten and avidly adhere to the endothelial surface. Further interaction results in the activation of cytoskeletal proteins, leading to active migration (diapedesis or transmigration) of the neutrophils through gaps between endothelial cells.

PECAM (platelet endothelial cell adhesion molecule–1; CD31) is expressed on the surface of both neutrophils and endothelial cells and provides the physical interaction that

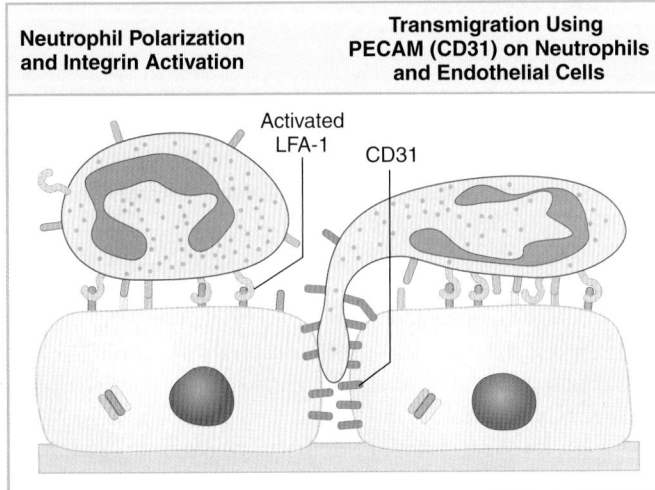

Early Neutrophil Interaction with Endothelial Cells

Rolling

A

Neutrophil Polarization and Integrin Activation

Transmigration Using PECAM (CD31) on Neutrophils and Endothelial Cells

Activated LFA-1

CD31

B

Figure 2-7. A, Early leukocyte interactions with activated endothelial cells. **B**, Leukocyte adhesion, activation, and transmigration.

BIOCHEMISTRY

CD31

CD31 (also called PECAM-1) is a single-chain transmembrane glycoprotein that is expressed on platelets, inflammatory cells, and endothelial cells. CD31 mediates homophilic interactions between neighboring endothelial cells and interacts with inflammatory cells to orchestrate diapedesis. CD99 cooperates with CD31 to manage the final phase of diapedesis of inflammatory cells between endothelial cells.

The extracellular domain of CD31 contains six immunoglobulin-like homology units of the C2 subclass. The CD31 cytoplasmic domain can be phosphorylated and may permit signal transduction through its Src (SH2) homology domain.

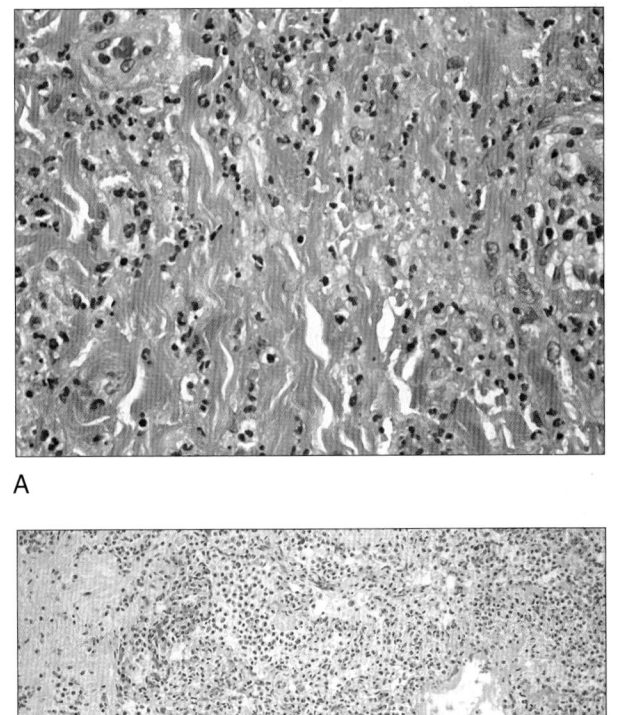

A

B

Figure 2-8. A, Acute inflammation. Predominance of neutrophils in the interstitium of inflamed soft tissue. **B**, Bacterial pneumonia. Confluent aggregates of granulocytes within alveolar spaces in this photomicrograph of lung tissue.

permits transmigration of neutrophils between endothelial cells into the interstitium (see Fig. 2-7B).

Proteases released by neutrophils then digest basement membrane material to allow access into the interstitium, where integrin binding domains on fibronectin and other extracellular matrix proteins facilitate the active movement of inflammatory cells. Chemotactic factors secreted by various inflammatory cells are important in directing the migration of neutrophils through the interstitial space to the precise location of inflammation. Formylmethionine, a unique bacterial product, also acts as a direct chemoattractant for neutrophils. As acute inflammatory cells, particularly neutrophils, migrate into tissue, they release additional inflammatory mediators that accelerate the accumulation and activation of additional inflammatory cells. As more and more acute inflammatory cells and proteins accumulate, the inflamed tissue takes on the features of an inflammatory exudate (Fig. 2-8A). If the inflammatory stimuli continue, this accumulation may progress to abscess formation with the confluent neutrophils. Hydrolytic enzymes, inflammatory mediators, and oxygen-derived free radicals released from active and dying neutrophils can cause severe tissue damage and result in marked organ dysfunction. The tissue life span of neutrophils is usually measured in hours, and this limits the time frame of an inflammatory response unless additional neutrophils are recruited.

Innate Immunity

Innate immunity comprises cellular and humoral processes that can respond to infection or other insults independently of antigen-specific recognition molecules (i.e., immunoglobulins or T-cell receptors). Adaptive (acquired) immunity depends on specific antigen-recognition molecules. Innate immunity is often less effective in killing pathogens than adaptive immunity but does not require priming to be effective. Innate immunity provides the initial response to most insults and may be fully effective. Even if innate immunity cannot eliminate a particular pathogen, it provides critical containment until an effective adaptive immune response can be primed and executed. Absence or deficiency of key innate immune mechanisms results in marked susceptibility to infection that may be fatal.

Neutrophils

Neutrophils derive from myeloid precursor cells in the bone marrow. Myeloid differentiation from committed myeloid progenitor cells progresses through promyelocytes, myelocytes, metamyelocytes, and band forms to produce mature neutrophils. Mature neutrophils are released into the systemic circulation and have a life span of less than 48 hours. Severe inflammatory responses can recruit immature myeloid cells from the bone marrow, and the presence of bands and metamyelocytes in the peripheral blood (a "shift to the left") is often a sign of severe acute inflammation (e.g., bacterial pneumonia; see Fig. 2-8B). Increased demand for neutrophils results in the expansion of myeloid progenitor pools and the generation of a much larger number of mature neutrophils over the course of hours to days.

Neutrophil killing of microorganisms involves three distinct steps. Neutrophils must first recognize bacteria through innate immune receptors on their surface or through specific antibodies or complement components bound to the microorganism. Once an activated neutrophil binds to a microorganism via these receptors, the action of cytoskeletal proteins results in its engulfment into a membrane-coated vesicle called a phagolysosome (Fig. 2-9). Following engulfment, there is further activation of the neutrophil and fusion of primary neutrophil granules with the phagolysosome. The primary granules of neutrophils contain myeloperoxidase (MPO), and fusion of these primary granules with phagolysosomes activates myeloperoxidase, which can convert hydrogen peroxide to hypochlorite, resulting in effective microbial killing. MPO reacts with hydrogen peroxide within the phagolysosome to form superoxide and hypochlorite, which are lethal to most microorganisms.

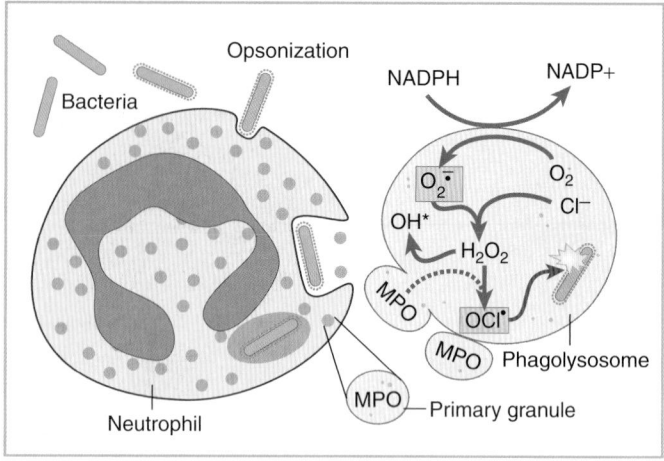

Figure 2-9. Neutrophil phagocytosis and intracellular killing of microorganisms.

The generation of superoxide depends on the reduction of NADPH and so requires the generation of large amounts of energy (the respiratory burst), which can only be accomplished by activated neutrophils. Tumor necrosis factor α (TNF-α) is important in priming neutrophils, making them more sensitive to activation by other cytokines. Leukocyte activation is mediated through several signaling pathways that interact to produce changes in the affinity of binding protein on the surface of neutrophils, to mobilize the cytoskeleton for chemotaxis and phagocytosis, and ultimately to trigger a respiratory burst and degranulation (Fig. 2-10). This high level of metabolic activity results in an anaerobic environment at the site of inflammation, and anaerobic glycolysis tends to lower the pH as well. Proteolytic enzymes and inflammatory mediators released from dying neutrophils can cause extensive tissue damage. Some microorganisms have developed protections from the cytotoxic mechanisms of neutrophils and can survive and persist as intracellular pathogens within neutrophils. Activated macrophages are more effective in killing some of these resistant intracellular pathogens (see Granulomatous Inflammation section).

Neutrophils have three types of cytoplasmic granules. Primary granules contain acid hydrolases, elastase, and serine proteases as well as myeloperoxidase and lysozyme. Proteases and elastases permit neutrophils to dissect the extracellular matrix and liquefy damaged tissue. Myeloperoxidase and lysozyme are directly involved in the killing of microorganisms. Secondary granules also contain proteases and have distinct staining characteristics. Tertiary granules contain proteases as well as gelatinase, which may be important in degrading basement membrane components to facilitate transmigration of neutrophils from blood into tissue. These enzymes may be released into the extracellular space at the leading front of inflammation and promote the invasion of tissues by other inflammatory cells. Neutrophils can also phagocytose some foreign material such as glass beads by undefined mechanisms. The limited life span of neutrophils limits the time scale of the initial inflammatory process to

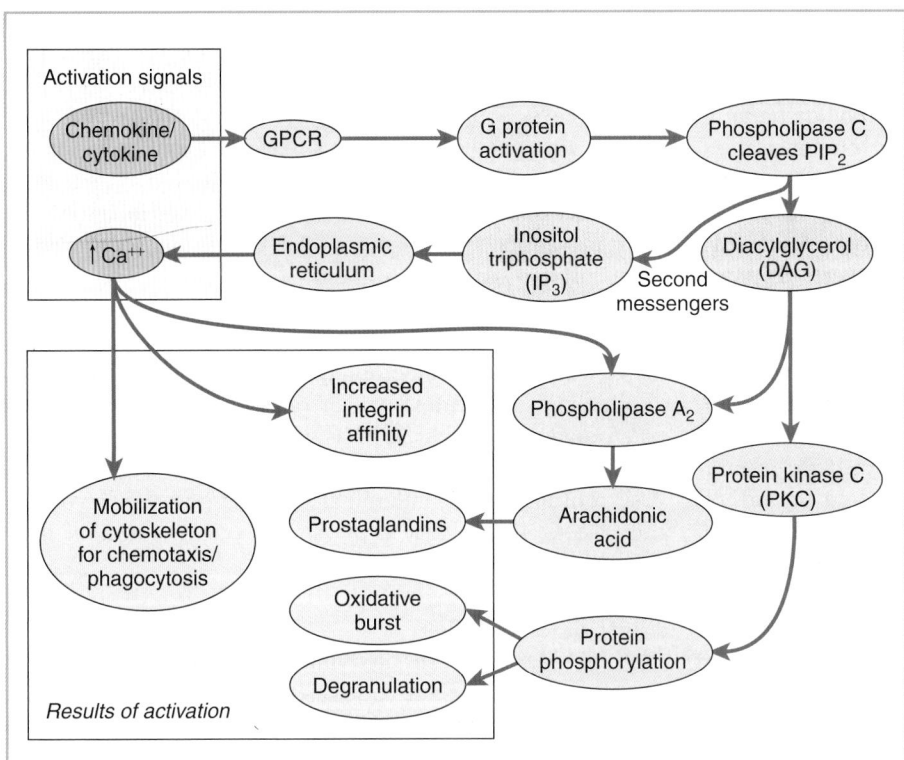

Figure 2-10. Cellular pathways for leukocyte activation.

hours. In most inflammatory reactions, there is a transition from acute to chronic inflammation over the course of days.

Multiple heritable defects in genes involved in leukocyte granule formation or function can result in immunodeficiency. Defects in leukocyte adhesion molecules (i.e., integrins such as LFA-1) impair the interaction of leukocytes with endothelial cells to block their transmigration into tissue and result in severe immunodeficiency.

A defect in the generation of oxygen free radicals to kill bacteria results in chronic granulomatous disease of childhood (CGD), in which patients are unable to effectively kill pyogenic bacteria such as *Staphylococcus aureus*. Without treatment, these children often succumb to bacterial infection. Defects in intracellular trafficking of phagosomes can also impair killing of bacteria.

Eosinophils

Eosinophils derive from myeloid progenitors in the bone marrow and are most important in the inflammatory response to parasites and also participate in many allergic reactions. The percentage of eosinophils in the peripheral blood can increase markedly during parasitic infection and in some types of allergic disease. The presence of numerous eosinophils in an inflammatory exudate can be a clue to the inciting agent. Since many parasites are larger than inflammatory cells, they cannot be effectively phagocytosed. Eosinophils attack these larger parasites by degranulating and releasing their granule contents into the extracellular space in the vicinity of the parasite. Eosinophil granules contain major basic and cationic protein as well as proteases that are cytotoxic to many parasites. Eosinophils are modulated by IL-5, which is secreted by the T_H2 subtype of $CD4^+$ T cells and

IMMUNOLOGY

Integrins

Integrins are transmembrane receptors composed of one α- and one β-chain. Eighteen α- and eight β-subunits are known that can form at least 24 specific integrins (not all α- and β-chains can functionally associate with each other).

Integrins have lower binding affinity than most cellular receptors but are expressed at higher concentrations (10 to 100 ×) on the cell membrane than are most other receptor molecules. Low integrin affinity requires the concentration of many integrins at a site of contact for effective binding. Clustering and activation of integrins requires redistribution of cytoskeletal proteins that activate focal adhesion kinase (FAK), MAP kinase, or phospholipase C to trigger cell activation (e.g., neutrophils) or changes in gene expression.

β-Chain	α-Chain	Ligands
1	1-11, v	Collagen, laminin, fibronectin
2	L, M, X, D	ICAM, VCAM, fibrinogen
3	IIb, v	Fibronectin, fibrinogen, von Willebrand factor, thrombospondin
4	6	Laminin
5	v	Vitronectin
6	v	Fibronectin, tenascin
7	4, E	Fibronectin, VCAM, E-cadherin
8	v	Collagen, laminin, fibronectin

mast cells. T_H2 cells also produce IL-4, which stimulates B cells to undergo a class switch from IgG to IgE. Eosinophils express large amounts of the Fc receptor for IgE on their surface and in this way can play a significant role in allergic reactions.

Basophils and Mast Cells

Basophils derive from myeloid precursors in the bone marrow and contain specific granules composed predominantly of histamine and serotonin. Basophils are relatively uncommon peripheral blood leukocytes under most circumstances (approximately 1%) but are present in most tissues, where they can rapidly trigger inflammatory responses by degranulating. Tissue basophils are usually referred to as mast cells and have typical morphologic features in tissue sections. Mast cells have a "fried egg" appearance in histologic sections with a central nucleus and basophilic cytoplasm. Many mast cells in tissue sections have undergone degranulation (in response to mechanical stimulation during the biopsy) and so no longer contain characteristic Giemsa-positive granules. Degranulation of mast cells results in the immediate release of preformed histamine and serotonin and is an important early inflammatory response that provokes vascular dilatation and edema. Degranulation can be triggered by antigen binding to IgE that is bound to Fc receptors on the surface of mast cells or by other stimuli such as heat, cold, or mechanical stimulation. Excessive activation of mast cells can result in systemic edema and vasodilation, which underlies much of the pathophysiology of anaphylactic shock (see Type I Hypersensitivity section). In addition to the virtually instantaneous release of preformed mediators, mast cell activation also triggers the production of prostaglandins and leukotrienes, which act as proinflammatory mediators.

Macrophages

Macrophages derive from myelomonocytic precursors in the bone marrow and are major effector cells in most chronic inflammatory reactions. Macrophages play an important role in phagocytizing microorganisms and other material but are also very important in coordinating inflammatory processes by virtue of cytokine secretion and cell-cell interactions. Macrophages have single, oval to kidney bean–shaped nuclei with vesicular chromatin and relatively abundant cytoplasm that is usually clear to gray-blue and may appear foamy. Macrophages derive from blood monocytes and are usually referred to as histiocytes when they are present in tissue. Macrophages have an essential role in clearing debris from sites of inflammation or infection. This phagocytic activity of macrophages is essential for the removal of damaged or necrotic material to allow the transition to healing and tissue repair. In some specific types of inflammatory reactions (see Granulomatous Inflammation section), macrophages are modified into epithelioid histiocytes, which play a key role in the killing of some types of microorganisms.

Macrophages are also responsible for producing key inflammatory mediators including IL-1 and TNF-α that have both local and systemic effects in stimulating and coordinating inflammatory reactions. Cytokines produced by macrophages also produce fever and other systemic inflammatory effects. Macrophages orchestrate inflammatory reactions by recruiting appropriate inflammatory cells and fibroblasts to sites of inflammation and stimulating these cells to effect an appropriate inflammatory response.

Macrophages are also important antigen-presenting cells (APCs) in terms of directing and coordinating the interactions of T and B cells to develop effective adaptive immunity. Macrophages constitutively express class II MHC molecules, which are necessary for this role in antigen presentation. Macrophages function in antigen presentation by ingesting and processing proteins (partial proteolytic degradation) and then presenting processed peptides in the context of class II MHC proteins to activate T cells (see T Cells, below).

Macrophages are the primary mediators of granulomatous inflammation, and secretion of interferon γ (IFN-γ) by T_H1 T cells can convert macrophages to activated histiocytes (epithelioid histiocytes), which can ingest and kill resistant microorganisms such as *Mycobacterium tuberculosis* by generating nitrous oxide and other potent oxygen-derived free radicals. Some inflammatory reactions also involve a subclass of T cells that express γ-δ T-cell receptor on their surface.

Natural Killer Cells

Natural killer (NK) cells are lymphocytes of intermediate size that form an important component of innate immunity. NK cells have cytotoxic mechanisms that are very similar to cytotoxic T cells (perforin and granzyme; see T Cells, below). NK cells have abundant granules and are often referred to as large granular lymphocytes. NK cells do not express T-cell antigen receptor on their surface and do not express CD8 or CD4 but are CD56-positive and express Fc receptors on their surface that can bind IgG. NK cells do not express antigen-specific recognition molecules on their surface as T cells do. NK cells do express innate immunity receptors (including Toll-like receptors) that can recognize generic epitopes present on the surfaces of many bacterial pathogens and virally infected cells. NK cells are thought to provide an important early response to viral infection before antigen-specific T cells have been induced to proliferate by antigenic stimulation. NK cells also express a receptor for generic class I MHC molecules (the receptor does not discriminate between self and foreign MHC molecules). Binding of this receptor inhibits NK cell activation. If NK cells encounter cells that do not express class I MHC, the lack of receptor binding triggers their activation and induction of a killing mechanism similar to that of cytotoxic T cells. This activity of NK cells may be important in immunosurveillance for tumors that could seek to evade T cells by ceasing MHC expression.

Platelets

Platelets are anucleate cell fragments that are derived from megakaryocytes in the bone marrow. Megakaryocytes are large cells with convoluted nuclei and abundant cytoplasm that shed small portions of their membrane with enclosed cytoplasm to form platelets. Platelets contain mitochondria and can generate energy by oxidative phosphorylation. They also contain messenger RNA and ribosomes and can synthesize protein but cannot transcribe new messenger RNA or modulate gene expression to replace damaged or altered proteins and so have a limited life span in blood (approxi-

IMMUNOLOGY

Natural Killer (NK) Cells

NK cells are large granular lymphocytes that express CD56 but do not express CD3 or T-cell receptor. They constitute up to 15% of peripheral blood lymphocytes but comprise a much smaller percentage of the lymphocytes in lymph nodes or spleen.

NK cells can be activated by T_H1 cytokines (e.g., IL-2 or IFN-γ) or by the binding of immunoglobulin attached to Fc receptors on their surface (antibody-dependent cellular cytotoxicity/cytolysis, ADCC).

Activated NK cells can produce cytokines including IL-2, IFN-γ, IFN-α, and TNF-α. NK cells can induce target cell lysis using the same mechanisms as cytotoxic CD8$^+$ T cells, including the release of granzyme and perforins. NK cells are inhibited by binding of MHC class I molecules of any haplotype, and this mechanism allows them to target tumor cells that have ceased MHC expression.

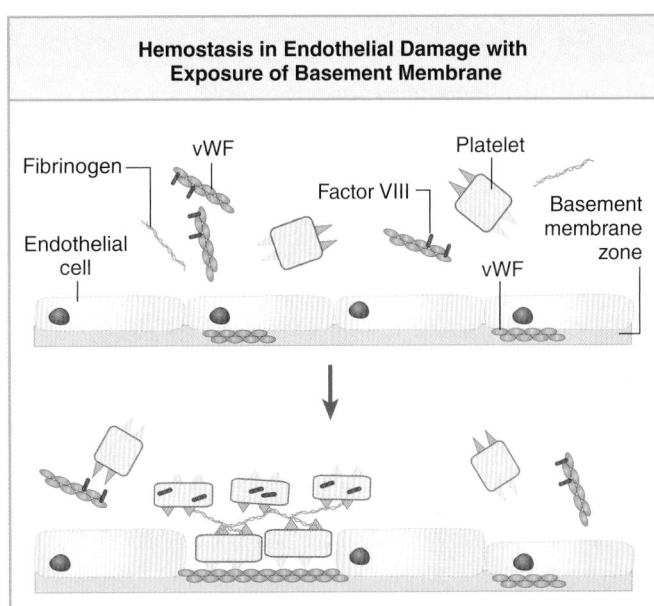

Figure 2-11. Initial hemostatic mechanisms in response to endothelial cell injury.

---

mately 2 days). Platelets contain abundant granules composed of ADP and serotonin and can also synthesize arachidonic acid–derived mediators (most importantly thromboxane) using the cyclo-oxygenase pathway (see Cyclo-oxygenase Pathway section).

Platelets function primarily as the initial hemostatic effectors at areas of vascular damage with exposed extracellular matrix. Platelet adhesion to the exposed basement membrane material is mediated by von Willebrand factor, which creates bridges between receptors on the platelet surface and the extracellular matrix. Von Willebrand factor exists in plasma as multimeric aggregates, and depletion or abnormalities of this protein can markedly reduce the effectiveness of platelets in early hemostasis (Fig. 2-11). Platelet binding to surfaces and secretion of tissue factor by damaged or activated endothelial cells stimulates platelets to undergo an activation reaction (so-called platelet release reaction) in which ADP is released from preformed granules. These stimuli also trigger platelet synthesis of thromboxane A_2, which causes vasoconstriction and accelerates the recruitment and activation of other platelets to initiate a chain reaction that leads to the formation of a platelet plug. Platelet membranes serve as substrates for the deposition and activation of coagulation factors and can greatly accelerate these reactions to facilitate the deposition of fibrin and maturation of the clot. Platelet activation also results in a conformational change in the membrane receptor GP that allows it to bind to fibrinogen and help coordinate the assembly of a platelet-fibrin plug that provides effective hemostasis.

Adaptive Immunity

Adaptive immunity requires the generation of antigen-specific receptor molecules (immunoglobulin or T-cell receptor) and so is not immediately available after initial challenge with antigen. Following exposure to antigen in the appropriate context (priming), effector cells that specifically bind antigen are stimulated to proliferate to a point at which they are sufficiently numerous to provide an effective immune response. Innate immune mechanisms must suffice to contain a pathogen until these antigen-specific effectors are available (days to weeks for an initial response and days for rechallenge with an antigen).

T Cells

Mature T cells express either CD4 (60% of T cells in peripheral blood) or CD8 (30% of T cells in peripheral blood). CD4$^+$ helper T cells are primarily responsible for interactions with B cells and CD8$^+$ T cells and promote their maturation and synthesis of antigen-specific receptors (antibodies and T-cell receptors). CD8$^+$ cells are prototypical cytotoxic T cells that interact with target cells and induce cell death by apoptosis or other mechanisms. The release of granzyme and other mediators by CD8$^+$ T cells induces apoptosis in sensitive host cells.

T cells derive from common lymphoid progenitor cells in the bone marrow. Progenitor T cells with germline T-cell receptor genes then migrate to the cortex of the thymus, where they first rearrange their γ- and δ-receptor genes. Most of these cells then undergo rearrangement of their α- and β-receptor genes. Progenitor T cells that have not yet expressed either CD4 or CD8 begin to express both of these receptors (i.e., they become "double-positive" cells). Double-positive T cells next undergo positive selection in the thymic cortex and are exposed to class I and II MHC molecules on the surface of thymic epithelial cells. Thymic epithelial cells present a variety of short peptides (6 to 8 amino acids in length) in the context of MHC, and pre–T cells that cannot bind MHC (the majority) trigger apoptosis and are eliminated.

IMMUNOLOGY

Major Histocompatibility Complex (MHC) Structure and Function

MHC class I and II molecules have little sequence homology, but both are members of the immunoglobulin superfamily and fold into similar three-dimensional structures.

Two extracellular domains in each molecule form a groove for antigen binding (α_1 and α_2 in class I molecules and α_1 and β_1 in class II molecules). These regions of the MHC genes show the most polymorphisms between different alleles.

MHC gene expression is codominant with expression of both maternal and paternal alleles on cells. The genotype inherited from one parent is called a haplotype and is usually inherited as a cassette without genetic recombination between individual MHC loci.

MHC class I α-chain binds β_2-microglobulin to form a functional receptor. MHC class II α- and β-chains dimerize to form a functional receptor.

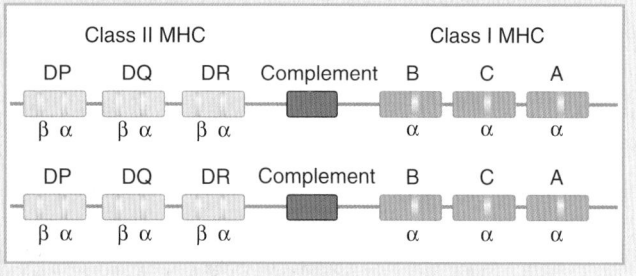

Double-positive cells that recognize class I MHC down-regulate expression of CD4 and migrate to the medulla. Conversely, cells that recognize class II MHC down-regulate CD8. These single-positive (CD4$^+$ or CD8$^+$) T cells then migrate to the thymic cortex, where they undergo negative selection. In the cortex, T cells that recognize self-antigens in the context of class I or II MHC trigger apoptosis and are eliminated. T cells that survive both positive and negative selection then exit the thymus and localize to lymph nodes and other lymphoid and nonlymphoid organs. Mature T cells can circulate between different lymphoid organs by virtue of specific integrins expressed on their surface that are recognized by specialized endothelial cells in lymphoid organs. Negative selection is critical in preventing the release of autoreactive T cells.

A small number of T cells that do not rearrange their α- and β-receptors (i.e., γ-δ T cells) do not express CD4 or CD8 on their surface. These γ-δ T cells tend to permanently localize in the skin and mucous membranes, where they recognize some protein antigens and appear to play a role in some infections (mycobacterial). γ-δ T cells may also play a role in immunosurveillance for tumors although their functions are less well understood than are those of more numerous α-β T cells.

Helper (CD4$^+$) and cytotoxic (CD8$^+$) T cells are key mediators and effectors of chronic inflammation. Both helper and cytotoxic T cells express a T-cell receptor complex (TCR) on their surface that includes multiple CD3 subunits (CD3

is common to all T-cell receptor complexes). The TCR also contains polymorphic proteins produced by somatic recombination of T-cell receptor α and α-β genes (or γ and δ genes in the case of γ-δ T cells) that are antigen specific. This complex is expressed in conjunction with CD4 on helper T cells and can act as a receptor for antigens presented in the context of MHC class II proteins by antigen-presenting cells. In this macromolecular complex, CD4 interacts directly with MHC proteins while the polymorphic α-β peptides interact with antigens that are held in the groove of the class II MHC molecules. Only cells that express class II MHC (e.g., APCs) can activate this receptor. A separate set of costimulatory molecules (CD28 and CD86) on the APC and T cell must also interact to effect signal transduction. This "double handshake" provides a fail-safe mechanism to prevent inappropriate activation of these highly active effector cells (Fig. 2-12). Signal transduction mediated through CD3 and other peptides associated with the TCR initiates cytokine synthesis to trigger division of the activated T cells (IL-2). Some of the progeny differentiate into CD8$^+$ effector cells and some become long-lived memory cells.

Helper T cells are typically categorized as having a T$_H$1 or T$_H$2 phenotype based on the types of cytokines they secrete. T$_H$1 and T$_H$2 T cells derive from uncommitted T cells under the stimulation of IL-4 (T$_H$2) or IL-2, TNF-δ, and IFN-γ (T$_H$1) (Fig. 2-13).

CD4$^+$ T cells of the T$_H$1 type tend to secrete primarily IL-2 and IFN-γ and are important mediators of type IV hypersensitivity (see Type IV Hypersensitivity section). These cytokines stimulate other T cells (particularly memory T cells) to proliferate and mature into effector cells (CD8$^+$ cells) that can attack cells expressing cognate antigen in the context of self class I MHC. IFN-γ is also a powerful activator of macrophages and can convert them to epithelioid histiocytes that are the major effector cells of granulomatous inflammation (see below). IFN-γ also up-regulates class II MHC expression in many cell types, enhancing the potential for antigen presentation to CD4$^+$ cells. Cytokines produced by T$_H$1 T cells also recruit other inflammatory cells and stimulate B cells to produce IgG and IgM, which can fix complement and act as effective opsonins for bacteria and other microorganisms. IL-2 also interferes with T$_H$2 reactions.

CD4$^+$ T cells of the T$_H$2 type produce IL-4 and IL-13, which stimulate B cells to undergo a class switch from IgM or IgG to IgE production. They also produce IL-5, which is an important activator of eosinophils, and IL-10, which interferes with T$_H$1 reactions. In this manner, T$_H$2 cells orchestrate and enhance allergic responses as well as inflammatory responses to some types of parasites. Some inflammatory reactions show combined features of classical T$_H$1 and T$_H$2 responses.

Antigen-specific T-cell receptors on the surface of CD8$^+$ T cells enable them to recognize virally infected cells in the context of class I MHC antigens. CD8$^+$ T cells are also important mediators of transplant rejection in response to foreign histocompatibility antigens. Some CD8$^+$ T cells can recognize foreign MHC class I molecules directly and can initiate cell-mediated cytotoxicity.

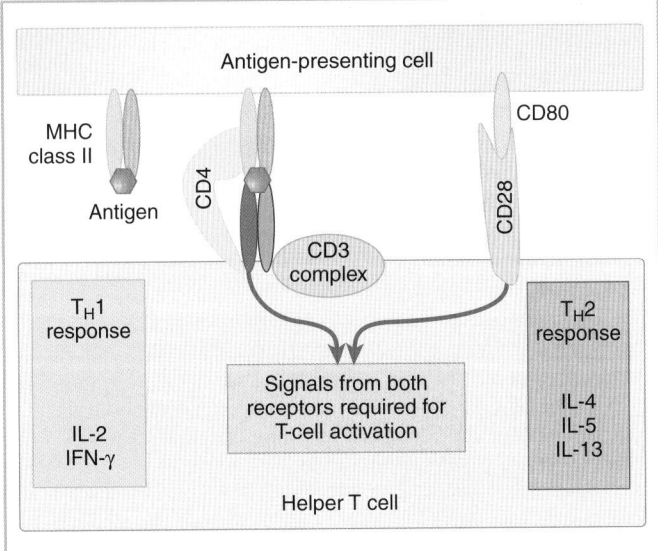

Figure 2-12. Activation of T_H1 and T_H2 CD4$^+$ T cells.

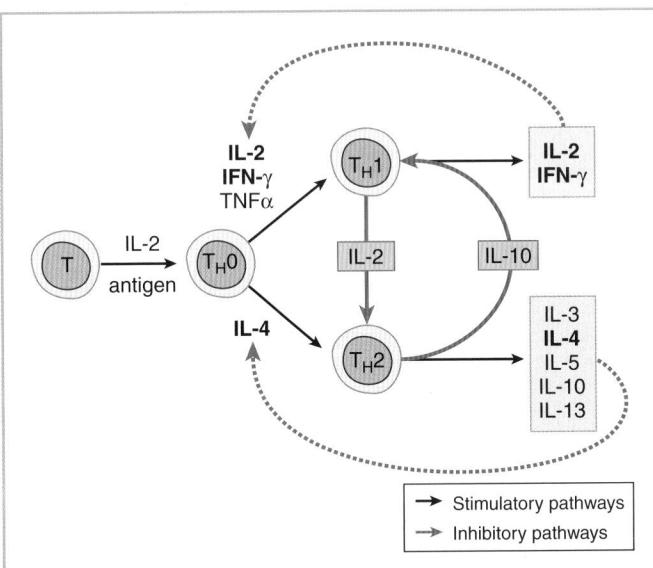

Stimulatory pathways
Inhibitory pathways

Figure 2-13. Maturation of T_H1 and T_H2 T cells and effector cytokines as produced by mature T_H1 and T_H2 cells.

B Cells

The primary function of B lymphocytes is to produce specific immunoglobulin molecules of high affinity that can react with exogenous antigens. B cells derive from common lymphoid progenitor cells in the bone marrow, where they begin to rearrange their immunoglobulin genes.

B cells that do not express a functional B-cell receptor on their surface undergo apoptosis. B cells that express surface immunoglobulin migrate to lymph nodes or extranodal lymphoid organs, where they undergo initial antigen stimulation in primary follicles. Interactions with CD4$^+$ T cells and APCs (dendritic cells and macrophages) select for the formation of cells expressing immunoglobulin that can functionally bind antigen. Signaling is mediated through a B-cell receptor

IMMUNOLOGY

Antigen Receptor Gene Rearrangement and Class Switching

Antigen receptor genes are composed of one or more constant regions (C), joining regions (J), and variable regions (V). Some antigen receptor genes also contain diversity regions (D) between the J and V regions.

Combinatorial recombination between V, D, and J segments creates substantial diversity for antigen recognition. Additional diversity results from random nucleotides incorporated by terminal deoxynucleotidyl transferase at the joining ends between DNA segments during antigen receptor gene rearrangement.

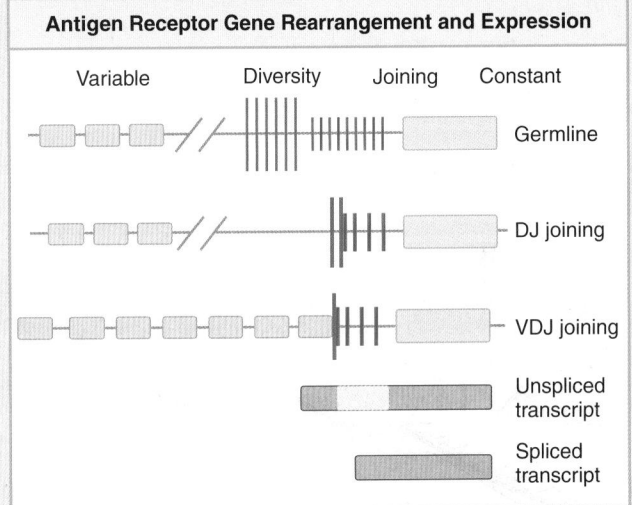

Antigen Receptor Gene Rearrangement and Expression

Class switching in the immunoglobulin heavy chain gene occurs in a similar manner to VDJ recombination by means of switch regions adjacent to each type of constant region to loop out and remove intervening DNA sequences.

Switching between IgM and IgD expression is accomplished by differential splicing rather than by gene rearrangement.

complex that is composed of immunoglobulin with associated Igα and Igβ proteins that are activated by antigen binding. A costimulatory signal is also required (similar to the activation of helper T cells) via interaction of CD40 with CD154 on helper T cells or by the binding of complement components to CD21 (Fig. 2-14). Some B cells that successfully bind antigen become memory cells, and others undergo a constant region class switch to from IgD to multimeric IgM that is very effective in fixing complement.

Secondary lymphoid follicles provide an environment for the selection of higher affinity antibodies by triggering hypermutation in the hypervariable regions of the heavy and light chain genes in B cells and setting up competition for antigen binding. B cells that express lower affinity immunoglobulin fail to compete for antigen binding and undergo apoptosis (Fig. 2-15). Post–germinal center B cells can undergo further maturation to form plasma cells that produce large quantities of immunoglobulin for secretion.

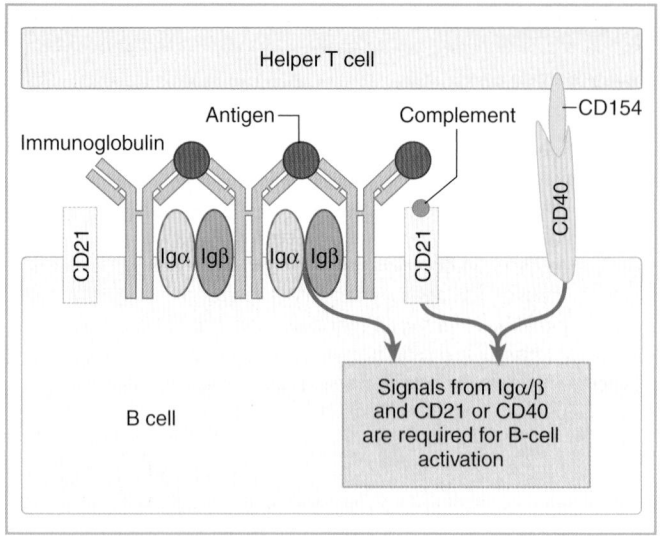

Figure 2-14. Activation of B cells by antigen and CD4+ T cells.

Immunoglobulin Structure

Immunoglobulin molecules have antigen recognition sites formed by the interaction of light chain and heavy chain variable regions.

Conserved framework regions in the variable portions of these genes provide canonical structure and orient the complementarity-determining regions (CDRs) around the antigen-binding pocket.

CDR III corresponds to the VDJ junction while CDR I and II show the most sequence variation between variable region family members.

Hypermutation during secondary antigen selection targets the three CDRs and allows selection for increased antigen-binding affinity ("affinity maturation").

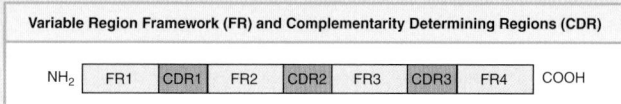

Variable Region Framework (FR) and Complementarity Determining Regions (CDR)

| NH$_2$ | FR1 | CDR1 | FR2 | CDR2 | FR3 | CDR3 | FR4 | COOH |

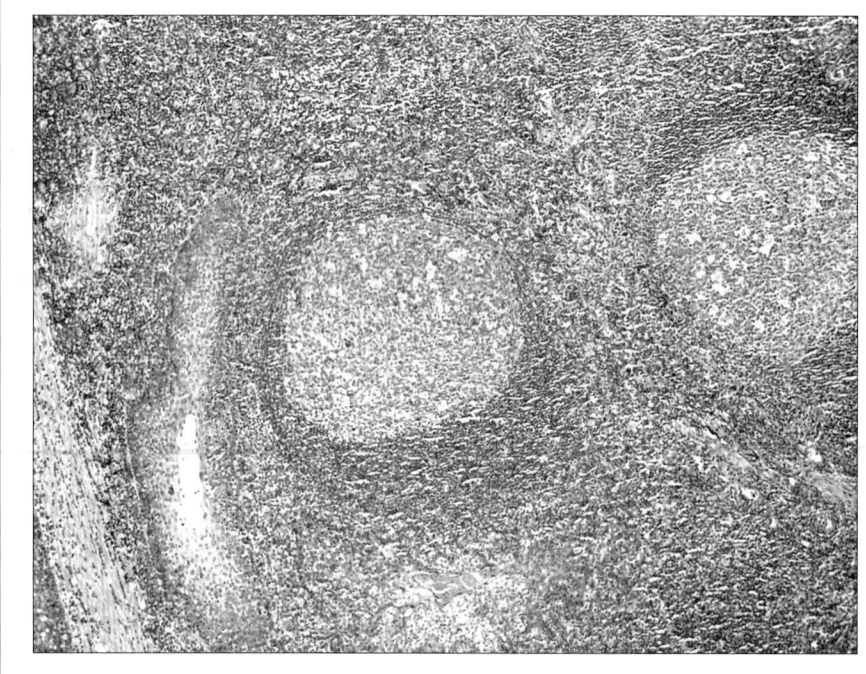

Figure 2-15. Reactive germinal center in a hyperplastic tonsil. Note the polarization of the germinal center with a well-organized mantle of small lymphocytes around it.

Most mature B cells undergo class switch to produce IgG, which accounts for 85% of the immunoglobulin in normal serum. IgG is not multimeric, and while it can fix complement, it is not so effective in this regard as IgM. The IgG constant region permits effective binding to Fc receptors on inflammatory cells that can enhance phagocytosis of microorganisms. Serum IgM antibodies are typical of an acute or subacute infection. The presence of serum IgG in the absence of IgM is evidence of prior infection. Mature B cells can also be induced to undergo class switch to IgA or IgE. Mucosa-associated B cells produce predominantly IgA in conjunction with secretory component, which allows IgA binding to mucosal surfaces in the gastrointestinal tract, providing an important barrier to some pathogens.

●●● INFLAMMATORY MEDIATORS

Inflammatory mediators are small molecules and proteins that are important for amplifying and terminating different types of inflammatory responses. These molecules are diverse in terms of their structure and are often pleiotropic in their effects. Almost all these mediators are short-lived in their activated state, and specific enzymes rapidly inactivate many of these compounds. Some of these mediators exist as preformed molecules that are activated by cleavage (e.g., complement components) or are sequestered in granules and become active on release (e.g., histamine). Inflammatory mediators act through specific receptors on target cells, and most mediators have effects on multiple cell types. Some inflammatory mediators trigger very different or even opposing effects when they stimulate different target cells. The simultaneous action of multiple mediators may result in enhanced or unique reactions in specific target cells (i.e., priming). Some mediators act predominantly as priming agents that increase the activation of target cells and cause them to have exaggerated responses if they are exposed to other mediators.

Some inflammatory mediators act alone, whereas others are part of highly organized, hierarchical cascades. These cascades (e.g., the complement and coagulation cascades) can result in massive signal amplification and permit the rapid activation of preformed effector molecules. Some inflammatory mediators are produced in very restricted cell types. For instance, thromboxane A_2 production is largely restricted to platelets. More often, inflammatory mediators are produced by a variety of different cell types.

The effects of different mediators in a single inflammatory response may be entirely contrary (e.g., one may have proinflammatory effects while others are anti-inflammatory). In this way, positive and negative regulators of inflammation can coordinate the rapid, orderly initiation of an inflammatory response as well as coordinate its cessation with a return to normal homeostasis. Some mediators, such as the anaphylotoxins (C3a and C5a) of the complement system, have predominantly chemotactic effects and specifically attract different types of inflammatory cells to a site of inflammation. Some inflammatory mediators act predominantly locally, whereas others produce a mixture of local and systemic effects. The balance between local and systemic effects can be shifted by the amount of mediators released (e.g., large amounts of IL-1 result in shock, with global activation of an inflammatory reaction).

Preformed mediators can be released and have effects within seconds while other mediators must be synthesized de novo by protein synthesis (e.g., cytokines) or after the induction of specific enzyme systems (e.g., prostaglandins). Some of these mediators (particularly cytokines) produce effects only after a lag time that is usually measured in hours rather than seconds or minutes. These temporal differences in the expression profile of different mediators are important for understanding the coordination of different inflammatory processes.

Vasoactive Amines

Vasoactive amines such as histamine and serotonin are important early mediators of inflammation, promoting vascular dilatation and increased vascular permeability that result in edema (increased fluid volume in interstitial tissue). Histamine is predominantly secreted by mast cells. Degranulation of mast cells occurs rapidly and can produce almost immediate changes in the vasculature. Histamine acts by binding to H1 receptors on endothelial cells and causes the dilatation of arterioles and the constriction of larger muscular arteries. This has the effect of increasing localized blood flow to the affected vascular bed. Histamine also results in increased vascular permeability through its action on venules and causes constriction of bronchial smooth muscle, which can result in bronchospasm.

Nitric Oxide

Nitric oxide (NO) is a reactive, small molecule with a very short half-life that has important effects on the microvasculature. Nitric oxide is generated by the specific enzymes called nitric oxide synthetases (NOSs). Two NOS isoforms can produce nitric oxide at sites of inflammation. Endothelial nitric oxide synthetase (eNOS) is expressed in activated endothelial cells and produces NO, which acts on vascular smooth muscle to promote relaxation and vasodilation (Fig. 2-16). Nitric oxide also has anti-inflammatory effects, inhibiting the adhesion of leukocytes and platelets to endothelial surfaces. Inducible nitric oxide synthetase (iNOS) is predominantly expressed in activated macrophages in which NO production is important for microbial cytotoxicity (generation of oxygen free radicals). Since activated macrophages are usually present at sites of inflammation, NO produced by macrophages can also have localized effects on vascular smooth muscle (promoting vasodilation) as well as effects on platelets and inflammatory cells. Because NO is a highly reactive and unstable compound, it also causes localized tissue injury by free radicals.

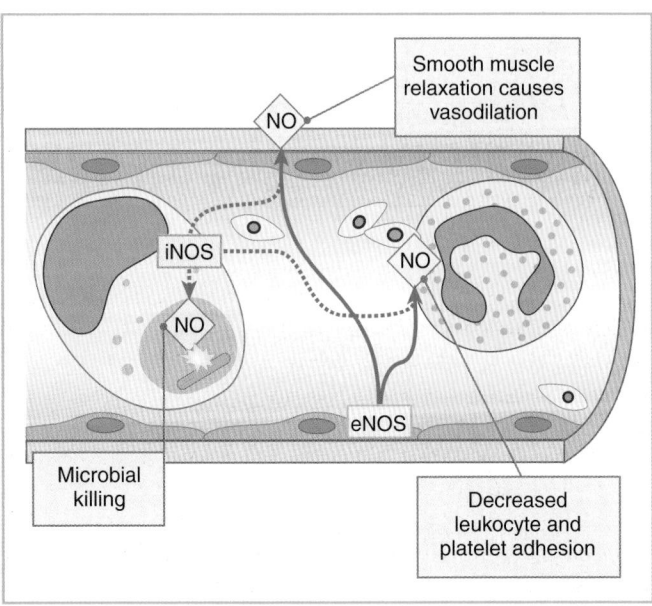

Figure 2-16. Endothelial and inducible nitric oxide synthase.

Neuropeptides

Some neuropeptides are expressed outside the central nervous system (CNS), where they can act as inflammatory mediators. Substance P is a small peptide that can be secreted by small nerves and neuroendocrine cells in various tissues to produce localized pain as well as mediate changes in vascular permeability.

Lipid-Derived Mediators

Many different inflammatory mediators are derived from membrane phospholipids through arachidonic acid intermediates.

These short-lived, small molecules can induce many different types of cellular responses by binding to specific G protein–coupled receptors (GPCRs) on target cells. Cleavage of linoleic acid by phospholipase A_2 and other phospholipases releases arachidonic acid that can be converted to multiple different effector molecules in cells that express the appropriate subset of enzymatic activities. Corticosteroids (endogenous and exogenous) inhibit phospholipase A_2 and can inhibit the formation of all arachidonic acid–derived mediators, providing a broad but blunt anti-inflammatory effect. Corticosteroids also act as immunosuppressive agents (inhibiting many actions of lymphocytes), and their therapeutic use is usually limited to serious pathologic conditions that cannot be effectively managed with more selective and less dangerous anti-inflammatory agents. There are two major enzymatic pathways for metabolism of arachidonic acid into inflammatory mediators (Fig. 2-17).

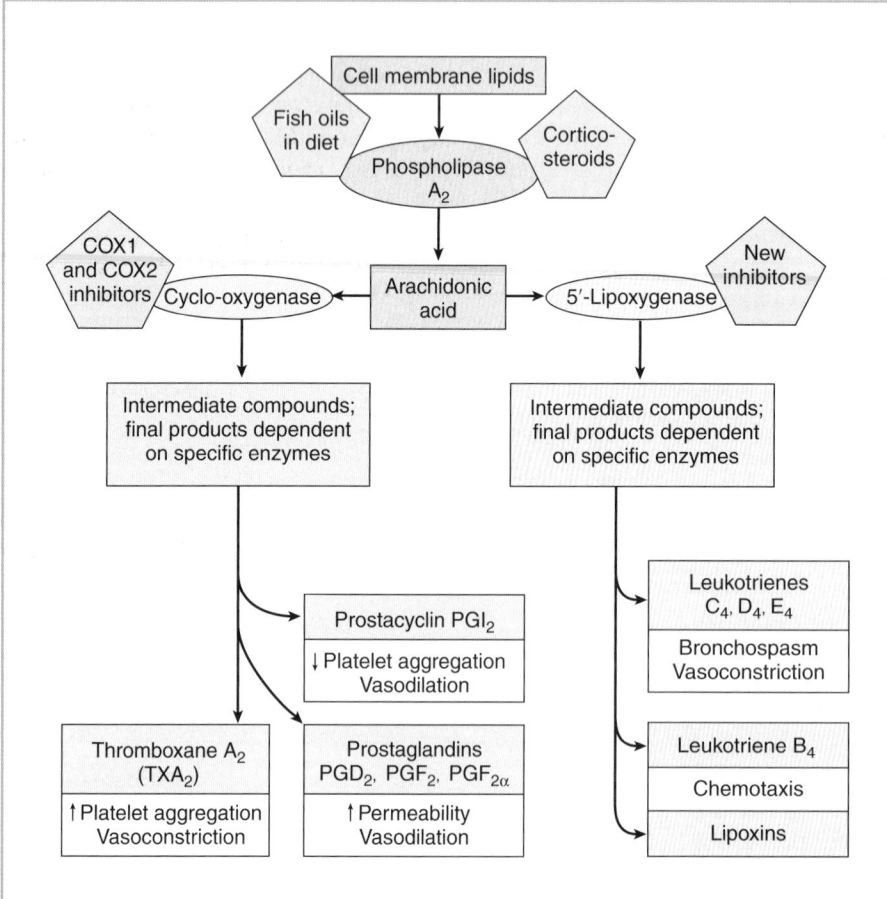

Figure 2-17. Arachidonic acid–derived inflammatory mediators.

Cyclo-oxygenase Pathway

The cyclo-oxygenase pathway is active in many different types of cells and results in the formation of prostaglandin and thromboxane precursors. The enzymatic pathways that form specific prostaglandins and thromboxane are usually expressed in different cell types. For instance, the enzyme required for thromboxane A_2 synthesis is expressed only in platelets while many prostaglandin synthases have a broader tissue distribution.

Two genetically distinct forms of cyclo-oxygenase are now recognized (COX1 and COX2) and are expressed in different types of cells. COX1 is expressed constitutively in many cell types including gastric epithelial cells. As a result, nonspecific COX1 inhibition often results in damage to gastric epithelium with mucosal erosion that can lead to ulcer formation. COX2 is predominantly expressed in activated inflammatory cells at sites of inflammation so that specific inhibition of COX2 has the potential to block inflammation without causing adverse effects on the stomach or other uninflamed tissues. Since platelets express COX1 rather than COX2, selective COX2 inhibition can result in the predominance of platelet-derived arachidonic acid mediators (particularly thromboxane A_2) at sites of inflammation. The effects of thromboxane A_2 (vasoconstriction and platelet aggregation) are normally opposed by prostaglandin (PG) I_2 (prostacyclin) produced by endothelial cells. Selective inhibition of COX2 blocks PGI_2 synthesis and can tip the balance in favor of thrombosis. In this way, targeted COX2 inhibition may produce a pro-thrombotic state that may accelerate atherosclerotic cardiovascular disease (Fig. 2-18).

Lipoxygenase Pathway

The other major pathway for the production of arachidonic acid–derived mediators is through the lipoxygenase pathway.

5′-Lipoxygenase is expressed predominantly in neutrophils and leads to the formation of leukotrienes and lipoxins. Many leukotrienes have prominent effects on bronchial smooth muscle and are important effectors of bronchospasm in the lung. Leukotrienes also have potent effects the vasculature. Lipoxins are another class of mediators that are produced through the metabolism of lipoxygenase products. Lipoxins predominantly promote chemotaxis, and the enzyme that forms lipoxin from 5′-lipoxygenase–derived intermediates is expressed only in platelets. Since platelets do not express 5′-lipoxygenase, the synthesis of lipoxin requires the transfer of precursor molecules from neutrophils to platelets (Fig. 2-19). Lipoxin production highlights the important interactions between different types of inflammatory cells to orchestrate an inflammatory response. It also provides a mechanism whereby the synthesis of some mediators is controlled by the interaction of two cell types. The required cooperation of activated neutrophils and platelets also provides an important control mechanism that tends to prevent the inappropriate synthesis of lipoxin in tissues that are not inflamed.

Platelet-activating Factor

Platelet-activating factor (PAF) is a lipid-derived mediator that is not derived from arachidonic acid precursors. PAF can be produced by platelets, leukocytes, and endothelial cells and is an extraordinarily potent mediator with effects similar to histamine but with up to 1000 times the potency of histamine.

Cytokines

Cytokines are protein mediators that are synthesized de novo in response to different stimuli. As a result, most cytokine effects occur hours after the inciting stimulus. Macrophages

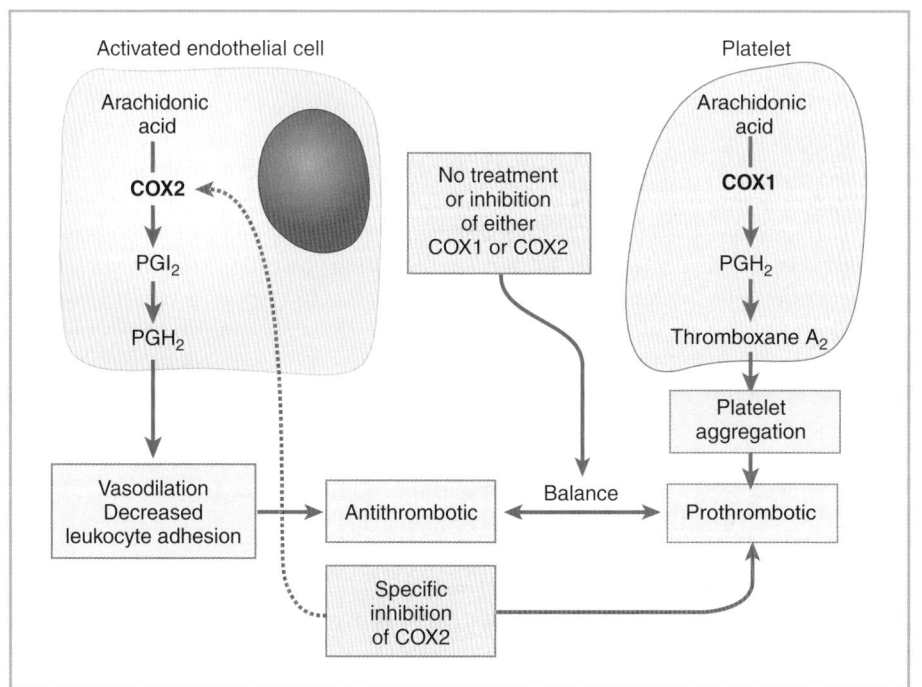

Figure 2-18. Cyclo-oxygenase (COX) 1 and 2 inhibition in endothelial cells and platelets.

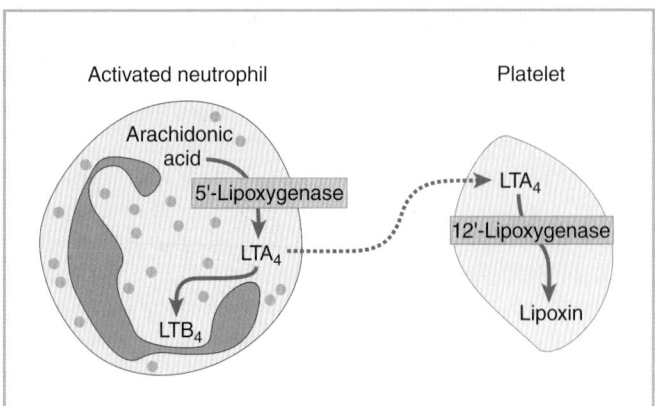

Figure 2-19. Lipoxin production requires cooperation between neutrophils and platelets.

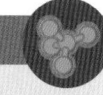

and lymphocytes produce many important cytokines, but other cell types produce some of these mediators as well. The most important inflammatory cytokines produced by macrophages are TNF-α and IL-1. These cytokines can produce both localized and systemic effects depending on the amount of cytokine released. IL-1 has a priming effect on many cell types including most inflammatory cells that results in increased sensitivity of other inflammatory mediators. For example, IL-1 induces changes in transcription in endothelial cells that result in endothelial activation and enhanced leukocyte adherence. Macrophage-derived IL-1 also results in autocrine signaling that promotes its own synthesis by binding to IL-1 receptors on the macrophages. TNF-α is critical for effective neutrophil activation and priming and can markedly increase the sensitivity of neutrophils to other inflammatory mediators. Both TNF-α and IL-1 can induce collagen synthesis by fibroblasts and are important in initiating the healing/repair response.

Large amounts of TNF-α and IL-1 can result in systemic effects including fever and decreased appetite. At even higher levels, IL-1 and TNF-α can cause shock. APCs produce IL-12, which is a potent stimulant for T_H1 responses. IL-12 can cause naïve CD4 cells to become T_H1 cells and enhances IFN-γ secretion by T_H1 cells. IFN-γ is an important mediator that can increase class II MHC expression and IL-12 production by macrophages. This effect can potentiate T_H1 immune responses by enhancing the activity of APCs. IFN-γ is also a potent stimulator of macrophages favoring granuloma formation (see Granulomatous Inflammation section) and can inhibit fibrosis in some inflammatory reactions. IL-2 is a potent growth factor for T cells that facilitates their clonal expansion after antigen stimulation.

Chemokines

Chemokines are small peptides (approximately 8 to 10 kDa molecular weight) that act predominantly as chemotactic factors for different classes of inflammatory cells. α-Chemokines have a characteristic peptide structure with a single amino acid separating conserved cysteine residues

(Cys-X-Cys). IL-8 is a prototypical α-chemokine that predominantly attracts neutrophils. β-Chemokines have no intervening amino acids between conserved cysteine residues (Cys-Cys). Monocyte chemoattractant protein (MCP-1) is an important β-chemokine that predominantly recruits mononuclear inflammatory cells to sites of inflammation.

γ- and δ-chemokines have slightly different structures and their activities are less well characterized.

Plasma Protein Cascades

Three plasma protein cascades are important in mediating inflammatory process and in maintaining hemostasis. There are significant interactions between these individual cascades, which include the complement system, the coagulation system, and the kinin system. The proteins that make up these cascades are synthesized predominantly by the liver and exist as inactive propeptides in the serum that can be activated by cleavage or binding of other cascade components. These preformed mediators can be activated very rapidly, and the hierarchical nature of these cascades can produce significant signal amplification. There are important interactions between these different cascades and receptors on endothelial and inflammatory cells and platelets. Endogenous inhibitors balance activation of these cascades. A fibrinolytic system is also important in terminating and removing blood clots formed by blood coagulation.

Complement Cascade

The complement system consists of 20 proteins and cleavage products. Three activation pathways converge to initiate a common pathway, which results in the formation of a mem-

BIOCHEMISTRY

Chemokines

Chemokines are 8- to 16-kD proteins that act predominantly as chemotactic agents by binding to and signaling through G protein–coupled receptors (GPCRs). GPCRs are members of a large family of receptor proteins with seven highly conserved membrane-spanning domains. Four chemokine receptors (CXCR1–4) have been identified for type A chemokines (e.g., IL-8).

Five chemokine receptors (CCR1–5) have been identified for type B chemokines (e.g., MCP-1, RANTES, and MIP-1a).

Chemokine receptor binding results in a rapid reconfiguration of adhesion molecules including β-integrins to facilitate endothelial cell binding, and activated leukocytes migrate up a chemokine concentration gradient.

A few chemokines appear to have actions other than chemotaxis (e.g., IL-8 stimulates endothelial cell proliferation, and IP-10, MIG, and PF-4 inhibit angiogenesis).

Disease	ENA-78	Exotoxin	IL-8	IP-10	MCP-1	MIP-1A	RANTES
Acute pneumonia	×		×		×		×
Asthma					×	×	×
Atherosclerosis			×		×	×	×
Contact dermatitis	×		×	×	×		×
Inflammatory bowel disease			×	×	×		×
Psoriasis	×		×	×	×		
Rheumatoid arthritis	×		×		×	×	
Wound healing					×	×	

MICROBIOLOGY

Lipopolysaccharide (LPS)

LPS is a major component of the outer membrane of gram-negative bacteria that is also shed into the environment.

LPS is a glycolipid composed of three parts:
- Lipid A is a glucosamine-based phospholipid that is inserted into the outer membrane and acts as an anchor for the other LPS components.
- Core polysaccharide is composed of keto deoxyoctulonate and heptulose.
- Side chains project from the core polysaccharide and vary in composition among different bacteria. O side chains are antigenic, and antibodies can provide protective immunity.

Release of even small amounts of LPS in the circulation can induce cytokine synthesis by macrophages and result in septic shock.

---

brane attack complex that can kill cells by creating a pore in bacterial or mammalian membranes that results in the loss of ion gradients (Fig. 2-20). Intermediate cleavage products of complement cascade also have important chemotactic and proinflammatory functions that often are more important than the formation of membrane pores.

Alternative Complement Pathway

The alternative pathway for complement activation can be directly activated by cleavage of the C3 molecule or by its interaction with bacterial products such as endotoxin.

C3b (one of the cleavage products of C3) can interact with the cleavage product of factor B (Bb) to form a heterodimer known as the alternate C3 convertase [C3bBb]. This protein complex can cleave additional C3 molecules to initiate the common complement pathway by forming alternate C5 convertase (by adding a second C3b molecule to the complex [C3bBb3b]). The other peptide fragment released from the cleavage of C3 (C3a) is called an anaphylatoxin because it has a number of proinflammatory activities including chemotaxis, the induction of mast cell degranulation (to release histamine and serotonin), and activation of 5′-lipoxygenase in neutrophils (to produce leukotriene mediators and to be a potent chemotactic factor for neutrophils and other leukocytes). In

addition to its role as a convertase, C3b can bind to cell membranes and act as an opsonizing agent that significantly promotes neutrophil phagocytosis.

Classical/Lectin Complement Pathway

The classical pathway of complement activation is initiated by the interaction of immunocomplexes (macromolecular aggregates of immunoglobulin bound to its antigen) with complement component C1. Immunocomplex binding activates C1 to cleave C4 and C2, forming a heterodimer composed of C4 and C2 cleavage products, which is called the classical C3 convertase [C4b2a]. This convertase can then cleave C3 and addition of C3b to the complex form the classical C5 convertase [C4b2a3b], which cleaves C5 to initiate the common pathway. Binding of plasma mannose-binding protein (MBP) to bacterial membrane proteins also can initiate the complement cascade via activation of C1. Additionally, the classical pathway produces C3a (anaphylatoxin) and additional C3b, which binds to cell membranes to act as an opsonin.

Common Complement Pathway

The classical, alternative, and lectin-binding pathways converge to activate the common pathway by cleaving C5 to release C5a and C5b. C5a is an anaphylatoxin with actions similar to C3a. C5b can bind to cell membranes and organize the assembly of complement components C6 through C9 into a so-called membrane attack complex. These proteins bind together and organize the formation of a pore in the cell membrane of bacteria or mammalian cells.

Low-level activation of the early complement components occurs in normal individuals by the actions of nonspecific plasma proteases. This low-level activation holds the complement system in readiness for rapid and sensitive activation if microorganisms or immunocomplexes are present. Other specific plasma proteases can cleave activated complement components (particularly C3 and C1) to terminate activation of the complement cascade. The balance between these

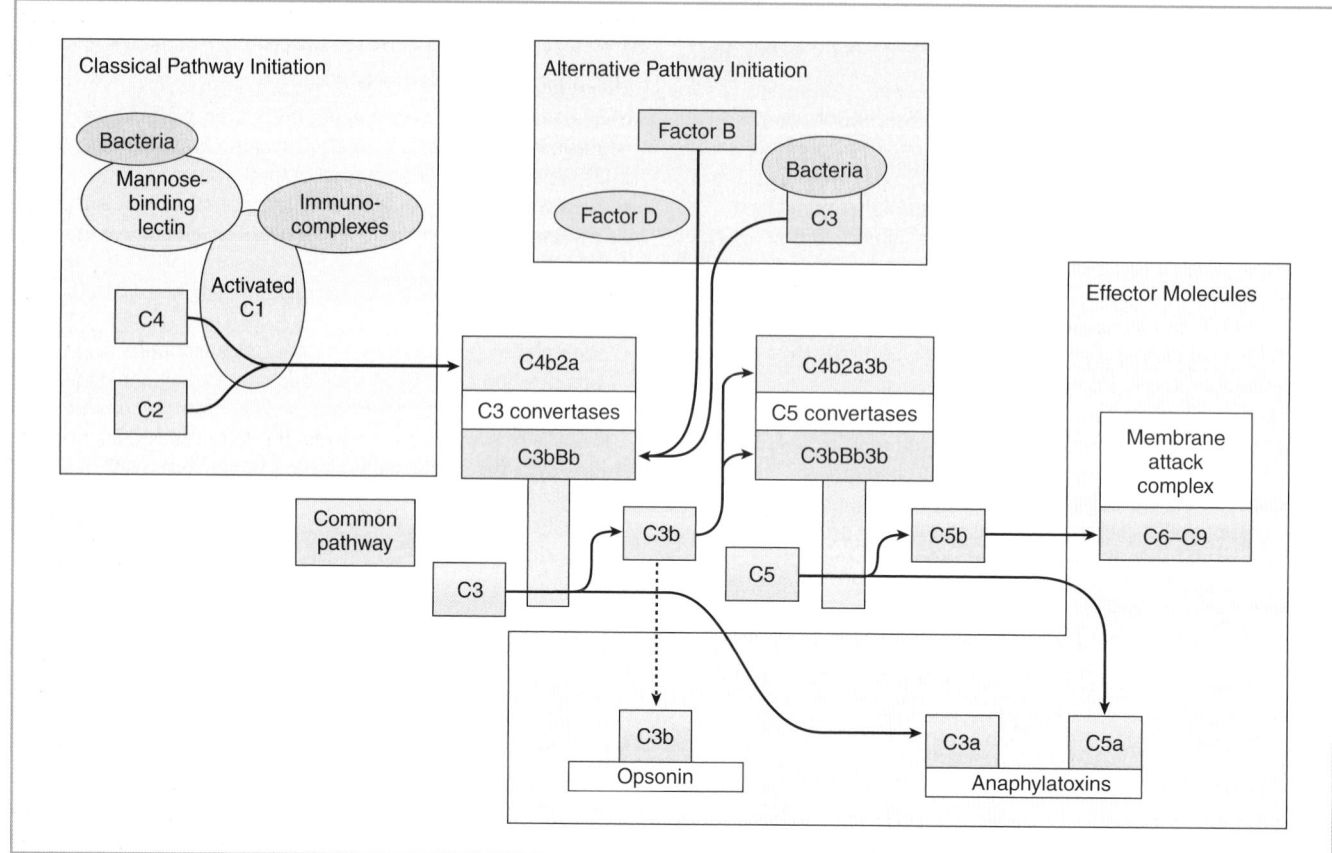

Figure 2-20. Complement cascade.

activating and inactivating factors is essential for normal homeostasis.

Deficiency of late complement components (C6–C9) prevents the formation of a functional membrane attack complex but does not cause severe immunodeficiency although individuals who are unable to form the membrane attack complex are more susceptible to infection by *Neisseria* species. Deficiency of C3 results in marked susceptibility to many different types of bacterial infection because of the failure to produce complement-derived opsonin (C3b) and anaphylatoxins (C3a and C5a). Genetic alterations in some of the early complement components (C2 and C4) are associated with autoimmune disease (remember that the complement genes are embedded in the MHC locus).

Coagulation Cascade

The main function of the coagulation cascade is to maintain hemostasis and prevent blood loss resulting from trauma or other types of injury. Two classical patterns of activation (intrinsic and extrinsic pathways) converge on a common pathway that results in the cleavage of fibrinogen to form a fibrin clot. The distinction between the intrinsic and extrinsic pathways is more related to laboratory testing than their role in vivo. In the laboratory, the intrinsic and extrinsic pathways are measured as the prothrombin time (PT) and partial thromboplastin time (PTT), respectively (Fig. 2-21). While this distinction is useful for the functional testing of different

complement components, both intrinsic and extrinsic pathways are simultaneously activated in response to almost all forms of vascular damage in vivo.

Activated Hageman factor (factor XII, intrinsic pathway) also cleaves prekallikrein to kallikrein, resulting in the activation of the kinin cascade and ultimately in the cleavage of plasminogen to form plasmin. Plasmin cleaves fibrin polymers to lyse formed clots and reestablish normal perfusion through thrombosed blood vessels. This fibrinolytic pathway is activated automatically by collaboration between the coagulation and kinin systems and illustrates the coordination of prothrombotic and antithrombotic mechanisms to achieve hemostasis. Plasmin also cleaves C3 and can thereby activate the complement cascade to initiate an inflammatory response at sites of thrombosis.

Intrinsic and Extrinsic Coagulation Pathways

The intrinsic pathway is activated by the cleavage of factor XII to form XIIa (Fig. 2-22). Factor XII can be activated by its interaction with subendothelial collagen or high-molecular-weight kininogen (HMWK). Factor XIIa cleaves prekallikrein to form kallikrein, which then cleaves additional factor XII molecules, resulting in the autocatalytic activation of factor XII. Factor XIIa cleaves factor XI to form active factor IXa, which can cleave factor X to initiate the common coagulation pathway. These reactions occur primarily in solution. Factor IX can also be activated by tissue factor from the extrinsic pathway.

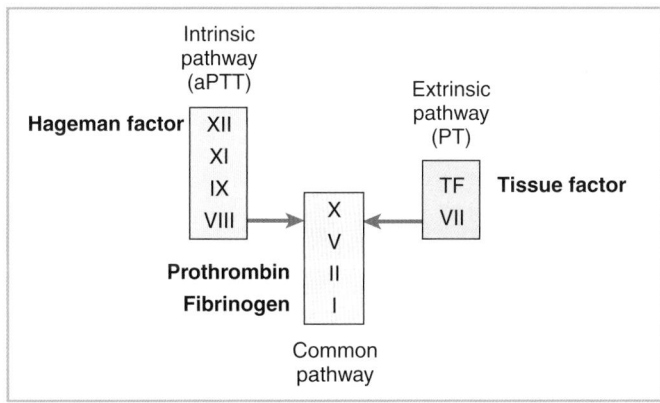

Figure 2-21. Intrinsic and extrinsic coagulation pathways.

CLINICAL MEDICINE

Laboratory Evaluation of Coagulation

The prothrombin time (PT) is measured by treating citrate-anticoagulated plasma with calcium and complete thromboplastin (usually a rabbit brain derivative). Coagulation is measured photometrically, and the time to completion is calculated by means of an algorithm.

Different lots of complete thromboplastin vary in activity, and all are compared with a common standard reagent to calculate the international normalized ratio (INR), which is normally between 0.9 and 1.2. The INR allows direct comparison of PT values measured in different laboratories.

Increased PT usually results from deficiency of factor I, II, V, VII, or X. The most common reason for increased PT clinically is treatment with warfarin, which blocks vitamin K metabolism and inhibits the formation of vitamin K–dependent factors, including factor VII.

The activated partial thromboplastin time (aPTT) is measured by adding a phospholipid activated with a negatively charged substance such as kaolin to citrate-anticoagulated plasma.

Increased aPTT (>35 seconds) can result from decreased activity of any coagulation factor to less than 30% of its normal level. aPTT provides a broader evaluation of the coagulation system than does the PT test (e.g., aPTT detects hemophilia and is used for monitoring heparin therapy).

Factor assays are designed to detect abnormalities of individual coagulation components by mixing patient serum with sera from patients with known coagulation defects. Mixed samples are then assessed in an aPTT assay to identify specific defects. Coagulation inhibitors can be identified by mixing patient serum with pooled normal sera.

The extrinsic pathway is initiated by the release of tissue factor by damaged endothelial cells that results in the cleavage of factor VII to form VIIa. VIIa can then cleave factor X to initiate the common pathway. Tissue factor can also activate factor IX in the intrinsic pathway.

Common Coagulation Pathway

The common pathway proceeds with the activation of factor X to form Xa, which can then interact with activated factor VIIIa to cleave prothrombin (factor II) to thrombin (factor IIa). Cooperation between factors IXa and VIIIa greatly speeds the cleavage of factor X and accelerates the coagulation reaction forward. Factor VIII is activated by thrombin (factor IIa), which is the terminal protease in the common pathway that also cleaves fibrinogen to form a fibrin clot. This complicated, nested pathway results in a situation in which the activation of earlier coagulation cascade components is regulated by activation of the terminal component. This mechanism tends to decelerate the cascade if thrombin is not produced and to accelerate the cascade if a localized clot is being formed by thrombin. This type of autocatalytic regulation is important to prevent an ineffective, partial activation of the coagulation cascade that could consume coagulation factors and cause injury without providing effective hemostasis.

Factor Xa interacts with factor Va to cleave prothrombin to produce thrombin. Factor V is activated in the same manner as factor VIII with thrombin cleaving factor V to form factor Va. This second nested activation step reinforces the control exerted by the interaction of factors VIIIa and IXa, resulting in an "on" or "off" setting for the terminal coagulation cascade and prevents ineffective, partial activation.

The activation of both factor X and prothrombin are calcium dependent and take place on membrane surfaces (usually platelet membranes) with factors VIIIa and Va acting as cofactors for factor IXa and Xa, respectively (Fig. 2-23). The membrane localization of these reactions serves to localize and focus the coagulation cascade and to prevent systemic activation of coagulation. Membrane localization also increases the rates of these reactions (two-dimensional rather than three-dimensional diffusion of reactants). Activated thrombin finally cleaves fibrinogen to fibrin, which forms a clot in cooperation with activated platelets. Thrombin also activates factor XIII to form factor XIIIa, which forms cross-links between linear fibrin polymers to enhance clot stability. Fibrinogen receptors on inflammatory cells and platelets facilitate their activation and recruitment to sites of vascular damage.

Fibrinolysis

Plasmin cleaves fibrin clot to form fibrin monomers that dissociate, resulting in clot lysis. Activation of the coagulation system indirectly results in the activation of plasmin through the kinin cascade so that even as a coagulation reaction is initiated, mechanisms are also put in place that can ultimately lyse the clot. Tissue plasminogen activator (t-PA) released by endothelial cells can also activate plasminogen to initiate clot lysis. Plasmin inhibitors (such as plasminogen inhibitor α-220 plasmin) provide a counterbalance to fibrinolytic activity.

Regulation of the Coagulation Cascade

Multiple specific inhibitors of coagulation cascade components are either present in plasma or are produced by activated endothelial cells. Antithrombin 3 is a plasma protein that is activated by binding to negatively charged polymers such as heparin. Antithrombin 3 can directly inhibit

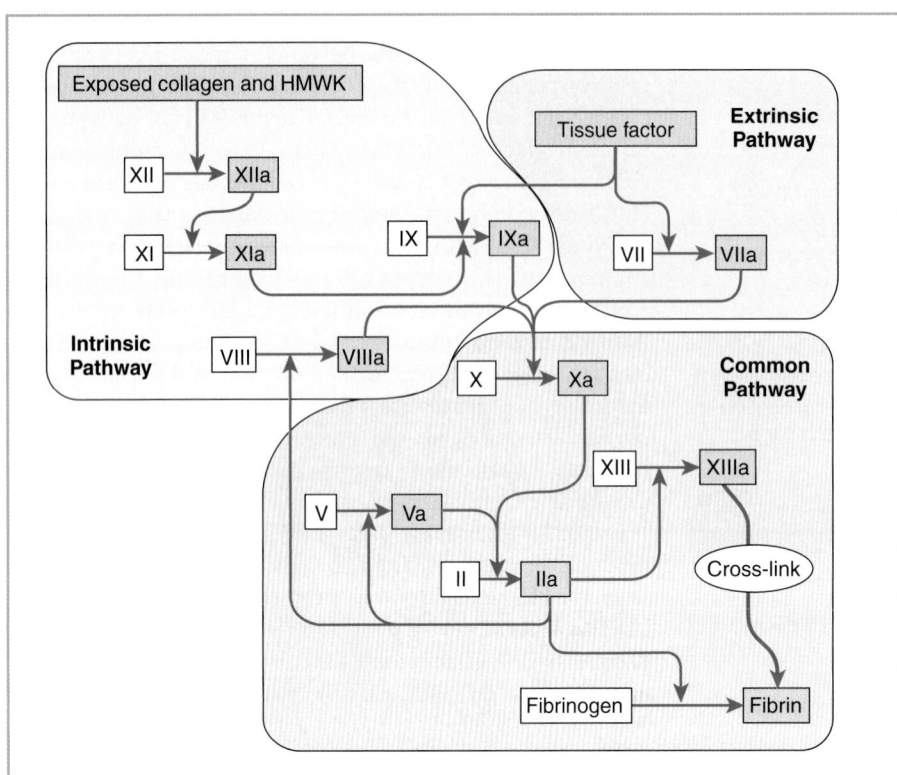

Figure 2-22. Coagulation cascade.

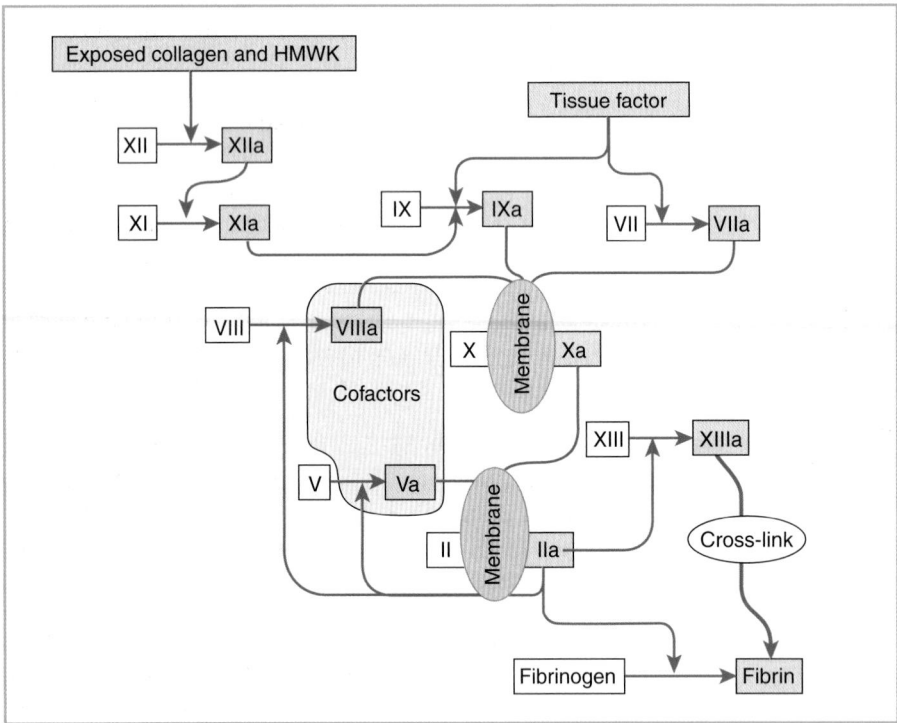

Figure 2-23. Role of cofactors and cell membranes in the coagulation cascade.

thrombin-meditated cleavage of fibrinogen as well as inhibit the actions of factors XIa and XIIa (Fig. 2-24). Protein C and protein S are vitamin K–dependent plasma proteins that can inactivate factors Va and VIIIa. Binding of thrombomodulin (produced by activated endothelial cells) to thrombin results in the activation of protein C, which cooperates with protein

S to cleave and inactivate factors Va and VIIa (Fig. 2-25). Plasmin and the fibrinolytic system ultimately terminate and reverse the actions of the coagulation cascade.

The interplay between soluble factors and factors synthesized by endothelial cells and platelets results in a coagulation cascade that is poised for rapid activation but can

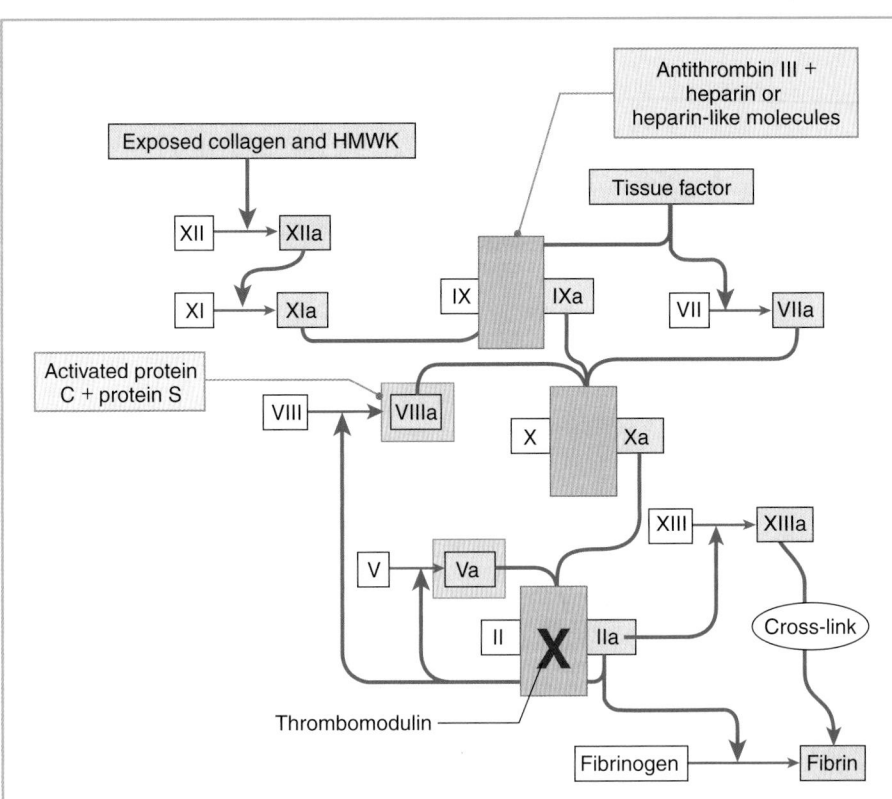

Figure 2-24. Inhibitors of coagulation.

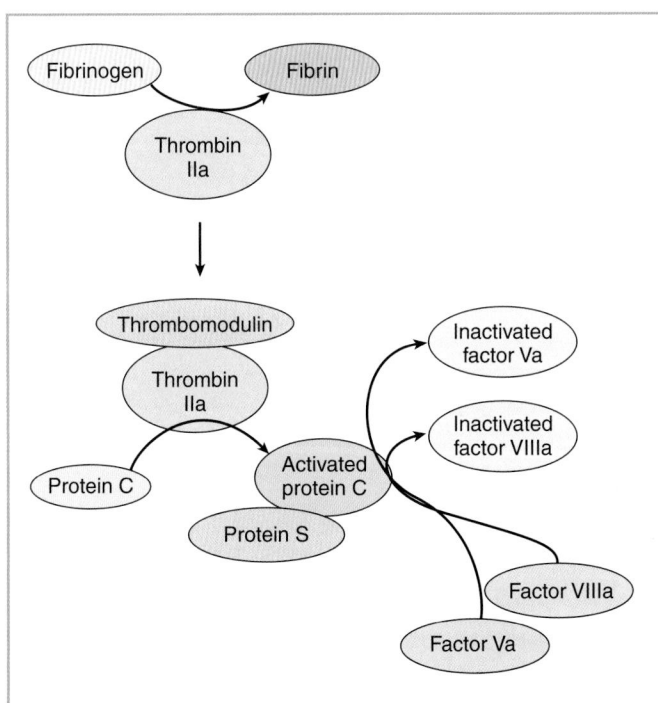

Figure 2-25. Activation of protein C.

platelet aggregation) are also key factors in modulating an appropriate hemostatic response.

Defects of the Coagulation Cascade

Genetic and acquired defects of the coagulation system are important causes of morbidity and mortality. Genetic abnormalities of coagulation proteins and positive or negative regulators of the coagulation cascade all can cause disease. Point mutations in the factor VIII gene that is located on the X chromosome causes classic hemophilia with diminished factor VIII function. Heterozygous females are usually normal, but affected males often have a severe bleeding tendency depending on the nature of the mutation.

Inherited or acquired deficiency of proteins C or S can result in a prothrombotic phenotype. Autoantibodies can sometimes activate various components of the coagulation cascade, resulting in hemorrhage or thrombosis. Nutritional deficiency, hepatic insufficiency, or both can result in inadequate quantities of coagulation factors in plasma. Deficiency of fat-soluble vitamin K results in diminished concentrations of functional vitamin K–dependent coagulation factors and regulatory proteins. These factors require vitamin K for carboxylation of specific glutamic acid residues that are essential for their interaction with calcium ions during activation (Fig. 2-27). Warfarin therapy takes advantage of this dependence on vitamin K by specifically blocking carboxylation to produce an "anticoagulated" state. Inhibitory proteins C and S are also vitamin K dependent, and warfarin therapy can occasionally result in a prothrombotic state owing to inactivation of these regulatory proteins.

also rapidly terminate clot formation and initiate clot lysis (Fig. 2-26). The interplay between PGI_2 produced by endothelial cells (vasodilation and inhibition of platelet aggregation) and platelet-derived thromboxane A_2 (vasoconstriction and

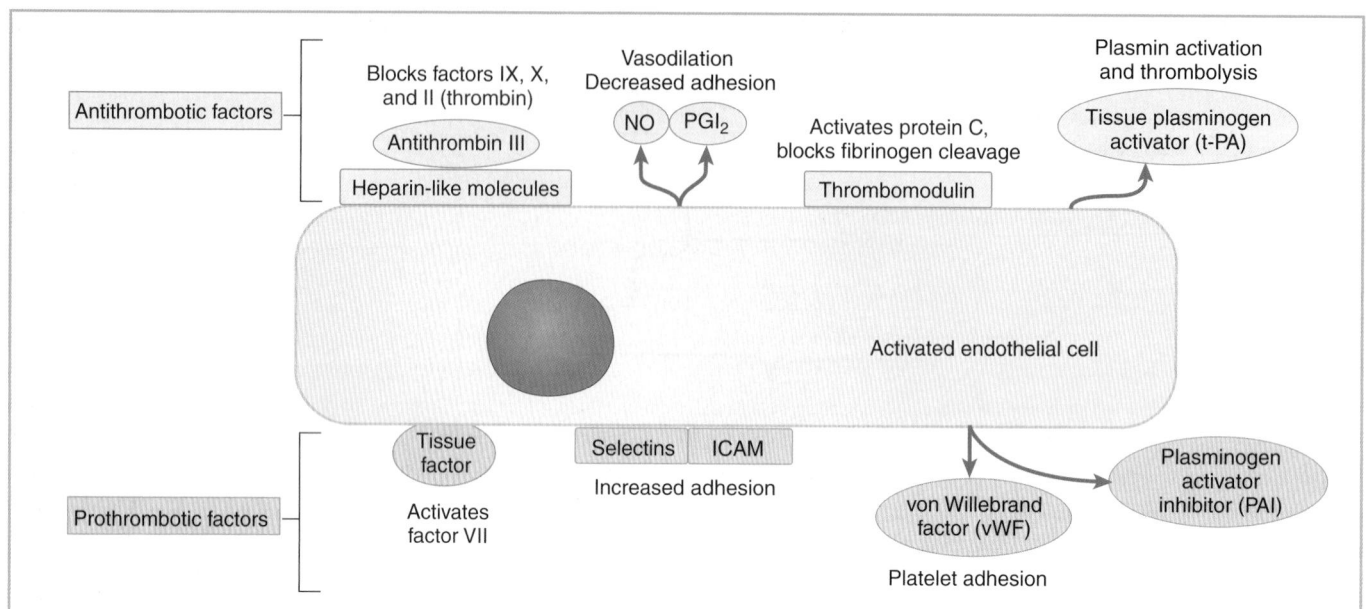

Figure 2-26. Role of endothelial cells in modulating hemostasis.

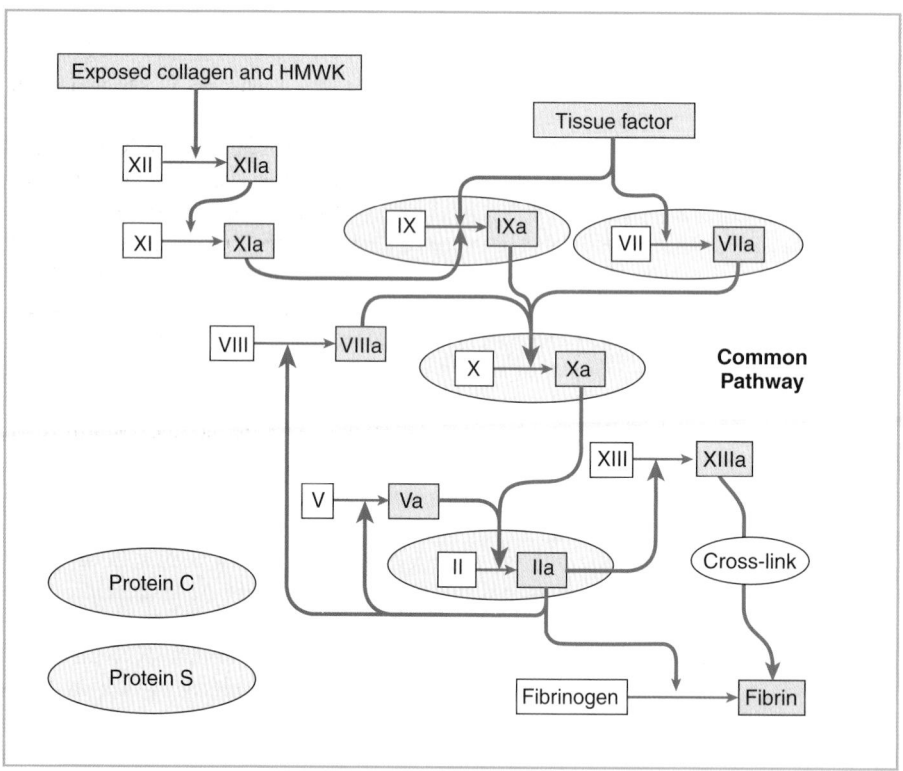

Figure 2-27. Role of vitamin K–dependent coagulation factors and inhibitors.

Heparin acts as an anticoagulant by activating antithrombin 3 (heparin is chemically similar to the normal binding partner of antithrombin 3—proteoglycan). Heparin-induced thrombocytopenia occurs in up to 5% of patients treated with unfractionated heparin. Susceptible individuals form antibodies against heparin that cross-react with platelet factor 4. Antibody binding to platelet membranes results in their rapid removal by the spleen, causing marked thrombocytopenia.

Thrombosis

Thrombosis is the abnormal or inappropriate activation of the coagulation system to form a clot. Thrombi may be intravascular or extravascular associated with hemorrhage. Both venous and arterial thrombi can form although the risk factors for each are largely different. Factors that predispose to thrombosis include endothelial injury, diminished blood flow, and a prothrombotic (hypercoagulable) environment (so-called Virchow's triad). Thrombosis is an important cause of morbidity and mortality (see Chapter 3).

Disseminated Intravascular Coagulation

Disseminated intravascular coagulation (DIC) is essentially the disordered systemic activation of the coagulation cascade. DIC results in the intravascular cleavage of fibrinogen to form small fibrin clots that lodge in the microcirculation and often cause severe renal and pulmonary dysfunction. Plasmin is also activated in DIC and cleaves fibrin microthrombi to release fibrin degradation products (so-called fibrin split products), which can be detected in the clinical laboratory. Intravascular fibrin deposits initiate platelet aggregation, endothelial activation, and inflammatory reactions that can produce additional tissue damage (e.g., adult respiratory distress syndrome, ARDS). The widespread activation of the coagulation cascade in DIC can rapidly deplete normal coagulation factors and consume platelets, resulting in a marked predisposition to life-threatening hemorrhage.

Kinin Cascade

The kinin cascade is activated by cleavage of prekallikrein by activated Hageman factor (factor XIIa) to form kallikrein. Kallikrein then cleaves HMWK to release the nonapeptide bradykinin (nine amino acids). Bradykinin causes localized pain and bronchospasm as well as increased vascular permeability and vasodilation. Bradykinin is rapidly degraded by kininase, which is present in most tissues. Any bradykinin that escapes into the systemic circulation is inactivated by angiotensin II in the pulmonary circulation, effectively preventing systemic effects from bradykinin release. Kallikrein can also cleave factor XII as part of an autocatalytic loop that can activate both the kinin and coagulation cascades. Another important action of kallikrein

is the cleavage of plasminogen to form plasmin. The thrombolytic activity of plasmin initiates clot lysis and facilitates the orderly termination of the blood coagulation.

Interactions Between Inflammatory Mediators

Interactions between different inflammatory mediators and pathways are critical in orchestrating an effective inflammatory response (Fig. 2-28). This regulation is complex, and small changes in various components can lead to abnormal inflammation and disease. Important connections between the intrinsic coagulation pathway and kinin activation can cause localized inflammation and favor thrombosis but also result in the activation of the plasmin to dissolve formed clots. Plasmin can also cleave early complement components to facilitate complement activation and release chemotactic anaphylatoxins (C3a and C5a). Some products of the coagulation cascade have important proinflammatory activities, and links between inflammation and coagulation permit the coordination of these processes. Activated thrombin binds to the protease-activated receptor (PAR-1), which is expressed on surface of platelets and endothelial cells as well as other cells. Activation of PAR-1 on endothelial cells results in the induction of COX2-mediated prostaglandin synthesis and the production of cytokines and nitric oxide (mainly antithrombotic effects). Conversely, thrombin binding to PAR-1 on platelets enhances thromboxane A_2 production to promote thrombosis.

At first glance, some of these interactions result in contrary effects, but the net result of these interactions usually is the rapid activation of inflammation and coagulation at sites of injury followed by a coordinated termination of this response and transition to tissue repair. The time scale of the generation, release, and inactivation of different inflammatory mediators and cellular activation pathways is

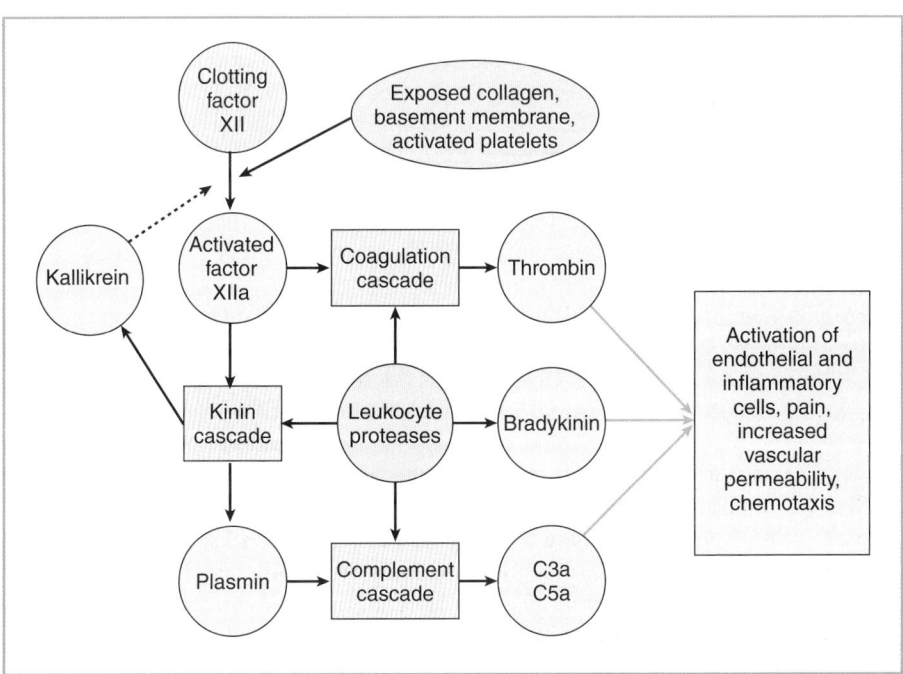

Figure 2-28. Interactions between inflammatory mediators.

important in coordinating these processes to orchestrate and appropriately localize a normal inflammatory response. Genetic and acquired abnormalities of any of these components can predispose to a pathologic deviation that can result in inappropriate activation or failure of one or more of these systems. Pharmacologic modulation of inflammatory reactions to minimize tissue damage and control symptoms comprises a significant portion of clinical medicine but can also result in serious adverse effects if the relationships between pathways are not carefully considered.

●●● PATTERNS OF INFLAMMATORY RESPONSE

Most inflammatory responses are complex and involve the interaction of multiple different cell types and soluble mediators. While most inflammatory reactions are in some sense unique, it is useful to consider four major types of inflammatory response—types I, II, III, and IV hypersensitivity—that are common mechanisms of disease. While these categories are useful constructs, it is important to remember that inflammatory reactions occurring in patients may incorporate features of several different types of hypersensitivity.

Type I Hypersensitivity

Type I hypersensitivity is synonymous with immediate type hypersensitivity and is almost always mediated through IgE antibodies that are bound to the surface of mast cells (Fig. 2-29A). Interaction of this IgE with antigen results in activation of mast cells and their rapid degranulation with the release of histamine, serotonin, and other inflammatory mediators. Type I hypersensitivity is dependent on the presence of preformed IgE antibodies. The release of large amounts of histamine and serotonin results in massive vasodilation, diminished blood pressure, and marked bronchoconstriction. Widespread activation of mast cells can result in a systemic response to antigen that can cause anaphylactic shock (see Shock section). Other mediators released by activated mast cells recruit eosinophils and other inflammatory cells (eosinophil and neutrophil chemotactic factors). Activated mast cells also produce PAF, prostaglandins, and leukotrienes. PGD_2 and leukotrienes are potent bronchospastic agents that can cause transient respiratory insufficiency in anaphylaxis. Production of cytokines such as TNF-α, IL-1, Il-3, and IL-5 result in a sustained inflammatory response while IL-4 facilitates IgE production by B cells.

Type II Hypersensitivity

Type II hypersensitivity is an antibody-dependent process in which specific antibodies bind to antigens, resulting in tissue damage or destruction (see Fig. 2-29B). If the antigen is present on cell surfaces, antibody binding can result in cell lysis through the in situ fixation of complement. IgM antibodies (multimeric) are often more effective in fixing complement than are than IgG antibodies (monomeric). Type II hypersensitivity is typified by a transfusion reaction in which mismatched red blood cells are rapidly destroyed by specific preformed antibodies (anti-ABO or -Rh) and complement. Although fixation of complement can result in direct cell lysis, opsonization and recruitment of inflammatory cells is often a more important cause of cell injury.

Type III Hypersensitivity

Type III hypersensitivity is caused by circulating immunocomplexes (see Fig. 2-29C) and is typified by serum sickness (a drug reaction in which multimeric drug-antibody aggregates form in solution). Preformed immunocomplexes deposit in various vascular beds and cause injury at these sites. Multimeric antigen-antibody complexes are efficient activators of the complement cascade through its classical pathway. The vascular beds in which immunocomplexes are deposited are determined in part by the physical nature of the complexes (their aggregate size, charge, hydrophobicity, etc.), and the specificity of deposition at particular locations can be surprisingly precise in some diseases. Typical sites of injury are kidney, skin, and mucous membranes. Type III hypersensitivity is common in systemic lupus erythematosus (SLE) and underlies most of the pathophysiology of this chronic autoimmune disease. Some inflammatory reactions may blend features of type II and III hypersensitivity with the formation of immunocomplexes in situ.

Type IV Hypersensitivity

Type IV hypersensitivity is also called delayed-type hypersensitivity (DTH) because the tissue reaction usually occurs 24 to 48 hours after exposure to antigen. Type IV hypersensitivity is a cell-mediated immunoreaction that is dependent on the presence of a significant number of primed, antigen-specific T cells (see Fig. 2-29D). This type of reaction is typified by the response to poison ivy, which typically reaches its peak 24 to 48 hours after exposure to antigen. Plant antigens (haptens) react with and modify cellular proteins that are then targeted by the sensitized T cells. Interaction of CD8+ T cells with antigen presented in the context of class I MHC results in the activation of these T cells and induces them to kill target cells displaying these antigens. APCs also display antigen in the context of class II MHC to activate CD4+ T cells to secrete cytokines, including IL-2, which result in the proliferation of CD8+ T cells. The result of these interactions is the amplification of antigen-specific T cells that initiate the hypersensitivity reaction over the course of a few days.

Delayed-type hypersensitivity also describes a positive response to the common test for tuberculosis (subcutaneous injection of mycobacterial purified protein derivative, or PPD). In this case, inactivated toxoid from mycobacteria recruits pre-primed T cells and macrophages, which initiate

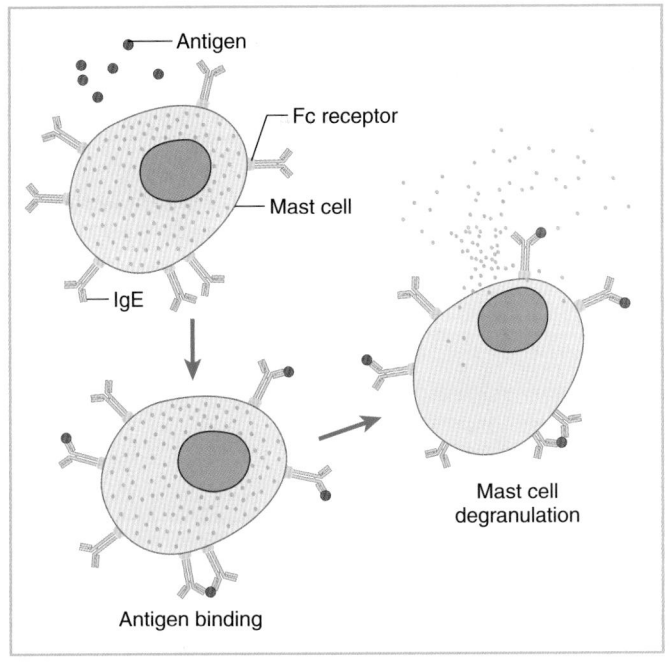

A

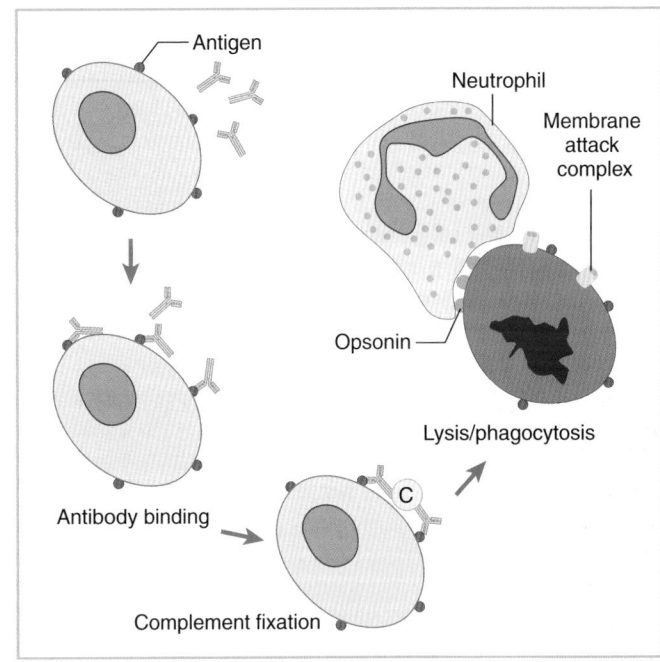

B

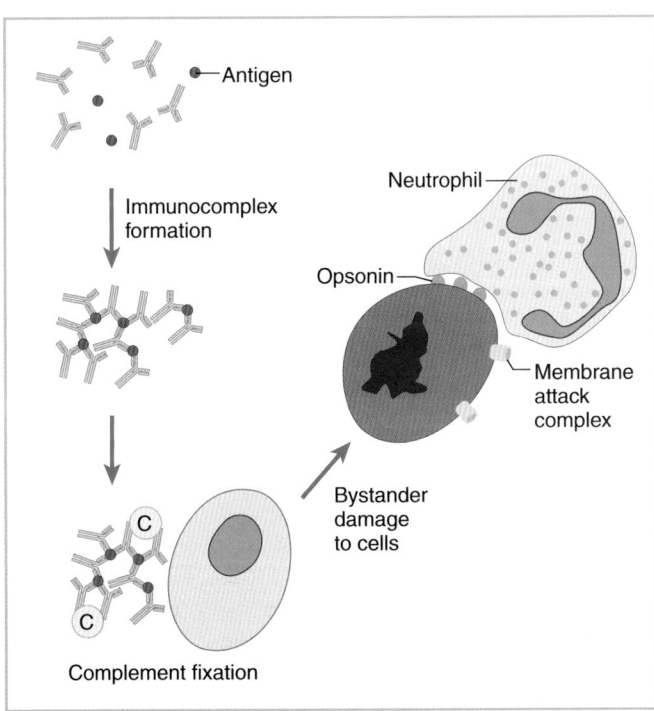

C

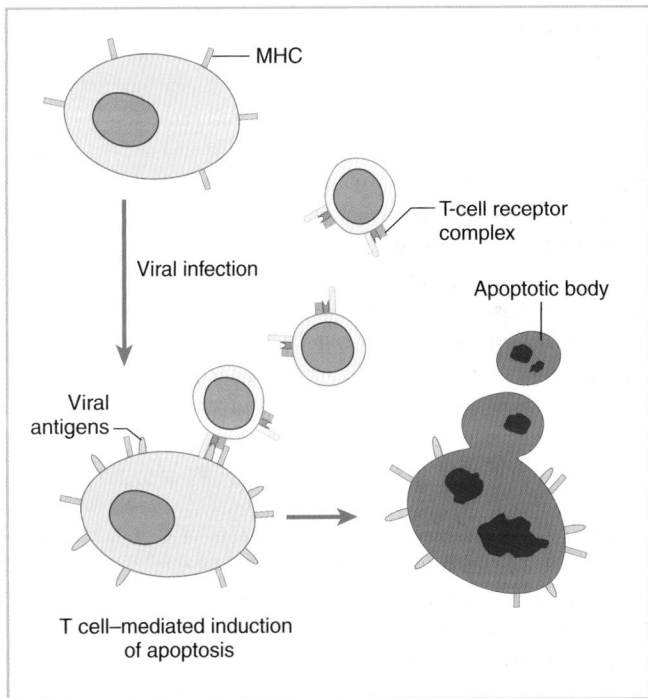

D

Figure 2-29. A, Type I hypersensitivity. **B**, Type II hypersensitivity. **C**, Type III hypersensitivity. **D**, Type IV hypersensitivity.

an inflammatory response. A positive test occurs only if a significant number of antigen-specific T cells are already present as a result of prior (or ongoing) exposure to mycobacterial antigens. Paradoxically, patients with disseminated tuberculosis may not respond to PPD because of significant immunosuppression produced by severe infection. The interaction of T cells and macrophages with antigen results in

the production of IFN-γ and TNF-α to orchestrate a strong inflammatory reaction that may be granulomatous in character (see below). Some types of natural killer cell inflammatory responses may be described as delayed-type hypersensitivity in that they are mediated exclusively by cellular components of the immune system but are not antigen specific.

Acute Inflammation

Acute inflammation implies an inflammatory reaction that develops over a rapid time scale (hours to days) and consists of a relatively stereotyped morphologic pattern. Acute inflammation is the initial response to many types of injury but is also characteristic of the response to most pyogenic bacterial infections. Neutrophils are the predominant cell type in almost all acute inflammatory reactions, sometimes in association with eosinophils. Most acute inflammatory reactions reach their peak after 48 to 72 hours and then transition to a mixed acute and chronic inflammatory cell infiltrate that may ultimately change to predominantly chronic inflammation. The time frame for this evolution depends on the nature and persistence of the injury, and pyogenic bacterial infections can result in prolonged acute inflammation if viable bacteria persist.

The earliest changes in acute inflammation are usually vascular rather than inflammatory cell infiltration. Most forms of injury result in damage to, and activation of, endothelial cells that release various inflammatory mediators that result in vasodilation and increased vascular permeability. These very rapid vascular changes produce the classical localized manifestations of acute inflammation (rubor, calor, tumor, and dolor). Increased redness (rubor) and warmth (calor) result from vascular dilatation. Swelling (tumor) or edema results from increased vascular permeability and the actions of inflammatory mediators. Pain (dolor) can result from the combined actions of neural stimulation and the release of substance P, bradykinin, and prostaglandins in affected tissues.

Some inflammatory mediators act as potent chemotactic agents that attract neutrophils and other inflammatory cells to sites of inflammation. Endothelial cell activation is also a key factor in recruiting inflammatory cells. Once inflammatory cells adhere to activated endothelial cells, they migrate between endothelial cells and digest through basement membrane using metalloproteinases to begin moving through tissue. During this process, neutrophils secrete additional inflammatory mediators that result in the recruitment of additional inflammatory cells as well as further activation of inflammatory cells already at the site of inflammation. Activation of neutrophils results in their polarization with mobilization of their cytoskeleton to promote active movement toward various chemoattractants. The complement components (C3a and C5a) and some lipoxygenase pathway products are important chemotactic factors for acute inflammation. Chemokines such as IL-8 and MCP-1 are also important chemotactic mediators for neutrophils and mononuclear cells, respectively. Lipopolysaccharide and formylmethionine (unique bacterial products) are also direct chemoattractants for neutrophils.

An acute inflammatory response may remain entirely localized but can also produce systemic symptoms. The recruitment of macrophages to a site of acute inflammation results in their activation and production of IL-1 and TNF-α, which cause fever through interaction with hypothalamic receptors. Release of cytokines such as IL-6 induces hepatocytes to increase production of acute-phase reactants including C-reactive protein (CRP). These acute-phase reactants cause increased stickiness of red blood cells, resulting in the laboratory phenomenon of increased erythrocyte sedimentation rate (ESR).

The consequences of an inflammatory reaction depend on the inciting stimulus as well as host-specific variations in inflammatory response. Phagocytosis and effective intracellular killing of microorganisms by neutrophils and macrophages may terminate an inflammatory response by removing the inciting stimulus. If viable microorganisms remain, the acute inflammatory response usually intensifies and may result in abscess formation.

An *abscess* is a collection of neutrophils, macrophages, and necrotic debris that has undergone liquefaction owing to the action of proteolytic enzymes released by inflammatory cells and bacteria (Fig. 2-30). Activated macrophages in and around an abscess produce cytokines resulting in fever and other systemic manifestations. If viable bacteria are present in the abscess, they may spread into the bloodstream (sepsis), since the hypoxic environment of an abscess cavity inhibits microbial killing (i.e., no respiratory burst is possible in this environment). If an abscess spreads to a body cavity such as the pleura or peritoneum, it can cause generalized inflammation and infection of the cavity with the formation of an empyema (pleural abscess) or intra-abdominal abscess with peritonitis.

The time scale of an acute inflammatory response is limited by the short life span of neutrophils (48 hours in the circulation but usually much less in inflamed tissues). Over time, most inflammatory reactions convert from acute to chronic inflammation with recruitment of longer lived mononuclear cells. Chronic inflammation often provides a transition to the tissue repair in which macrophages engulf cellular debris to facilitate repair by fibroblasts and other cell types.

Chronic Inflammation

Chronic inflammation is characterized by a predominantly mononuclear inflammatory cell infiltrate with few neutrophils present. Chronic inflammation often develops during the transition from acute inflammation to tissue repair. Chronic inflammation may also develop de novo in response to certain types of insults. In particular, viral infections (as well as a few specific types of bacterial infections) preferentially induce a chronic inflammatory response with minimal acute inflammation. Chronic inflammation is typically much longer lasting than acute inflammation and may persist for weeks, months, or even years (Fig. 2-31). Different types of chronic inflammatory reactions may be characterized by the predominance of T cells, B cells, plasma cells, or macrophages. In prolonged chronic inflammation, plasma cells are often prominent in the inflammatory infiltrate, and localized immunoglobulin secretion may be important in the pathophysiology in this type of inflammatory reaction.

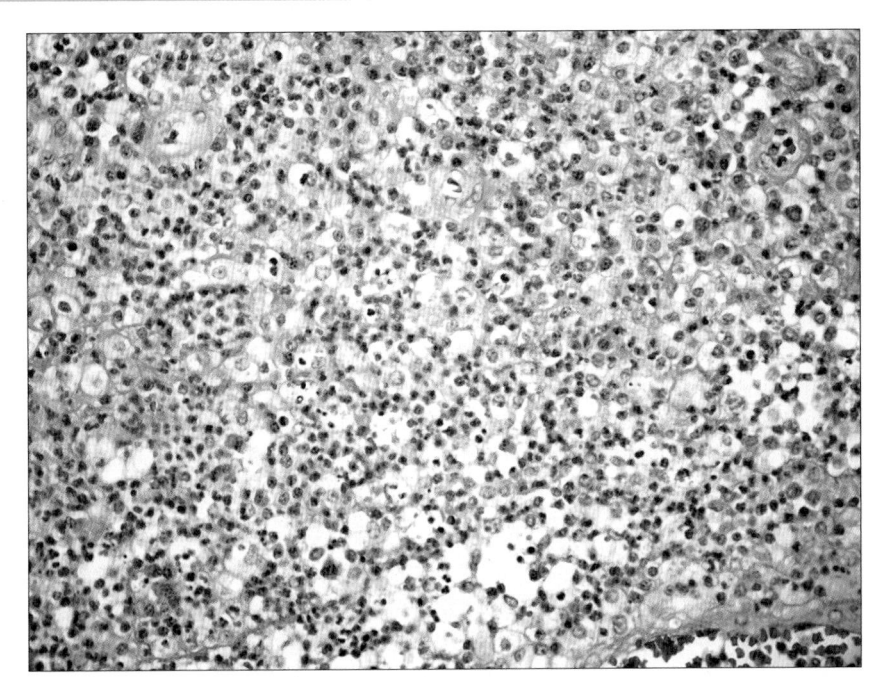

Figure 2-30. Abscess. Photomicrograph from the central portion of an abscess showing confluent granulocytes with prominent apoptosis. Occasional histiocytes phagocytize cellular debris.

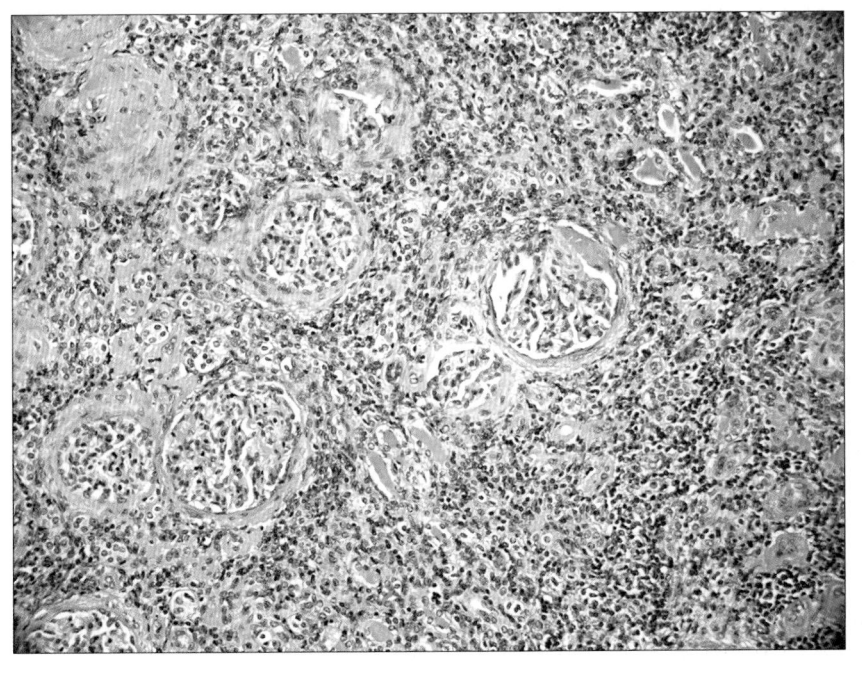

Figure 2-31. Chronic pyelonephritis. Photomicrograph of a kidney with marked chronic inflammation and periglomerular fibrosis as a result of repeated bacterial infection.

In some individuals, genetic polymorphisms in inflammatory mediators or cellular receptors may favor an exuberant chronic inflammatory reaction that results in tissue injury. Chronic inflammation often occurs as a physiologic response to various kinds of infection or injury but may also be a primary pathologic process that causes tissue injury in the setting of autoimmune disease.

Granulomatous Inflammation

Granulomatous inflammation is a specific form of chronic inflammation that results from cell-mediated hypersensitivity in response to certain types of antigens. Macrophages are the predominant effector cells in most types of granulomatous inflammation, but T cells are an essential component and recruit and stimulate the macrophages to form granulomas. In particular, T_H1 T cells mediate most granulomatous inflammatory reactions after they are activated by antigen presented in the context of class II MHC molecules present on macrophages. T_H1 cells secrete IFN-γ and other cytokines that convert macrophages to epithelioid histiocytes (activated tissue macrophages), which are much more effective in killing intracellular pathogens than are other macrophages. These epithelioid cells often fuse together to form multinucleated giant cells. In most types of granulomatous inflammation, histiocytes form concentric nodules called granulomas (Fig. 2-32A). Granulomas may develop central necrosis, and the morphologic features of a granuloma are often helpful in identifying the cause of the inflammation. Granulomatous inflammation is the characteristic response to certain bacterial and protozoal infections. Necrosis in granulomas is

often described as caseous (meaning "cheese-like") necrosis. Caseous necrosis was originally a gross pathologic term, and the use of this term to describe microscopic features is a misnomer, but it is now understood to describe a central focus of necrosis consisting of eosinophilic debris without residual nuclear or cytoplasmic outlines.

Caseous necrosis is suggestive of infection with *M. tuberculosis* infection, but necrosis in granulomas can be seen with other pathogens and in the absence of invading microorganisms and in some autoimmune diseases (see Fig. 2-32B).

Granulomas also can develop in response to exogenous foreign material (i.e., foreign body giant cell response to damaged tissue components) and some drugs (small granulomas in the liver are relatively common manifestations of drug reactions). Foreign body reactions typically do not

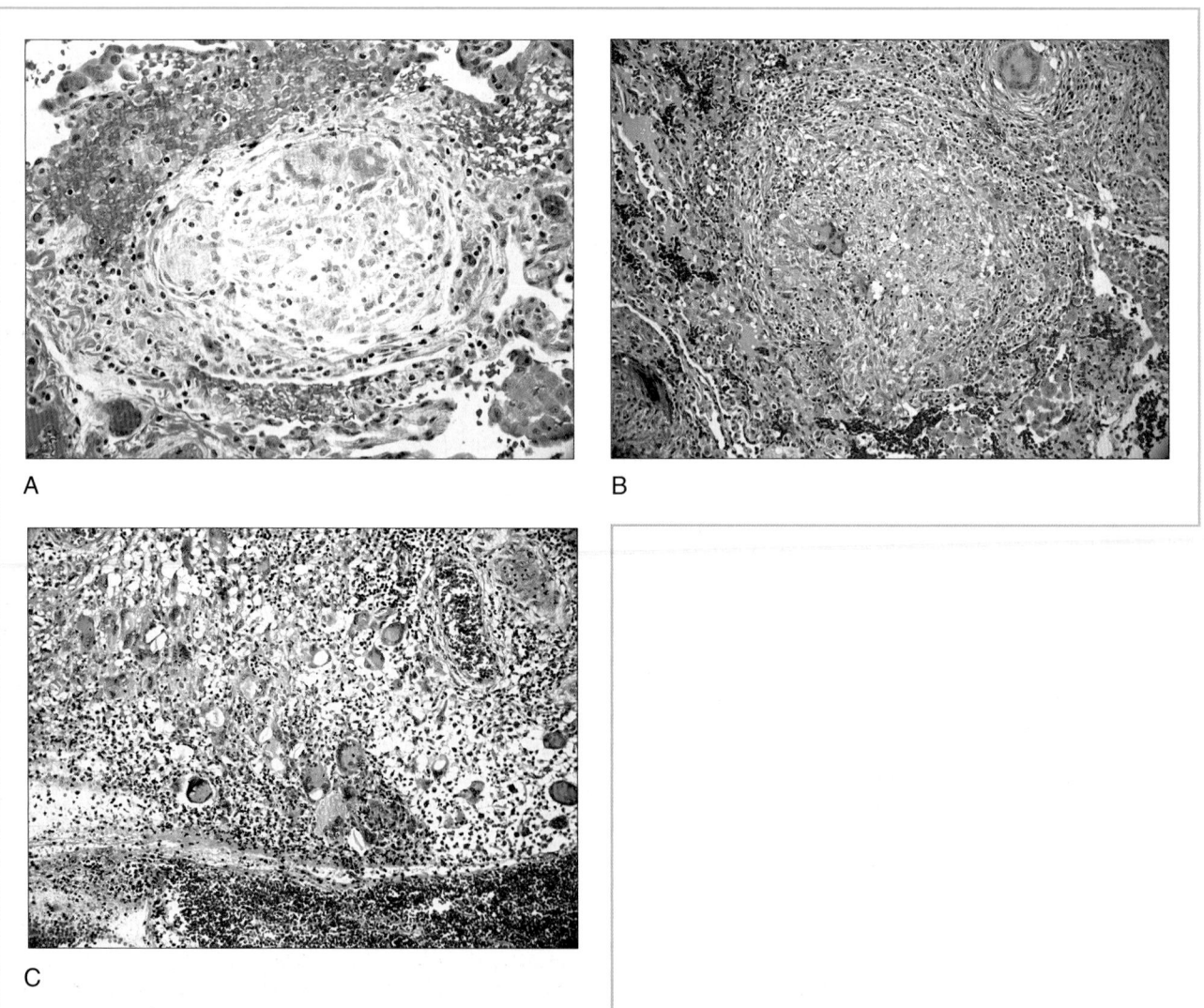

Figure 2-32. A, Pulmonary granuloma. Note the circumscription and compact organization of this granuloma, which is composed predominantly of histiocytes. Multinucleated giant cells have formed by fusion of individual histiocytes. **B**, Pulmonary granulomas with central necrosis. Well-formed granulomas with central necrosis (eosinophilic area at the center) with a prominent T-cell infiltrate about its periphery. **C**, Foreign body reaction. Note the lack of organization and circumscription of this foreign body reaction to exogenous material. Numerous multinucleated giant cells are present, and many of these contain ingested foreign material.

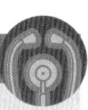
form tightly organized granulomas and usually are dominated by multinucleated giant cells that often contain ingested foreign material in their cytoplasm (see Fig. 2-32C). Granulomas are the main pathologic manifestation of sarcoidosis, which is an inflammatory disease of unknown cause that often responds to immunosuppressive therapy with corticosteroids.

Granulomatous inflammation is strongly promoted by the secretion of IFN-γ by T cells, but cross-talk between T cells and macrophages via cytokine secretion is required to orchestrate this type of highly organized tissue reaction. Granulomatous inflammation can be effective in killing or containing some types of microorganisms that are not killed effectively by other inflammatory cells.

T cells that express γ-δ T-cell receptors on their surface may play a role in granulomatous reactions. Most γ-δ T cells reside in the skin and mucous membranes. Some γ-δ T cells can recognize protein antigens independently of MHC molecules, and their role in different disease conditions remains incompletely understood.

Shock

Shock is a systemic pathologic process that results in inadequate blood flow to sustain normal organ function. Shock can result from acute blood loss due to depletion of intravascular volume (e.g., rapid blood loss of more than 1 L is usually sufficient to induce shock). Shock can also occur because of inadequate blood volume due to systemic vasodilation or increased vascular permeability, as occurs in anaphylactic shock.

In addition, shock can result from inadequate blood flow due to severe heart failure after myocardial infarction. Less commonly, shock can result from abnormalities of the nervous system that result in marked loss of vascular tone.

Hypoperfusion of tissues in shock results in hypoxia and ischemia in multiple organs. Most forms of shock are associated with a high mortality rate depending on the inciting stimulus and the presence of comorbid disease. The initial manifestations of shock are produced by compensatory responses that attempt to maintain blood pressure. These neural and hormonal (predominantly glucocorticoids and catecholamines) responses cause marked vasoconstriction and reduction of blood flow to noncritical tissues. Because of these changes, patients typically appear cold and clammy because of redistribution of blood flow from the skin to the CNS and other vital organs. This phase of shock is associated with a marked increase in heart rate in an attempt to increase perfusion. If these compensatory mechanisms do not reverse tissue hypoxia, shock moves to a "progressive" phase in which these compensatory mechanisms are overwhelmed. Progressive shock frequently transitions to an "irreversible" phase in which failure of multiple organ systems dominates the clinical course.

Septic Shock

Shock can result from the systemic activation of inflammatory mediators that usually occurs as a result of bacterial infection of the blood (hence the name *septic shock*). Septic shock is usually caused by the massive release of cytokines from inflammatory cells in response to the exposure to specific bacterial products. In contrast to other forms of shock, septic shock does not result in peripheral vasoconstriction (compensatory mechanism) because vasodilation is driven by the release of inflammatory mediators. Patients with septic shock are typically warm and dry and lack the cold, clammy appearance usually associated with hypovolemic shock.

Gram-negative Septic Shock

Bacterial endotoxin (lipopolysaccharide, LPS) is a component of the bacterial cell wall of gram-negative bacteria (lipid A and polysaccharide) that can directly activate macrophages to produce IL-1 and other cytokines.

The release of large amounts of LPS into the circulation results in massive secretion of the cytokines by macrophages throughout the body with the initiation of a systemic inflammatory reaction. LPS in plasma interacts with CD14 on the surface of macrophages, which facilitates LPS-mediated activation of Toll-like receptor 4 (TLR-4; innate immunity), resulting in transcriptional activation of cytokine synthesis (Fig. 2-33). The changes induced are similar to those produced in a localized acute inflammatory reaction, but the greater amount of LPS results in systemic changes with massive vasodilatation and permeability changes in numerous vascular beds. Systemic vasodilation causes a drop in systemic blood pressure and circulatory volume. Septic shock can be produced by injection of bacteria-free LPS, which results in the sequential release of TNF, IL-1, and IL-6 over the course of a few hours. Direct effects of these cytokines on endothelial cells and other tissues also result in cell damage and the priming and activation of inflammatory cells. Large amounts of nitric oxide produced by endothelial cells and macrophages may further enhance systemic vasodilation and cause additional free radical–mediated damage to endothelial and parenchymal cells. Widespread endothelial cell damage and activation can inappropriately activate the coagulation cascade, resulting in disseminated intravascular coagulation.

Gram-positive Septic Shock

Gram-positive organisms do not contain large amounts of LPS but can produce a similar pattern of shock by several different mechanisms. Staphylococcal toxic shock syndrome results from the release of a protein superantigen that can bind to all T cells expressing a particular subclass of T-cell receptor variable regions.

T-cell receptor binding results in the promiscuous activation of T cells that secrete IL-2, leading to a chain

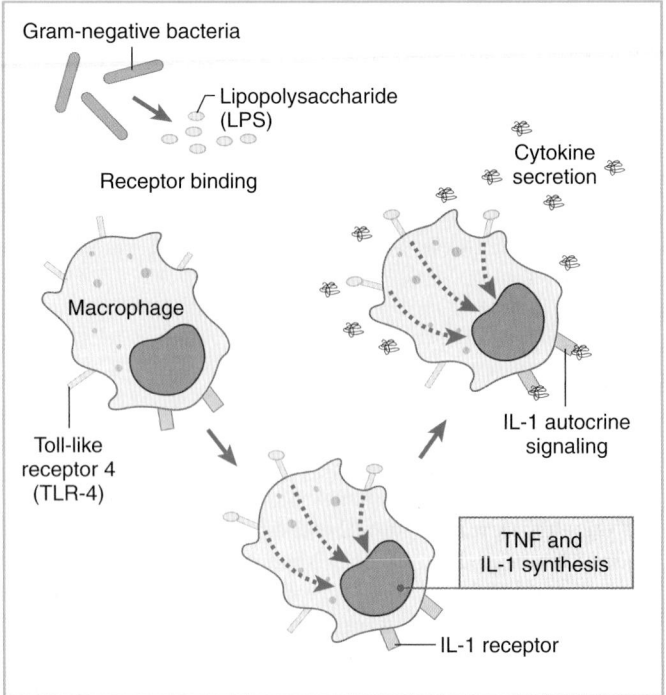

Figure 2-33. Pathogenesis of gram-negative septic shock.

IMMUNOLOGY

Superantigens

Superantigens are unusual microbial toxins that can interact with a large number of different CD4$^+$ T cells (up to 20% of T cells can be activated by a single type of superantigen).

Most known superantigens are peptides of between 22 and 29 kD that are resistant to proteases and heat inactivation and share common structural features.

Superantigens can bind directly to MHC class II molecules and T-cell receptors on CD4$^+$ T cells to cause T-cell activation without prior processing.

Superantigen binding is predominantly controlled by the shape of the TCR-β variable region, and superantigens typically bind to all T-cell receptors that derive from a single family of TCR-β variable region gene segments (e.g., the Vβ8).

Most known superantigens are produced by streptococci and staphylococci. Superantigens are thought to play important roles in the pathophysiology of some forms of bacterial food poisoning, toxic shock syndrome, Kawasaki's disease, psoriasis, and possibly some autoimmune conditions.

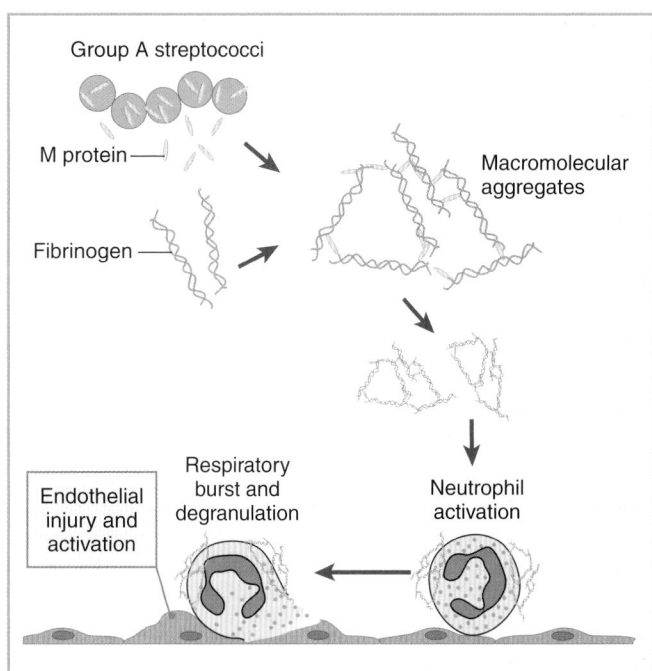

Figure 2-34. Pathogenesis of streptococcal septic shock.

reaction of cytokine synthesis that terminates in the production TNF-α and IL-1 (similar to gram-negative septic shock).

Streptococcal M protein can act as a superantigen in some pathologic conditions (see rheumatic heart disease in Chapter 7) but can also bind directly to fibrinogen in plasma (Fig. 2-34). Streptococcal M protein and fibrinogen can form multimeric complexes that bind to and activate fibrinogen receptors on inflammatory and endothelial cells, activating them to cause cell injury. Multimeric fibrinogen induces neutrophils to undergo a respiratory burst and degranulation that results in severe endothelial damage. Widespread endothelial injury can initiate disseminated intravascular coagulation as well as increased vascular permeability.

●●● IMMUNE DISORDERS

Immune-mediated diseases can usually be classified as immunodeficiency (with increased susceptibility to infection) or autoimmunity processes (in which normal cellular components act as antigens). Some disease states show overlap between these two paradigms.

Autoimmune Disease

Autoimmunity can result from the failure of immune regulation or the abnormal presentation of endogenous antigens to the immune system (or both). The majority of autoimmune diseases are significantly more common in women than in men, and most tend to present in adolescence or young adulthood. The predisposition to various autoimmune diseases is strongly linked to specific major histocompatibility antigens (class I and II antigens are implicated in different diseases). Genetic changes in complement components and in

other inflammatory mediators are important risk factors for the development of some types of autoimmune disease. Cells that express class II MHC molecules are essential to initiate a humoral or cellular autoimmune response. Class II expression is restricted to APCs and a limited number of parenchymal cells under normal conditions, but some types of inflammation or other stimuli (particularly IFN-γ produced by T$_H$1 cells) can induce class II MHC expression in other cell types. Activated cells that express class II are likely important in the initiation of many autoimmune phenomena.

External antigens are thought to act as triggers that can unmask or activate a genetic susceptibility to autoimmune disease. This idea is clearly true for some transient autoimmune diseases such as rheumatic fever in which streptococcal bacterial infection initiates an autoimmune reaction against components of the cardiovascular system. Viruses have been suspected as environmental triggers for many other types of chronic autoimmune disease; however, a viral link has not been documented for the most common, serious autoimmune diseases despite exhaustive investigation.

Laboratory evidence of serum autoantibodies (e.g., a positive ANA, see below) is not sufficient to make a diagnosis of autoimmune disease. The diagnosis of autoimmune disease requires that the patient manifest clinical signs of disease that are causally related to autoimmunity. Indeed, transient expression of some types of autoantibodies is relatively common in genetically susceptible individuals who never manifest clinical signs and symptoms of disease. Exposure to tissue antigens as a result of tissue damage (e.g., myocardial infarction) can also cause transient expression of antibodies to intracellular antigens (usually without clinical consequence). Indeed, autoantibodies resulting from tissue destruction or in response to tumors are quite common. These antibodies are usually present in low concentrations and do not produce clinical symptoms. Clinical laboratory detection of some of these antibodies may be useful diagnostically in classifying some disease processes, however.

Some autoimmune diseases persist throughout life although most wax and wane in severity. Less commonly, patients with autoimmune disease have a rapidly progressive course while others appear to have only a single episode of clinical disease. A few types of autoimmune disease are clearly transient and are directly related to exogenous antigen exposure. The pathophysiology of many autoimmune diseases can be characterized as type II, III, or IV hypersensitivity reactions, although some diseases manifest different patterns of immune disease at different times during their clinical course.

Systemic Lupus Erythematosus

SLE occurs much more commonly in women than in men and is more common among African American and Hispanic women. SLE has protean disease manifestations and is associated with the formation of numerous different types of autoantibodies at different times. These antibodies tend to form antigen-antibody complexes that are responsible for most of the pathologic features of SLE (type 3 hypersensitivity).

SLE tends to have a waxing and waning course typical of many autoimmune diseases with flares of disease activity induced by various stresses including pregnancy. Deposition of immune complexes in the kidney results in inflammation of glomeruli (glomerulonephritis), usually with the accumulation of proteinaceous material between endothelial cells and their basement membrane. These deposits can be detected by immunofluorescent staining of renal biopsies with diagnostic antibodies directed against human immunoglobulin or complement components (Fig. 2-35). Complement-induced inflammation and chronic accumulation of proteinaceous electron-dense deposits composed of immunocomplexes can ultimately result in renal failure.

Deposition of immune complexes in the skin (in the basement membrane zone) causes the typical rash of SLE that is characteristically located over the malar eminence on the face, termed a *butterfly rash*. Not all patients with lupus have a skin rash, but almost all develop some form of renal disease, which is the most important cause of morbidity and mortality in most patients. SLE can affect almost any organ system, and patients may develop vascular inflammation (vasculitis) that may result in hemorrhage or vascular occlusion. Ongoing endothelial cell injury from immune complexes in SLE also predisposes to accelerated atherosclerosis.

Most patients with SLE will have a positive ANA test at some time during their clinical course.

A positive ANA test is not specific for SLE and is observed in patients with other forms of autoimmune disease and in some individuals without evidence of autoimmune disease (usually at low titers). A homogenous nuclear staining pattern is typical of SLE and often correlates with the presence of antibodies directed against double-stranded DNA. Most patients with SLE have anti-double-stranded DNA antibodies, and this serologic test can be used to help confirm the diagnosis. Demonstration of so-called anti-Smith antibody is also relatively specific for SLE.

While most disease processes in SLE result directly from type III hypersensitivity, patients with SLE can also develop complications from direct antibody binding to cells (such as

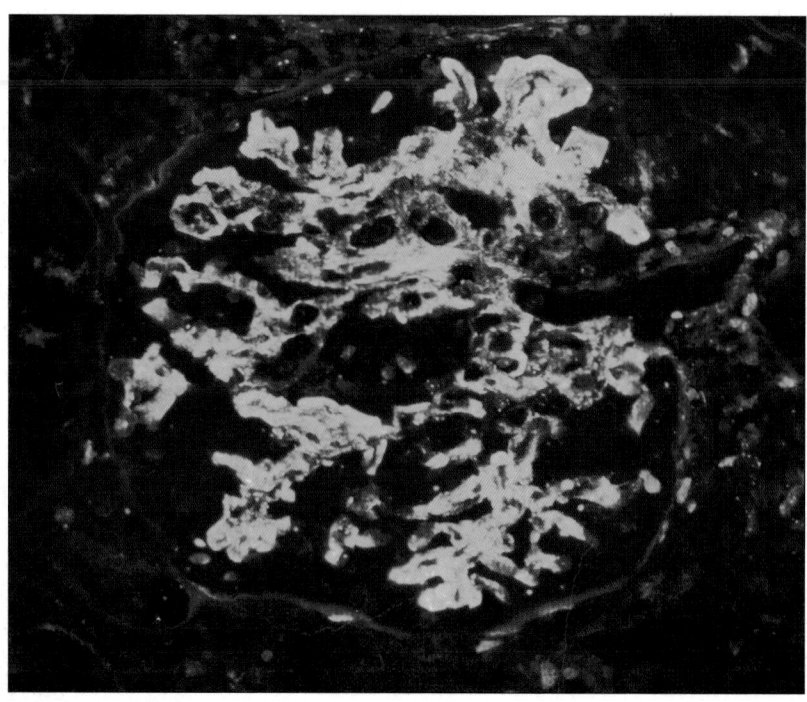

Figure 2-35. Immune-complex glomerulonephritis. Immunofluorescence stain of glomeruli for IgG. The bright green, granular staining of the glomerular tuft is indicative of immunocomplex deposition. A similar staining pattern would be observed for complement components C3 and C4.

IMMUNOLOGY

Antinuclear Antibody (ANA) Test

ANA tests are performed by incubating patient sera with human epithelial cells that have been grown in vitro on glass slides. After washing, these cells are stained with an anti-IgG antibody labeled with fluorescein (green fluorescence), washed to remove unbound antibody, and viewed under ultraviolet light. A positive result (particularly at a high serum titer) is suggestive of autoimmune disease.

A number of different ANA staining patterns can be observed. The homogeneous pattern (see figure) consists of diffuse nuclear staining with intense staining of metaphase chromosomes in the cell undergoing mitosis (bright bars in two cells in the figure). The homogeneous pattern often results from anti-double-stranded DNA antibodies and is the most common pattern observed in patients with SLE.

The speckled pattern shows absence of staining of metaphase chromosomes and may occur in SLE or other autoimmune diseases.

The anticentromere pattern shows dot-like staining that marks the centromeres of individual chromosomes and is strongly associated with the CREST syndrome (a subtype of systemic sclerosis).

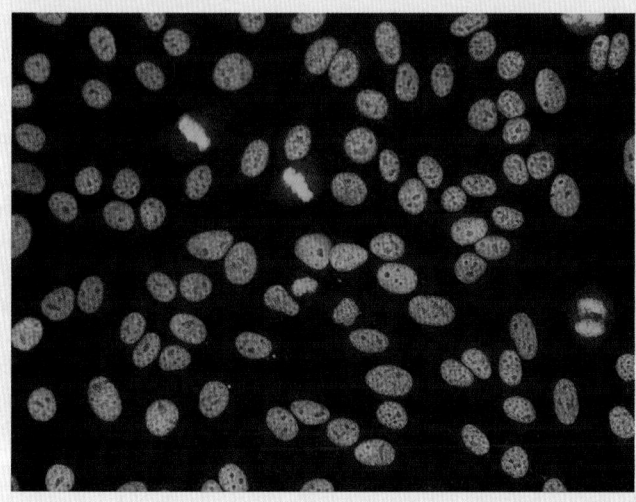

red blood cells to produce hemolytic anemia), which corresponds to type II hypersensitivity. So-called "lupus anticoagulant" is another form of type II hypersensitivity in which antibodies to phospholipids result in a markedly prothrombotic state that shares many clinical features with DIC and thrombotic thrombocytopenia purpura (TTP). Paradoxically, the blood of patients with lupus anticoagulant appears "anticoagulated" in laboratory assays because anti-phospholipid antibodies interfere with in vitro coagulation assays.

Rheumatoid Arthritis

Rheumatoid arthritis (RA) is a severe, deforming, inflammatory arthritis that is more common in women than men and tends to develop at a much younger age than osteoarthritis. Patients with RA often have an autoantibody in their serum that reacts with their own IgG (so-called rheumatoid factor, RF), but the pathophysiology of joint inflammation and destruction is complex and probably involves a combination of cellular and humoral mechanisms. Rheumatoid arthritis is discussed in more detail in Chapter 6.

Systemic Sclerosis

Systemic sclerosis (SS) is a fibrosing disorder that can be associated with autoantibodies that react with ribonucleo-protein particles and produce a "nucleolar staining pattern" in the ANA assay. Patients tend to have a variable clinical course with progressive fibrosis of the skin as well as other organs. Systemic sclerosis often involves the esophagus, where fibrosis results in dysmotility and dysfunction with marked difficulty in swallowing (dysphagia). Inflammatory cells are generally sparse in the lesions of systemic sclerosis, and abnormalities of the microvasculature resulting from chronic endothelial injury are thought to be the underlying cause. Microvascular disease causes tissue ischemia and promotes abnormal fibrosis. Some patients with systemic sclerosis have cryoglobulins (antibodies that precipitate at low temperature that can cause vascular sludging in the reduced temperature environment of the extremities). These cryoglobulins may produce Raynaud's phenomenon (pain and color change in the digits on exposure to cold or other stimuli) and exacerbate ischemia, leading to digital infarction. A subset of patients with systemic sclerosis (CREST syndrome) have a limited pattern of involvement (usually restricted to the skin) and characteristic associated disease phenomena. Patients with CREST syndrome typically show a characteristic anticentromere pattern on ANA.

Transplant Rejection

Transplant rejection is a normal immune response against foreign antigens on transplanted tissue. Transplant rejection is classified according to whether the response occurs very soon after transplantation (hyperacute rejection), over the course of weeks to months to years (acute rejection), or over the course of multiple years (chronic rejection) (Fig. 2-36). These three forms of rejection are caused by distinct mechanisms. Graft-versus-host disease occurs when transplanted lymphoid cells respond to host antigens, resulting in a systemic inflammatory process similar to acute transplant rejection.

Hyperacute Rejection

Hyperacute rejection results from the interaction of preformed antibodies with proteins on the surface of transplanted cells. A simple example of hyperacute rejection is a transfusion reaction occurring with ABO incompatible blood (e.g., type A blood transfused in a type O recipient). In this case, preformed antibodies result in a type II hyper-sensitivity reaction with complement-mediated lysis and opsonization of transfused red blood cells. This pattern of rejection can also occur with solid organ transplants. In that

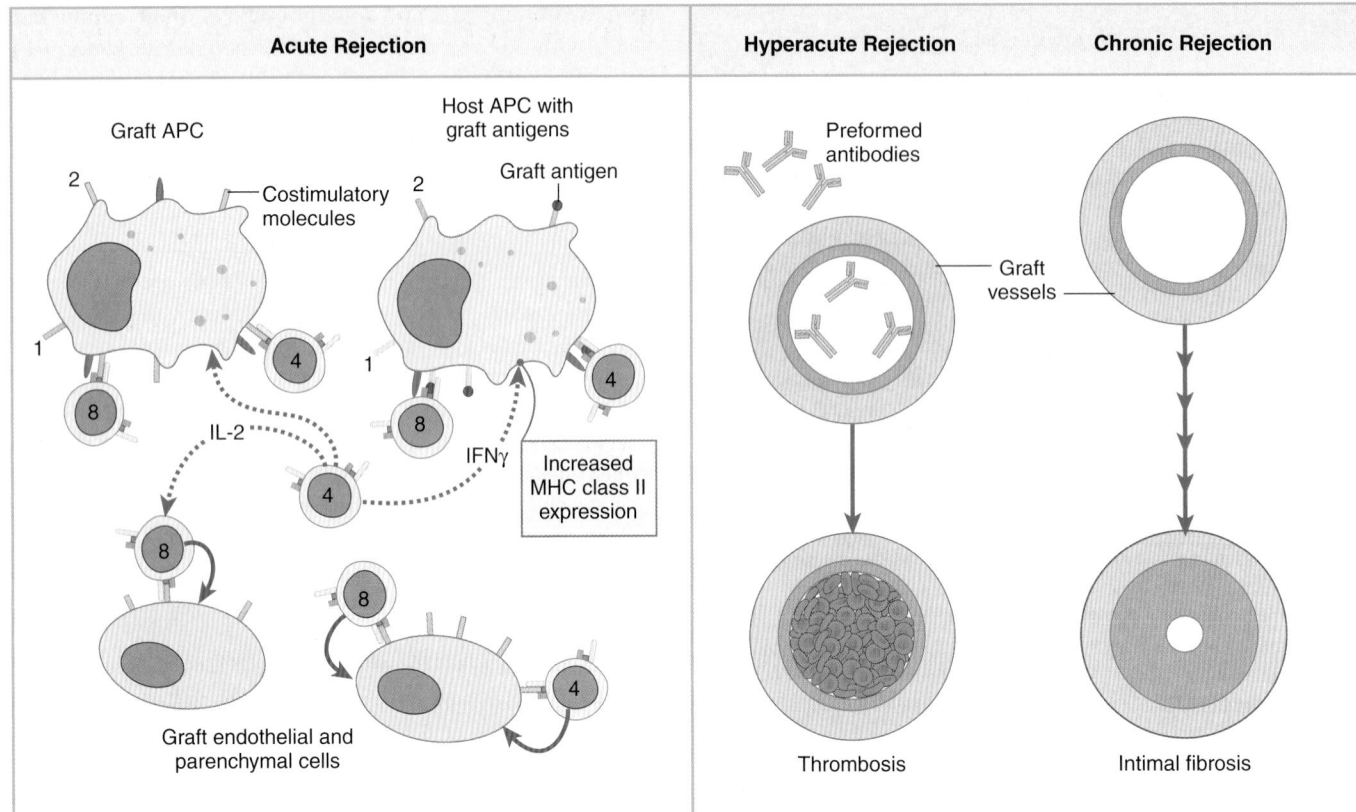

Figure 2-36. Pathogenesis of transplant rejection.

case, antibodies reactive against ABO and other transfusion antigens expressed on endothelial cells result in vascular inflammation with secondary thrombosis and ischemic necrosis, causing graft destruction over the course of hours (Fig. 2-37A).

Acute Rejection

Acute rejection is a cell-mediated inflammatory reaction that can be initiated within days of an organ transplant and may persist for the life of the transplant depending on the degree of immunosuppressive treatment and the extent of MHC mismatch between donor and host. In acute rejection, T cells recognize foreign major histocompatibility antigens on the graft and initiate a type IV hypersensitivity reaction against cells expressing these foreign proteins. In immunocompetent individuals, this immune response is usually able to destroy a graft over the course of weeks in the absence of immunosuppressive therapy. Modulation of this immune response with immunosuppressive agents can result in long-term graft survival if acute rejection is effectively controlled. The intensity of acute rejection depends on the degree of mismatch between host and donor major histocompatibility antigens as well as other transplantation antigens. Acute rejection is characterized by the presence of abundant lymphocytes (predominantly T cells) and macrophages. Neutrophils do not play a significant role in acute rejection unless graft infarction occurs. Acute rejection can produce various forms of immune-mediated injury to vascular and

parenchymal cells, and the details of the morphologic changes vary among different types of organ transplants (see Fig. 2-37B).

CD8$^+$ T cells are the main effectors of acute rejection and can respond directly to foreign class I MHC molecules on graft cells to induce apoptosis. CD4$^+$ T cells also participate by stimulating CD8$^+$ T cells to proliferate and in some cases by recruiting other types of inflammatory cells to the graft via cytokine secretion. CD4$^+$ cells can be stimulated by host APCs that present ingested graft proteins in the context of class II MHC. CD4$^+$ T cells may also be activated by APCs that accompany the graft. Depletion of APCs from grafts may slow or diminish some manifestations of acute rejection. Conversely, active graft inflammation that results in IFN-γ release by T cells can induce class II MHC expression in graft endothelial and parenchymal cells, which may enhance their ability to activate CD4$^+$ T cells. In this manner, prompt treatment of acute rejection may diminish the expression of class II MHC on graft cells and prevent the full activation of a type IV hypersensitivity reaction.

Chronic Rejection

Chronic rejection is a vascular process in which intimal hyperplasia gradually develops in graft blood vessels. This hyperplasia results in the progressive narrowing of graft vessels over the course of years. Chronic rejection is not usually retarded by immunosuppression, and the underlying pathophysiology is not well understood. Chronic rejection is

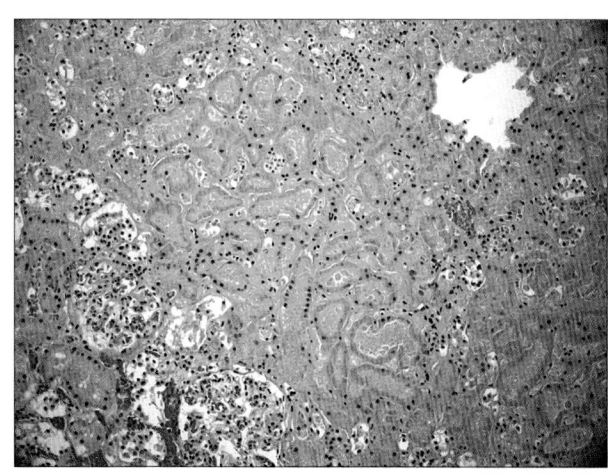

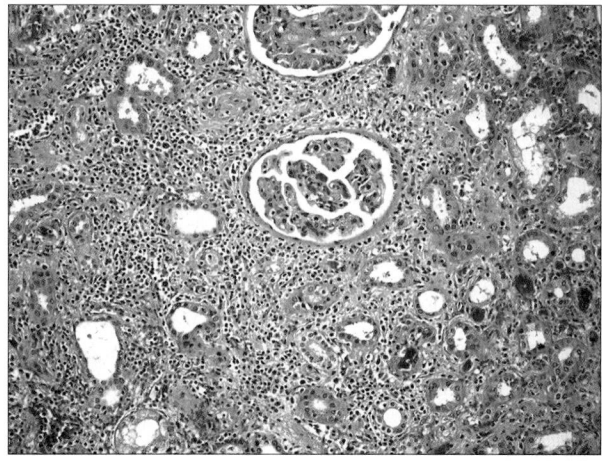

Figure 2-37. **A**, Hyperacute rejection in a renal transplant. There is a prominent hemorrhage and coagulation necrosis. **B**, Acute rejection in a renal transplant. There is a prominent chronic inflammatory cell infiltrate in the interstitium with associated evidence of cell injury in glomeruli and tubules.

now the major cause of long-term graft failure secondary to vascular stenosis and ischemia.

Graft-Versus-Host Disease

Graft-versus-host disease (GVHD) can occur when donor lymphocytes respond to host MHC antigens expressed on host cells. Limited GVHD can sometimes occur with the transfer of passenger lymphocytes in solid organ transplants if the recipient is profoundly immunosuppressed. More commonly, GVHD develops in patients who have undergone bone marrow transplantation because of aplastic anemia or as a component of cancer therapy. In this case, the host immune system is largely or completely destroyed (as part of the bone marrow transplantation procedure) and donor immune cells partially or completely reconstitute the host's immune system. GVHD can result in significant morbidity but can also have therapeutic effects by attacking residual

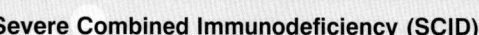

IMMUNOLOGY

Severe Combined Immunodeficiency (SCID)

SCID is a genetic disease in which both T and B cells are severely deficient. SCID occurs in approximately 1 in 80,000 live births and usually presents at 6 months of age (loss of maternal antibodies) with infection. Untreated, most infants die of intractable infections within the first year of life.

Many genetically different forms of SCID exist, but the most common is inherited as an X-linked recessive trait resulting from mutations in the γ_c chain of the IL-2 gene on the X chromosome. Adenosine deaminase or purine nucleoside phosphorylase deficiency results in purine metabolism causing an accumulation of deoxynucleotides that is toxic to lymphoid progenitor cells in the bone marrow. SCID can also result from mutations in the γ_c chain of interleukins 4, 7, 9, and 15 that signal through JAK3 or from JAK3 mutations. Mutations in the RAG-1 or RAG-2 genes that prevent normal VDJ recombination also can produce a SCID phenotype.

SCID patients can be effectively treated with bone marrow transplantation (if matched donor stem cells are available). Gene therapy to replace specific genetic defects has been successful in some patients but has been complicated by leukemia in other patients.

host tumor cells. This antitumor effect is an important component of allogeneic bone marrow transplantation therapy for acute leukemia.

Immunodeficiency

Immunodeficiency can result from defects in multiple aspects of the immune system and can be inherited or acquired. Immune defects may be subtle and result in only a slight predisposition to specific types of infection. Conversely, some disease results in immunodeficiency with uncontrollable infection and early death. Some forms of immunodeficiency also predispose to the development of autoimmune disease.

Congenital Immunodeficiency

Heritable abnormalities of the innate and adaptive immunity are rare but can result in severe immunodeficiency. Chronic granulomatous disease of childhood results from a genetic defect in NADPH oxidase that prevents a normal respiratory burst by activated neutrophils, resulting in defective bacterial killing. Affected patients tend to develop recurrent infections with pyogenic bacteria. Other immunodeficiency syndromes can impair chemotaxis of neutrophils (e.g., bare lymphocyte syndrome, in which integrin expression is genetically defective). Deficiency of key complement components such as C3 and C5 can result in marked susceptibility to many types of infection while deficiency of late complement components (i.e., the membrane attack complex) is associated with increased risk of infection by *Neisseria* species.

Genetic diseases of adaptive immunity have been very important in elucidating the physiology of the normal immune system. Severe combined immunodeficiency can result from a deficiency of the recombinase that normally catalyzes the rearrangement of antigen receptor genes in T and B cells.

Affected individuals have a very limited ability to produce antigen-specific T cells or immunoglobulin and usually succumb to infection early in life. Other genetic defects can block later steps in either T- or B-cell differentiation or maturation and predispose affected individuals to different types of the infections.

Acquired Immunodeficiency

Acquired defects of the immune system may result from therapeutic immunosuppression (iatrogenic) or viral infection (e.g., HIV) or be secondary to cancer or cancer therapy. Cancer chemotherapy can result in profound immunosuppression that predisposes to infection with low virulence pathogens that are ubiquitously present in the environment. The major immunosuppressive effect of most forms of chemotherapy is to reduce bone marrow production of neutrophils, resulting in a markedly impaired innate immune response to a wide variety of pathogens. If the absolute neutrophil count drops below 500/mm^3, the likelihood of developing infection from microorganisms in normal flora or the environment is substantial. Chemotherapy also tends to result in more subtle, long-term abnormalities of adaptive immunity that may persist throughout life. Treatment of autoimmune diseases or of transplant rejection with immunosuppressive and anti-inflammatory agents such as corticosteroids can also result in significant immune dysfunction with susceptibility to specific types of infection.

Human Immunodeficiency Virus Infection (HIV) and Acquired Immunodeficiency Syndrome (AIDS)

HIV preferentially targets CD4 T cells for infection and ultimately results in marked decreases in the number of CD4$^+$ cells.

As the CD4 count diminishes, patients are at risk for infection with organisms that are ubiquitous such as *Pneumocystis carinii*, fungi, protozoa, and some mycobacterial species. Absolute CD4 counts of less that 500/mm^3 are associated with an extremely high risk of opportunistic infection. Prophylactic treatment of immunocompromised individuals with drugs such as trimethoprim-sulfamethoxazole can diminish the risk of some types of infections (e.g., *Pneumocystis* pneumonia). Immunodeficient patients are also at increased risk for a more virulent infection by usual pathogens. In addition to exogenous pathogens, latent viruses such as cytomegalovirus (CMV) may reactivate and produce serious dysfunction of the lung and other organs. Although HIV preferentially infects CD4$^+$ T cells, other cell types may be infected later in the clinical course of HIV infection, leading to additional dysfunction. Specific treatment of HIV with antiretroviral agents may allow significant reconstitution of the immune system.

MICROBIOLOGY

Human Immunodeficiency Virus 1 (HIV)

HIV is an enveloped RNA virus that is very sensitive to inactivation by environmental exposure or disinfectants. Viral particles contain reverse transcriptase and integrase that permit the synthesis of cDNA after a viral infection followed by viral integration into the host genome (provirus).

The viral envelope contains a viral attachment glycoprotein (gp120) that usually binds to the CD4 molecule in conjunction with a chemokine receptor (usually CXCR4 or CCR5). The CD4 interaction underlies the tropism of HIV for helper T cells, and chronic infection results in marked depletion of CD4$^+$ cells in untreated patients.

In productive infection, structural viral proteins are synthesized as pro-proteins that are cleaved by viral protease to form functional viral subunits. Host cells can also be latently infected with minimal transcription of proviral genes. Activation of latently infected cells or NFκB signaling tends to reactivate viral gene transcription and induce viral replication.

Many of these steps are unique to retroviral replication and offer possible targets for chemotherapy.

Complications

The major complications of immunosuppression and immunodeficiency are infections as well as an increased risk for neoplasia. The types of infections occurring in immunosuppressed patients are often different from those that occur in immunocompetent individuals and vary geographically. The type of immunosuppression or nature of the immunodeficiency may predispose to specific types of bacterial, viral, protozoal, or fungal infections (Fig. 2-38). Established infections usually progress more rapidly and behave more aggressively than in immunocompetent patients.

Patients with high-level immunosuppression and advanced AIDS are at significantly increased risk for the development of multiple different types of malignancies. In some cases, defects in immunosurveillance may allow tumors to develop. Some otherwise unusual neoplasms are strongly associated with HIV infection including primary CNS lymphoma and Kaposi's sarcoma. Coinfection with other viruses (e.g., human herpes virus 8 [HHV-8] in Kaposi's sarcoma) may cooperate in tumor development.

Abnormal proliferations of B lymphocytes (monoclonal or polyclonal) can also occur in patients with profound immunosuppression due to HIV or after organ transplantation. These so-called posttransplant lymphoproliferative disorders (PTLDs) are often associated with Epstein-Barr virus (EBV) infection. Transactivating proteins produced by EBV may facilitate the autonomous replication of B-cell clones, resulting in a lymphoma-like illness. PTLDs often regress if the level of immunosuppression is diminished or reversed.

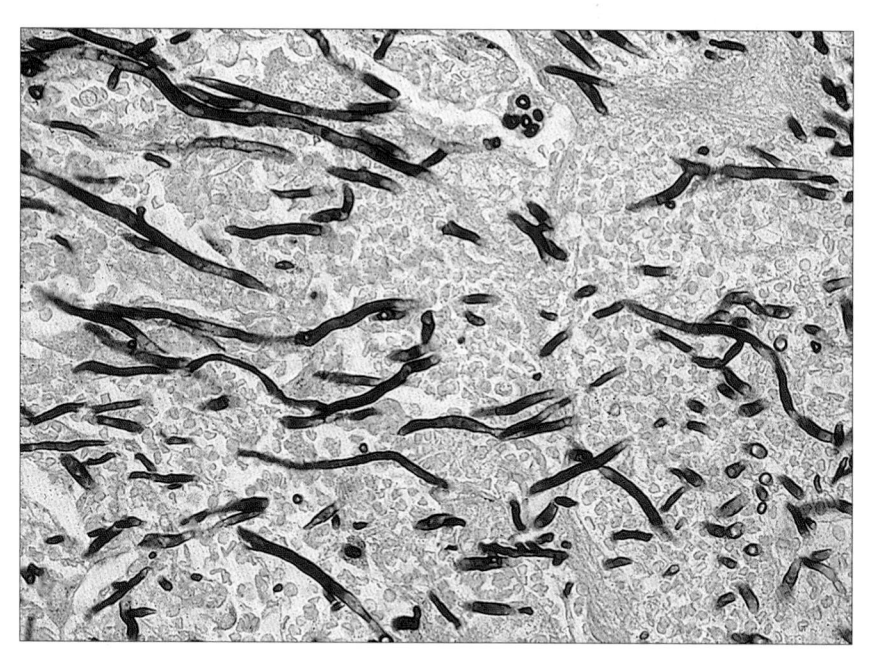

Figure 2-38. *Aspergillus* infection. Special staining (Gomori methenamine silver, GMS) of lung tissue demonstrates septate hyphae of *Aspergillus* (black). The green counterstain shows some details of lung tissue.

Tissue Homeostasis, Damage, and Repair

3

●●● TISSUE HOMEOSTASIS

Homeostasis is the situation in which an organ or tissue is at steady state. For some tissues such as the central nervous system (CNS), steady state reflects the persistence of essentially all cells with virtually no cell death or cell division. In other tissues such as the gastrointestinal tract, epithelial lining cells are replaced every 1 to 2 days under normal conditions so that steady state reflects an active balance between cell division and cell loss. The CNS is by and large a "permanent" tissue, implying that it has essentially no ability to replace parenchymal cells in response to injury or adverse conditions. The intestinal mucosa is a "labile" tissue, which normally renews itself on a rapid basis. One consequence of the rapid cell turnover in labile tissues is a robust capacity to respond to many forms of injury with replacement of damaged or destroyed cells. Conversely, labile tissues are more sensitive to some types of injury that preferentially

damage dividing cells (e.g., ionizing radiation), since precursor cells are constantly undergoing DNA replication to maintain steady state.

Other tissues such as the liver have a relatively low turnover of parenchymal cells under normal conditions but can respond to many forms of injury by inducing the proliferation of precursor cells that can differentiate into mature parenchymal cells to restore tissue homeostasis. In most solid organs, the ability of precursor cells to proliferate and effectively replace damaged parenchymal cells is dependent on the secretion of appropriate growth factors and on the interaction of proliferating cells with extracellular matrix components. In most organs and tissues such as the liver, this dependence on extracellular matrix scaffolding for the normal replacement of parenchymal cells is critically important. Repeated injury that damages the extracellular matrix tends to result in the regeneration of architecturally abnormal parenchyma that is dysfunctional (e.g., hepatic cirrhosis).

If the extracellular matrix is completely destroyed by severe injury, normal regeneration of tissue is usually impossible. In this situation, the only option for tissue repair is the proliferation of fibroblasts and the deposition of collagen to form a scar that can maintain the structural integrity of the tissue or organ but does not replace the function of lost parenchymal cells. Scar formation is always a departure from normal homeostasis and often results in significant loss of organ or tissue function.

Stem Cells

Stem cells are precursor cells that retain the ability to proliferate and differentiate into different types of mature cells. There are different classes of stem cells that reside in different compartments in the body. Some stem cells can migrate to areas of tissue damage through the circulation and then proliferate to assist in restoration of normal function. This type of long distance migration has been demonstrated for endothelial cell precursors and is probably a more common and important phenomenon than was previously recognized.

Embryonic stem cells have unlimited proliferative capacity and have the potential to differentiate into all types of fetal and adult tissue (Table 3-1). This class of stem cell

TABLE 3-1. Properties of Stem Cells

Cell Type	Number of Possible Cell Divisions	Totipotential Differentiation
Embryonic stem cells	Unlimited	Yes
Nonembryonic stem cells	Unlimited	No
Lineage-committed progenitor cells	Limited	No
Terminally differentiated cells	None or minimal	No

corresponds to germ cells, and true embryonic stem cells probably do not normally exist in the human body outside the setting of sexual reproduction. Manipulation of some stem cells in vitro may permit them to undergo a wider range of differentiation, and this potential is being actively investigated as a possible therapeutic intervention.

Other types of stem cells present in adults also have an unlimited (or nearly unlimited) replicative capacity but are constrained to differentiate along particular pathways to form a limited spectrum of mature cell types. The best studied example of this class of stem cells is the pluripotent hematopoietic stem cell. These stem cells can divide innumerable times but normally differentiate only into cells of the hematopoietic lineage and a few other specific cell types. Normal differentiation of these cells is dependent on the presence of cytokines and growth factors as well as appropriate cell-cell interactions that provide a suitable microenvironment.

As pluripotent hematopoietic stem cells divide, the vast majority of their progeny become progenitor cells so that the total number of pluripotent stem cells remains quite low under most conditions. Progenitor cells have a somewhat more limited spectrum of possible differentiation than do pluripotent hematopoietic stem cells and have a significant, but limited, replicative capacity. Such committed progenitor cells eventually give rise to progeny that differentiate into mature red blood cells, white blood cells, or other specialized cells. In general, more differentiated progenitor cells have lower replicative capacity than do less differentiated progenitor cells. In this way, the number of stem cells with unlimited replicative capacity remains small while the number of mature cells that can be generated is enormous and can be adjusted by small changes in the pool size of progenitor cells at various stages of differentiation (Fig. 3-1). This paradigm provides for an ample supply of inflammatory cells at times of injury or infection, since expansion of the progenitor cell pools can markedly increase the number of mature or inflammatory cells produced over a relatively a short period of time. Conversely, limiting the proliferative capacity of more differentiated cells is a fail-safe mechanism to prevent somatic mutations in these cells from giving rise to neoplasms (tumors).

ANATOMY AND EMBRYOLOGY

Stem Cells

Human embryonic stem cells reside in the inner cell mass (ICM) of the blastocyst among primitive ectodermal cells, blastomeres, and primordial germ cells. It is not clear how embryonic stem cells are created from gametes and what the exact precursor of embryonic stem cells is. Embryonic stem cells are essential for maintaining the high rate of cell division that is needed during embryogenesis.

Human embryonic stem cells can be derived from the in vitro culture of 5-day-old blastocysts under highly specialized tissue culture conditions that usually require a feeder layer of mouse embryo cells. These cells are defined experimentally by the expression of a unique set of markers that can be detected with monoclonal antibodies. These markers include alkaline phosphatase, DAZL, ERG, $HMGA_1$, Nanog, OCT_4, POU_5F_1, Sox-2, $SSEA_{3\&4}$, STELLAR, and Trafalgar.

Treatment of embryonic stem cells with specific growth factors can induce them to differentiate into neurons, myocytes, hematopoietic cells, etc.

A few stem cells can be isolated from blood remaining in umbilical cords after birth. These cells can be banked and expanded in vitro for therapeutic purposes. They represent a potentially rich source of therapeutic stem cells.

Pluripotent hematopoietic stem cells reside in the bone marrow, and in vitro culture of these cells under proper conditions can produce colonies of myeloid, erythroid, and lymphoid cells but usually not other cell types such as epithelial or muscle cells.

The balance between proliferation and differentiation is mediated through soluble growth factors, inhibitory factors, and epigenetic changes in differentiating cells as well as cell-cell and cell–extracellular matrix interactions. Collectively, these interactions constitute the hematopoietic microenvironment. Many of these interactions critically control the cell cycle, which is responsible for accurately replicating cellular DNA. Removal of key growth factors can result in failure of cell division and may trigger apoptosis of progenitor cells.

Cell Cycle Regulation

Most cells in the body are at the G_0 stage of the cell cycle (Fig. 3-2). These cells are quiescent and are not engaged in DNA replication or cell division. Stimulation of sensitive cells by appropriate growth factors can induce them to migrate from G_0 to G_1 phase. The growth factors and cell interactions that propel a cell from G_0 to G_1 vary greatly among different tissues and different cell types. Some cells cannot be induced to leave G_0 phase and so have no replicative capacity (e.g., permanent tissues such as neurons in the adult CNS). Cells in G_1 phase are preparing for DNA replication and undergo many changes in gene expression including the synthesis of cyclin proteins that are essential for initiating normal DNA replication. Multiple sensor/effector molecules are also active during this phase of the cell cycle and can detect and repair

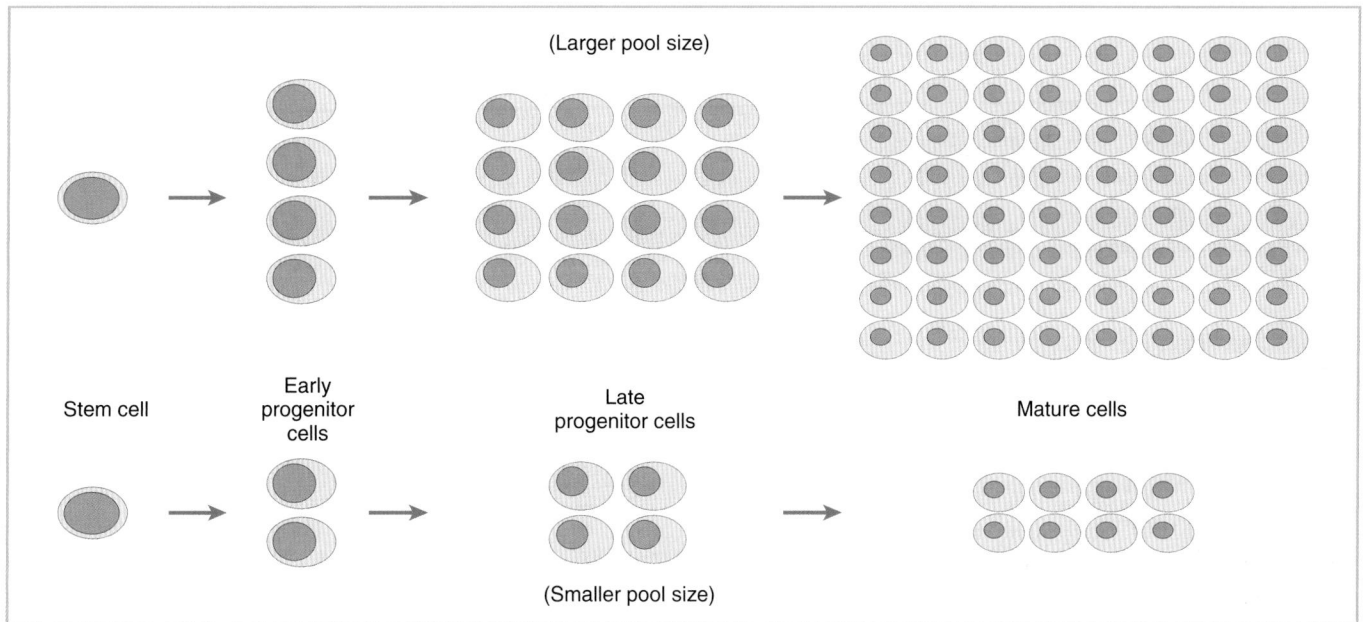

Figure 3-1. Changes in the size of progenitor cell pools control the number of mature cells produced.

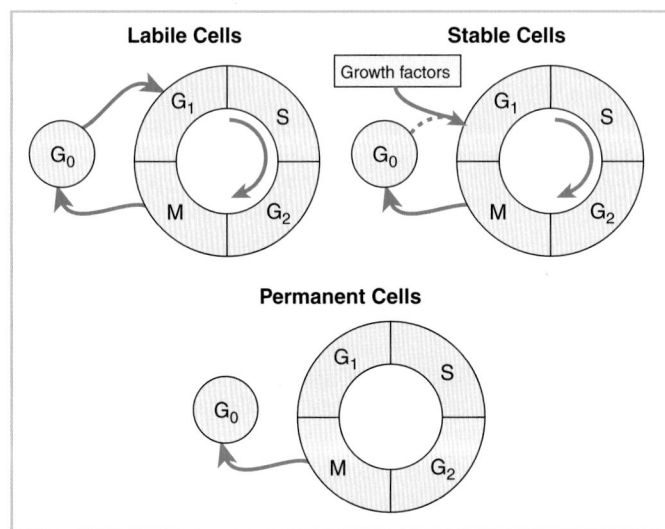

Figure 3-2. Cell cycle entry in different cell types.

If growth factor stimulation is sufficient and G_1 phase progresses without detection of mutations, cyclins bind to and activate cyclin-dependent kinases (CDKs). This activation step triggers CDKs to phosphorylate the retinoblastoma (Rb) protein. Rb phosphorylation releases bound transcription factor E2F from Rb so that it can interact with DNA binding sites to initiate DNA replication. DNA replication begins at numerous sites throughout the chromosome (Fig. 3-3).

As the cell cycle progresses through S phase, the cyclins synthesized during G_1 are degraded and different cyclin proteins are produced that trigger other CDKs that manage the transition from G_2 phase to M phase. G_2 is a resting phase in which cells prepare for division and chromosomal segregation. Nuclear chromatin is condensed during prophase so that individual chromosomes can attach to the mitotic spindle, which will guide distribution of chromosomes between daughter cells. Specific inhibitors of cell cycle progression at G_2M can also be triggered by various internal and external stimuli, and some of these signals may initiate apoptosis in sensitive cells. These mechanisms further enhance the stringency of control over DNA replication to prevent the propagation of genetic errors. If no mutations are detected, cell division progresses to the separation of daughter chromatids and the creation of two daughter cells. Chromosomal integrity during M phase is maintained by repetitive sequence elements at the ends of chromosomes called telomeres. In normal replicating cells, these telomeres consist of long stretches of DNA repeats that tend to prevent adherence between chromosomes that could lead to chromosomal translocations or loss or gain of genetic material during mitosis. At the conclusion of M phase, most cells return to G_0 phase either permanently (if appropriate growth factors are not available) or until appropriate stimuli allow reentry into the cell cycle.

DNA damage. One of the most important of these factors is the p53 protein. Detection of DNA damage or mismatched DNA base pairs at G_1S phase can trigger various nuclear sensor proteins that signal through p53 to either block the initiation of DNA synthesis or initiate apoptosis to remove the damaged cell from the proliferative pool. These functions are essential to maintain genetic stability in cells and prevent the accumulation of mutations in labile and stable tissues. Many of these genetic control functions are targeted for disruption in tumor cells. Activation of cyclin-dependent kinases can be blocked by a number of other inhibitory proteins, which can be activated by various intracellular and extracellular signals (e.g., TGFβ).

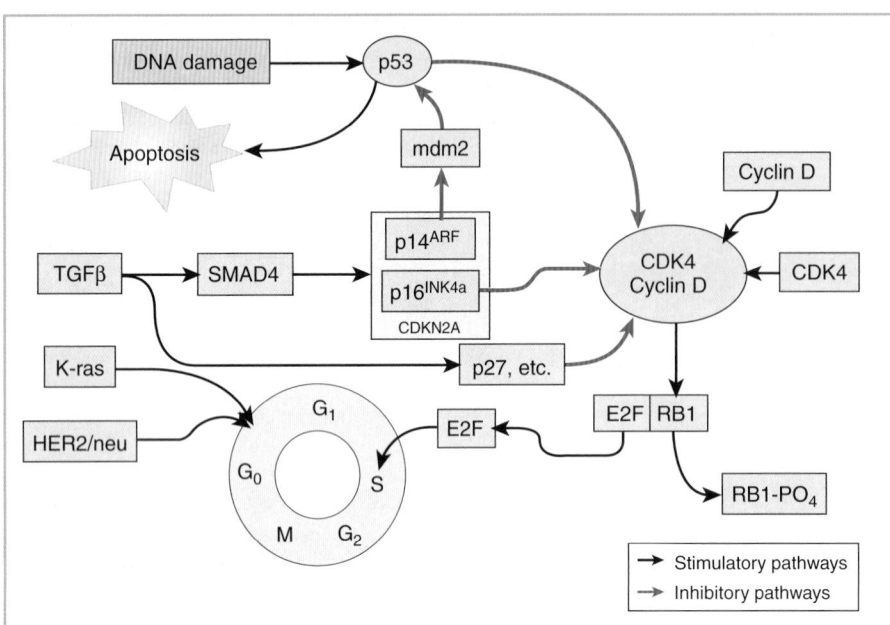

Figure 3-3. G_1S cell cycle checkpoint.

Signal Transduction

Multiple different types of signaling apparatus transduce the signals that trigger cells to divide or undergo differentiation. Some of these systems are interconnected, allowing functionally important cross-talk between them. Several classes of transmembrane protein receptors transduce the majority of signals that help modulate cellular function and direct changes in transcription. NFκB signaling is important in many inflammatory cells, and modulation of this pathway by different classes of membrane receptors is important in many cellular reactions.

A major class of these signal transduction molecules is ion channels (Fig. 3-4). These are membrane-spanning proteins that can facilitate entry of calcium or other ions into cells. The binding of a specific ligand to these channels causes them to open, permitting passive calcium entry into the cytoplasm. Cytoplasmic calcium concentration is normally kept very low by the action of energy-dependent plasma membrane pumps and by the active sequestration of calcium in organelles such as mitochondria. Calcium is an important regulator of cellular function, and increased calcium concentrations can produce diverse changes in different cell types (e.g., immediate contraction of sarcomeres in muscle cells and modulation of gene expression in other cells).

Another important class of signal transduction molecules is the receptor tyrosine kinases (RTKs). Binding of specific ligand to the extracellular portion of these transmembrane proteins activates an intrinsic tyrosine kinase activity. The activated kinase autophosphorylates the receptor protein, causing structural changes that activate it to signal through a variety of second messengers that are specific to individual RTKs. Phosphorylation of RTKs is transient and is usually rapidly reversed by the actions of phosphatases that convert them to their inactive state. Some RTKs signal through the RAS proteins that are activated by binding GTP. Activated

RAS signals through RAF proteins that ultimately activate MAP kinase. Activated MAP kinase can phosphorylate specific nuclear targets, resulting in changes in gene expression or cell cycle progression. Some RTKs signal via the IP_3 pathway, which mediates increases in intracellular calcium similarly to ion channel receptors. Some RTKs can also signal through the PI3 kinase pathway, which results in the phosphorylation of Akt that modulates gene expression and cell replication as well as influencing apoptotic signaling. Other regulatory molecules modulate the activity of the second messenger pathways. For instance, the neurofibromatosis (NF) protein can inactivate RAS by converting its bound GTP to GDP.

G protein–coupled receptors (GPCRs) are a large family of membrane receptors that share a conserved structure with seven membrane-spanning domains. There are numerous GPCRs encoded by separate genes that can bind to a wide variety of diverse ligands including small molecules (e.g., prostaglandins) and intermediary metabolites. Indeed, GPCRs in olfactory epithelium bind to exogenous substances to mediate olfactory sensation. A considerable number of GPCRs are still "orphans," since their specific ligands have not yet been identified. GPCRs trigger changes in gene transcription by interacting with G proteins that signal through the cyclic AMP (cAMP) pathway. The sensitivity of some GPCRs can be modified by their dimerization, which can be induced by some physiologic stimuli (e.g., dimerization of adrenergic receptors in vascular smooth muscle cells can occur in response to chronic hypertension; Fig. 3-5).

Integrins are a class of surface receptors that are important in cell-cell adhesion but are also connected to cytoskeletal proteins and can directly induce changes in cell conformation. Integrin binding can also result in signal transduction with activation of inflammatory cells. Integrins are heterodimers composed of one β-chain (usually CD18 in inflammatory cells) and a variety of different α-chains. Binding of integrins

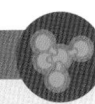

BIOCHEMISTRY

NFκB Signaling Pathway

NFκB is an important signal transduction system for immune and inflammatory cells and helps modulate most inflammatory responses. The actions of NFκB can be blocked by the binding of its specific inhibitor (IκB). IκB binding prevents recognition of the nuclear localization signal on NFκB so that it is not translocated to the nucleus and remains sequestered in the cytoplasm, where it cannot interact with target genes.

Signaling through Toll-like receptors or other membrane receptors can result in the phosphorylation and subsequent ubiquitination of IκB, which directs it to the proteasome for destruction. Release of NFκB from IκB exposes its nuclear localization signal, which then allows NFκB to translocate to the nucleus, where it binds to consensus sequences in the promoters of proinflammatory genes to help activate an inflammatory response.

NFκB is a multimeric protein complex that can be formed with several different protein components. Three isoforms of IκB (α, δ, and ε) can be expressed in different cells. The molecular heterogeneity of NFκB and IκB isoforms provides a versatile but complex signal transduction mechanism. NFκB can also interact with other signal transduction systems (e.g., Erk) in addition to the "classical" NFκB signaling pathway described here. IKK, IκB kinase.

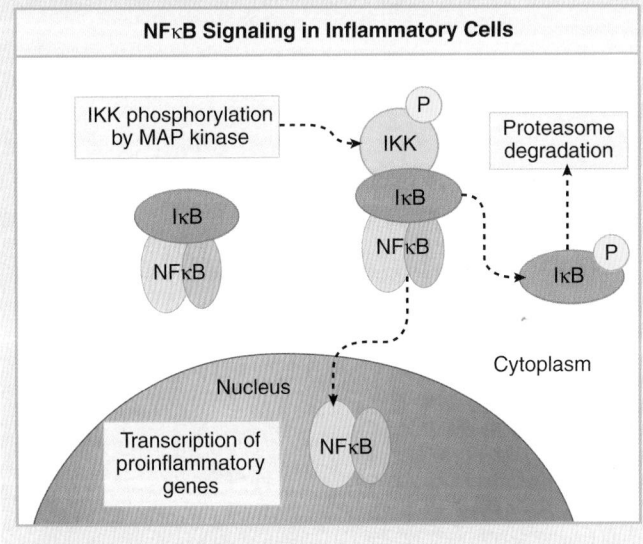

NFκB Signaling in Inflammatory Cells

IKK phosphorylation by MAP kinase
IKK
P
Proteasome degradation
IκB
NFκB
IκB
P
IκB
Cytoplasm
Nucleus
Transcription of proinflammatory genes
NFκB
NFκB

can allow inflammatory cells to recognize specific receptors on endothelial cells and initiate transmigration from the vascular space into tissue.

Some transmembrane receptors that transduce signals from cytokines lack intrinsic tyrosine kinase activity. Binding of specific ligands to these receptors enables their interaction with intracellular JAK proteins, which can then interact with STAT proteins, which ultimately mediate changes in gene transcription.

Cell-Signaling Growth Factors

The presence of appropriate concentrations of specific growth factors is necessary for normal cells to initiate DNA replication. Homeostasis of some stable and permanent cells is dependent on growth factor stimulation, and some cells may initiate apoptosis unless a minimum level of growth factors is maintained. Growth factors and other types of mediators can be delivered to cells in multiple different ways. Four general types of cell signaling—autocrine, paracrine, endocrine, and specialized—are utilized in various situations to control replication, differentiation, and function of different cell types under normal conditions and in disease states (Fig. 3-6).

Autocrine Signaling

Autocrine signaling means the production and secretion of an extracellular mediator by a cell followed by the binding of that mediator to receptors on the same cell to initiate signal transduction. A well-characterized form of autocrine signaling is the secretion of IL-1 by macrophages. Binding of IL-1 by receptors on macrophages further activates these cells and triggers the secretion of additional cytokines (including additional IL-1). This type of pure autocrine signaling in which one cell type stimulates itself is relatively uncommon in normal physiology but can be an important feature of some pathologic conditions such as cancer in which tumor cell proliferation may be driven by autocrine signaling. Signaling between two different types of cells is much more common in normal physiology, where the required interaction of different cell types provides an element of regulatory control for critical processes.

Paracrine Signaling

Paracrine signaling means secretion of mediators by one cell that acts on other cells in its immediate vicinity. This type of signaling is common, since many mediators have a relatively short half-life and so must act quickly after they are secreted if they are to have an effect. Paracrine signaling facilitates the organization of localized tissue responses such as inflammation or angiogenesis by focusing the action of mediators within a small geographic area.

Endocrine Signaling

In endocrine signaling, effector molecules secreted by cells are released into the bloodstream and then diffuse into different tissues to affect target cells at a great distance from the cell that produced the mediator. Mediators that function in an endocrine mode are typically relatively long lived (half-life measured at least in minutes) and may have specific binding proteins in plasma that modulate their half-life and concentration. Endocrine and paracrine signaling reflect two extreme paradigms, and many mediators may show features that are intermediate between paracrine and endocrine signaling. Cytokines such as IL-1 and TNF-α are good examples in that they mediate both paracrine (neutrophil priming) and endocrine (induction of fever by stimulation of hypothalamic receptors) signaling. Even mediators that predominantly mediate paracrine effects may have endocrine-like actions if they are released in large amounts (e.g., nitric oxide can have systemic effects in septic shock because of the large amount released).

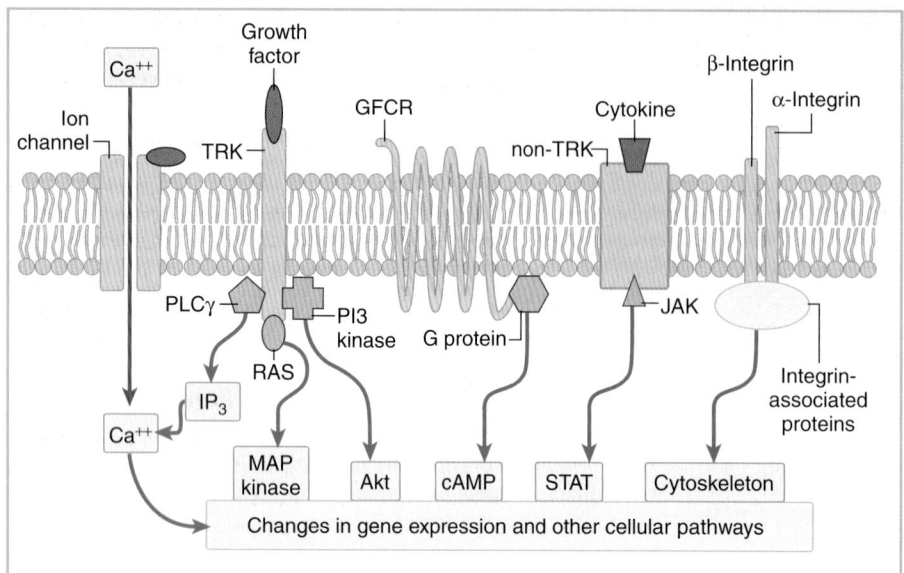

Figure 3-4. Signal transduction mechanisms.

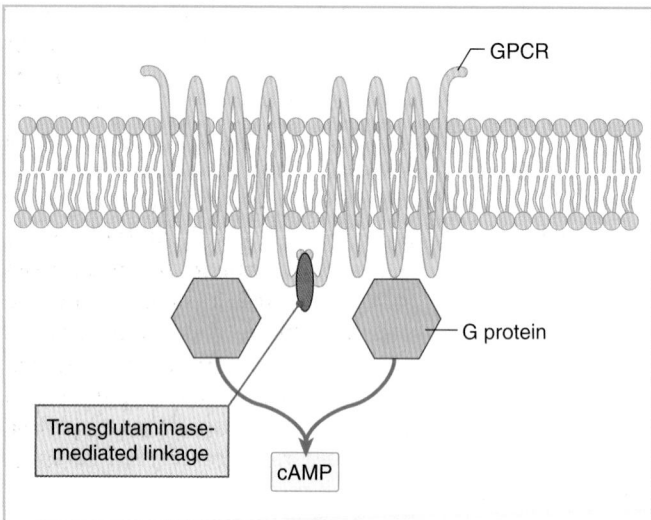

Figure 3-5. Covalent modification of the angiotensin receptor (GPCR) in hypertension.

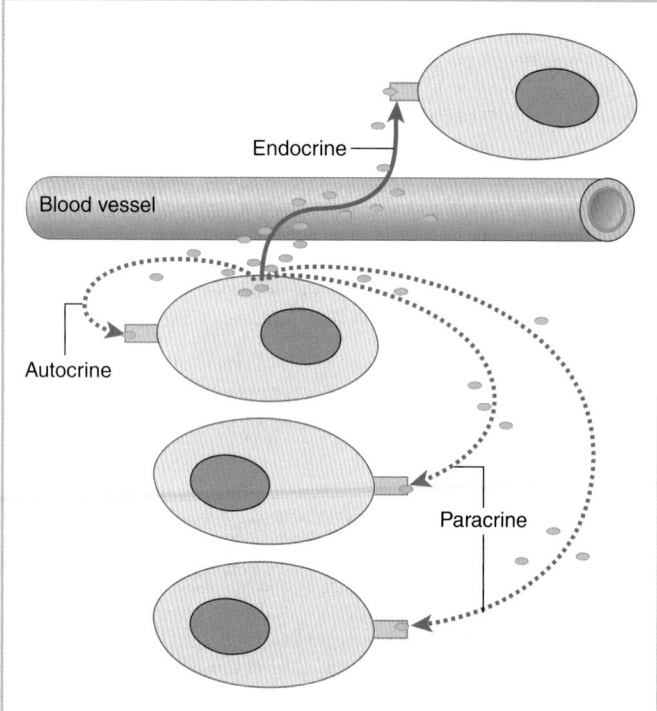

Figure 3-6. Autocrine, paracrine, and endocrine signaling mechanisms.

Specialized Signaling

Neural signaling shares some features of endocrine and paracrine signaling in that actions directed by the axon body may have effects on distant target cells (Fig. 3-7). Neural signaling may also result in the release of paracrine or endocrine mediators by neuroendocrine cells. Cells in some tissues have extensive gap junctions between them, and these junctions permit intercellular signaling via second messengers (e.g., Ca^{++}, which is not possible in cells without this specialized feature).

●●● TYPES OF INJURY

Different types of injury pose different challenges for tissue repair and reestablishment of homeostasis. The severity of the injury, regenerative capacity of the injured tissue, and overall health of the organism all are important factors in determining the response to various injuries.

Physical Injury

Physical injury results from the transfer of energy from an external source to tissue. The simplest form of physical injury in everyday life is trauma, in which mechanical energy is transferred to tissue. Energy transfer from solar and ionizing radiation also is categorized as physical injury. Most types of

Gap Junctions

Gap junctions allow adjacent cells to communicate with each other and share very-low-molecular-weight metabolites.

Gap junctions can form between cells that are held together by desmosomes and consist of protein channels formed by six connexon subunits in each cell's membrane.

Gap junctions allow passage of molecules, including small proteins up to the size of 1 kDa, but organelles and very large proteins cannot pass through them.

Gap junctions also allow electronic coupling between cells and are prominent in features in growing cells.

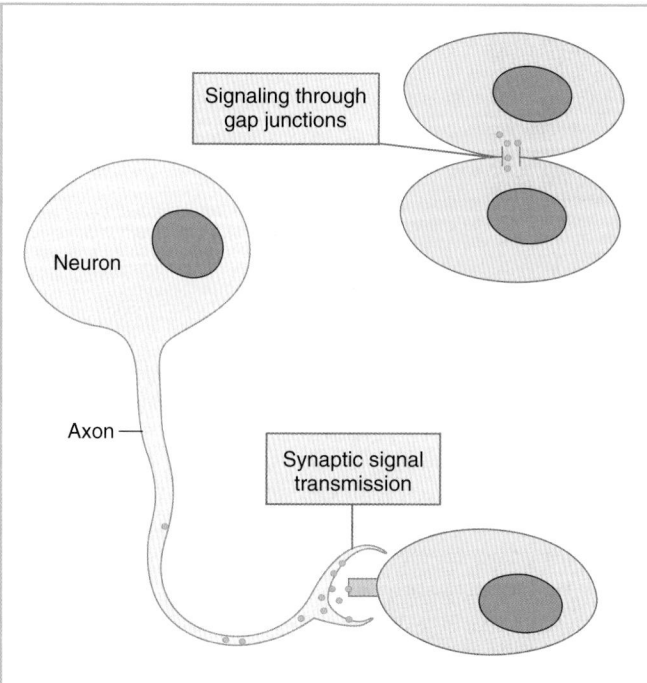

Figure 3-7. Specialized signaling mechanisms.

physical injury result in the release of inflammatory mediators, which may produce additional injury as part of the inflammatory process.

Trauma

Trauma can take many different forms and produce primary tissue damage as well as many secondary effects. In most forms of traumatic injury, the extent of tissue damage depends on the amount of energy transferred and the nature of the tissue injured. The structure of the extracellular matrix facilitates its deformation and absorption of energy to protect parenchymal tissue. Similarly, adipose tissue cushions and protects many organs. Cerebrospinal fluid provides a liquid cushion for the brain, but powerful acceleration/deceleration of the cranium can result in damage to the brain at the site of contact (coup injuries) or at a point opposite the contact because of deceleration of brain tissue against bone (contra-

coup injury). Damage to the vasculature by blunt or penetrating trauma can cause hemorrhage, hematoma, or both. More severe vascular injury may result in interruption of the blood supply, causing ischemia and necrosis.

Penetrating injury results when the external pressure exceeds the physical strength of the skin. Objects with a very small surface area (e.g., a scalpel blade) can penetrate tissue with very little applied force. Projectiles such as bullets can cause penetrating injury but also transfer a large amount of their kinetic energy to tissue, resulting in a large amount of tissue destruction. Since kinetic energy is proportional to the square of velocity, higher velocity bullets (military weapons and high-powered rifles) can produce an enormous amount of severe tissue damage that radiates outward from the bullet track. Most penetrating injuries also have the potential to inoculate microbial pathogens and can result in sepsis or abscess formation.

Thermal Injury

Heat and cold both can result in tissue injury or death. If the source of heat or cold is external to the body, the damage is greatest at the skin surface (burn injury or frostbite). If the injury is severe or prolonged, progenitor cells in the epidermis may be destroyed, so that normal regeneration of the epidermis is not possible. More extensive injury can result in damage to the extracellular matrix underlying the epidermis as well as irreversible damage to nerves and skin appendages. Overheating the whole body (heat stroke or malignant hyperthermia) can result in the widespread denaturation of protein and the induction of heat-shock proteins. This type of injury typically induces seizures because of CNS dysfunction. Although hypothermia does not result in protein denaturation, the cardiovascular system eventually ceases to function as core temperature drops well below normal, resulting in death unless the patient is resuscitated and warmed.

Radiation Injury

Tissue damage due to irradiation depends on the form of irradiation and the proliferative state of the cells damaged. Ultraviolet light has limited ability to penetrate the dermis but can cause severe injury to the epidermis and superficial dermis, resulting in free radical damage to collagen and other proteins as well as the formation of thymidine dimers in cellular DNA that are potentially mutagenic. Melanin pigment in the basal layer of the epidermis can absorb much of this type of irradiation, and induction of melanin by prior sun exposure can have a marked protective effect (Fig. 3-8)

Ionizing radiation is more penetrating than ultraviolet light and can damage tissue deep within the body. Irradiation can cause damage by producing free radicals but can also directly interact with DNA to produce alterations in DNA bases or double-strand breaks in the DNA chain. Radiation dose is important in determining the type of injury and the organism's response. At lower doses, proliferating cells are affected most because DNA damage during cell replication can trigger apoptosis or result in mutations in daughter cells.

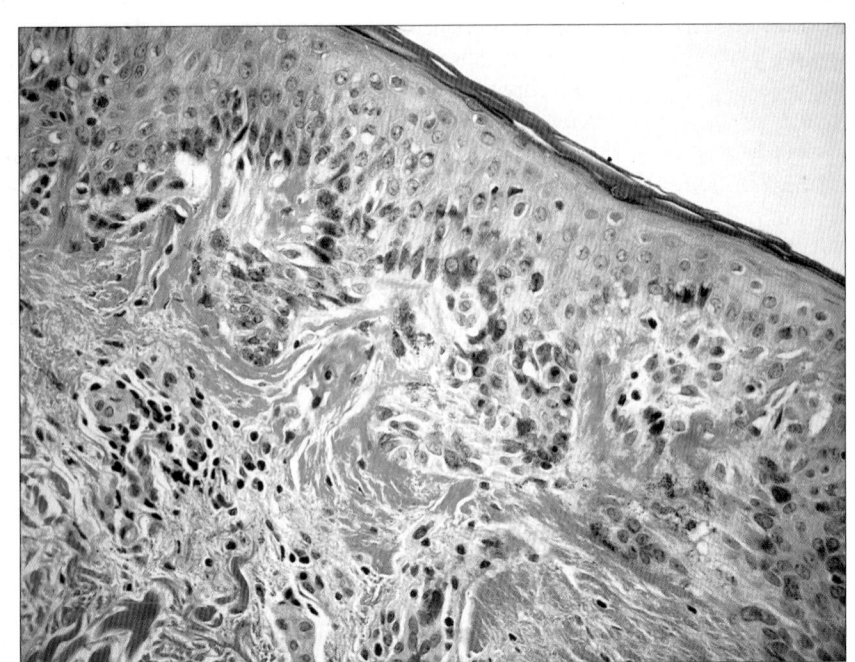

Figure 3-8. Melanin pigment in the cytoplasm of basal keratinocytes in skin.

BIOCHEMISTRY

Melanin Synthesis

Melanin refers to a family of biologic molecules that cause pigmentation of different structures and tissues. Melanin pigment consists of aggregates of monomers that form a biopolymer.

Most melanin is produced by melanocytes that reside along the dermal-epidermal junction in the skin. Melanin pigment is transferred from melanocytes to the cytoplasm of keratinocytes. Melanin pigment is important in preventing damage from solar ultraviolet radiation. Skin inflammation can result in the extravasation of melanin pigment in the epidermis, where it is ingested by macrophages. Eumelanin is the most abundant melanin in the body and is the predominant melanin pigment in hair and skin. Pheomelanin is reddish and is more prominent in red-haired individuals.

Melanin is formed by specialized organelles in melanocytes called melanosomes that can be specifically identified by electron microscopy. Melanocytes are embryologically related to nerve cells, and melanin can influence neural activity. Malignant transformation of melanocytes results in the aggressive tumor melanoma that is often darkly pigmented but may be amelanotic (containing no melanin pigment).

Neuromelanin is a by-product of dopamine metabolism that is present in neurons in the substantia nigra and locus ceruleus in the brain.

Inflammation triggered by radiation exposure can result in significant additional tissue damage. At very high doses (e.g., nuclear fallout, >10,000 cGy), free radical damage to the CNS is acutely fatal.

Chemical Injury

Chemical injury can be produced by the direct action of caustic materials (acids and bases) that damage cells by directly reacting with cellular components to alter or destroy their structure. Toxins typically cause the stimulation or blockade of specific enzymes or receptors or interfere with intermediary metabolism (e.g., cyanide poisons oxidative phosphorylation in mitochondria). Drugs can produce cell injury as a direct consequence of their intended pharmacologic action, by interfering with other target molecules, or as idiosyncratic reactions.

Toxins

Toxins are organic or inorganic substances that can disrupt normal cellular function. Chemicals such as cyanide can directly poison oxidative phosphorylation and result in the rapid loss of ATP by cells with the conversion to anaerobic glycolysis. Some toxic compounds preferentially target specific organs (e.g., mercury toxicity to the kidney). Protein toxins such as snake venom can result in the cleavage of specific coagulation factors that can block normal blood coagulation and so result in vascular injury. Bacterial toxins can bind to specific cell receptors and mimic physiologic stimuli (e.g., cholera toxin induction of adenylate cyclase in colonic epithelium to induce watery diarrhea) or induce a systemic inflammatory response (e.g., lipopolysaccharide from gram-negative bacteria producing septic shock).

Drug Toxicity

Drugs can cause tissue damage via exaggeration of their intended pharmacologic effect. Most types of drug toxicity are dose dependent, being more severe at higher doses.

Dose-dependent toxicity may result from effects on the intended drug target but also from effects on other targets. Different individuals may respond very differently to drugs because of dissimilarities in cellular receptor proteins or drug metabolism. The metabolism of drugs can be affected by changes in renal or hepatic function or by polymorphisms in cytochrome P-450 enzymes, which activate or metabolize various drugs.

In addition to dose-dependent effects, some drugs may result in severe toxicity in small numbers of individuals (i.e., idiosyncratic drug reactions). Idiosyncratic reactions may result from an unusual interaction between the drug and a specific genotype or from an allergic reaction to the drug or carrier molecules, or the mechanism of injury may remain unexplained.

Environmental Injury

Environmental factors can adversely affect specific organs and tissues and often affect organs with a greater exposure to the environment (e.g., the lung in the context of most types of air pollutants). The accumulation of toxic environmental compounds over a long period of time can also result in damage to many different types of tissues (e.g., renal toxicity from mercury may develop only after years of accumulation).

Air pollutants comprise a wide variety of different types of materials. Ozone and sulfur dioxide are respiratory irritants that can activate inflammatory cells in the respiratory tract and result in inflammation and dysfunction particularly in patients with reactive airway disease (asthma). Environmental air pollutants include heavy metals such as lead that can accumulate, resulting in systemic toxicity (e.g., brain damage in children and anemia in adults).

Particulates are larger fragments of material that can cause damage in different ways. Particulates that are small enough to be inhaled beyond the mucociliary blanket (i.e., into alveolar spaces) are not effectively removed from lung tissue. Accumulation of particulates in alveoli can result in the persistent activation of inflammatory cells with resultant fibrosis that can cause significant lung dysfunction. Some particulates are present as a component of global air pollution, for instance anthracotic (carbon) pigment from the burning of hydrocarbons is deposited in the lungs of cigarette smokers and city dwellers (Fig. 3-9). Some particulates are related to occupational exposure and can produce specific disease syndromes (e.g., silica particles in unprotected sandblasters).

Immune/Inflammatory/Infectious Injury

Immune and inflammatory cells are essential for defense against microorganisms and actively participate in the response to most types of tissue damage. Most inflammatory processes generate free radicals and other substances that can damage nucleic acids, protein, and membrane lipids. Many inflammatory mediators released by inflammatory cells produce tissue edema and promote thrombosis and so may lead to vascular insufficiency, ischemia, and fibrosis.

Host Barriers

Host barriers provide essential protection from pathogens and noxious materials in the environment as well as protecting from excessive water loss to the environment. The skin and mucous membranes form the largest external barriers. The keratinized layer of the skin furnishes an essential vapor barrier that retards water loss and provides significant protection from various agents, microorganisms, heat and cold, and radiant energy. Like the gastrointestinal tract, the skin has an associated immune system that is composed predominantly of T lymphocytes.

Mucosal surfaces are protected by a layer of mucin throughout most of the gastrointestinal tract. Mucosa-associated lymphoid tissue (MALT) is closely juxtaposed with the mucosa so that it can respond rapidly to infection or other stimuli. MALT provides specific acquired immunity with the secretion of IgA on mucosal surfaces. In addition to acquired immune effector molecules, multiple innate immune receptors are expressed along mucosal surfaces that help to modu-

---

PHARMACOLOGY

Cytochrome P-450

Cytochrome P-450 enzymes (CYPs) are a superfamily of microsomal enzymes that are very important in the metabolism of most drugs. CYPs are prominently expressed in the liver as well as in some other tissues. CYPs normally participate in the biosynthesis and degradation of steroid hormones, lipids, and vitamins. CYP action can markedly reduce or alter the pharmacologic activity of many small-molecule drugs and is required for the elimination of many endogenous and exogenous substances. Fifty-seven CYP genes are known in humans, but a smaller number of proteins in the CYP1, CYP2, and CYP3 subfamilies are predominantly involved in drug metabolism.

Individual CYPs have substrate specificity for a particular region of a drug molecule, for an enantiomer, or for both. There is significant overlap in substrate specificity of some CYPs, and so the metabolism of one drug may depend on more than one CYP.

The expression of many CYPs is induced by exposure to their substrate so that induction of CYPs can be important in controlling therapeutic drug levels. Some drugs are extensively inactivated during their absorption and initial passage through the portal circulation (e.g., approximately 90% of the antipsychotic fluphenazine is metabolized before reaching the systemic circulation), and so inhibition of CYPs can result in extreme changes in drug levels. Since many drugs are metabolized by the same CYP, induction or competitive inhibition can also affect drug metabolism.

CYP3A is involved in the metabolism of up to half of therapeutic drugs, and differences in its expression level can result in variation in drug activity of up to 400-fold in different individuals. Functionally significant CYP polymorphisms are present in at least 1% of the general population.

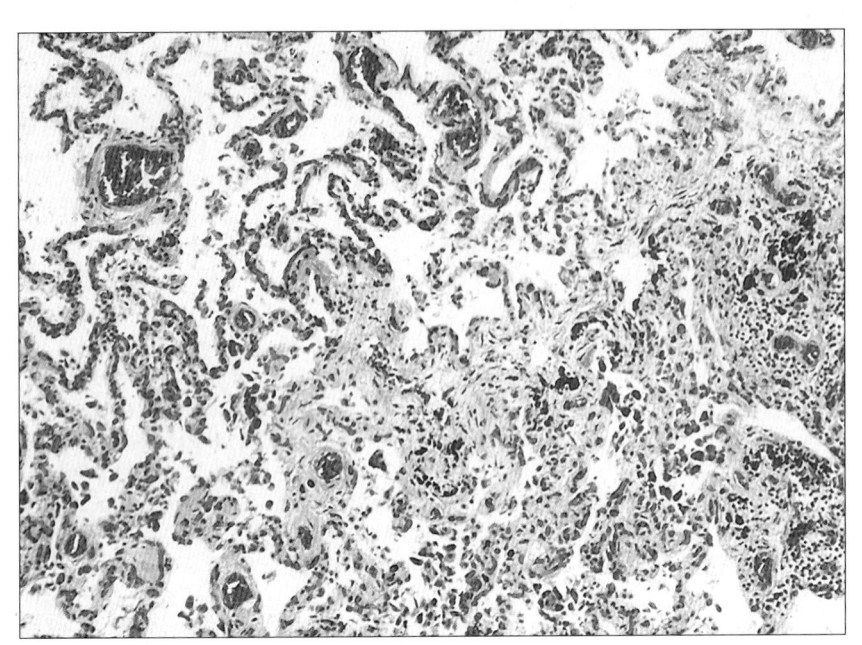

Figure 3-9. Anthracotic pigment in lung tissue. Inspired carbon (anthracotic) pigment has collected in alveolar macrophages and the lung interstitium.

late interactions between the gastrointestinal mucosa and luminal bacteria. These receptors, including Toll-like receptors, can trigger activation of epithelial and endothelial cells and recruit inflammatory cells to areas in which the mucosal barrier is compromised. Inappropriate or excessive activation of these receptors can trigger chronic diseases such as inflammatory bowel syndrome. The presence of beneficial commensal bacteria in the gastrointestinal tract is important to maintain the integrity of these mucosal barriers by inhibiting the growth of potentially pathogenic organisms. Commensal bacteria also produce substances important for nutrition.

The mucociliary blanket of the lung is an effective defense mechanism against many inhaled microorganisms as well as larger particulates that tend to become trapped in mucin and swept outward by cilia. Dysfunction of this system in smoking (ciliated epithelial cells are replaced by squamous metaplasia), genetic abnormalities of cilia (e.g., immotile cilia syndrome), and abnormal mucus (e.g., cystic fibrosis) result in increased risk of pulmonary infection.

Host-Parasite Interactions

Some bacteria are specialized to live in the environment of the gastrointestinal tract. They may have pili that help them to adhere to mucosal surfaces so that they are not swept out by the flow of luminal contents.

Viruses may exploit surface receptors on epithelial and lymphoid cells to gain entry to these cells and initiate infection. In the absence of specific antibodies or effector T cells, innate immunity provides an early response to viral infections with the synthesis of IFN-α and possibly micro-RNAs (miRNAs) in infected cells that can interfere with viral replication.

BIOCHEMISTRY

Microtubule Structure, Function, and Abnormalities

Microtubules have a critical role in maintaining cell structure and shape (e.g., neuronal axons) and in moving material about within cells (e.g., mitotic spindle).

Microtubules form from heterodimers composed of α- and β-tubulin monomers that are associated with two GTP molecules. Microtubules initially form in the MTOC (microtubule organizing center), where addition of heterodimers to protofilaments results in longitudinal growth. Microtubules initially form as a ring composed of 13 tubulin monomers that is 24 nanometers in diameter. Addition of more dimers creates a polar helical microtubule. One end of the microtubule is usually anchored and grows slowly while the unanchored end can grow rapidly by the addition of heterodimers.

Microtubule-associated proteins (MAPS) are tissue- and cell-specific and include dynein and kinesins, which can "walk" along microtubules in an energy-dependent fashion. Kinesins walk toward the plus end and dyneins toward the minus end of the microtubule.

Cilia and flagella are composed of axonemes surrounded by plasma membrane. Axonemes are composed of a ring of nine doublet microtubules with attached dynein arms with two central microtubules forming the core. The dynein arms are located at periphery of the axoneme and allow rhythmic beating of the cilia or flagella. Axonemes are connected to centrioles near the plasma membrane. Genetic abnormalities of microtubules and associated motor proteins can cause immotile cilia syndrome with infertility and recurrent respiratory infection.

MICROBIOLOGY

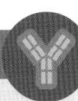

Bacterial Pili

Pili are thin tubes formed of protein (pilin) that originate from the cytoplasmic membrane of bacteria.

Pili are present in almost all gram-negative bacteria but rarely in gram-positive bacteria. The tips of pili are adhesive and are capable of binding to glycoproteins or glycolipids on the surface of host enterocytes (luminal epithelial cells in the gastrointestinal tract). These adhesive ends can be exchanged to adapt to different hosts. Binding of pili to enterocytes prevents bacteria from being swept out in the fecal stream. After their initial attachment to enterocytes, pili may depolymerize to allow more intimate adherence of bacteria to the epithelium.

Attachment pili (also called fimbriae) are short and tend to be numerous on the bacterial surface. Conjugation pili (also called F or sex pili) are much longer and are used for DNA transfer between bacteria.

Some viral infections produce characteristic cytopathic effects in cells that allow recognition of the viral pathogen in cytologic or biopsy specimens (e.g., herpesvirus infection) (Fig. 3-10).

Metabolic/Nutritional Injury

Metabolic diseases can occur as a result of inadequate caloric nutrition or a diet that is deficient in essential nutrients or vitamins. Abnormalities in host enzymes in which important enzymatic activities are absent as a result of genetic mutation (e.g., inborn errors of metabolism) can cause severe dysfunction. Defective secretion or release of various mediators and hormones can also cause metabolic disease. For example, insulin deficiency or resistance in types 1 and 2 diabetes mellitus results in the abnormal regulation of plasma glucose levels and in abnormal glucose and lipid uptake and metabolism by target tissues. Diabetes and its complications are considered in detail in Chapter 10.

Nutritional Deficiency

Relative deficiency of carbohydrates, protein, or lipids tends to result in different forms of nutritional deficiency that differentially affect specific tissues and organs. The consequences of malnutrition are different in children (growth retardation) than in adults (e.g., loss of muscle mass due to atrophy). A diet deficient in high-quality protein results in the deficiency of essential amino acids that blocks new protein synthesis (e.g., kwashiorkor in which decreased plasma protein synthesis results in diffuse edema from loss of oncotic pressure). Caloric restriction induces gluconeogenesis by the liver, and this stress may unmask subtle genetic abnormalities of various metabolic pathways. Malabsorption resulting from primary gastrointestinal disease (e.g., celiac disease, see Chapter 9) or intestinal parasites can also cause nutritional deficiency. Malabsorption of fats due to deficiency of pan-

GENETICS

Micro-RNAs and Small Interfering RNAs

Several different classes of small, noncoding RNA molecules (endogenous miRNA and synthetic siRNA) can modulate gene expression posttranscriptionally. Both micro-RNA (miRNA) and small interfering RNA (siRNA) molecules have short regions of sequence homology with specific mRNA molecules and under some conditions are capable of silencing or attenuating the translation of these mRNAs in a sequence-dependent manner.

siRNAs can be produced experimentally by introducing short, double-stranded RNA (RNAi) into the cytoplasm of target cells. Double-stranded RNAi is cleaved to form short RNA fragments (21 to 25 nucleotides in length) by a specific cytoplasmic endonuclease called Dicer. The RNA cleavage fragments (siRNA) are incorporated into a multiprotein complex called the RNA-induced silencing complex (RISC). Once incorporated in RISC particles, siRNAs are unwound and converted to single-stranded form by an ATP-dependent helicase. The single-stranded siRNA molecules in RISC particles can then base-pair with homologous mRNAs in the cytoplasm. RISC binding results in mRNA cleavage by Slicer (an endonuclease contained within RISC), which irreversibly blocks mRNA translation.

RNA interference (RNAi) is thought have evolved as a cellular defense mechanism against viruses and is conserved across a wide range of organisms, including mammals. Introduction of longer double-stranded RNAs in cells induces interferons (as an antiviral response) that trigger large-scale RNA degradation and inhibition of protein synthesis.

In model systems, RNAi techniques have been used to specifically target and "knock down" the expression of many genes. The therapeutic potential of RNAi (delivered in liposomes or in a viral expression vector) for infectious and neoplastic disease is being actively investigated.

Micro-RNAs are small, cellular RNAs that are also processed by Dicer cleavage and incorporated into RISC particles. miRNAs are transcribed from unique cellular genes (200 to 1000 are now thought to exist in the human genome). miRNAs have only recently been discovered, and one miRNA may target up to 200 individual mRNAs, making these molecules potentially powerful regulators of gene expression. miRNA expression is altered in some tumors, and tumor-specific inactivating mutations have been identified in some miRNAs, suggesting that they may act similarly to tumor suppressor genes (see Chapter 5).

creatic enzymes or bile produces steatorrhea (abnormal fat content in the feces), leading to bacterial overgrowth that can cause diarrhea with preferential loss of fat-soluble vitamins. Diets rich in fish oils (eicosapentaenoic acids) can alter the prostaglandin and leukotriene pathways, resulting in a different mix of products that may slow atherosclerosis.

Vitamin and Mineral Deficiency

Minute amounts of most essential vitamins provide adequate nutrition in adults although children and pregnant women require larger amounts of some vitamins. Vitamins serve

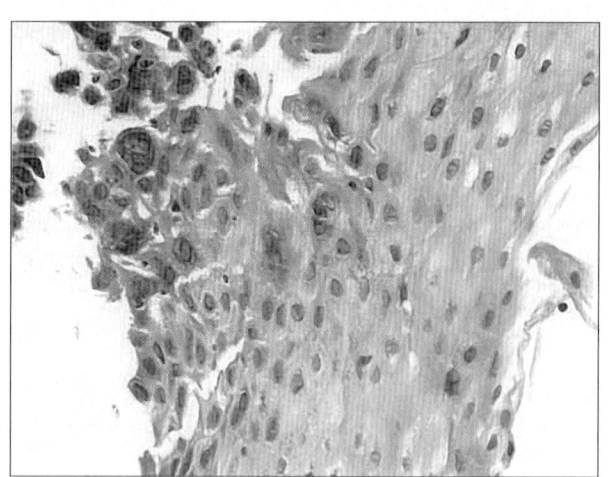

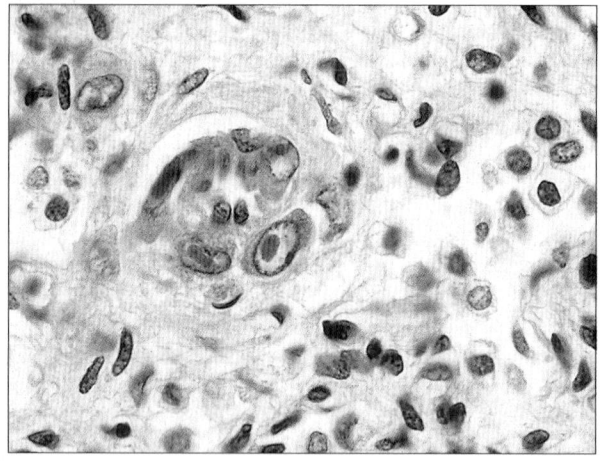

Figure 3-10. A, Herpes simplex virus infection of esophageal squamous mucosa. Note the multinucleation, nuclear clearing, and nuclear molding in infected squamous cells. **B**, Cytomegalovirus infection. An area of nuclear clearing surrounds large intranuclear eosinophilic inclusions. Cytoplasmic inclusions are barely visible in infected cells.

a number of different purposes in cells as cofactors for specific enzymes.

Water-soluble Vitamins and Minerals

Some essential water-soluble vitamins are not produced by the human body and must be acquired from the environment. A large variety of processed foods in developed countries are supplemented with water-soluble vitamins so that deficiency of these vitamins is very unusual in individuals with adequate nutrition (except for vitamin B_{12} and folate; see below). Limited diet diversity in developing countries can result in deficiency of these vitamins. Dietary deficiency of some essential minerals such as calcium is relatively common in some developed countries. Environmental deficiency of some rare minerals (e.g., selenium, copper, and zinc) is a cause of endemic disease in some areas of the world.

MICROBIOLOGY

Herpesviruses

The family Herpesviridae all share structural characteristics including a lipid envelope that surrounds a nucleocapsid with icosahedral symmetry. The nucleocapsid has a diameter of 200 nm and contains a single double-stranded DNA molecule that is approximately 125 kb in length.

All herpesviruses tend to produce lifelong latent infection that may reactivate under some conditions. The prevalence of infection for some herpesviruses in many adult populations (e.g., Epstein-Barr virus [EBV] and varicella-zoster virus [VZV]) exceeds 50%.

Different herpesviruses are trophic for specific cell types. Some produce one or more specific clinical scenarios while others usually result in subclinical infections or in nonspecific symptoms. Some herpesviruses produce *trans*-activating proteins or proteins that mimic cytokines and hormones. Some of these proteins can cause abnormal cellular growth and contribute to some forms of neoplasia (e.g., EBV is involved in the genesis of some cases of Burkitt's lymphoma, and human herpes virus 8 [HHV8] is involved in all cases of Kaposi's sarcoma).

BIOCHEMISTRY

Vitamins

Vitamins are chemicals that can act as cofactors for chemical reactions or have hormonal effects. They are typically active at very low concentrations so that only minimal amounts are required in the diet. Vitamin supplementation of processed foods has largely eliminated deficiencies in industrialized countries, but vitamin deficiency remains prevalent in the developing world.

Vitamin A deficiency is endemic in developing countries and contributes to increased mortality in young children. Delivery of 100,000 IU of vitamin A twice a year could lower this death rate.

Folic acid deficiency during gestation is associated with an increased rate of neural tube defects.

B vitamin supplementation can lower serum homocysteine levels and may reduce the risk of atherosclerotic heart disease. Supplementation with vitamins C and E and carotene and zinc may diminish the rate of progressive macular degeneration.

Vitamin C deficiency results in scurvy with defective cross-linking of collagen fibers and severe abnormalities of the extracellular matrix that prominently affect the skin and skeletal system. Niacin (vitamin B_3) deficiency produces pellagra with diarrhea and dementia. High doses of niacin cause vasodilation with flushing and may be toxic. Thiamine deficiency (vitamin B_1) can cause beriberi with heart failure or may result in neuropathy and hemorrhage into the mamillary bodies, resulting recent memory dysfunction (e.g., Wernicke-Korsakoff syndrome can occur in malnourished alcoholics). Deficiency of riboflavin (vitamin B_2) or pyridoxine (vitamin B_6) causes cheilosis (ulcerations and tears at the corners of the mouth) and atrophy of the tongue as well as interstitial keratosis in the cornea.

Vitamin B_{12} absorption requires intrinsic factor secreted by parietal cells in the stomach to protect it from gastric acid and mediate its uptake by specific receptors in the terminal ileum. Abnormalities of the stomach or ileum can each result in B_{12} deficiency that can produce anemia (megaloblastic anemia; see Chapter 11) and irreversible neurologic damage. Folate deficiency can also produce anemia but does not result in neurologic complications in adults. Maternal folate deficiency early in gestation can predispose to neural tube defects early in human embryogenesis.

Fat-soluble Vitamins

Deficiency of fat-soluble vitamins is much more frequent in developed countries than deficiency of water-soluble vitamins. Intestinal malabsorption with steatorrhea can result in the rapid depletion of some fat-soluble vitamins through the gastrointestinal tract. High intake of fat-soluble vitamins can result in toxicity because they are excreted only through bile and the capacity for hepatic excretion of these compounds is limited.

Deficiency of vitamin D results in abnormal skeletal development in children (rickets) and abnormal calcium metabolism in adults (see Metabolic Bone Disease section in Chapter 6). Since the active form of vitamin D can be formed by the action of ultraviolet light on 7-dehydrocholesterol, individuals with limited exposure to sunlight are at increased risk for developing significant deficiency (Fig. 3-11).

Vitamin K deficiency results in defective formation of critical blood coagulation factors that require carboxylation of conserved glutamic acid residues to create calcium-binding sites that are necessary for their normal function. Inhibition of vitamin K by warfarin provides an important pharmacologic means of anticoagulation.

Vitamin A deficiency results in abnormal rhodopsin pigment in retinal cells that causes diminished night vision. Continued deficiency results in squamous metaplasia of ocular tissues resulting in drying of the cornea (xerophthalmia) that can lead to corneal destruction and blindness.

Vitamin E is an antioxidant and deficiency may enhance oxygen damage to various tissues. Vitamin E deficiency increases red blood cell fragility and may produce neuropathy.

Obesity

Obesity in adults is defined as a body mass index (BMI) >25 (BMI >30 is severe obesity) and is associated with significant morbidity and excess mortality.

Obesity is epidemic in the United States and is a major contributing factor to death from atherosclerotic cardiovascular disease and diabetes mellitus. Abnormal deposits of adipose tissue in obese patients are important causes of insulin resistance, which is a major factor in the development of type 2 diabetes. Obesity is also associated with increased levels of low-density lipoprotein cholesterol and triglycerides in the blood, which are major risk factors for atherosclerosis. Nonalcoholic steatohepatitis (NASH) is much more likely to develop in obese individuals and diabetics (Fig. 3-12). The incidence of NASH is increasing rapidly and in some patients evolves to hepatic cirrhosis with liver failure. Obese

PHYSIOLOGY

Body Mass Index (BMI)

BMI is calculated as the ratio of an individual's weight in kilograms divided by the height in meters squared (BMI = kg/m^2). BMI provides a useful measure of body fat percentage and obesity.

BMI in Adults	Weight Status
<18.5	Underweight
18.5–24.9	Normal
25.0–29.9	Overweight
>30.0	Obese

BMI has different normal ranges in children than in adults. Children are considered underweight if their BMI is less than the 5th percentile of BMI for their age. Similarly, children are considered overweight if their BMI is more than the 95th percentile of BMI for their age. Children are considered at risk for being overweight if their BMI is more than the 85th percentile but less than the 95th percentile of BMI for their age.

Women usually have more body fat than men of the same age with the same BMI.

Older individuals may have more body fat than young adults with the same BMI.

Age (yr)	95th Percentile BMI for Boys
2	19.3
4	17.8
9	21.0
13	25.1

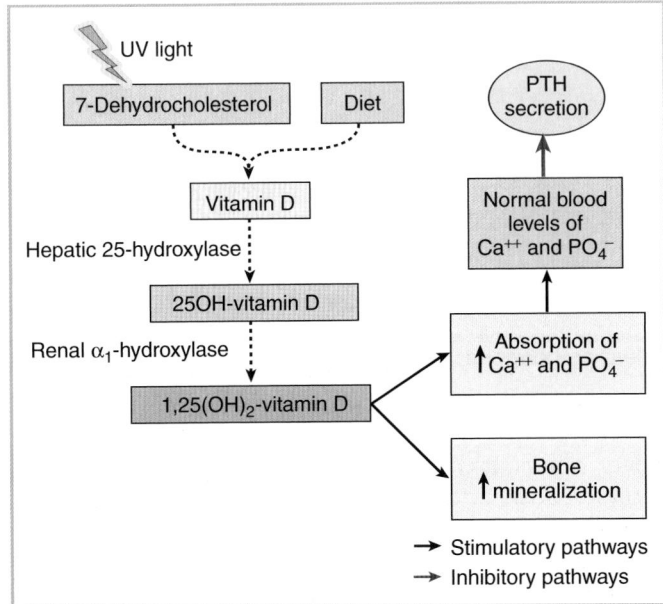

Figure 3-11. Vitamin D metabolism.

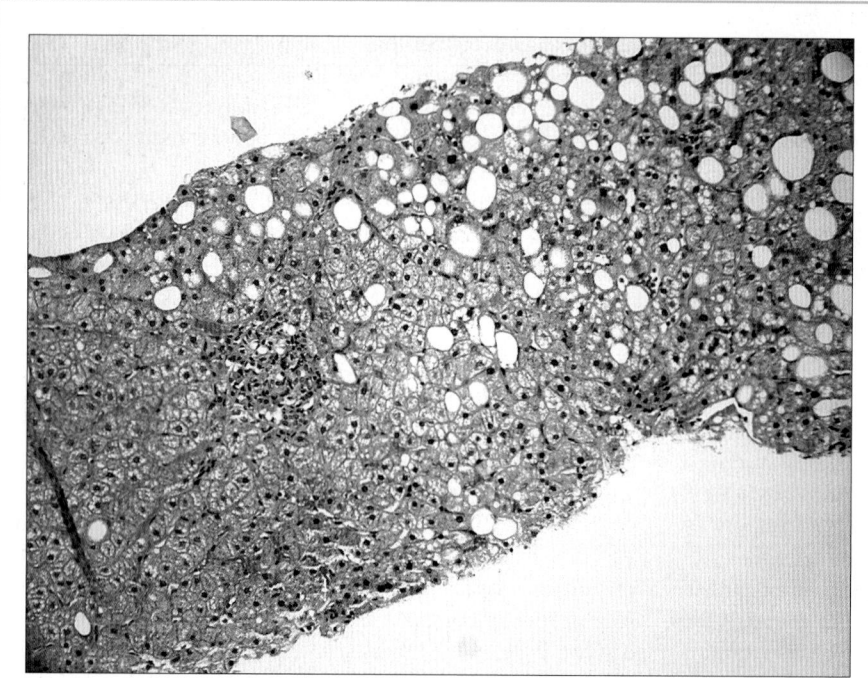

Figure 3-12. Nonalcoholic steatohepatitis (NASH). Photomicrograph of liver needle biopsy specimen showing prominent accumulation of fat droplets (steatosis) in hepatocytes with an associated chronic inflammatory reaction.

individuals are also at increased risk for the development of colon and prostate cancer as well as other forms of malignancy. The mechanisms underlying increased cancer risk are less clear, but increased oxidative stress (free radicals produced by a high-calorie diet and excess oxidation of fatty acids in adipose tissue) may contribute to carcinogenesis.

Although the excess morbidity associated with obesity is clear, the causes of obesity are much less well understood. Leptin is a protein hormone produced by adipocytes that interacts with hypothalamic receptors to decrease appetite (Fig. 3-13). Rare patients with genetic leptin deficiency are morbidly obese, but most obese patients have relatively high levels of leptin, suggesting that their hypothalamic receptors are resistant. Leptin is also important in modulating sensitivity to insulin in target tissues, and high leptin levels can result in marked resistance to some insulin effects. Ghrelin is secreted by the stomach in response to gastric distention by food and is important in appetite control. The presence of multiple redundant systems to ensure that appetite drives adequate nutrition emphasizes the evolutionary importance of adequate food consumption (to prevent starvation during interruptions in food supply). This redundancy may be responsible for the difficulty in designing effective strategies to block appetite in obese individuals.

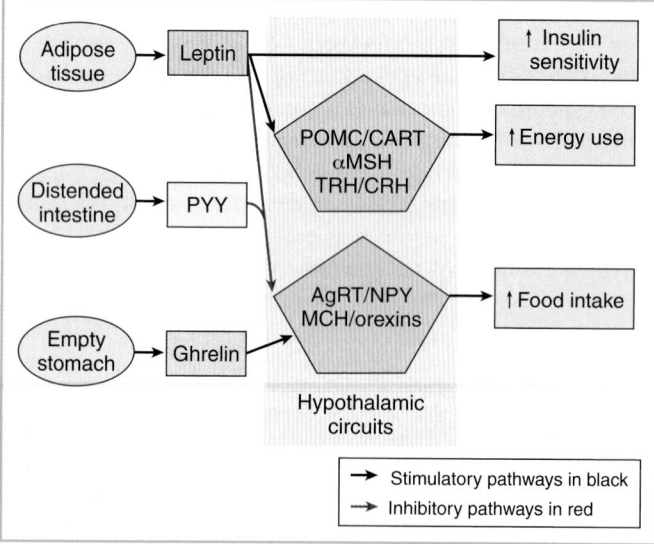

Figure 3-13. Hormonal control of energy balance and appetite. AgRT, Agouti-related peptide; CRH, corticotropin-releasing hormone; MCH, melanin-concentrating hormone; αMSH, alpha melanocyte-stimulating hormone; NPY, neuropeptide Y; orexins, orexigenic peptides; POMC, pro-opiomelanocortin; PYY, peptide YY; TRH, thyrotropin-releasing hormone.

●●● PATTERNS OF INJURY

A small number of relatively stereotyped patterns of response to injury occur in most organs and tissues. These patterns evolve over relatively characteristic time scales and have predictable consequences in most settings. Understanding these basic patterns of response to injury allows prediction of the natural course of many diseases based on observable morphologic features. Examination of tissue grossly and microscopically to assess these changes is the main substance of anatomic pathology. Gross and microscopic examination of tissue usually allow pathologists to characterize the acuteness or chronicity of different insults, and this temporal information is often important in arriving at a correct diagnosis and in choosing optimal therapy.

Edema

Edema is increased interstitial fluid in the extracellular tissue space. The accumulation of edema fluid results in increased organ and tissue weight, and the cut surfaces of edematous tissues tend to weep fluid. Histologically, intercellular edema can result in separation between cells and the expansion of the extracellular matrix (Fig. 3-14A). Intracellular and extracellular edema may coexist. Fluid accumulations are usually characterized as transudates or exudates. An exudate is actively induced by inflammatory mediators and contains relatively large amounts of protein, which can be assessed by measuring its specific gravity. Exudates are usually defined as fluids with specific gravity greater than 1.020 g/mL. Edema is one of the earliest responses to many inflammatory mediators and is induced by loosening of junctions between endothelial cells in venules.

Transudates have relatively low protein content and low specific gravity, usually less than 1.012 g/mL. Transudates are usually not associated with large numbers of inflammatory cells and result from the passive movement of water from the vasculature into the interstitium. This can occur because of increased hydrostatic pressure in blood vessels, decreased oncotic pressure in plasma, or increased osmotic pressure in tissues (e.g., sodium retention in congestive heart failure). Plasma proteins are responsible for the bulk of the intra-vascular oncotic pressure. Markedly decreased serum protein concentrations (renal protein loss, decreased hepatic synthesis due to liver disease, or malnutrition) can result in anasarca, with severe edema involving most organs and tissues.

When excess fluid is present in the extracellular matrix, it increases tissue volume, resulting in swelling. The tissue distribution of edema may suggest the nature of the abnormality. For instance, in congestive heart failure, increased central venous pressure results in the transudation of fluid-producing edema that is most severe in dependent areas (i.e., where venous pressure is highest because of gravity). In ambulatory patients with congestive heart failure, edema typically develops in the lower extremities, whereas in nonambulatory patients, it is usually presacral in location. This type of dependent edema is often described as pitting because sustained digital pressure on the affected tissue can redistribute some the excess fluid, resulting in depressions (pits) when the pressure is removed (see Fig. 3-14B). Edema fluid can also collect in body cavities such as the pleural space or the peritoneum, where it is referred to as an effusion.

Edema is a useful sign of inflammation, but it can result in significant morbidity and even mortality. The accumulation of large amounts of fluid in the pleural space can compress the lung, resulting in decreased oxygenation. Intra-alveolar edema in the lungs (pulmonary edema; see Fig. 3-14C) can cause even more serious impairment of gas exchange, producing severe hypoxemia. Brain edema results in increased

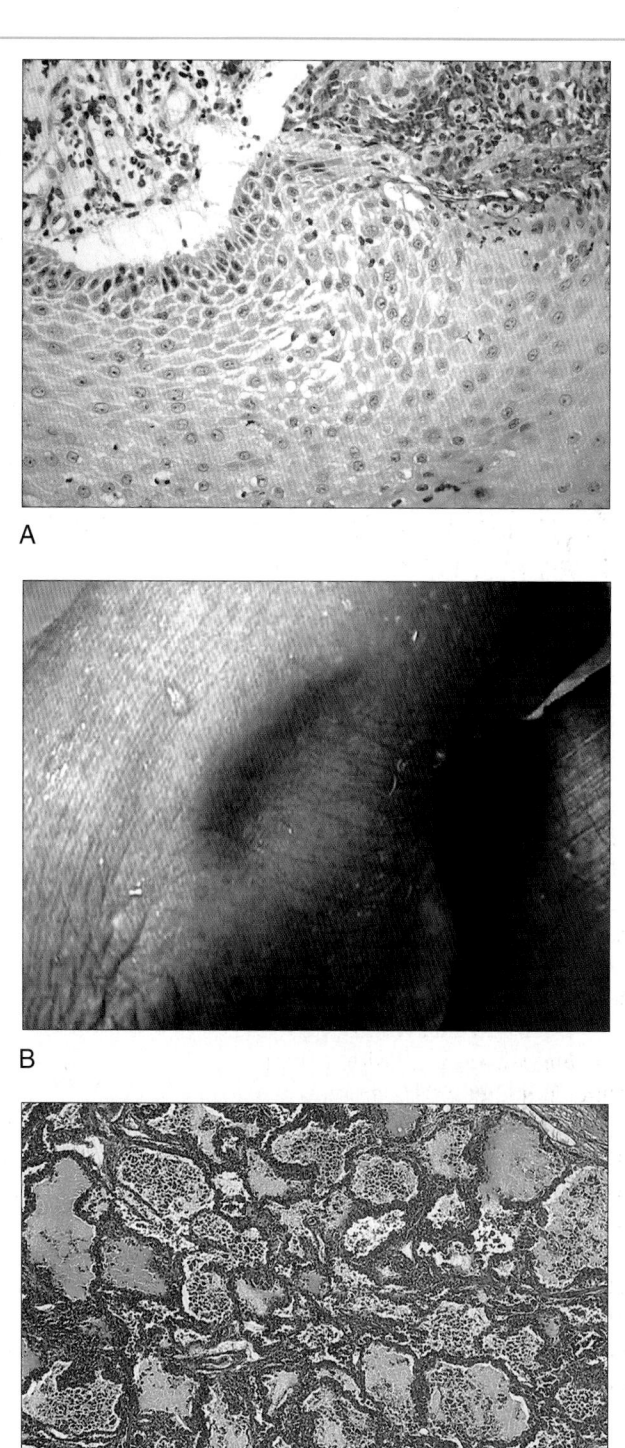

A

B

C

Figure 3-14. A, Spongiosis. Microscopic section of skin showing intercellular edema causing visible separations between keratinocytes (spongiosis). **B**, Skin with pitting edema. **C**, Pulmonary edema. Note that alveolar spaces are filled with eosinophilic proteinaceous material, which is a component of the edema fluid in this clinical setting.

brain volume that can result in herniation (i.e., the brain stem is forced through the foramen magnum, resulting in vascular occlusion because of the closed nature of the cranial compartment).

Hemorrhage

Hemorrhage is the extravasation of blood due to loss of vascular integrity. Hemorrhage can be either external (into the environment) or internal, forming a hematoma in tissue or filling a body cavity (e.g., hemothorax, hemopericardium, hemoperitoneum, or hemarthrosis). Acute hemorrhage of more than 20% of blood volume (approximately 1 L) usually causes hypovolemic shock. Hemorrhages in tissue are characterized clinically in terms of their gross morphologic appearance, which often suggests the cause of the hemorrhage.

Petechiae are 1- to 2-mm hemorrhages in the skin, mucous membranes, or serosal surfaces that result from minute defects in the microvasculature (typically capillaries) (Fig. 3-15A).

Since erythrocytes are extravasated into the extracellular space, petechiae do not blanch when pressure is applied. These areas of hemorrhage are so small that they cannot be felt (palpated) on clinical examination. Petechiae are usually caused by abnormalities in platelets or in elements of the coagulation cascade. A decreased platelet count (thrombocytopenia) is the most common cause of petechiae. Normal body movements produce wear and tear that causes microscopic defects in the microvasculature on a minute-by-minute basis. These microscopic defects are normally immediately plugged by platelets, preventing hemorrhage. In individuals with very low platelet counts ($<5000/mm^3$), this homeostatic mechanism is ineffective, and hemorrhage from innumerable microscopic defects in the vasculature can lead to serious or fatal hemorrhage.

Purpura describes hemorrhages in the skin or mucous membranes that are greater than 3 mm in diameter and form plaque-like lesions that are palpable on clinical examination. Purpura often results from vascular inflammation (vasculitis),

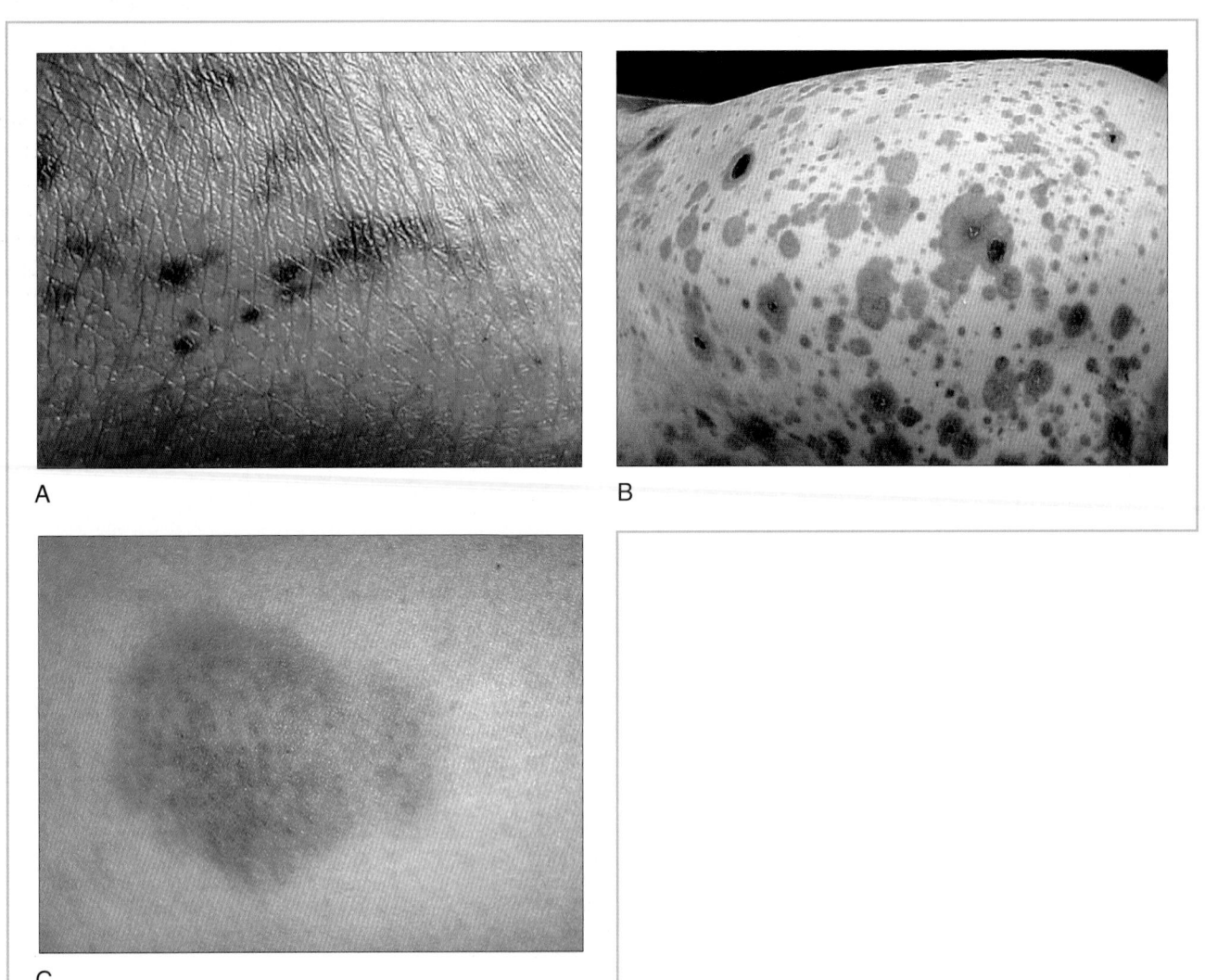

Figure 3-15. A, Skin with petechiae. **B**, Skin with purpura. **C**, Skin with ecchymoses.

which can cause functional breaks in blood vessels (see Fig. 3-15B). Purpura develops when vasculitis involves small blood vessels (venules or small arteries) beneath mucosal surfaces or in the dermis of the skin.

Ecchymoses are larger extravasations of blood into tissue and are synonymous with "bruises." Ecchymoses tend to be >10 mm in diameter and are almost always caused by trauma (see Fig. 3-15C). *Hematomas* are solid collections of coagulated blood that can form by blood dissecting through tissue under pressure or by hemorrhage filling spaces in tissue created by penetrating trauma or surgery.

Thrombosis

Thrombosis is the inappropriate activation of normal hemostasis within vascular spaces to form a thrombus (blood clot). Normal hemostasis is essential to maintain vascular integrity even in the absence of significant trauma. For this reason, the coagulation system must be poised for rapid activation. Three critical factors can predispose to thrombosis and are often referred to as Virchow's triad: endothelial injury, abnormal blood flow, and hypercoagulability (Fig. 3-16).

Endothelial injury results in endothelial cell activation, and the exposure of basement membrane collagen is a strong stimulus for the normal initiation of the coagulation cascade. Endothelial cell activation results in increased adherence of platelets and inflammatory cells, favoring platelet activation that may be sufficient to initiate the coagulation cascade. Even subtle endothelial cell dysfunction can predispose to thrombosis, and ongoing endothelial injury associated with atherosclerotic plaques is a major contributing factor to most arterial thromboses. Tissue inflammation (e.g., infection or trauma) also activates endothelial cells to recruit inflammatory cells to the site of injury, resulting in an increased tendency to thrombosis.

Alterations in blood flow additionally can predispose to thrombosis. Flow within the vascular system is typically laminar with the slowest flow rate immediately adjacent to endothelial surfaces.

This arrangement minimizes shear stress on the endothelium and decreases the likelihood of endothelial cells becoming activated. Abnormalities in the blood vessels (e.g., atherosclerotic plaques) or in cardiac valves can result in abnormal (turbulent) flow, which can subject endothelial cells to excessive shear stress and result in their activation.

Stasis or pooling of blood promotes thrombosis in several different ways. Diminished blood flow results in oxygen depletion of red blood cells, which causes hypoxia of adjacent endothelial cells, resulting in endothelial cell injury and activation. Since the coagulation system normally has a low level of intrinsic activation (for rapid response to vascular damage), blood pooling can result in the accumulation and concentration of activated coagulation factors that may be sufficient to cause thrombosis. Conversely, blood pooling may block the access of normal inhibitors of coagulation to favor thrombosis.

Blood pooling is much more common in veins than in arteries. This is particularly true in the veins of the leg, which depend on skeletal muscle contraction and intrinsic venous valves to return blood against gravity. Leg veins often become fibrotic and dilated in older individuals (varicose veins) making their valves ineffective so that stasis develops. Immobilization of the extremities (e.g., bed rest) decreases muscle contraction and can further predispose to stasis and thrombosis. In patients with atrial fibrillation, the lack of coordinated atrial contraction also causes stasis and favors

Figure 3-16. Virchow's triad.

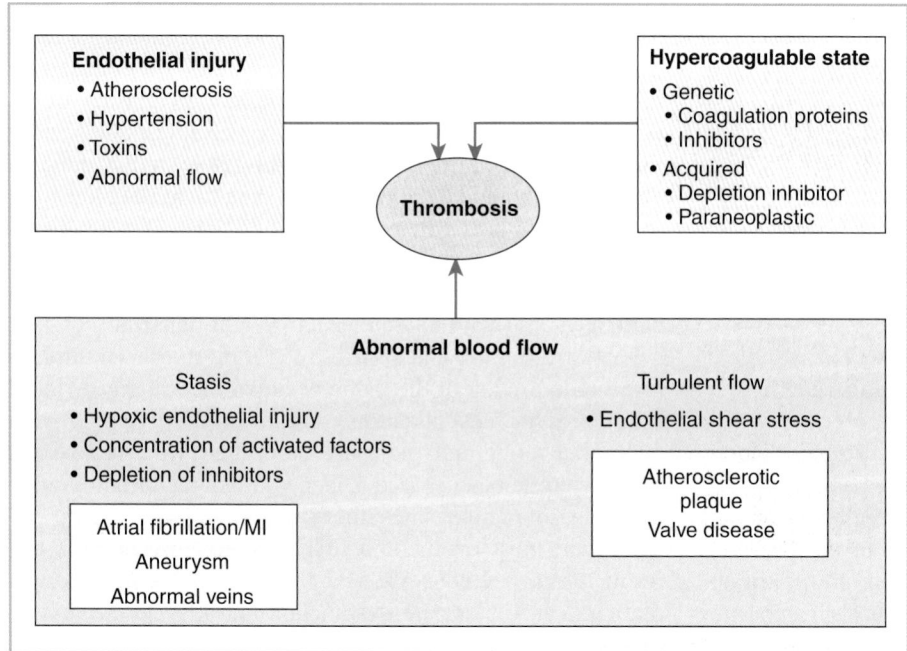

PHYSIOLOGY

Laminar and Turbulent Blood Flow

Laminar flow is a condition of any liquid flowing through a tube in which there is a parabolic distribution of flow velocity with the most rapid flow at the center of the tube. In laminar flow, liquid flows in layers (laminae) with progressively slower flow at the periphery (adjacent to the endothelial surface of blood vessels), which minimizes shear stress.

Laminar flow tends to keep cellular elements in the blood separated from the endothelial surface but allows blood cells at the periphery to move more slowly and interact with endothelial cells (margination).

Turbulent flow occurs if the flow velocity is too great for the size of the vessel and can cause cellular injury and obstruct flow. Turbulence develops when the Reynolds number exceeds a critical value that is proportional to the flow velocity, vessel diameter, and fluid density and inversely proportional to fluid viscosity. Turbulent flow in the circulation is often audible as a murmur on auscultation.

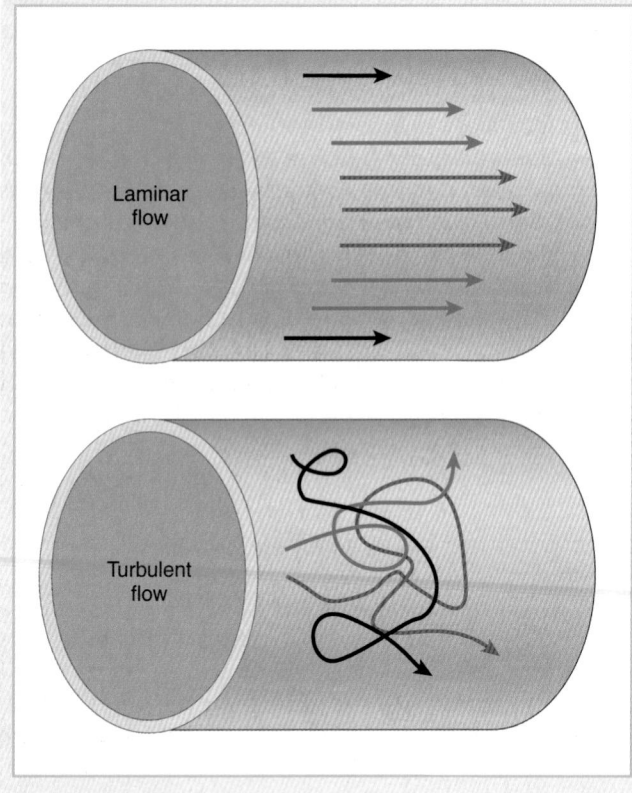

the formation of mural thrombi (thrombi adherent to the endocardial surface of the heart).

Hypercoagulability means an abnormal tendency for blood to clot and can result from genetic or acquired abnormalities of the coagulation cascade, inhibitors of coagulation, or the thrombolytic system. Depletion of protein S or protein C in disease states can produce a markedly prothrombotic condition in which both arterial and venous thrombosis may occur. Rare abnormalities in a few other genes can also result in a

marked predisposition to thrombosis. Conversely, several common genetic variations are clearly associated with a mildly increased risk of thrombosis.

A single amino acid substitution in the factor V protein (factor V Leiden) makes it slightly more resistant to inactivation by activated protein C, resulting in a mild increase in risk for venous thrombosis. Factor V (Leiden) is quite prevalent (present in a heterozygous state in >5% of individuals in some populations in the United States and Europe). The combination of a mild genetic predisposition to thrombosis with other host (e.g., stasis) or environmental factors (e.g., bed rest) is a common mechanism underlying venous thrombosis. A polymorphism in the 3' untranslated region of the prothrombin gene also results in slightly higher levels of prothrombin in blood and is associated with a small increased risk of venous thrombosis. Coinheritance of several different mild genetic risk factors for thrombosis may result in a severe phenotype. Genetic risk factors for arterial thrombosis are less clearly defined at this time.

Arterial and venous thrombi have somewhat different morphologic appearances on pathologic examination and have greatly different clinical consequences. Arterial thrombi that form while blood is actively flowing tend to have laminations composed of alternating layers of fibrin and red blood cells (so-called lines of Zahn; Fig. 3-17). In contrast, venous thrombi typically lack prominent lines of Zahn because they form all at once in the setting of blood pooling or stasis. Arterial thrombi tend to extend (propagate) in retrograde direction extending backward from the thrombus toward the heart. Arterial thrombi usually contain relatively more fibrin and fewer red blood cells than venous thrombi contain and so have a pale appearance on gross examination. Venous thrombi are referred to as red thrombi because they contain many red blood cells and tend to have a gelatinous consistency. Ninety percent of clinically significant venous thrombi develop in leg veins and form an occlusive cast of the vessel lumen over a long distance. Deep venous thrombi (DVTs) are often asymptomatic but are the predominant cause of pulmonary emboli (see Emboli, below). The risk of DVTs may be assessed by measuring the concentration of D-dimer in plasma or by assessing venous flow by means of Doppler ultrasound. Venous thrombi extend in the direction of blood flow so that clot may eventually extend all the way to the vena cava. The likelihood of an immobilized patient developing a clinically significant DVT (and so being at risk for pulmonary embolism) can be markedly reduced by prophylactic treatment of hospitalized patients at risk with low-molecular-weight heparin.

Most arteries are end arteries so that most arterial thrombi result in infarction of the tissue or organ they supply. Arterial thrombi occur most commonly in the coronary, cerebral, and femoral arteries and most are associated with preexisting atherosclerotic plaques (see Chapter 7). Venous thrombi rarely result in infarction, since there are extensive venous collaterals in most organs and tissues. Venous thrombosis can result in marked congestion of the affected tissue or organ that can cause pain and dysfunction and may predispose to infection (infectious thrombophlebitis). Venous thrombosis

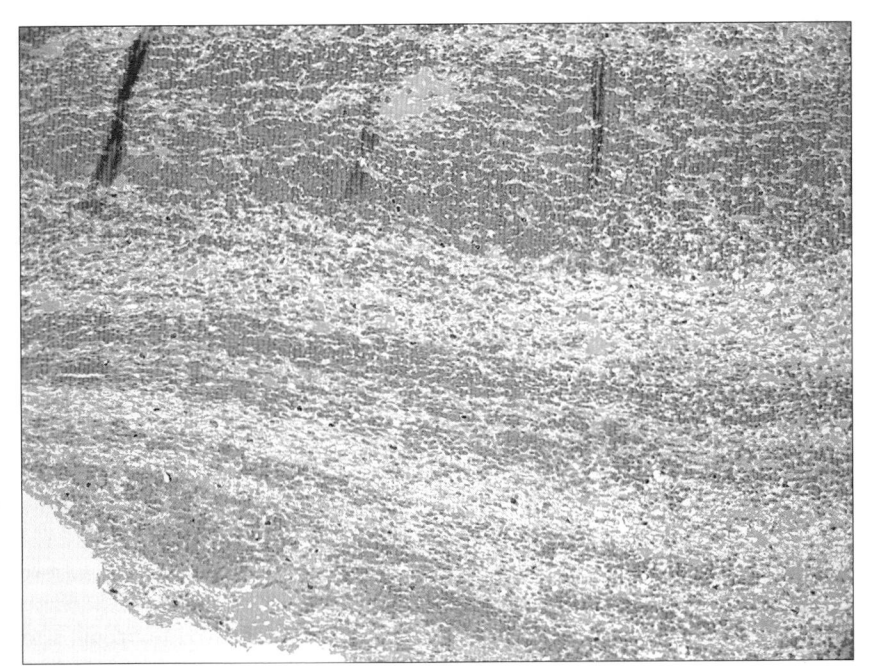

Figure 3-17. Lines of Zahn. Microscopic section of arterial thrombus with alternating lamina composed of red blood cells or fibrin.

affecting the ovary, testis, or in some cases the kidney can result in hemorrhagic infarction, since these organs have a single conduit for venous drainage without significant collateral vessels. Infarcts resulting from venous thrombosis are always hemorrhagic, whereas arterial thrombi tend to cause pale infarcts. DVTs in the larger veins of the leg are usually asymptomatic because of collaterals but are an important cause of morbidity and mortality, since they give rise to most pulmonary emboli.

Embolus

Emboli are detached, intravascular solid, liquid, or gaseous materials that are transported intravascularly from their site of origin to a distant site. The vast majority of emboli are thrombi (or *thromboemboli*) that have dislodged from their site of formation in the arterial or venous system. The most common type of thromboembolism results from dislodgment of venous thrombi in deep leg veins, which travel through the vena cava and right heart to lodge in the lungs (pulmonary thromboemboli; Fig. 3-18). Pulmonary emboli result in blockage of a portion of the pulmonary circulation, causing a mismatch between ventilation and perfusion that results in hypoxemia (in proportion to the amount of pulmonary circulation affected). Normal individuals have a large pulmonary reserve, and loss of up to half of lung function does not result in life-threatening sequelae. In contrast, patients with significant comorbid pulmonary or cardiovascular disease can develop significant hypoxemia as a result of small pulmonary emboli. Over time (weeks), pulmonary emboli are recanalized by tissue repair, which may leave an eccentric scar in the vessel wall or a web of fibrous tissue in the lumen as a marker of prior pulmonary emboli.

Large or extensive pulmonary emboli acutely increase pulmonary artery blood pressure, exerting strain on the right ventricle that may result in failure or compensatory hypertrophy of the right ventricle. If pulmonary hypertension is severe and prolonged, right heart failure (cor pulmonale) may result. Very large pulmonary emboli that arise in the deep veins of the leg can completely block the bifurcation of the pulmonary artery (so-called saddle embolus); this is almost instantly fatal because complete blockage of the pulmonary circulation results in the abrupt loss of cardiac output. Pulmonary infarction is a relatively rare complication of pulmonary emboli because the lung has a dual circulation (bronchial arteries in addition to pulmonary arteries). Repeated episodes of pulmonary emboli (chronic pulmonary emboli) can degrade the pulmonary circulation to a point at which additional emboli result in pulmonary infarcts.

Most arterial thromboemboli result from dislodgment of thrombi adherent to atherosclerotic plaques. Arterial thromboemboli typically result in infarction of the tissue or organ supplied by the involved artery. A "paradoxical embolus" is a venous thromboembolus that crosses into the arterial circulation through a persistently patent foramen ovale or through an atrial or ventricular septal defect. Paradoxical emboli are rare but tend to cause end-organ infarction, as do other arterial emboli. Septic thromboemboli (containing live bacteria or other pathogens) typically occur in bacterial endocarditis (infection of the heart valve) and can develop from infected venous thromboemboli.

Several different types of nonthrombotic emboli are clinically important. Atheroemboli result from the disruption of an atherosclerotic plaque and the release of lipid material (cholesterol crystals) from the center of the plaque. This cholesterol material is highly thrombogenic and tends to lodge

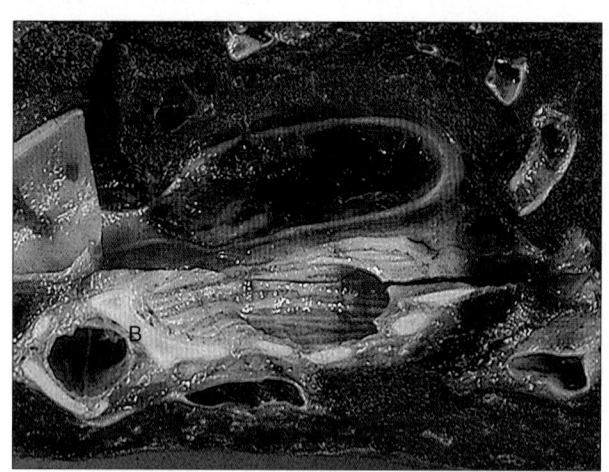

A

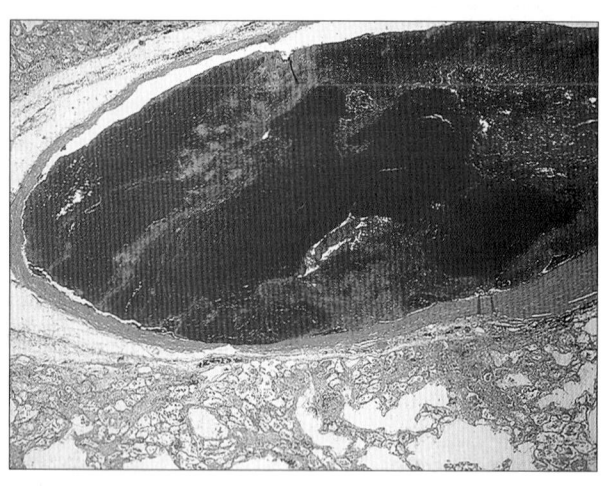

B

Figure 3-18. A, Pulmonary embolus. Gross section through lung hilum showing a large pulmonary embolus distending a major pulmonary artery branch. An adjacent, unremarkable bronchus is evident ("B"). **B,** Pulmonary embolus. Microscopic section of an acute pulmonary embolus.

in the microvasculature of organs and can result in widespread thrombosis. A shower of atheroemboli to the kidneys can cause acute renal failure.

Traumatic fracture of bones can result in the release of bone marrow fat into the vasculature, producing fat emboli that lodge in the lung. Fracture of multiple bones can result in fat embolism syndrome, which is caused by the release of inflammatory mediators in response to the intravascular adipose tissue. These mediators cause respiratory distress, neurologic complications, and endothelial injury similar to that occurring in septic shock.

Amniotic fluid embolism is a rare complication of pregnancy (1 in 50,000 deliveries). Increased amniotic fluid pressure during labor and delivery can occasionally force amniotic fluid into the maternal venous circulation, where squamous and cellular debris lodge in the pulmonary

circulation inciting widespread activation of inflammatory mediators and activation of the coagulation cascade (80% mortality).

Air embolism can occur with thoracic trauma or surgery but must be large (>100 mL) to cause significant symptoms. Gaseous nitrogen microemboli occur as a consequence of rapid decompression in deep-sea divers and result in severe pain in multiple organs.

Hypoxia and Ischemia

Tissue and organ hypoxia can result from decreased oxygenation of blood or defective delivery of oxygen to tissues caused by anemia, decreased respiratory function, or decreased blood flow. Decreased blood flow also results in ischemia with combined hypoxia and acidosis of the involved tissue (diminished blood flow results in the accumulation of acidic waste products from oxidative phosphorylation and anaerobic glycolysis). Decreased tissue pH can exacerbate damage caused by hypoxia. Ischemic injury is more common than pure hypoxic injury, since it results from arterial blockage, which is a frequent complication of atherosclerosis.

Tissue hypoxia is a relative term, since more oxygen is required for metabolically active tissues than for resting tissues. Hypoxia initially results in depletion of cellular ATP, which can occur within seconds. If hypoxia is prolonged, most cells switch from oxidative phosphorylation to anaerobic glycolysis in an attempt to maintain energy charge. Glycogen stores are rapidly consumed, and there is a marked increase in the amount of lactic acid produced. The lack of ATP and cellular acidosis result in dysfunction of cellular proteins and eventually lead to the loss of integrity of cell membranes and cell death. If the oxygen supply is restored, reversibly injured cells can restore normal function although they may remain "stunned" and incapable of some of their normal functions for hours. Most irreversibly injured cells undergo coagulative necrosis, but some injured cells may initiate apoptosis and may complete this process if sufficient energy stores are available.

Infarction and Necrosis

Most infarcts result from vascular occlusion in the involved tissue or organ. The venous supply to most organs and tissues has significant collaterals to allow sufficient venous return if venous thrombosis occurs. When venous occlusion results in infarction, the infarcted tissue is usually hemorrhagic owing to marked vascular congestion.

Since most arteries are end arteries, arterial thrombosis usually results in infarction. Organs with a dual blood supply (e.g., the lung and liver) are an exception. Infarction produces the typical changes of coagulative necrosis in most organs and tissues (Fig. 3-19). Essentially all parenchymal cells supplied by the affected artery undergo necrosis or trigger apoptosis. The geometry of infarcts is determined by the geography of the vascular supply. For this reason, most infarcts in solid organs are wedge shaped (characteristic triangular shape with

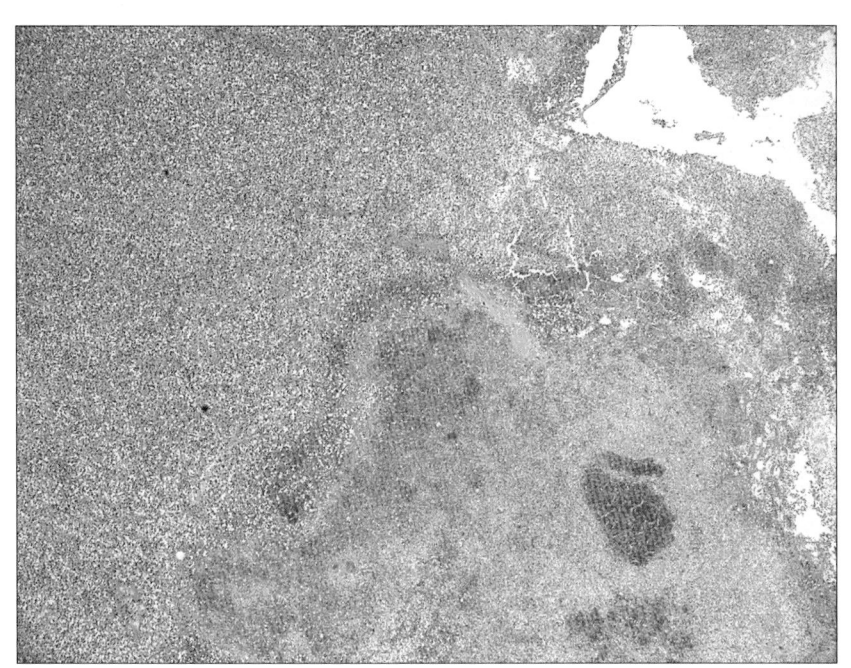

Figure 3-19. Acute infarct. Wedge-shaped infarct in splenic parenchyma secondary to vascular thrombosis. The typical features of coagulation necrosis are evident with hypereosinophilia and loss of nuclear staining.

the base of the triangle at the serosal surface) and extend to the serosal surface of the affected organ.

Tissue necrosis results in the robust recruitment of inflammatory cells that aid in the digestion and removal of necrotic cellular material. The initial inflammatory response to necrosis is composed almost exclusively of acute inflammatory cells (neutrophils). In most infarcts, the peak of neutrophilic infiltration occurs between 24 and 48 hours after infarction. Neutrophils do not arrive in areas of infarction until well after the parenchymal cells have undergone irreversible injury. Parenchymal cells at the margin of the infarct may be reversibly injured and may ultimately recover. As an infarct ages, there is a transition from acute inflammation to chronic inflammation followed by the ingrowth of granulation tissue and tissue repair with fibrosis. Loss of dead parenchymal cells and contraction of the fibrous scar result in a diminished volume that tends to pucker the surface of an organ over a healed infarct (Fig. 3-20).

The evolution of infarcts can be altered if blood flow is restored to the tissue soon after infarction has occurred (so-called reperfusion injury). Reperfusion usually causes hemorrhage because of damage to endothelial cells and blood vessels within the infarct. Reperfusion may allow the recovery of reversibly injured parenchymal cells that would otherwise have undergone coagulative necrosis.

Different organs typically have somewhat different morphologic patterns of infarction. In soft organs (e.g., the lung and liver) and organs with a dual blood supply (e.g., the lung and liver), infarcts are typically hemorrhagic because a small amount of blood flow from the alternative blood supply continues after infarction. The spongy nature of soft organs (e.g., the lung) and tissues permits fairly extensive extra-

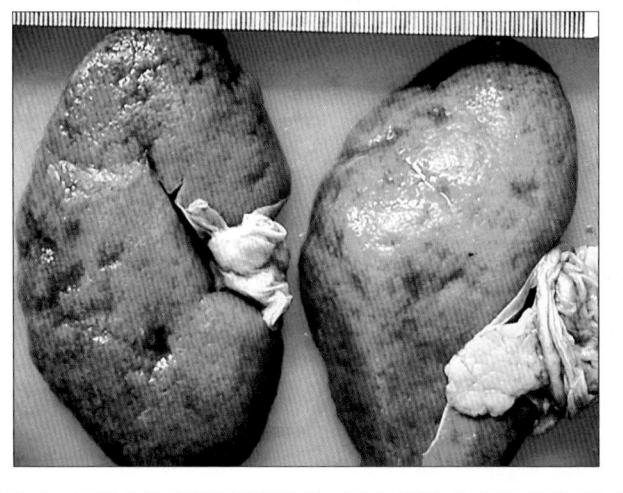

Figure 3-20. Healed renal infarcts. Gross image of renal surface with the renal capsule removed. The depressed areas correspond to healed microinfarcts with associated fibrosis and tissue loss.

vasation of red blood cells from damaged veins under low hydrostatic pressure. Infarcts in more solid organs (e.g., the kidney) tend to be pale with little extravasated blood.

In most organs, sufficient extracellular matrix is present to prevent tissue liquefaction so that the infarct remains relatively solid. In the CNS, infarction tends to produce "liquefactive" rather than coagulative necrosis because the minimal extracellular matrix present in the brain is insufficient to maintain infarcted tissue in a solid or semisolid state. Secondary infection of any infarct can result in liquefaction of the necrotic tissue with abscess formation.

Gangrene is a distinct form of necrosis that typically develops in extremities in individuals with severe atherosclerotic cardiovascular disease or diabetes mellitus. Dry gangrene results when the blood supply to the extremity is incrementally decreased over a long time interval, resulting in the dehydration (mummification) of the tissue with relatively little associated inflammation (Fig. 3-21). Wet gangrene corresponds to the rapid onset of necrosis of a large portion of an extremity that can be caused by infection (e.g., gas gangrene caused by *Clostridium perfringens*).

In some tissues with minimal supporting extracellular matrix, necrosis and associated inflammation result in liquefaction with the formation of a liquid composed of cell debris and inflammatory cells. This process can be referred to descriptively as liquefactive necrosis and it is typical of ischemic necrosis in the CNS.

Other descriptive terms are applied to some patterns of necrosis. Fibrinoid necrosis is a descriptive term for necrosis with amorphous necrotic debris that appears brightly eosinophilic (i.e., fibrin-like) in routine tissue sections. Fibrinoid necrosis can be associated with some specific pathologic processes (e.g., vasculitis in polyarteritis nodosa or malignant hypertension). Caseous necrosis is discussed in Chapter 2 in relation to necrotizing granulomatous inflammation. Lytic necrosis is often used to describe the destruction of individual hepatocytes in the setting of hepatitis due to virus infection. Lytic necrosis in this setting may actually combine some features of necrosis and apoptosis.

●●● TISSUE REPAIR

Tissue repair is an orchestrated process that may restore normal function after injury or may result in the formation of a fibrous scar with loss of normal tissue function. Tissue repair is coordinated by cell-cell interactions, cell–extracellular

MICROBIOLOGY

Clostridium Species

Clostridia are large, anaerobic, gram-positive, sporulating bacterial rods that are ubiquitous in the environment.

C. perfringens is the agent of traumatic gas gangrene (infection is usually acquired from wounds contaminated with bacterial spores). Gas gangrene is an acute infection of muscle and soft tissue that grows explosively. Foul-smelling gas produced by *C. perfringens* creates bubbles in infected tissue that help the organism rapidly dissect along tissue planes over the course of minutes to hours. Gas gangrene is always associated with extensive necrosis and tissue destruction. Toxins produced by clostridia impede the action of neutrophils, exacerbating infection that is frequently fatal. *C. perfringens* can also cause infectious or toxic gastroenteritis.

C. septicum is more resistant to oxygen than is *C. perfringens* and is a major cause of nontraumatic gas gangrene. *C. septicum* may gain access to tissue through ulcerations in colonic mucosa (the classic presentation in a patient with occult colon cancer).

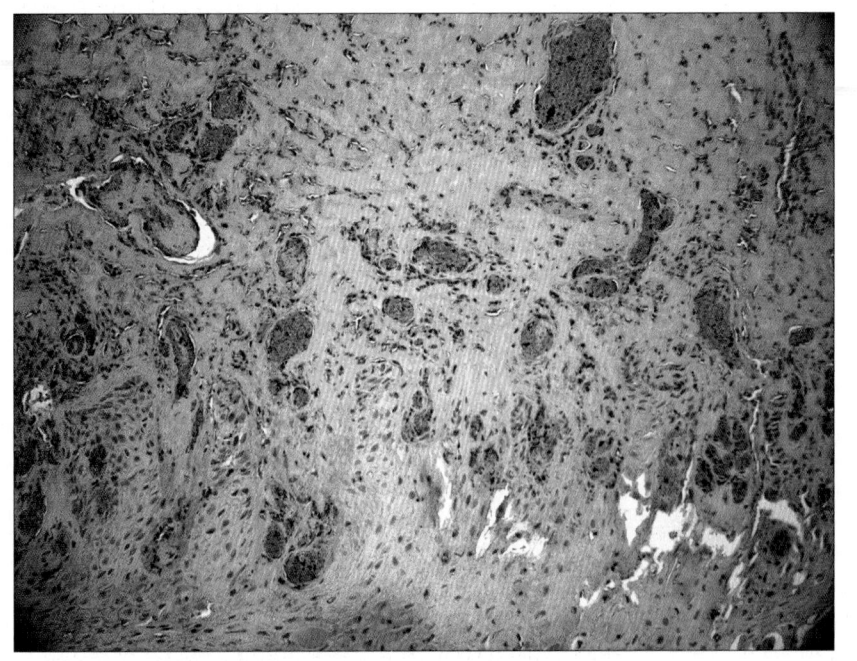

Figure 3-21. Gangrene. Microscopic section of gangrene in the lower extremity secondary to peripheral vascular disease.

matrix interactions, and secretion of growth factors and other mediators by endothelial cells, damaged parenchymal cells, and inflammatory cells (Fig. 3-22). The degree to which normal function can be restored is dependent on the nature and extent of the injury, the tissue injured, the genetic make-up of the patient, and the presence of comorbid conditions. Most tissue repair processes attempt to restore mechanical stability to tissues and to prevent loss of blood or other fluids. The end result of tissue repair may be the restoration of normal function, diminished normal function, abnormal function, or total loss of function. Tissue repair may also have marked deleterious effects (e.g., in some situations exuberant fibrosis may damage or destroy the normal function of a minimally damaged tissue). In this situation, limiting the extent of fibrosis by use of corticosteroids may help preserve normal tissue function.

Restoration of Normal Function

The restoration of normal function by tissue repair depends on the presence of functional precursor cells and an appropriate microenvironment in which they can divide and differentiate to replace parenchymal cells that have been irreversibly injured or killed (Fig. 3-23). In the CNS, precursor cells capable of replacing damaged neurons do not exist and the restoration of normal function is not possible (i.e., adult neurons are permanent cells). In most tissues, reestablishment of normal function is highly dependent on the integrity of the extracellular matrix that normally supports parenchymal cells. Arterial infarction of a portion of the kidney results in a wedge-shaped area with destruction of both parenchymal cells and extracellular matrix. The loss of extracellular matrix prevents tubular regeneration by precursor cells. In contrast, renal acute tubular necrosis (ATN) (usually resulting from transient hypoxia/ischemia) irreversibly injures tubular epithelial cells but leaves the extracellular matrix intact. Since the extracellular matrix is intact, proliferation of precursor cells can restore normal

renal function over the course of a few days with little or no permanent loss of function.

Some organs such as the liver have an even more marked capacity for regeneration. In some species, partial hepatectomy results in regrowth of an entire liver lobe with regeneration of extracellular matrix and parenchymal cells. In the human liver, repeated cycles of tissue damage and regeneration ultimately result in abnormal architecture with increased fibrosis and improper organization of parenchymal cells that causes severe hepatic dysfunction (i.e., cirrhosis; Fig. 3-24). Most tissues that can replace damaged parenchymal cells (i.e., stable cells) behave similarly (i.e., repeated cycles of injury and repair eventually result in abnormal architecture and dysfunction).

Role of the Extracellular Matrix

The extracellular matrix (ECM) is composed of a complex mixture of fibrillary proteins (collagen and elastin) and proteoglycans that bind to each other and to the surface of cells via adhesive glycoproteins (e.g., fibronectin and laminin; Fig. 3-25A). These components provide structural integrity (collagen), elasticity (elastin), and tissue turgor (proteoglycans). Together, these materials provide a microenvironment in which cells can function normally and are shielded from mechanical forces by the elastic and deformable components of the ECM. The ECM also serves as a reservoir for growth factors and cytokines and provides a matrix in which cells can live and actively migrate from place to place (e.g., inflammatory cells).

Two qualitatively different types of extracellular matrix exist: the basement membrane zone and the interstitial matrix zone. The basement membrane zone is composed of a layer of type IV collagen complexed with adhesive glycoproteins, the most important of which is laminin.

Laminin has binding sites for type IV collagen and proteoglycans as well as a cellular binding domain. Laminin acts like

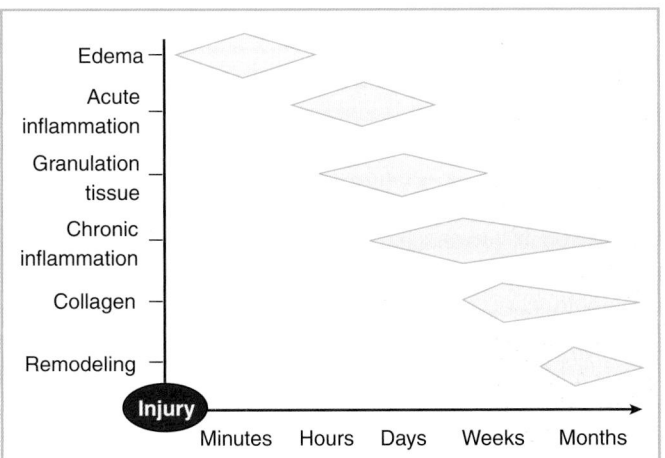

Figure 3-22. Time scale of tissue responses to injury.

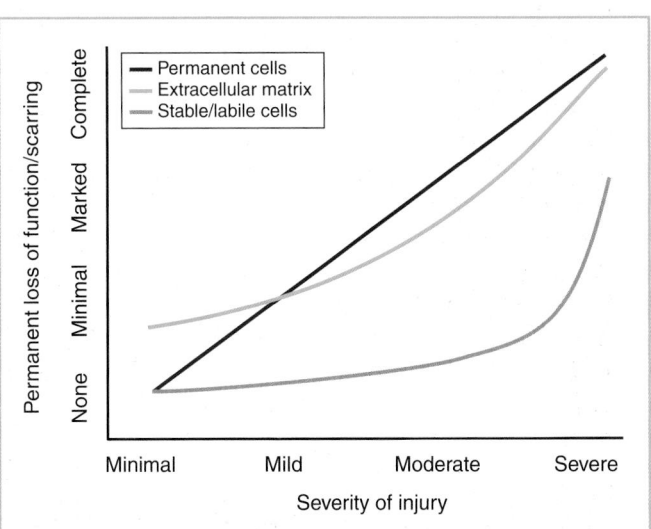

Figure 3-23. Consequences of injury to permanent and stable/labile cells and the extracellular matrix.

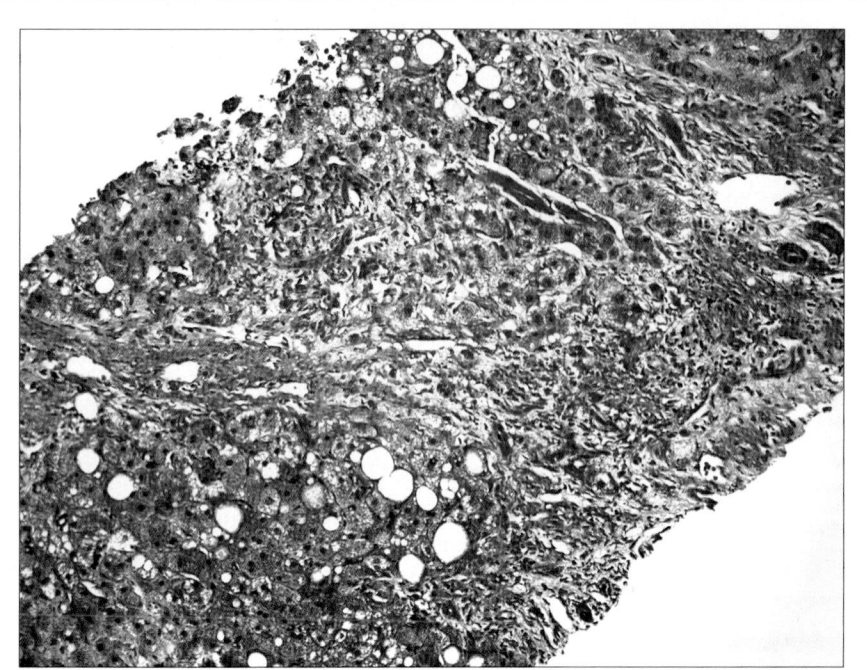

Figure 3-24. Hepatic cirrhosis. Microscopic section of liver tissue stained with a trichrome stain (collagen stained blue) showing severe disruption of normal architecture and extensive fibrosis.

glue, allowing interactions between cells and all other basement membrane zone components. Endothelial cells and epithelial cells interact directly with the basement membrane zone via membrane proteins on their basolateral surfaces (see Fig. 3-25B). The basement membrane zone provides orientation for these cells as well as structural support, and it is porous so that nutrients and oxygen diffuse through it to nourish epithelial cells.

The interstitial matrix zone is not normally in direct contact with epithelial or endothelial cells, but fibroblasts are embedded in it and are responsible for the synthesis of many of its components. Many other cell types including inflammatory cells are normal residents of the interstitial matrix and may alter its composition in response to various stimuli. The interstitial matrix is composed of proteoglycans that are complex polymers that bind water molecules and provide much of the turgor that is normally present in interstitial tissue.

Elastin fibers in the extracellular matrix provide elastic recoil that in combination with turgor allows the extracellular matrix to deform in response to stress and then return to its original shape.

Much of the tensile strength of the extracellular matrix derives from fibrillar collagen (types I and II) arranged in parallel arrays that are cross-linked (see Fig. 3-25C). Adhesive glycoproteins including fibronectin have domains that can bind to fibrillar collagen as well as proteoglycans such as heparin sulfate and chondroitin sulfate. This allows critical interaction between structural components of the extracellular matrix and receptors on cell surfaces. Integrin-binding sites on fibronectin provide essential scaffolding for inflammatory cells to attach to and use as anchors for locomotion during inflammatory processes.

Wound Healing (Repair with Diminished Function)

In situations in which restoration of normal function is not possible because of lack of precursor cells or loss of extracellular matrix, wound healing typically supervenes to fill defects resulting from injury and provide a functional barrier to restore the structural integrity of the damaged tissue or organ. This form of tissue repair is typified by healing after myocardial infarction, which results in the replacement of necrotic myocytes with a dense, hypocellular scar of great tensile strength. Cardiac myocytes do not have the capacity to proliferate so that scar formation is the only option available to maintain the physical integrity of the ventricular wall after infarction. Enzymes released by acute and chronic inflammatory cells digest necrotic myocytes. This cellular debris is then ingested and cleared by macrophages. Macrophages also produce key growth factors including FGF, PDGF, and TGF, which stimulate endothelial cells and fibroblasts to proliferate and migrate to the area of infarction. These cells proliferate and synthesize collagen that is deposited in the ECM (Fig. 3-26A). Over time, this extracellular collagen is remodeled and cross-linked to form a mature scar (see Fig. 3-26B).

This repair process has three relatively distinct but overlapping stages. The initial phase is the recruitment and proliferation of fibroblasts. The second stage is the preliminary deposition of extracellular collagen to form a crude scar. The third stage is a remodeling process in which extracellular collagen is remodeled and arranged into parallel arrays of highly cross-linked collagen fibers that provide marked tensile strength and assure the physical integrity of the ventricle during contraction. Since scar tissue is not contractile, the end

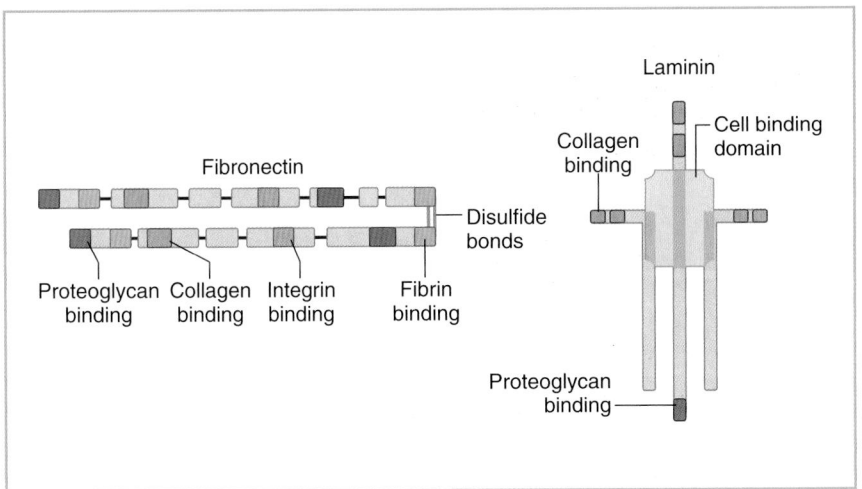

A

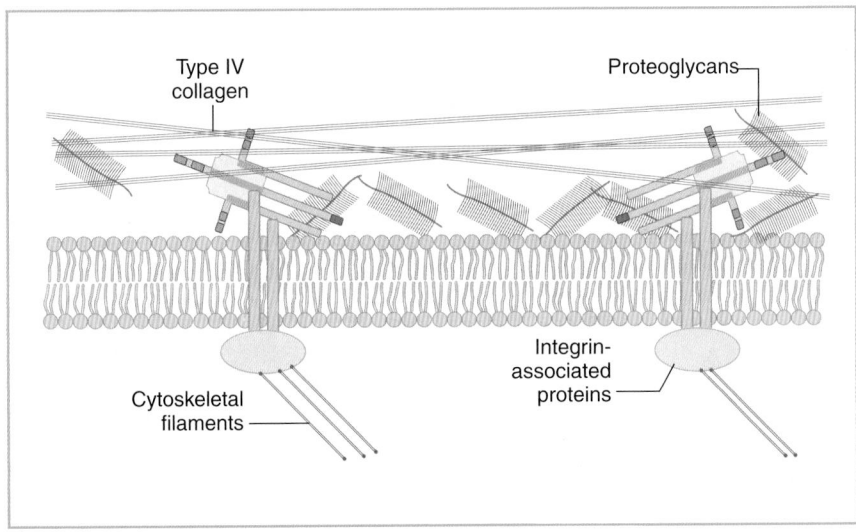

B

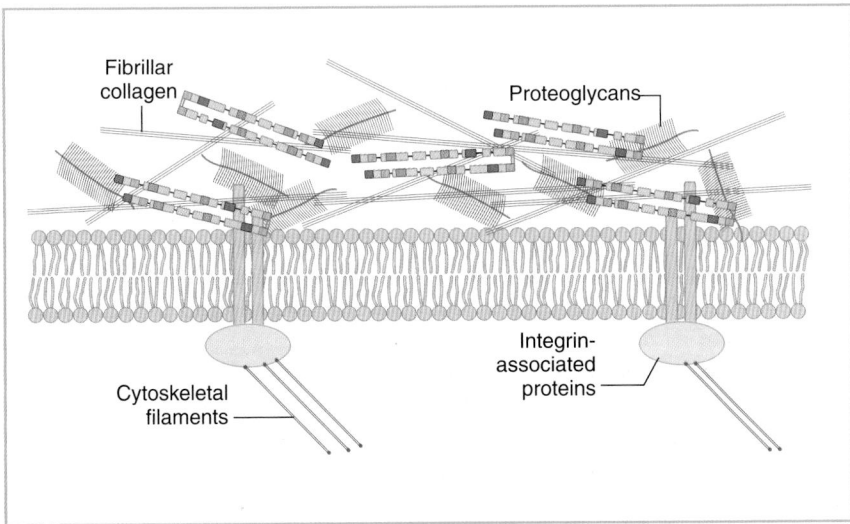

C

Figure 3-25. **A**, Extracellular matrix components. **B**, Basement membrane zone of the extracellular matrix. **C**, Interstitial zone of the extracellular matrix.

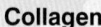

BIOCHEMISTRY

Collagen

Collagens are structural proteins that form a major part of the extracellular matrix. The fibrous collagens (types I and II) are formed by the assembly of three amino acid chains, each of which is more than 1000 amino acids in length. This unique triple helix structure depends on the presence of glycine residues at every third position in each protein molecule. Mutations that result in substitution of a bulky amino acid for glycine usually result in severe disease (e.g., osteogenesis imperfecta).

Type I collagen is the most abundant protein in bone and other connective tissues.

Type II collagen is a major component of cartilage and traps proteoglycans within its structure to produce the elasticity of normal cartilage.

Type III collagen provides structural integrity for the intestine, uterus, and arteries.

Type IV collagen forms a key component of the basement membrane zone beneath epithelial and endothelial surfaces, which also include collagens V and VI. A meshwork of type IV collagen forms a critical component of the glomerular basement membrane filter in the kidney.

Other low-abundance collagens exist, but their specific functions are unknown. Collagen transcription is activated by vitamin C (types I and III) and inhibited by glucocorticoids.

BIOCHEMISTRY

Proteoglycans

Proteoglycans are a special class of highly glycosylated glycoproteins that make up a large portion of the extracellular matrix. Glycosaminoglycan chains are covalently added to a protein core to form proteoglycans. These side chains are long, linear carbohydrates with a strong negative charge due to attached sulfate and uronic acid groups.

The protein core of proteoglycans is produced in the rough endoplasmic reticulum of fibroblasts, and individual sugars are added in the Golgi apparatus. Completed polymers are secreted via vesicles. Three major types are distinguished based on their glycan chains: chondroitin sulfate and dermatan sulfate, heparan sulfate, and keratin sulfate.

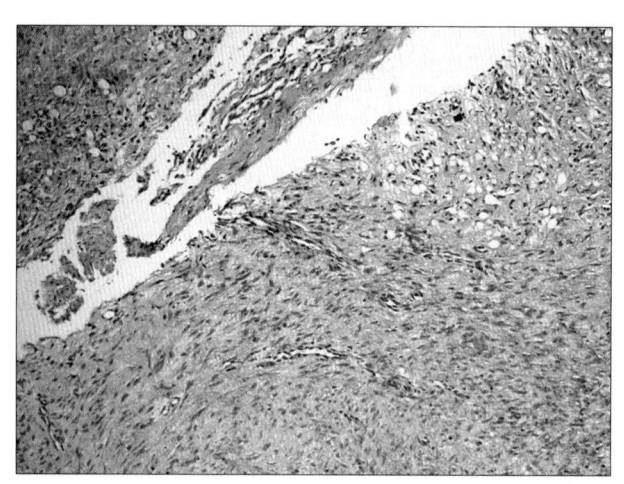

A

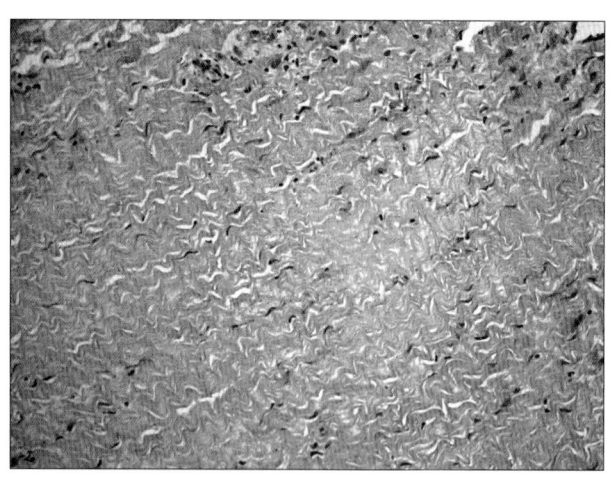

B

Figure 3-26. A, Active fibrosis. Fibroblasts are prominent in this focus of tissue repair with associated small blood vessels and a small amount of extracellular collagen. **B,** Mature scar. Remodeled hypocellular scar (mature scar) with parallel collagen fibers. Scattered fibroblasts and inflammatory cells are also present.

result is a structurally sound ventricle with permanent loss of some of its normal contractile function and diminished compliance because of the rigidity of the scar tissue.

Angiogenesis

An essential component of scar formation is the ingrowth of small blood vessels to supply nutrition and building blocks (cellular and metabolic) for wound healing. Endothelial cells are induced to proliferate through the secretion of angiogenic factors such as vascular endothelial growth factor (VEGF) and platelet-derived growth factor (PDGF). The ingrowth of small

blood vessels in the area of tissue damage is referred to as angiogenesis, and the resulting tissue response is termed *granulation tissue* (Fig. 3-27). Some endothelial cells in granulation tissue migrate from adjacent existing blood vessels while others arrive as progenitor cells carried through the bloodstream from other locations (Fig. 3-28). Endothelial cells digest through basement membrane and migrate into the extracellular matrix, forming small vascular lumens. Over time, these new blood vessels are remodeled into functionally mature vascular networks in much the same manner that collagen is remodeled to form a mature scar. Some of the newly formed blood vessels that are no longer needed

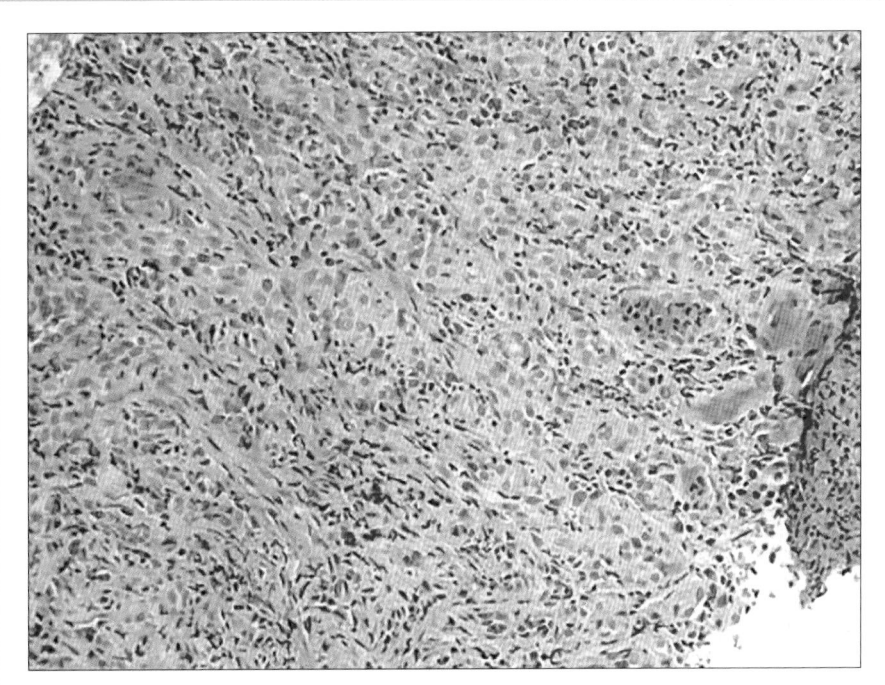

Figure 3-27. Granulation tissue. Numerous small, newly formed blood vessels with prominent, reactive fibroblasts and a mixture of chronic inflammatory cells.

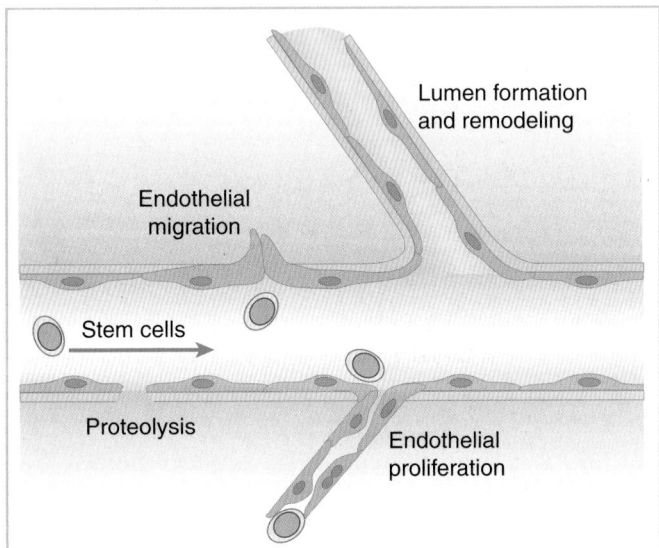

Figure 3-28. Angiogenesis.

undergo apoptosis, triggered by a decrease in the concentration of angiogenic factors as blood flow is restored to hypoxic tissue.

Healing by First and Second Intention

Wounds in the skin are classically described as healing by primary or secondary intention. These processes are analogous to tissue repair with nearly complete restoration of normal function (primary intention) and repair with loss of function (secondary intention). Injury to the skin (both traumatic and surgical) is sufficiently common and clinically important that it deserves further consideration as a special case. Wound healing in skin has been extensively studied as a model of healing so that the details are well understood and demonstrate important principles about tissue repair in general.

Wounds in which the two epithelial surfaces are closely opposed (e.g., a small cut or close surgical reapposition of the two sides of a wound) tend to heal by primary intention (Fig. 3-29). In this setting, a fibrin clot initially forms to fill the small epithelial defect. Next, angiogenesis begins with ingrowth of granulation tissue from the periphery of the defect. Fibroblasts and epithelial cells proliferate at the edges of the defect and reestablish the continuity of the basement membrane zone across the defect. Macrophages and other inflammatory cells participate by ingesting and destroying microorganisms and digesting cellular debris resulting from tissue damage at the site of injury. Over time, fibroblasts synthesize collagen to repair the ECM with the formation of a scar that is remodeled through the actions of fibroblasts and macrophages. The extent of scar formation depends on a number of factors including (1) the size of the original defect, (2) whether secondary injury resulting from infection or installation of foreign material complicates the healing process, and (3) host factors. Systemic hormones such as corticosteroids can influence the extent of collagen deposition and the tensile strength of the scar that is ultimately formed. Corticosteroids tend to inhibit collagen synthesis while TGF-β may enhance fibrosis and collagen formation in some situations.

Larger defects in which the epithelial surfaces are far apart or in which a large portion of skin has been destroyed (e.g., burns) are healed by secondary intention. In this setting, fibrin fills the initial defect (Fig. 3-30) and is slowly replaced by granulation tissue growing inward from the edges of the defect. Fibroblasts produce extracellular matrix with

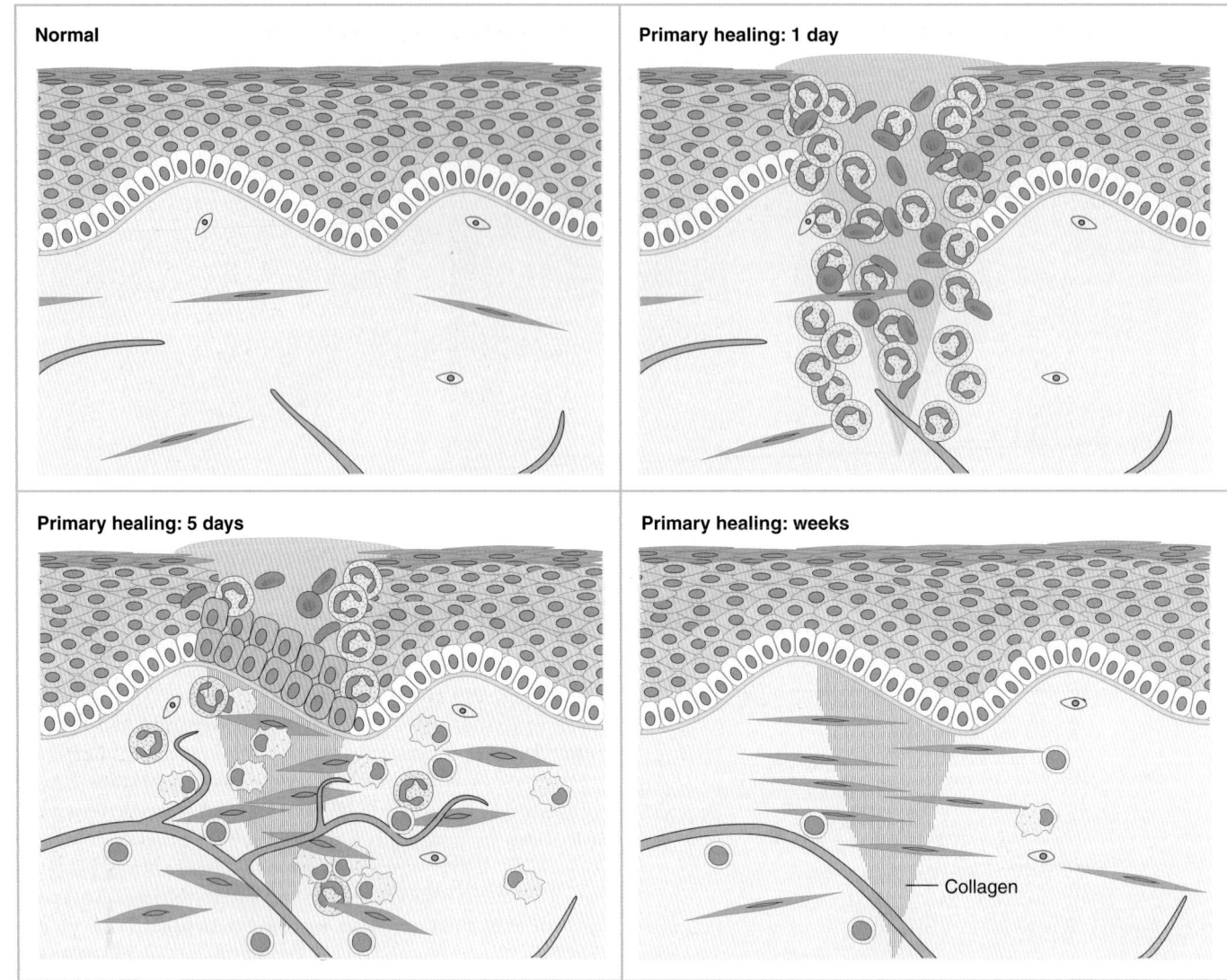

Figure 3-29. Healing by primary intention.

extensive collagen to provide mechanical strength. Over time, epithelial cells migrate inward from the edges of the defect toward its center. Ultimately, a continuous epithelial layer is reestablished with the loss of normal skin appendages. The resulting surface is hard and inelastic and has a flattened structure that lacks the typical rete ridges of normal skin. Myofibroblasts contract to bring the edges of the defect closer to their original location, resulting in a raised scar. Defective repair mechanisms and secondary infection can result in chronic ulceration with more severe scaring (Fig. 3-31).

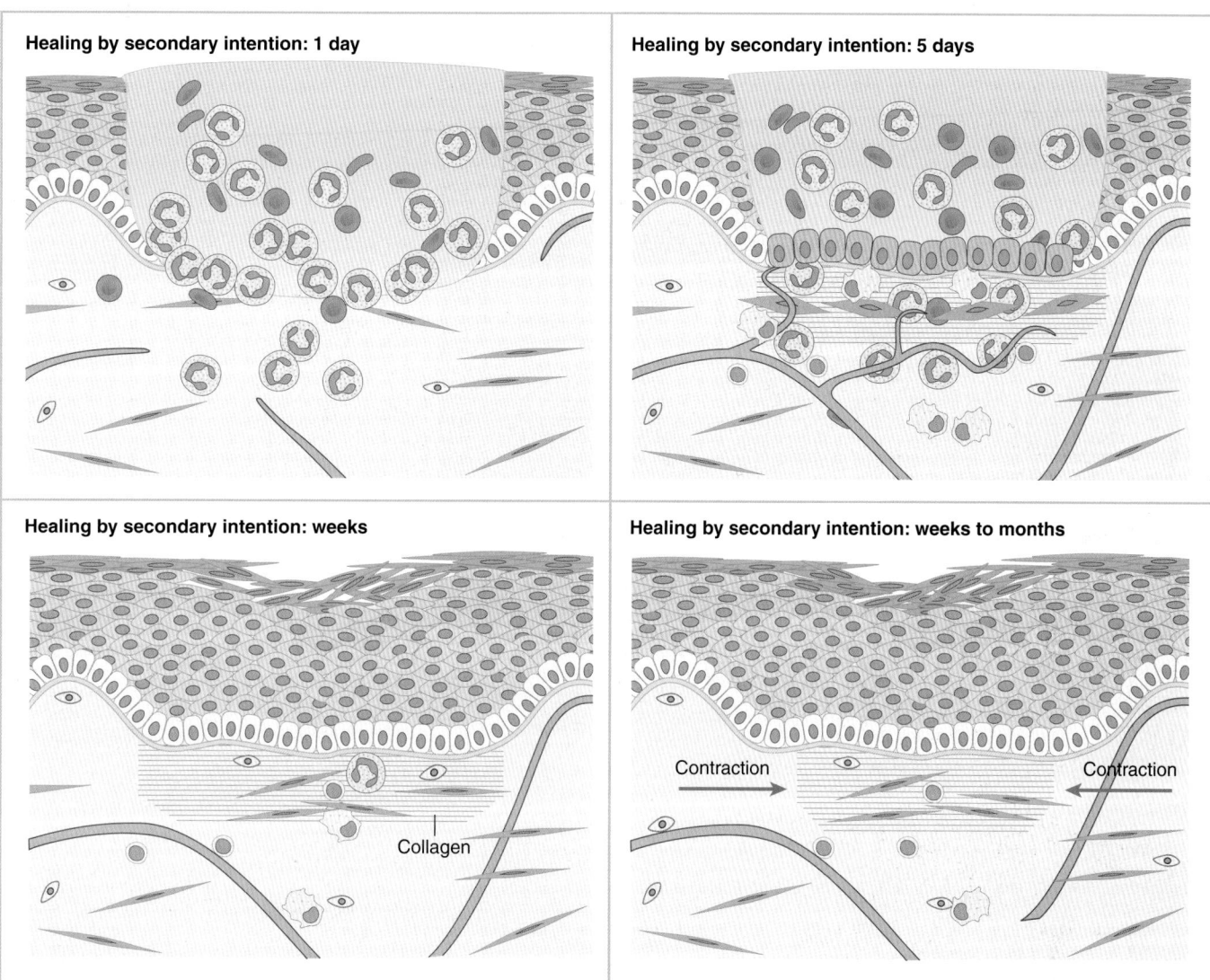

Healing by secondary intention: 1 day

Healing by secondary intention: 5 days

Healing by secondary intention: weeks

Collagen

Healing by secondary intention: weeks to months

Contraction

Contraction

Figure 3-30. Healing by secondary intention.

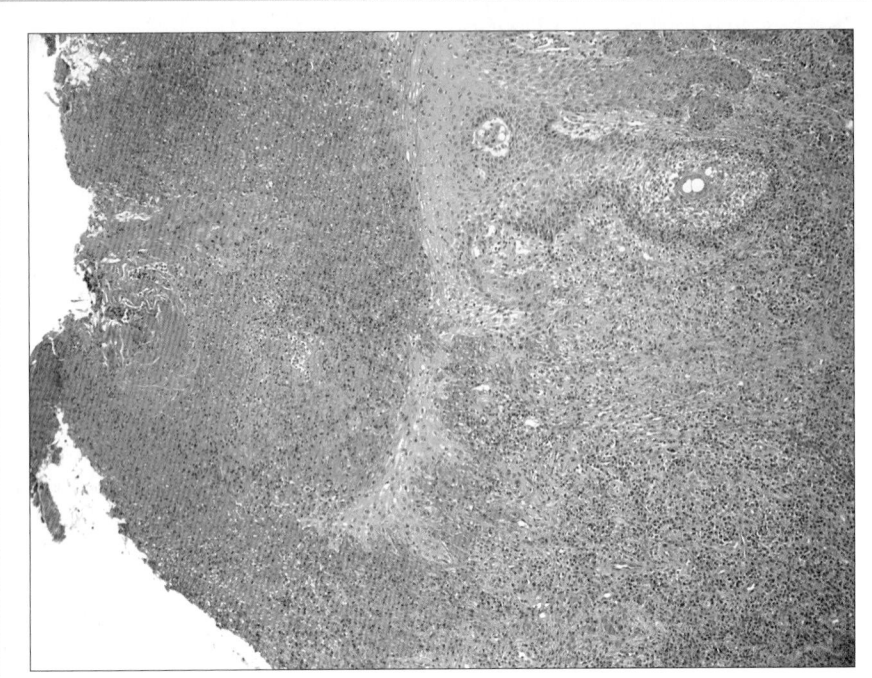

Figure 3-31. Chronic ulcer. Granulation tissue and proliferating fibroblasts fill the gap between opposing surfaces of the wound in healing by secondary intention.

Genetic and Perinatal Disease

4

CONTENTS

Genetic and perinatal diseases are considered together here because many genetic diseases present in the perinatal period. Indeed, a significant proportion of perinatal diseases are genetic in origin. Genetic disease is usually defined as an illness that arises predominantly because of changes in one or a few genes or chromosomes. Multifactorial (polygenic) disorders result from changes in many different genes and have a familial pattern of inheritance that does not correspond to simple mendelian genetic segregation.

The development of most human disease is intimately related to an individual's precise genotype. Predisposition and resistance to many types of disease are controlled by sequence variations in many different genes (polygenic trait). On the other hand, some genetic changes result in a sufficiently severe negative phenotype that they are regarded as mutations (i.e., they are always deleterious). Mutations are responsible for most genetic diseases that follow simple mendelian inheritance. Mutations are distinguished from genetic polymorphisms, which are genetic variations that may cause quantitative or qualitative differences in phenotype but are not consistently associated with the development of a disease. The distinction between mutations and polymorphisms is operational in many situations, and some polymorphisms may be advantageous or detrimental in different contexts. In an individual patient, genetic polymorphisms can interact with other genes, the environment, and comorbid disease to produce small or large, positive or negative effects. Our understanding of the significance of different genetic variations will continue to be refined as information from the human genome project is further integrated with clinical medicine.

Genetic disease can result from alterations in any portion of a gene or chromosome. Many common genetic diseases result from point mutations (single nucleotide changes) in the coding region of a gene that results in altered protein structure with the substitution of one amino acid for another (missense mutations). In some cases, the severity of missense mutations can be predicted by whether or not the amino acid substitution is conservative (i.e., replacement with a chemically similar amino acid) or nonconservative (e.g., substitution of glycine for phenylalanine). Other single base changes create premature stop codons (nonsense mutations), which result in a truncated protein that lacks normal amino termini.

The phenotype produced by nonsense codons is not always easy to predict. Some nonsense mutations result in a peptide fragment that is rapidly degraded and has no function. Alternatively, partially formed peptides may be partially functional or may interfere with the normal function of the full-length protein or other cellular proteins. Genetic alterations can also result in the insertion or deletion of segments of DNA into the coding region of a gene. Most insertions and deletions result in frame-shift mutations that disrupt the amino acid reading frame, resulting in premature termination of translation (similar to nonsense point mutations). In-frame insertions and in-frame deletions occur less frequently and can result in the gain or loss of one or more amino acids in an otherwise full-length protein. The phenotype of small in-frame deletions and insertions may be similar to that of point mutations in the coding sequence.

Sequence variation outside the protein-coding region of a gene can also influence its expression. Base changes that disrupt consensus splice donor or splice acceptor sequences can block pre-mRNA splicing so that no protein is made.

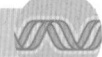

Mutations

There are two major classes of DNA mutations: point mutations (in which one base pair is replaced by another) and insertions or deletions (in which nucleotides are added or removed).

Point mutations can be described as transitions (when one purine replaces another purine or one pyrimidine replaces another pyrimidine) or transversions (when a purine replaces a pyrimidine or vice versa). Overall, transitions occur more frequently than transversions.

Most point mutations result from the misincorporation of single nucleotides by DNA polymerase during replication. Point mutations can also occur spontaneously or as a result of exposure to substances that chemically alter individual bases. Spontaneously occurring mutations can also result from tautomerization of bases, depurination (leading to loss of A or G), deamidation (C → uracil; $^{5\text{-methyl}}$C → T), and oxidative damage. Induced mutations can result from exposure to alkylating agents (e.g., nitrosourea), base analogs (e.g., BrdU), polycyclic hydrocarbons, methylation, DNA cross-linking agents (e.g., platinum), and irradiation.

Point mutations can also be described as missense (resulting in the substitution of one amino acid for another) or nonsense (in which a stop codon is created that causes premature termination of translation).

Insertions and deletions usually result from errors in DNA replication or from the treatment of DNA with intercalating agents (such as acridine orange or proflavin). Insertions and deletions often alter the reading frame for translation and cause premature termination of translation.

True reversion mutations are rare and convert the altered base back to the original sequence, whereas second site revertants are mutations elsewhere in the DNA sequence that restore gene function.

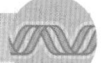

Splice Donor and Acceptor Sites

The spliceosome is a multimeric complex composed of proteins and 5 small nuclear RNA molecules (snRNA U1, U2, U4, U5, and U6) that mediate splicing of pre-mRNA in the nucleus.

The spliceosome recognizes introns by consensus donor (agGTa/gagt) and acceptor (c/tAGgt) sequences at each end of the intron (invariant nucleotides are capitalized in the consensus sequences). A branch point signal (c/tta/gAc/t) is also present approximately 25 nucleotides upstream of the splice acceptor site. A polypyrimidine tract is typically present between the branch point signal and the splice acceptor site.

These consensus signals provide essential information for splicing, but adjacent sequences (splicing enhancers and splicing silencers) as well as trans-acting factors and intron tertiary structure are also important in controlling these events. Up to 30 proteins that regulate splicing have been identified in *Drosophila*.

snRNAs in the spliceosome bind to donor sites and branch signals and bring the ends of the exons together. Cleavage at the splice acceptor site generates a free 3′ end that is ligated to the invariant A residue in the branch signal to form a "lariat" RNA out of the intron. The lariat sequence is ejected as the two exons are fused together.

Alternative splicing allows the production of multiple different mRNAs and proteins from a single gene. Alternative splicing was once thought to be a relatively uncommon form of gene regulation, but recent evidence suggests that it is much more common and occurs in up to 75% of human genes. Splice variants are often expressed in a tissue-specific manner.

Splice site mutations may also result in the utilization of alternative splice sites to form a protein containing fewer or different exons than would normally be expressed in that cell type.

The precise nature of the base changes in splice consensus sequences determines the "leakiness" of the phenotype (complete blockage of normal splicing or an incremental reduction in efficiency). Single base changes in the promoter region or 3′ untranslated region of a gene may also have significant effects on the level of gene transcription and messenger RNA stability. Either of these can affect the amount of protein expressed in cells. The effects of such single base changes are usually difficult to predict. Most single base changes (polymorphisms) in untranslated regions are phenotypically silent, however. Disruption of a consensus transcription factor-binding site may suggest an effect on gene transcription, but the ability to accurately predict the consequence of changes in promoter sequence in silico (i.e., based on computer analysis of DNA sequences) is limited. Even gene transfection experiments may be inconclusive if it is not possible to test promoter sequence variations in a cell type that expresses all the relevant transcription factors. Segregation analysis of the disease phenotype and the sequence variation within an affected family may be helpful in establishing that a specific genetic change is causal.

● ● ● MENDELIAN DISORDERS

Mendelian disorders result from alterations in single genes that are inherited through the germline. The extent to which a disease phenotype develops in genetically affected individuals is a measure of the penetrance of the mutation. Most diseases that are considered mendelian have relatively strong (complete) penetrance (i.e., the majority of genetically affected individuals manifest disease) although other genes and environmental factors are important in modulating phenotype. Mendelian disorders are often suspected because of the clustering of one unusual disease in a family, and evaluation of the family pedigree may suggest a specific pattern of inheritance: autosomal recessive, autosomal dominant, or sex-linked inheritance (for genes on the X or rarely on the Y chromosome). For some genetic diseases, new mutations are quite rare so that the family pedigree is very helpful in establishing a specific diagnosis. In other diseases, new mutations are sufficiently common that many individuals with disease represent new germline mutations so that analysis of parents and siblings is not helpful in clarifying the nature of their illness (e.g., in Duchenne's muscular dystrophy, up to 40% of newly diagnosed cases are new mutations because of chromosomal instability at this locus).

Autosomal Recessive Disorders

Diseases that have an autosomal recessive pattern of inheritance almost always result from the loss of function of the affected gene. Most homozygotes have a severe phenotype as a result of loss of function mutations in both alleles of the affected gene. Depending on the type of mutation (missense, nonsense, or frame shift), homozygotes may have no, limited, or significant residual gene function. Individuals who are heterozygous for a specific loss of function mutation usually do not have overt disease, but phenotypic abnormalities may be detectable by laboratory testing. In a minority of autosomal recessive diseases, heterozygotes have a definite phenotype that is less severe than that of homozygotes. Some recessive genetic diseases (in which heterozygotes often manifest a phenotype) overlap with dominant genetic diseases (see below).

Some autosomal recessive diseases result from unique mutations in the affected gene (e.g., sickle cell [SC] anemia defined by A → T causing a glutamic acid → valine substitution at amino acid 6 in the β-globin gene) while others result from two different abnormal alleles (i.e., compound heterozygotes). In some cases, inheritance of two different mutant alleles results in a different phenotype. For instance, in SC disease, individuals inherit one allele coding for hemoglobin S and one allele coding for hemoglobin C (glutamic acid → lysine also at amino acid 6 in β-globin). These compound heterozygotes with SC disease have a qualitatively different and milder form of anemia than do hemoglobin S homozygotes.

Autosomal recessive diseases are more frequently observed in inbred populations, and recessive genetic disease should be suspected if the children of a consanguineous marriage are affected. Family trees are very helpful in assessing the possibility of autosomal recessive disease (Fig. 4-1). The number of affected individuals in a family (homozygotes) is always much smaller than the number of carriers (heterozygotes). Autosomal recessive disease is usually inherited equally in males and females (although the manifestation of disease may be sex limited, e.g., a gene that causes ovarian cancer can manifest only in females). If both parents are carriers of the disease, one fourth of their offspring will be homozygotes (unless homozygosity results in excess fetal loss). Recessive diseases may appear to skip generations. The identification of an individual with genetic disease (proband) usually leads to an evaluation of family members (either by laboratory testing or genetic analysis), which may allow the identification of phenotypically normal heterozygotes and permit clear delineation of the pattern of inheritance. These studies may provide useful information for reproductive counseling and identify individuals who may benefit from therapy or close clinical monitoring.

Lysosomal Storage Disease

Lysosomal storage diseases can result from loss of function mutations in individual lysosomal enzymes or from mutations that cause defective targeting of these enzymes to the lysosomal compartment (more than 30 different forms have been identified). Affected individuals lack a specific enzymatic activity and so are incapable of degrading some types of macromolecules that accumulate in lysosomes. In Hunter's and Hurler's syndromes (so-called mucopolysaccharidoses), deficiency of different lysosomal enzymes required to degrade mucopolysaccharides (critical components of the extracellular matrix) result in the accumulation of mucopolysaccharides in lysosomes. Over time, lysosomes expand and eventually impinge on normal cellular components, resulting in cellular dysfunction. Since the genetic changes are present in every cell in the affected individual's body, all organs and tissue can potentially be affected. Because mesenchymal cells produce most mucopolysaccharides, these cells are preferentially affected in mucopolysaccharidoses. The skin and musculoskeletal system are most severely affected, with prominent growth retardation and coarse facial and skeletal

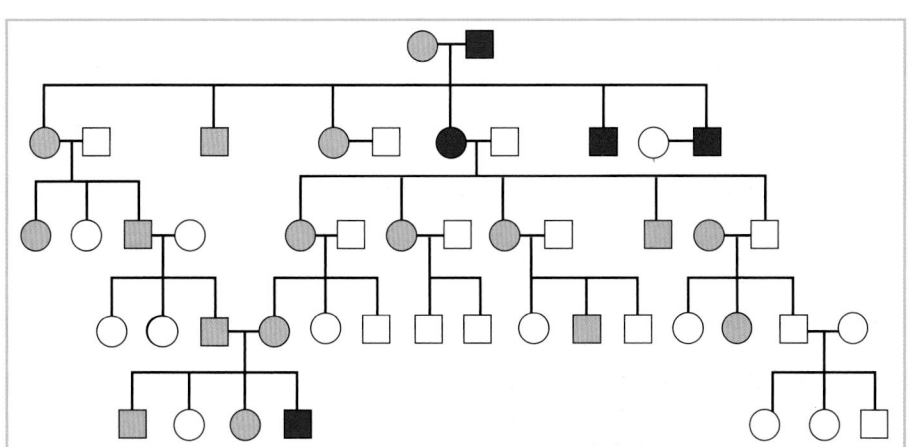

Figure 4-1. Typical pedigree showing autosomal recessive inheritance. Males are squares, and females are circles. Individuals with disease (homozygotes) are dark purple, and heterozygotes are light purple.

features that are characteristic of these conditions. Patients with mucopolysaccharidoses also develop important abnormalities of cardiac myocytes, with displacement of normal contractile proteins by dilated lysosomes. Other types of lysosomal storage disease can result from genetic defects in trafficking of lysosomal enzymes to lysosomes (e.g., the addition of glucose 6-phosphate [G6P] to carbohydrate residues on glycoproteins is required to target them to lysosomes) as well as in the enzymes themselves.

Glycogen Storage Disease

Glycogen polymers are an important mechanism for glucose storage in some tissues including the liver and muscle. Multiple different enzymes are involved in glycogen synthesis and glycogen degradation and specific isoforms of some of these enzymes are preferentially expressed in different tissues. As a result, multiple different forms of glycogen storage disease can occur, depending on which enzyme (or isoenzyme) is affected.

In von Gierke's disease, inheritance of two defective copies of glucose-6-phosphatase results in the accumulation of glycogen that ultimately impinges on normal organelles (similar to lysosomal storage diseases). This enzyme is expressed in liver (as well as in other tissues), and deficiency results in massive glycogen accumulation in hepatocytes and

hypoglycemia because hepatic glycogen stores cannot be mobilized to maintain blood glucose levels.

Hemoglobinopathy and Sickle Cell Disease

Hundreds of different structural variants of hemoglobin have been identified in different populations. Most of these variants differ by a single amino acid, and many result in only mild changes in hemoglobin structure and function.

Some hemoglobin variants cause disease only in selected situations or under unusual patterns of stress, while a few hemoglobin variants produce severe disease. Hemoglobin S produces sickle cell disease in homozygous individuals and is common in African and African American populations (1/500 blacks are homozygotes). Hemoglobin S is composed of two normal α-globin chains and two mutant β-globin chains with

---

BIOCHEMISTRY

Glycogen Storage Disease

Glycogen is the main storage form of glucose in cells and can be rapidly depolymerized to generate energy. Polymerization of glucose to glycogen is essential to prevent the osmotic swelling of cells that would occur if glucose were stored as a monomer.

Glycogen is formed by a series of discrete enzymatic steps: first, hexokinase phosphorylates glucose to form glucose 6-phosphate (G6P), which is converted to glucose 1-phosphate (G1P) and then to uridine diphosphoglucose by the addition of uridine. Glycogen synthetase combines these building blocks into highly branched chains composed of G1P with α-1,4-glycoside bonds.

Degradation of glycogen by various phosphorylases in the cytoplasm regenerates G1P. Debrancher enzymes are required to split branched chains of less than four residues in length. Glycogen can also be degraded by acid maltase in the liver, and the expression of enzymes that modulate its metabolism is strongly regulated by hormones.

Type	Affected Tissue(s)	Enzyme Deficiency
I	Multiple	Glucose-6-phosphatase
II	Heart, liver	Acid maltase
III	Multiple	Glycogen debrancher
IV	Multiple	Glycogen branching enzyme
V	Muscle	Muscle glycogen phosphorylase
VI	Liver	Hepatic phosphorylase
VII	Muscle	Muscle phosphofructokinase
IX	Multiple	Phosphorylase kinase

BIOCHEMISTRY

Hemoglobin Synthesis and Structure

Hemoglobin synthesis utilizes different genes during embryogenesis and fetal life and switches from hemoglobin F (HbF) to predominantly α- and β-globin synthesis (hemoglobin A) at the time of birth. These changes are necessary for adaptation to the different oxygen tensions in the placenta and postnatal lungs. Sometimes fetal hemoglobin synthesis is incompletely suppressed, but this is usually not of functional consequence.

Functional hemoglobin molecules are composed of two α-chains and two β-chains. If significantly more α- or β-chains are produced, there is a tendency for homopolymers to form that can aggregate and cause apoptosis of erythroid precursors (e.g., thalassemia).

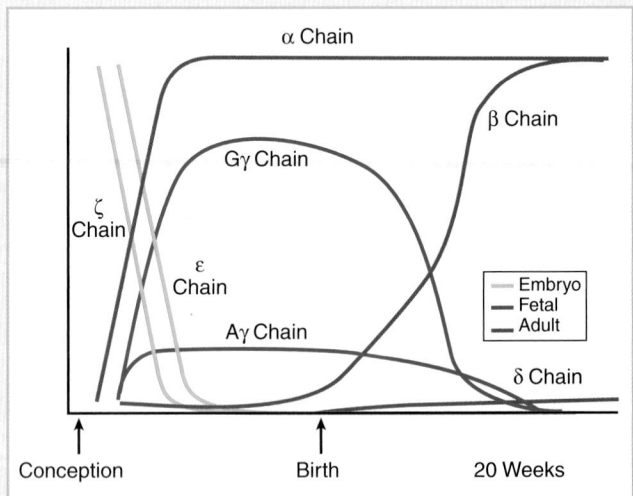

Globin Chains	Hemoglobin	Normal Expression
$\alpha_2\beta_2$	A	Adult
$\alpha_2\delta_2$	A_2	Adult
$\alpha_2{}^A\gamma_2$	F	Fetus
$\alpha_2{}^G\gamma_2$	F	Fetus
$\alpha_2\epsilon_2$	Gower2	Embryo
$\zeta_2\epsilon_2$	Gower1	Embryo

a nonconservative substitution of valine for glutamic acid at position 6. Sickle cell disease and other hemoglobinopathies can usually be diagnosed by a combination of hemoglobin electrophoresis (as a screening and diagnostic test) and DNA sequence analysis.

Hemoglobin S has an abnormal tendency to self-associate, particularly under conditions of low oxygen saturation. As a result, hemoglobin S can form long homopolymers that can disrupt red blood cell structure (sickled red blood cells) and cause plasma membrane breaks that shorten their life span. Chronic damage to red blood cells (RBCs) results in hemolytic anemia, which is compensated by increased RBC production. Increased RBC turnover and blood transfusions can lead to iron overload and pathologic changes related to iron deposition in tissue (see Hereditary Hemochromatosis section). Interruption in the production of new RBCs causes a rapid drop in hematocrit in patients with sickle cell disease because of the short half-life of their RBCs (so-called aplastic crisis). Aplastic crises can result from a transient viral infection that disrupts RBC formation in the bone marrow (parvovirus is frequently implicated) or from nutritional deficiency (e.g., of B_{12} or folate). Aplastic crisis can be fatal if lost RBCs are not promptly replaced by transfusion.

PHYSIOLOGY

Hemoglobin Electrophoresis

Hemoglobin electrophoresis is commonly used to screen for mutations in hemoglobin. Electrophoresis can be carried out under acid or alkaline conditions, using isoelectric focusing (separation by protein pH) or by electrophoresis of separated globin chains. Alkaline electrophoresis is the most popular technique used in clinical laboratories and is performed using cellulose acetate as an electrophoresis medium.

All hemoglobin molecules have a net negative charge and migrate toward the anode. Their rate of migration is determined by their net charge so that amino acid substitutions frequently result in charge differences that can be detected by electrophoresis.

Alkaline electrophoresis is a good screening test for hemoglobinopathy, but many hemoglobin variants migrate to the same position. These comigrating bands can often be distinguished by the other electrophoresis methods.

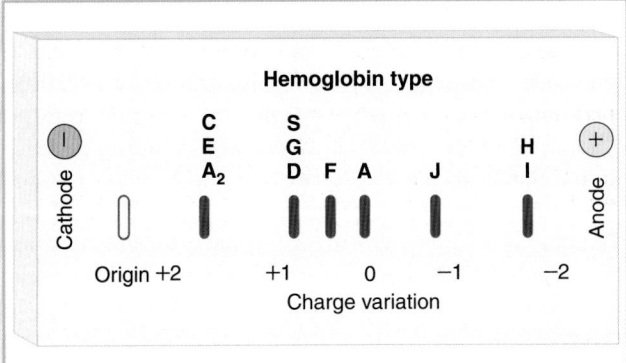

In patients with sickle cell anemia, RBCs sickle in capillary beds, where oxygen tension is low, and their rigid structure tends to obstruct these small blood vessels. Capillary blockage results in increased tissue hypoxia, which may initiate a chain reaction in which many more RBCs sickle. The resulting ischemia causes microinfarcts, which produce severe pain in the involved organ (so-called pain crisis). Decreased hematocrit increases tissue hypoxia and further promotes sickling of residual RBCs. Since oxygen tension in the spleen and long bones is lower than in most other organs, sickling and infarction preferentially affect these sites. Repeated infarction of bones predisposes patients to bacterial infection of bone (osteomyelitis), particularly with *Salmonella* species.

The severity of sickle cell disease depends in large part on the degree to which fetal hemoglobin is produced during erythropoiesis. Fetal hemoglobin ($\alpha_2 \gamma_2$) synthesis is normally switched off (by hypermethylation of the γ-globin promoter) soon after birth, but a small amount is produced in most adults. Some patients with sickle cell anemia produce greater amounts of fetal hemoglobin and this decreases the severity of their anemia and the frequency of pain crises. The only currently approved pharmacologic therapy for sickle cell anemia is hydroxyurea, which is designed to the derepress synthesis of fetal hemoglobin genes by decreasing global DNA methylation.

Thalassemia

Thalassemia is another type of hemoglobin abnormality that shows recessive inheritance. In thalassemia, there is a quantitative abnormality in the amount of β- or α-globin chains produced, which interferes with the assembly of normal hemoglobin molecules. β-Thalassemia results from a variety of different mutations in the β-chain gene (mainly point mutations) that result in diminished synthesis of normal β-globin protein. β^0 mutations completely block synthesis of β-globin protein (most are splice junction mutations or nonsense mutations) while β^+ mutations (often promoter mutations and some splice junction mutations) allow diminished protein production (about 25% of normal). Inheritance of two β^0 alleles causes thalassemia major with severe anemia that requires frequent blood transfusions. Some individuals who inherit two β^+ alleles also have thalassemia major, and others have thalassemia intermedia (significant anemia that does not require regular transfusions). Some heterozygotes with one normal and one β^0 allele also have thalassemia intermedia while others have thalassemia minor (mild morphologic abnormalities of RBCs only). Individuals with one normal and one β^+ allele also have thalassemia minor. Deficiency of β-globin blocks normal assembly of hemoglobin A (two α- combined with two β-chains) during erythropoiesis. Newly formed RBCs are deficient in hemoglobin, and excess α-chains aggregate and adhere to erythroid membranes, causing hemolysis. In thalassemia major, extensive destruction of RBC precursors (ineffective erythropoiesis) results in a high level of iron turnover, which predisposes to iron overload. Expansion of erythroid progenitors in the bone marrow can expand the

GENETICS

Gene Therapy

The goal of gene therapy for inherited diseases is to deliver a functional copy of a specific gene to target cells whose own copies of the gene are abnormal or nonfunctional. Successful delivery of replacement genes allows cells to produce some normal protein that may significantly reduce symptoms. Gene therapy is currently an experimental protocol largely because targeted delivery of DNA to specific cell types remains a significant challenge.

Gene therapy has had beneficial effects in a few patients but has also produced leukemia in some patients with hereditary immunodeficiency in whom vector integration activated a proto-oncogene. In a highly publicized case, a strong immunologic response against the modified virus used to deliver the gene caused a patient to die. Partially because of these issues, progress with gene therapy has remained relatively slow, particularly with vectors that can produce stable (i.e., long-lasting or permanent) expression.

Gene therapy has been explored in cancer with the goal of delivering a gene that can kill cancer cells or render them more susceptible to chemotherapy. As with other forms of gene therapy, a major objective is to utilize vectors that specifically target tumor cells.

Various vectors have been used for delivery of replacement genes, and some of their properties are summarized in the following table.

Vector	Maximum DNA Insert (kb)	Persistence of Expression	Cells Infected
Retrovirus	7	Stable	Dividing cells
Adenovirus	7	Transient	Most
Lentivirus	7	Stable	Most
Herpes simplex	30	Unknown	Most, including neurons
Liposomes with oligonucleotides	10	Transient	Most

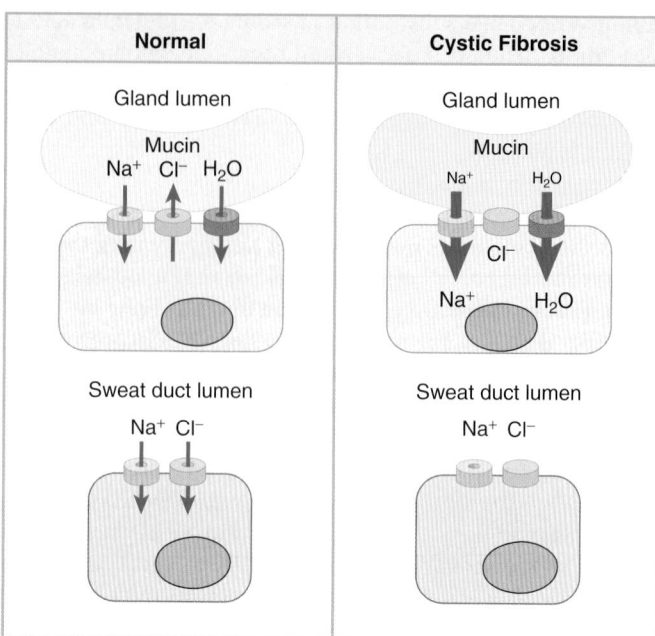

Normal	Cystic Fibrosis

Figure 4-2. Chloride conductance in glandular and ductal cells in a normal individual and in a patient with cystic fibrosis.

marrow space and cause deformity of the facial bones (so-called chipmunk facies).

Most cases of α-thalassemia result from deletions of one or more α-globin alleles (normally four alleles, two per haploid genome). Loss of a single allele does not produce symptoms. Loss of two alleles (one maternal and one paternal, two paternal, or two maternal) causes α-thalassemia trait with phenotypic features similar to those of β-thalassemia minor. Loss of three alleles causes hemoglobin H disease with significant anemia, similar to β-thalassemia intermedia. Loss of all four alleles is not compatible with life and results in death in utero with hydrops fetalis (see below).

Phenylketonuria

Most cases of phenylketonuria (PKU) result from homozygous deficiency of phenylalanine hydroxylase. Affected individuals cannot convert excess dietary phenylalanine into tyrosine, resulting in the accumulation of phenylalanine in the blood and tissues that ultimately produces neurologic toxicity and metal retardation. Since phenylalanine freely crosses the placenta, maternal phenylalanine hydroxylase prevents damage in utero. Shortly after birth, plasma concentrations of phenylalanine increase in homozygotes and if not corrected cause abnormal neural development with severe mental retardation. Institution of a diet low in phenylalanine can ameliorate abnormalities in central nervous system development. PKU is the only genetic disease for which widespread screening of asymptomatic neonates is commonly practiced.

Cystic Fibrosis

Cystic fibrosis (CF) is caused by mutations in an integral plasma membrane protein that normally functions as a major chloride transport protein (CTFR) in glandular and ductal cells of different organ systems. The CTFR gene is large and many different mutations or short deletions can cause cystic fibrosis, with the phenotypic severity varying with different mutations. Alterations in the CTFR gene are relatively common in the white population (2% to 4% are heterozygotes) so that homozygotes occur with an appreciable frequency (approximately 1/3000 live births) in nonconsanguinous marriages. Defective chloride transport in homozygotes results in decreased water content in secreted mucin (Fig. 4-2). This viscous mucin plugs the ducts and tubules of glands in many organs. Up to 10% of cases may present in infancy with intestinal obstruction caused by inspissated (dehydrated) meconium (so-called meconium ileus). Recurrent pancreatitis occurs in most patients because blockage of the pancreatic ducts results in the inappropriate release and activation of digestive enzymes (zymogens) within the pancreas. Most patients lose pancreatic acinar function over time and develop intestinal malabsorption unless digestive enzymes are supplemented.

Most importantly, mucous plugging in bronchi in the lungs results in defective clearing of bacteria and a marked predisposition to bacterial infection. Repeated cycles of infection cause chronic inflammation that further degrades lung structure and defense mechanisms. These abnormalities can lead to the development of bronchiectasis (abnormal bronchi that extend all the way to the pleural surface). Eventually, these changes result in respiratory failure, which is the cause of death in most patients. Infections with specific strains of *Pseudomonas aeruginosa* that are trophic for the abnormal mucin in the airways of these patients cause virtually incurable infection. Therapy is predominantly supportive and is aimed at clearing inspissated secretions from the respiratory tract. Meticulous chest physical therapy and antibiotics now allow many patients to live into the third decade.

Most patients have manifestations of cystic fibrosis early in life, but milder disease (missense rather than nonsense mutations) may initially present in adolescence or young adulthood with recurrent respiratory tract infections. Diagnosis can be made by genetic analysis although this is complicated by the large size of the CTFR gene and by the large number of genetic alterations that can produce disease (more than 1000 different mutations are known). Functional testing by analyzing chloride levels in sweat still is a useful diagnostic test because of the diversity of CTFR gene alterations. The CTFR gene is expressed in the ducts of sweat glands and manifests as abnormally high concentrations of NaCl in sweat because of the blockage of passive chloride reabsorption.

Familial Hypercholesterolemia

Familial hypercholesterolemia is caused by mutations in the low-density lipoprotein (LDL) receptor. The LDL receptor is expressed on the surface of hepatocytes (as well as adipose and muscle cells), and binding of LDL and intermediate-density lipoprotein (IDL) triggers receptor (and ligand) internalization by endocytosis in clathrin-coated pits (Fig. 4-3). The endocytosed LDL and IDL are then transferred to lysosomes while the LDL receptor is recycled to the cell surface. Digestion of LDL and IDL releases triglycerides and cholesterol into the cytoplasm of hepatocytes, where some is repackaged to form very low density lipoprotein (VLDL) in conjunction with triglycerides delivered from the intestine via chylomicrons. The free cholesterol in hepatocytes inhibits HMG-CoA reductase to shut down endogenous cholesterol synthesis by hepatocytes and stimulates cholesterol acyltransferase (ACAT) to form cholesterol esters for long-term storage in hepatocytes. Cholesterol also inhibits the production of new LDL receptors (to prevent lipid overload of individual hepatocytes).

Various mutations of the LDL receptor gene can result in receptors that are dysfunctional in substrate binding, receptor internalization, or receptor recycling to the cell surface. Any of these changes inhibit delivery of cholesterol to hepatocytes and increase serum cholesterol (predominantly LDL cholesterol). Loss of LDL receptors also results in the inappropriate activation of hepatic HMG-CoA reductase (loss of normal inhibition by cholesterol) and constitutive cholesterol synthesis by hepatocytes that further increase serum cholesterol. High cholesterol levels favor the uptake of cholesterol via another receptor (scavenger receptor) that is expressed on

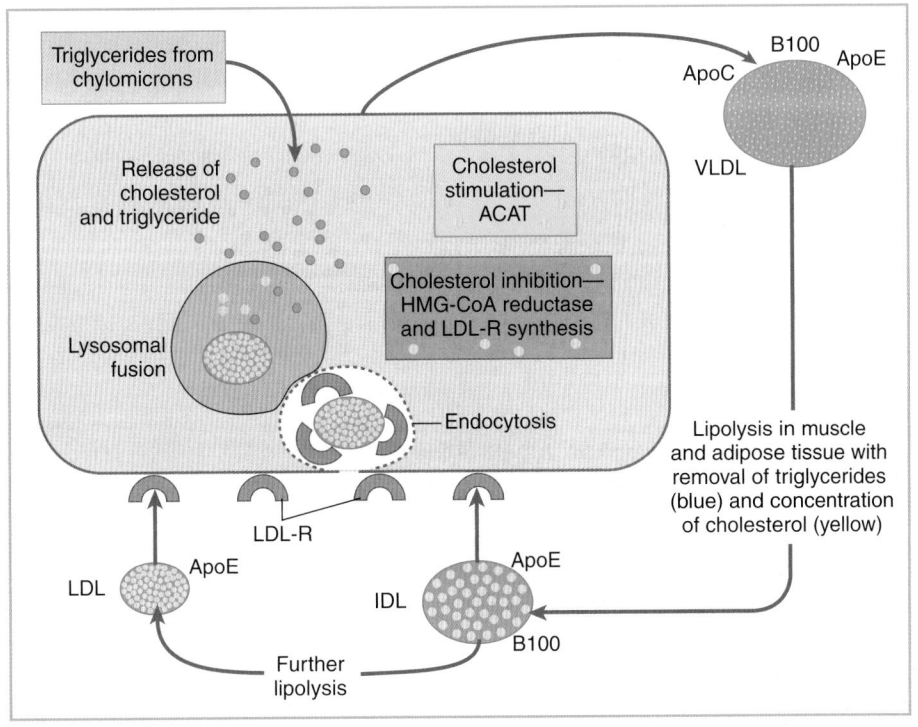

Figure 4-3. Normal cholesterol metabolism.

histiocytes as well as other cells. These changes contribute directly to the development of atherosclerosis (see Chapter 7) as well as to deposition of cholesterol in tissue (xanthomas).

Individuals with homozygous deficiency of functional LDL receptors have a marked increase in serum cholesterol and LDL and develop severe atherosclerosis with myocardial infarction well before 40 years of age. Individuals who are heterozygotes for LDL receptor mutations (approximately 1/500 in the general population) tend to have significantly higher than normal serum cholesterol (roughly two to three times normal) and are at substantially increased risk for atherosclerotic cardiovascular disease. In this sense, familial hypercholesterolemia merges features of autosomal recessive and autosomal dominant genetic disease.

Hereditary Hemochromatosis

Most cases of hereditary hemochromatosis result from mutations in the HFE gene. Two point mutations are common in the white population (1 in 15 individuals are heterozygous for H63D or C282Y). These mutant alleles are much less common in nonwhites, and hemochromatosis in some other ethnic groups is caused by mutations in other genes. Individuals with homozygous HFE mutations (1/500 in the white population) are at substantially increased risk for developing iron overload although disease penetrance is quite variable (Fig. 4-4). Iron homeostasis involves active absorption of iron in the duodenum and recycling of endogenous iron (predominantly from the breakdown of senescent or damaged RBCs). Iron is transported in the blood bound to transferrin and is targeted to the liver as well as other tissues (predominantly erythroid progenitors in the bone marrow) via transferrin receptors.

Hepatocytes produce the hormone hepcidin and are key regulators of iron homeostasis. Hepcidin inhibits the iron transport protein ferroportin, which is expressed in enterocytes (in the duodenum), macrophages (RBC catabolism), and hepatocytes. Hepcidin release decreases iron concentration in the blood, and persistent hepcidin action results in iron loss through the gastrointestinal tract as enterocytes (and their iron stores) are shed into the gut lumen. Since iron can be eliminated only by the gastrointestinal tract (or by external hemorrhage or phlebotomy), this control mechanism is essential to maintain iron homeostasis. Hepcidin release by hepatocytes is modulated by the transferrin receptor 2 (depending on the level of transferrin saturation with iron), HFE (possibly by sensing the level of free iron), and hemojuvelin (control mechanism not known).

Common mutations in HFE apparently disrupt the appropriate release of hepcidin in response to increased iron and result in iron accumulation. Mutations in transferrin receptor 2 and hemojuvelin have been identified in nonwhites with iron overload and likely are responsible for some cases of hemochromatosis that are not associated with HFE mutations. Other control mechanisms modulate the active absorption of iron by enterocytes, and these genes may be responsible for some cases of hemochromatosis, particularly in nonwhites.

Excessive iron accumulation is more frequent in men with hemochromatosis than in women because menstrual blood loss mitigates the tendency to absorb and retain excessive amounts of iron. Conversely, comorbid diseases requiring transfusion therapy can greatly accelerate iron accumulation in patients with HFE mutations and may result in symptoms in heterozygotes (or even in individuals with no genetic pre-

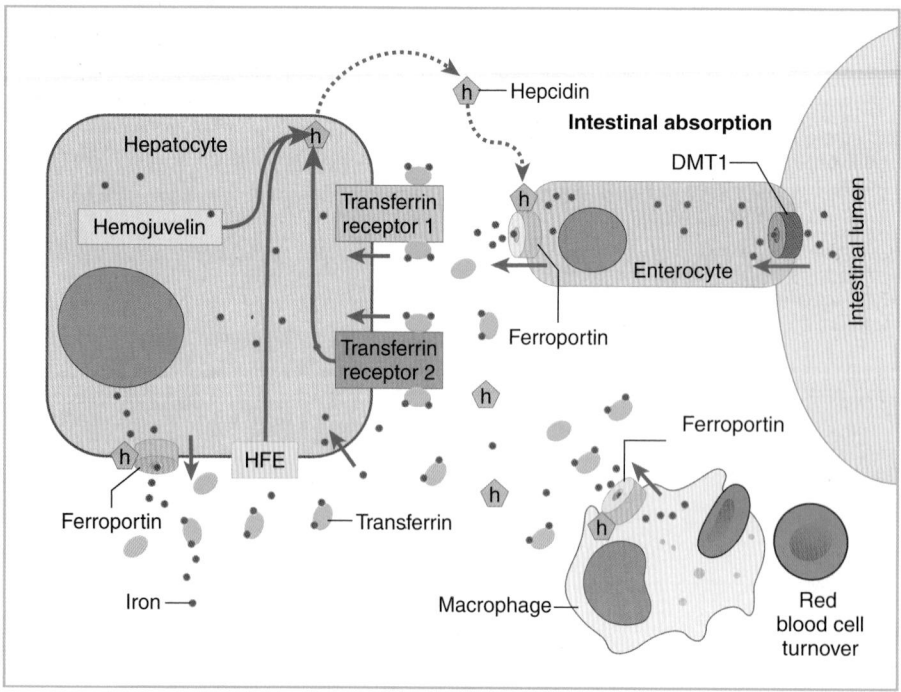

Figure 4-4. Normal control of iron absorption and recycling.

disposition to iron overload). Alterations in other genes (e.g., hemojuvelin) clearly can influence iron homeostasis, and variations in these genes may contribute to the differences in disease penetrance observed in individuals with homozygous HFE mutations. Deposition of iron in tissue (Fig. 4-5) causes cellular toxicity that can result in dysfunction of the liver (causing cirrhosis), the endocrine pancreas (causing diabetes), the gonads (causing infertility), and the heart and joints.

Chelation therapy (to remove excess iron) may slow or reverse early disease but cannot reverse many of the complications of hemochromatosis (e.g., tissue damage and fibrosis) once they have developed.

Von Willebrand's Disease

Von Willebrand factor is a critical plasma protein that facilitates platelet adherence to subendothelial collagen at sites of vascular injury (see Chapter 2). Mutations in the gene are common (up to 1% of the population). Most mutations show an autosomal dominant pattern of inheritance, but some show a recessive pattern. Affected individuals tend to have excessive (but not life-threatening) bleeding from wounds and spontaneous bleeding from mucous membranes. The bleeding time (a functional test that measures the time required to stop bleeding from a wound of standard size) is elevated in affected patients.

Autosomal Dominant Disorders

Autosomal dominant genetic diseases are usually caused by point mutations in one allele of the affected gene which produces an abnormal protein that interferes with normal cellular function. Proteins that function as homodimers are particularly susceptible to this type of pathology because binding of the abnormal protein to the normal protein may inactivate it by formation of nonfunctional heterodimers. Accumulation of abnormal or misfolded proteins can also result in cellular dysfunction or toxicity. It is uncommon for the simple numeric deficiency of the normal gene (gene dosage) to cause a severe enough phenotype to produce an autosomal dominant genetic disease.

Autosomal dominant diseases tend to be represented in all generations in an affected family and can be passed from mothers or fathers to sons or daughters (Fig. 4-6). If one parent is affected, typically half the children will have disease. Different point mutations may result in different phenotypic effects so that different kindreds may show qualitatively distinct phenotypes. Penetrance may be quite variable (even in single kindred) if environmental or genetic cofactors are required to manifest clinical disease.

Marfan Syndrome

Marfan syndrome results from point mutations in the fibrillin 1 gene on chromosome 15 (incidence approximately 1/10,000). Fibrillin is an extracellular matrix protein that coordinates the deposition of elastin fibers in the extracellular matrix. Abnormalities of fibrillin result in deficient deposition of elastin fibers in the extracellular matrix, causing it to be structurally defective. Specific point mutations tend to differentially affect the extracellular matrix in different organs and are associated with different levels of disease severity. Affected individuals in one family typically show a similar phenotype, but penetrance is variable and some diagnoses may not be able to be made on clinical grounds.

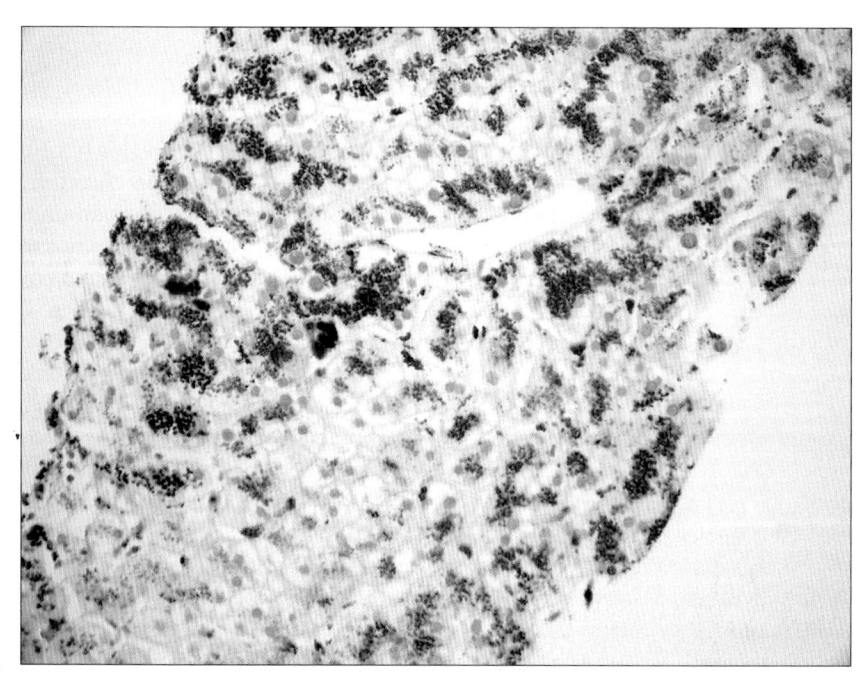

Figure 4-5. Hemochromatosis of the liver. Microscopic section of a liver needle biopsy stained with Prussian blue (iron appears as blue granules) showing extensive intracellular iron accumulation.

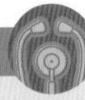

CLINICAL MEDICINE

Diagnosis of Iron Overload

Free iron is toxic to cells, and iron is normally complexed with proteins such as ferritin, hemosiderin, or transferrin to prevent toxicity. Hemochromatosis results when excess free iron causes significant cell or tissue toxicity. Iron is not normally excreted so that the only means of elimination is decreased intestinal absorption or blood loss. Since one unit of red blood cells contains 200 to 250 mg of iron, multiple transfusions can rapidly cause iron overload.

Serum iron level is a measure of the amount to iron bound to transferrin (normally between 50 and 100 µg/dL). Under steady-state conditions, the serum iron is a useful measure of total body iron stores.

Total iron-binding capacity (TIBC) is an indirect measure of the amount of transferrin in the circulation (normally between 300 and 360 µg/dL). Transferrin saturation is a percentage calculated as the ratio of serum iron and TIBC (normally 25% to 50%). Transferrin saturation greater than 50% is suggestive of iron overload.

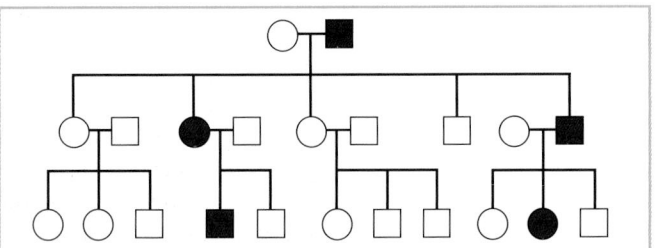

Figure 4-6. Typical pedigree showing autosomal dominant inheritance. Males are squares, and females are circles. Individuals with disease are purple.

Individuals with Marfan syndrome tend to be quite tall with a scaphoid chest and elongated fingers that are often double jointed. These and other features are not specific for Marfan syndrome but are sometimes described as marfanoid body habitus. Many have speculated that President Abraham Lincoln had this syndrome, but this remains unproved. Individuals with Marfan syndrome tend to have lax connective tissue, which predisposes to musculoskeletal injury. More significantly, they are at markedly increased risk for aortic dissection, which can be rapidly fatal. In this condition (see Chapter 7), blood dissects into the arterial media and may rupture (dissect) through the aortic wall, resulting in massive hemorrhage. Other common complications of Marfan syndrome include recurrent pneumothorax (defective extracellular matrix in the lung pleura predisposes to rupture).

Von Hippel–Lindau Disease (VHL)

Von Hippel–Lindau disease results from point mutations in one copy of the VHL tumor suppressor gene (see Chapter 5). The VHL protein is normally involved in modulating angiogenesis in response to cellular hypoxia. Defective VHL protein

tends to cause overexpression of angiogenic cytokines and growth factors, which can result in overgrowth of blood vessels and in the development of unusual benign tumors of different tissues. Most of these tumors have a very prominent vasculature and are characteristic of this genetic disease.

Huntington's Disease

Huntington's disease results from the elongation of a tract of triplet repeats in the Huntington gene. Normal individuals have between 11 and 34 copies of the nucleotide triplet CAG in the coding region of the Huntington's gene that encode a stretch of repeated glutamine residues. Individuals with more than 40 copies of the repeat usually develop dementia and loss of fine motor control in middle adulthood. The dementia is progressive, leading to death within 10 to 15 years. The age at onset of symptoms is related to the number of glutamine residues, with a larger number of repeats causing disease earlier in life. Individuals with 35 to 40 copies may or may not develop clinically recognizable dementia. The abnormal protein accumulates as aggregates in neurons and results in neuronal toxicity and eventually cell death. The preferential loss of neurons in the basal ganglia results in characteristic neurologic symptoms with progressive loss of higher cerebral functions and choreiform movements (delicate, involuntary, repetitive movements). Although the number of CAG repeats in this disease is a quantitative abnormality, disease-causing alleles are inherited as an autosomal dominant trait in most families.

Huntington's disease was targeted for genetic analysis early in the development of molecular genetics because the late age of disease onset did not allow for reproductive counseling in affected families. Genetic diagnosis was initially accomplished through linkage studies in each affected family but can now be performed by direct sequence analysis of the Huntington gene.

X-linked Recessive Disorders

X-linked recessive diseases result from abnormalities in genes carried on the X chromosome. Since males have only one copy of the X chromosome, they are functionally hemizygous for most X chromosome genes (a small number of X chromosome genes are present on the Y chromosome). As a result, inheritance of one defective X chromosome allele can result in total loss of function for that gene (Fig. 4-7). X-linked diseases always show a maternal pattern of inheritance in which females are carriers who pass the disease on to their sons but not to their daughters. In some forms of X-linked recessive disease, female heterozygotes may have some symptoms. In females, one X chromosome is randomly inactivated by hypermethylation during embryogenesis. As a result, females are mosaics with some cells expressing one X chromosome and some the other (i.e., lyonization, the same process responsible for stripes on a cat). Since X inactivation occurs early in embryogenesis, large patches of tissue may carry the abnormal X allele, which can produce disease symptoms under some conditions. Expression of the

GENETICS

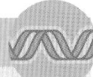

Linkage Analysis

Before the human genome project, detailed knowledge of gene sequences was limited to a small number of genes, and the sequences of most intragenic regions were unknown.

Classical genetics utilizing mendelian laws of segregation and recombination allowed the provisional mapping of genes based on the relative rates of recombination between different loci (usually expressed in centiMorgans). Using this type of information in families with a genetic disease, it was possible to infer the location of an unknown disease-causing gene relative to known genes. Genetic information from a number of different families was combined using LOD scores, which are statistical measures of the likelihood of association between a disease phenotype and marker genes.

This information was then used for genetic counseling (e.g., in Huntington's disease) by assessing the transmission of disease-linked genes in different individuals using restriction fragment linked polymorphism (RFLP) analysis or other techniques. Since there is always a chance that recombination has occurred between the marker and the disease gene (particularly if the distance between them is large), this technique provides a statistical likelihood that a disease gene is present rather than a certain diagnosis.

This type of linkage analysis is no longer commonly employed diagnostically, since molecular technology allows direct assessment of most genetic alterations.

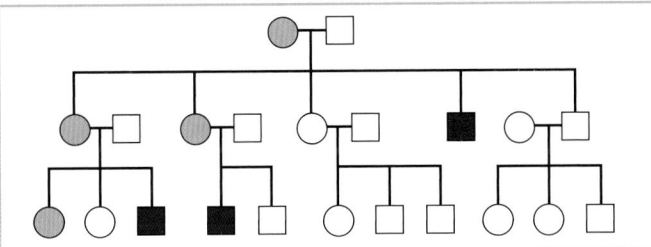

Figure 4-7. Typical pedigree showing sex-linked recessive inheritance. Males are squares, and females are circles. Individuals with disease are dark purple (hemizygous), and heterozygotes are light purple.

normal allele in many other cells usually prevents a severe phenotype, however.

Duchenne's Muscular Dystrophy (DMD)

Duchenne's muscular dystrophy results from alterations in the dystrophin protein, which is a very large intracellular protein that normally associates with other proteins (so-called dystrophin-associated proteins) at the inner surface of the plasma membrane of muscle cells. Dystrophin is essential for assembly of these proteins into a transmembrane complex that functionally and mechanically connects muscle cells to the extracellular matrix. Because skeletal and cardiac muscle function by exerting mechanical force on the extracellular

matrix, this transmembrane connection is critical for the normal transfer of mechanical force. The amino terminus of the dystrophin protein is required to assemble the transmembrane complex, so patients without a functional dystrophin protein have defective links between their muscle cells and the extracellular matrix. As muscle cells contract, these abnormal connections result in repeated microtrauma, producing minute plasma membrane tears that allow extracellular calcium to flow into damaged muscle cells. This calcium influx directly activates sarcomeres, triggering hypercontraction of the muscle fibers, which causes additional damage and eventually causes necrosis of individual myocytes. Over time, accumulated damage results in the replacement of muscle fibers by fibroblasts and adipocytes, which give rise to the pseudohypertrophic appearance of muscles in these patients. Since dystrophin is located on the X chromosome, muscular dystrophy is inherited as an X-linked recessive disorder. Female heterozygotes occasionally have very mild symptoms. Male patients typically have muscle weakness in early childhood that progresses to severe loss of strength and inability to ambulate. Patients usually die as a result of failure of the muscles of respiration or loss of function of cardiac muscle, which causes dilated cardiomyopathy.

Most of the genetic alterations in the dystrophin gene that cause Duchenne's muscular dystrophy are deletions (large or small) within the coding region of the gene. Another clinical form of X-linked muscular dystrophy (Becker's muscular dystrophy) causes only mild muscle weakness that is not progressive. Surprisingly, patients with Becker's dystrophy were found to have deletions in the dystrophin gene that are similar to those in Duchenne's patients (Fig. 4-8). Further analysis showed that patients with Becker's dystrophy had in-frame deletions that allow synthesis of dystrophin's amino terminus. The shortened dystrophin protein in patients with Becker's dystrophy can direct assembly of the dystrophin-associated protein transmembrane complex to form a functional junction with the extracellular matrix. Most deletions in patients with Duchenne's dystrophy cause frame shifts, resulting in premature termination of translation. The absence of dystrophin's amino terminus prevents assembly of the transmembrane complex in these patients, resulting in markedly dysfunctional attachment of muscle cells to the extracellular matrix.

The large size of the dystrophin gene (>100 kb) provides a challenge for molecular diagnosis using standard DNA sequencing technology. Since most gene alterations are deletions, a multiplex PCR assay that utilizes dystrophin cDNA as a template can detect most such deletions efficiently by employing exon-specific primers that span exons (Fig. 4-9). Loss or size change of individual PCR bands in this type of assay is diagnostic of a deletion in affected males. Molecular assays are helpful for genetic counseling and prenatal diagnosis in affected families. Unfortunately, up to 40% of cases of Duchenne's muscular dystrophy result from new germline mutations and are not detectable by focused prenatal genetic testing. The high forward mutation rate

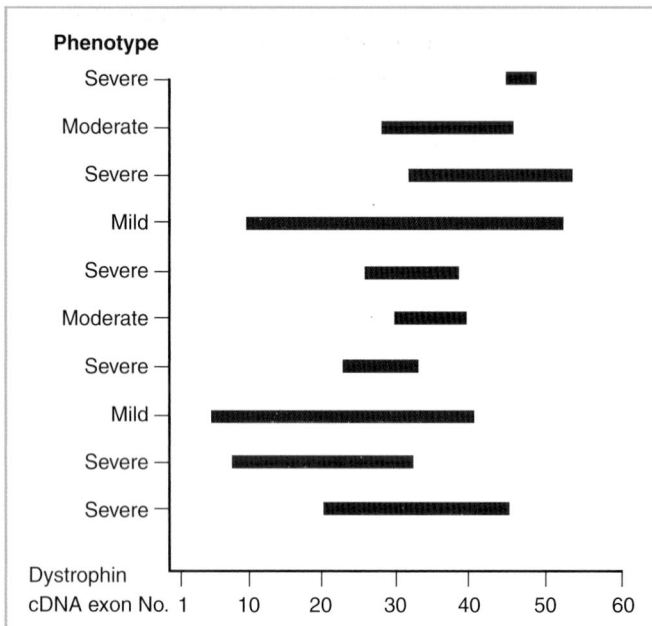

Figure 4-8. Dystrophin gene deletions in Duchenne's and Becker's muscular dystrophy.

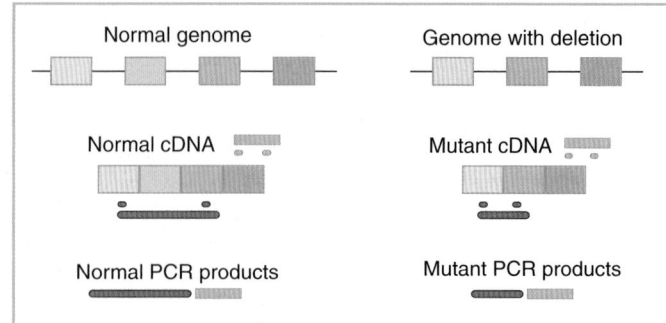

Figure 4-9. Detection of dystrophin gene deletions by multiplex PCR.

apparently results from structural instability in this region of the X chromosome.

Hemophilia

Hemophilia A and B result from deficiency of clotting factors produced by the liver. Hemophilia A is caused by point mutations in the factor VIII gene on the X chromosome. Hemophilia B results from mutations in factor IX (an autosomal gene) and so is inherited as an autosomal recessive disease (Fig. 4-10). Different mutations result in different levels of disease severity, and up to 30% of patients have a new germline mutation. Patients with either type of hemophilia are at markedly increased risk for some types of bleeding, particularly internal hemorrhage. Hemorrhage into joints (hemarthrosis) is particularly common, and chronic injury can result in severe joint deformity. Treatment with purified factor VIII to a critical level can dramatically decrease the risk of life-threatening hemorrhage in hemophilia A patients. Female heterozygotes may manifest some level of disease if X inactivation in the liver results in predominant expression of the mutant allele (so-called unfavorable lyonization).

X-linked Dominant Disorders

X-linked dominant disorders are uncommon relative to other types of mendelian diseases and show an excess of affected females in a family, since women have two X chromosomes (Fig. 4-11). X-linked dominant disorders do not show father to son transmission, and affected males (hemizygous for the mutant allele) are usually more severely affected than female heterozygotes.

Renal phosphate transport disorder is an X-linked dominant disease that results in abnormalities of bone and teeth due to abnormal vitamin D metabolism, resulting in impaired resorption of phosphate by renal tubules. Patients have defective bone mineralization and, if untreated, show failure to thrive and short stature with thin, curved bones (rickets). The defective gene PHEX is located on the short arm of the X chromosome, but its normal function is not clearly defined. Patients respond to treatment with hydroxylated vitamin D.

NONMENDELIAN DISORDERS

Nonmendelian disorders include multifactorial (polygenic) diseases that have a familial tendency but show a varied pattern of inheritance. These diseases are by far the most common type of genetic disease and underlie increased risk for some of most common and serious diseases such as diabetes mellitus and atherosclerotic heart disease. In most cases, the precise genes and alleles involved in causing disease are either not known or are incompletely characterized.

Although most genes are inherited as two allelic copies on autosomes, some genes are present in the genome in more than two copies. The number of gene copies (gene dosage) is a heritable genetic trait for at least a small number of genes. Only a few studies have evaluated the phenotypic effects of such alterations in gene dosage, and it remains to be seen whether they contribute significantly to human disease. The phenotypic effects are likely to be modest based on experience with recessive mendelian disorders but may add an additional level of complexity to multifactorial genetic diseases.

Nonmendelian disorders also include a number of rare conditions that result from quantitative (rather than qualitative) alterations in nuclear genes or involve changes in chromatin structure that do not alter DNA sequence. Rare alterations in the mitochondrial genome are included in this category.

Fragile X Syndrome

Fragile X syndrome results from an abnormally large number of copies of a trinucleotide repeat in the X chromosome that can cause defective chromosome segregation during mitosis in somatic cells. Some daughter cells have abnormal chro-

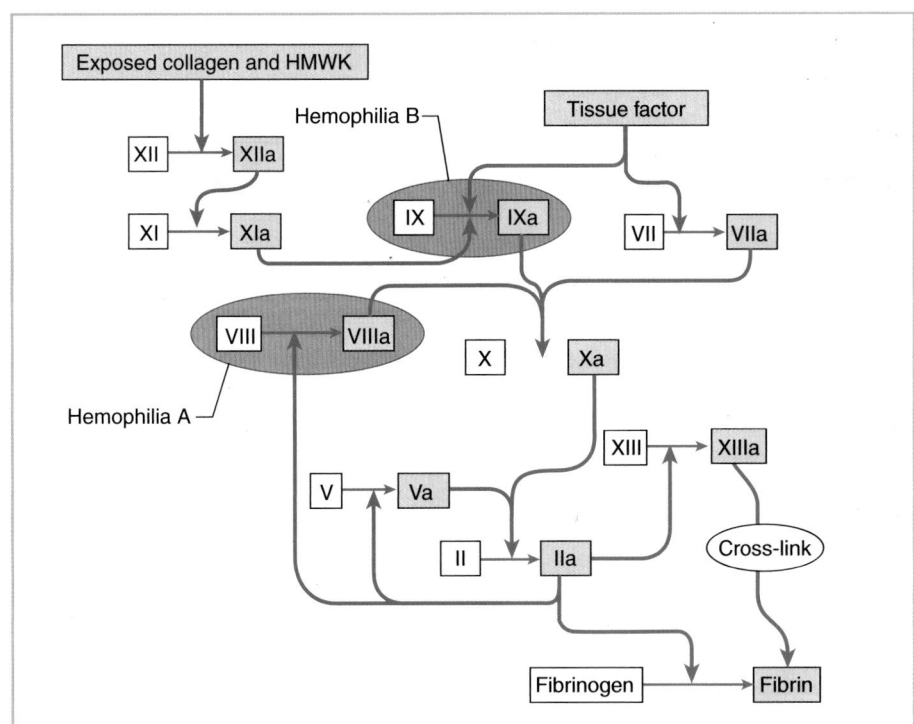

Figure 4-10. Coagulation cascade defects in hemophilia A and hemophilia B.

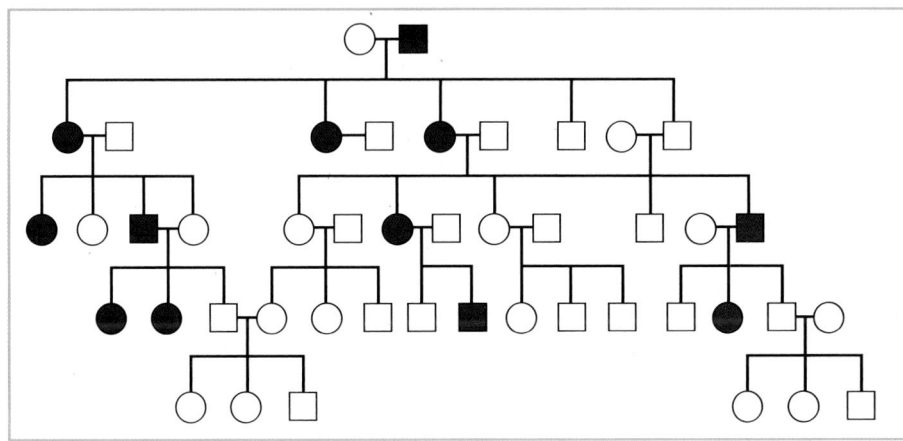

Figure 4-11. Typical pedigree showing sex-linked dominant inheritance. Males are squares, and females are circles. Individuals with disease are purple.

mosomal content that usually results in cell dysfunction or death. Fragile X syndrome predominantly impacts the central nervous system, causing mental retardation (neurons have essentially no capacity for hyperplasia to replace genetically damaged cells). Patients with longer repeats tend to have more severe retardation. This condition is unusual in that the degree of genetic defect is quantitative (longer repeats cause a more severe phenotype) and the tendency to lengthen these repeats is heritable so that the disease tends to amplify within a family until the repeats reach a critical length and produce overt disease.

Mitochondrial Disorders

Mitochondria contain a small circular chromosome that codes for tRNAs and a small number of proteins that are expressed in mitochondrial oxidative phosphorylation.

Most mitochondrial proteins derive from nuclear genes that are translated by cytoplasmic ribosomes and are specifically targeted to mitochondria. Mitochondria are preferentially or exclusively inherited from maternal oocytes with no (or minimal numeric contribution) from paternal sperm. Since mitochondria control their own replication, this large maternal contribution tends to persist throughout life and is passed on in the maternal germline. Unlike in mendelian genetic diseases, the percentage of mitochondria with abnormal DNA can vary continuously from 0% to 100%, resulting in a wide spectrum of disease severity.

Since most proteins encoded by mitochondrial DNA are involved in oxidative phosphorylation, mutations tend to result in abnormalities in energy generation. The severity of disease is determined both by the type of mutation and by the percentage of mitochondria that carry the mutation in different tissues. Some affected individuals have metabolic

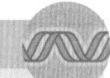

GENETICS

Mitochondrial DNA

Mitochondrial DNA exists as a small circular chromosome within mitochondria. The small number of genes encoded by mitochondrial DNA are separated by transfer RNAs which serve as cleavage signals for endoribonucleases that process long RNA transcripts for translation within the mitochondria.

Transcriptional promoters (one for each strand) and the origins of DNA replication are located in the D loop, which is a novel DNA sequence that usually exists as a short, single-stranded DNA segment hybridized to one strand of mitochondrial DNA that displaces the complementary strand (i.e., the D loop).

Control of mitochondrial replication is modulated through this D loop and is nominally under the control of nuclear genes. Mutations in mitochondrial DNA can result in defective energy metabolism often presenting as muscle dysfunction (myopathy) or metabolic acidosis.

Some theories of cellular senescence suggest that accumulated mitochondrial DNA mutations result in a failure of energy generation as individuals age. Alternatively, mitochondria are exposed to significant oxidative stress, which can result in release of mitochondrial proteins including cytochrome *c* to trigger apoptosis.

Mitochondrial DNA sequence changes are a convenient marker for population genetic studies that measure population migration or the relationships of different ethnic groups. Because mitochondrial genes follow maternal inheritance, they are not subject to founder effect mutations that can skew analyses based on mendelian genes.

GENETICS

CpG Islands and DNA Methylation

CpG islands are short stretches of palindromic DNA with the sequence "CpG" that code for the same sequence in the complementary strand (i.e., repeated cytosine and guanine nucleotides with the "p" representing the linking phosphate). CpG islands are often present around the promoters of housekeeping genes and other actively expressed genes.

Methylation of cytosines in CpG islands in promotor regions can prevent transcription factors to effectively block gene expression, and CpG islands are frequently methylated in genes that are not actively expressed. CpG methylation also attracts methyl-binding proteins and other protein complexes that chemically acetylate histones associated with chromosomal DNA to alter chromatin structure and further silence transcription.

These patterns of gene inactivation are usually passed on to daughter cells through the action of maintenance methylases which methylate only CpG sequences that are base-paired with methylated CpG sequences (remember that CpG islands are palindromic sequences with the same sequence in each DNA strand).

Methylated cytosines can be converted to thymidine by deamidation, and this type of mutation is inefficiently repaired by mismatch repair enzymes. Methylated DNA is therefore prone to somatic mutation so that over evolutionary time, deamidation results in a gradual shift from CpG to TpG sequences.

---

acidosis in childhood that may be triggered by infection or other stress that increases energy demands. If a significant percentage of mitochondria in critical tissues have defective oxidative phosphorylation, relatively minor stress may result in ATP depletion, triggering a switch to anaerobic glycolysis that leads to acidosis. Some mitochondrial DNA mutations primarily affect skeletal muscle or the nervous system.

Epigenetic Disorders

Epigenetic disorders result largely from changes in the methylation patterns of chromosomal DNA that result in gene silencing (blockage of transcription). DNA methylation patterns in somatic cells are inherited from progenitor cells (imprinting) during DNA replication.

While the methylation pattern is not so tightly controlled as DNA sequence, daughter cells usually follow the parental pattern closely. Propagation of epigenetic changes in somatic cells is important for maintaining normal cellular differentiation and in determining the phenotypic characteristics of neoplasms (see Chapter 5). Other changes in chromatin structure (e.g., histone acetylation) are also at least partially heritable. Identical twins have very similar genomic methylation patterns at birth, but these patterns may diverge with increasing age, particularly if they live in different environments.

In contrast to somatic cells, embryonic stem cells do not normally retain the methylation pattern of their progenitors and are functionally "reset" so that all genes are potentially expressible. A few genes may escape demethylation in gametes and cause loss of gene function in affected embryos. The Prader-Willi and Angelman syndromes result from inheritance of an epigenetically inactivated region of chromosome 15 (q11-q13) in combination with a corresponding small deletion of this portion of the other parental chromosome. Alternatively, methylated DNA from the silenced chromosome may replace a portion of the normal chromosome (probably by mitotic recombination). Affected individuals have marked mental retardation. Diseases caused by this type of imprinting are thought to be quite unusual in human beings but may be facilitated by in vitro manipulation of gametes for in vitro fertilization.

Multifactorial (Polygenic) Disorders

Inherited predisposition to many types of diseases involves multifactorial inheritance. The combined effect of different alleles in many genes is ultimately responsible for most of our genetic identity but can also predispose to (or protect from) various types of diseases. In contrast to the genetic diseases discussed thus far, the combination of different normal alleles for various genes may result in an individual who is predisposed to (or protected from) various disorders. Diabetes mellitus, hypertension, and atherosclerotic cardiovascular disease show a multifactorial pattern of inheritance in most patients. While mutations in some single genes can greatly accelerate the development and progression of selected diseases (e.g., LDL receptor mutations that cause familial hypercholesterolemia result in severe cardiovascular disease regardless of other genetic or environmental risk factors), most polygenic diseases result from small, incremental contributions from a number of different alleles at different loci. The interaction of these genetic variations with each other and with environmental factors ultimately determines the likelihood of disease development. Some alleles may be adaptive in one environment and deleterious in another (e.g., hemoglobin S confers a degree of resistance to malarial parasites that gives heterozygotes a significant survival advantage in areas where falciparum malaria is a major cause of death). In addition to determining the likelihood of developing different diseases, some genetic changes have marked effects on drug metabolism (e.g., hepatic cytochrome CYP450 enzymes) that can alter a drug's therapeutic index or result in unexpected toxicity.

Polygenic diseases tend to run in families but do not show the typical pattern of mendelian inheritance. The likelihood of developing an index disease in an affected family usually diminishes progressively for second- and third-degree relatives of the index cases (gene dilution effect). Because the involved genes are unknown in most familial diseases, SNP (single nucleotide polymorphism) based approaches have been employed to track involved genes through families and within populations.

SNPs are polymorphic nucleotides that have been mapped in the human genome relative to their chromosomal location. Most SNPs are not in coding regions so that variations in their sequence do not usually cause significant genotypic or phenotypic changes. SNPs are convenient linkage markers that can be used to identify disease-causing genes. Analyzing the sequence of many SNPs in diseased and normal (control) populations can allow inferences about the chromosomal location of genes that may cause or protect from disease. SNP genotyping can be done rapidly and economically so that hundreds or thousands of potential markers can be interrogated in a population.

Chromosome Abnormalities

Gross chromosomal abnormalities cause most spontaneous abortions early in pregnancy and are common events during human embryogenesis. Aneuploidy (abnormal chromosome number) for larger autosomes is usually lethal because variance in gene dosage for some of the thousands of genes encoded on each chromosome is generally incompatible with life. Less severe chromosomal abnormalities can result from abnormal reassociation between different chromosomes (translocations) and may be balanced or unbalanced. In balanced translocations, all the normal chromosomal material is maintained in normal copy number but some genes

GENETICS

Single Nucleotide Polymorphisms (SNPs)

SNPs are defined as single base differences at specific locations that are present in more than 1% of the population (in practice, useful SNPs are present in at least 5% to 10% of a study population). SNPs make up 90% of the sequence differences between individual human beings and occur at 200 nucleotide intervals (on average) in the human genome.

SNPs are inherited in the same way as classical mendelian genes (i.e., SNPs are stably inherited from parent to child), and their high frequency in the genome makes them an ideal tool for precise genetic mapping of different diseases or traits. Although most SNPs have no direct effect on cell function (i.e., they do not change protein sequence or alter transcription), many are closely associated with disease-causing alleles or genes that control how an individual responds to specific drugs.

SNPs are usually measured using PCR to amplify DNA encompassing specific SNPs, followed by sequencing to identify the genotype of each SNP. Newer technology may allow very high throughput assays (hundreds to thousands) that bypass individual PCR amplification of sequences and directly assess numerous SNPs by primer extension.

SNP haplotypes can be inferred statistically based on known population frequencies of different SNP alleles.

reside on different chromosomes (Fig. 4-12). Individuals with balanced translocations may be phenotypically normal but are usually infertile because recombination during meiosis produces unbalanced translocations in gametes. Individuals with unbalanced translocations typically lose or gain some portion of one or more chromosomes, causing changes in gene dosage that result in hemizygosity for many genes, which may expose nonfunctional alleles (similar to X-linked recessive disorders).

Some chromosome abnormalities are associated with specific phenotypes that correspond to various congenital anomaly syndromes. Some of these syndromes result in abnormalities in utero that cause morphologic changes which are evident at birth. For instance, oligohydramnios of any cause (decreased amniotic fluid volume) results in the typical facial features of Potter's syndrome of beaklike nose, low-set ears, etc.

Most significant gains or losses of autosomal chromosomes result in severe mental retardation and abnormal development if the affected embryo survives to term. A few specific numeric chromosome abnormalities are sufficiently common to merit individual attention and are discussed below.

Down Syndrome

Down syndrome occurs in 1 in 1000 live births and results from the presence of three copies of chromosome 21 (trisomy 21), which is one of the smallest autosomes. The likelihood of producing a baby with Down syndrome increases steeply with maternal age over 35 years. Affected individuals have some degree of mental retardation, which may be relatively

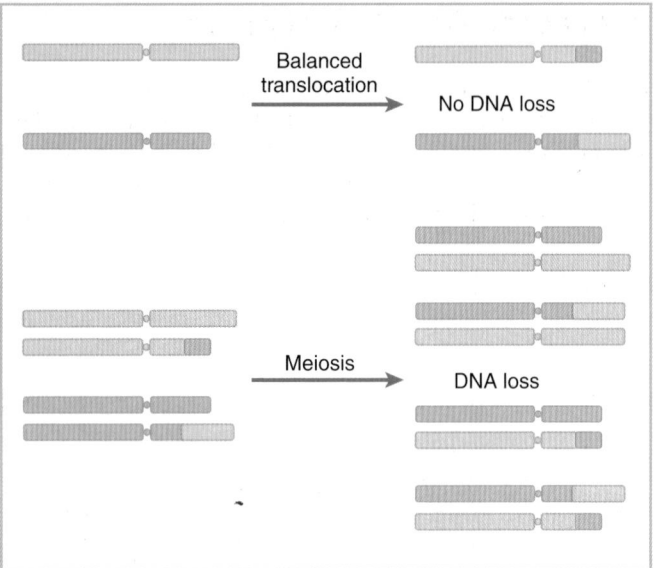

Figure 4-12. Balanced chromosomal translocations.

EMBRYOLOGY

Oligohydramnios

Amniotic fluid is essential for normal fetal growth and development and provides a cushion from physical trauma. Amniotic fluid is required for the formation of pulmonary alveoli, and fetal breathing of amniotic fluid is an essential physiologic stimulus for this process. Oligohydramnios is defined as an amniotic fluid index of less than 5 cm by ultrasound and affects approximately 4% of pregnancies in the United States.

Membrane rupture is the most common cause of oligohydramnios late in pregnancy, and it can lead to cord compression and fetal distress. Oligohydramnios can also be caused by maternal use of angiotensin-converting enzyme (ACE) inhibitors or prostaglandin synthase inhibitors.

The most common causes of oligohydramnios early in pregnancy are bilateral renal agenesis (Potter's syndrome), autosomal recessive polycystic kidney disease, and various forms of obstructive uropathy that prevent the passage of urine to replenish inspired and swallowed amniotic fluid.

Deficient amniotic fluid during pregnancy results in characteristic abnormalities of the external features (including hypertelorism, low-set ears, micrognathia, bowed legs, and narrow chest) that result from fetal compression in utero.

mild or severe. Patients with Down syndrome also have an increased frequency of other congenital abnormalities such as congenital heart disease (tetralogy of Fallot is the most common; see Chapter 7). Many phenotypic consequences of Down syndrome appear to be related to gene dosage. Down syndrome patients are at significantly increased risk for myeloid leukemia, which is thought to be related to the additional copy of the bcr gene on chromosome 21 (the bcr gene is the translocation partner of the abl proto-oncogene in

most cases of chronic myeloid leukemia). Gene dosage also results in the onset of Alzheimer's disease at an early age because of the inheritance of three copies of the amyloid precursor protein gene on chromosome 21 (see Chapter 14).

Klinefelter's and Turner's Syndromes

Klinefelter's and Turner's syndromes result from abnormalities in the number of the sex chromosomes. Patients with Turner's syndrome have one X chromosome and no Y chromosome (some patients have one normal X chromosome and one X chromosome lacking its short arm). Patients with Turner's syndrome are phenotypically female but are infertile and most have significant growth retardation. Some patients with Turner's develop lymphangiomas of the head and neck region called cystic hygromas that may suggest the diagnosis. Analysis of buccal smears stained to assess the number of Barr bodies (inactivated X chromosomes, one present in somatic cells from normal females) is diagnostic.

Patients with Klinefelter's syndrome are phenotypically males but typically have two X chromosomes and at least one Y chromosome. Most patients are infertile, but some are mosaics and may have a normal karyotype in some of their germ cells. Klinefelter's syndrome is associated with increased maternal age, and patients may have a characteristic body habitus but tend to have few other abnormalities.

●●● PERINATAL DISEASES

Congenital Anomalies

Congenital anomalies are morphologic abnormalities that are evident at the time of birth or in the prenatal or perinatal period. A few congenital anomalies are associated with single gene alterations. Alterations in genes that coordinate embryogenesis can also result in complex morphologic abnormalities (e.g., situs inversus in which the right and left viscera are reversed in orientation). Many severe congenital abnormalities are associated with chromosomal abnormalities and may include translocations, additions, deletions, or differences in the number of chromosomes (Fig. 4-13). The most frequent congenital anomalies affect the cardiovascular system (see Chapter 7). Some of these are associated with chromosomal syndromes but most are sporadic and are not associated with identified genetic alterations. Urogenital abnormalities are also relatively common. Bladder extrophy results from a failure of closure of the anterior abdominal wall so that the bladder mucosa is exposed to the external environment, resulting in infection and squamous metaplasia. Posterior urethral valves result in congenital hydronephrosis owing to blockage of urine flow out of the bladder in utero. Unilateral or bilateral renal dysplasia can occur sporadically or in combination with specific genetic and chromosomal abnormalities.

TORCH Syndrome

Maternal infection with a number of different microorganisms during gestation can result in spontaneous abortion or in abnormalities in the fetus. Transplacental spread of infection with *t*oxoplasmosis, [*o*ther infections], *r*ubella, *c*ytomegalovirus, *h*erpes simplex virus (TORCH syndrome), and syphilis all can cause severe malformations of the fetus and may produce active infection at the time of birth. Infection with other viruses can result in more subtle abnormalities. For instance, prenatal infection with mumps virus is associated with fibrosis of the endocardium and heart valves, which can cause restrictive cardiomyopathy and heart failure (Fig. 4-14). Infection of neonates with herpes simplex virus during passage through the birth canal results in a disseminated infection that is almost always fatal.

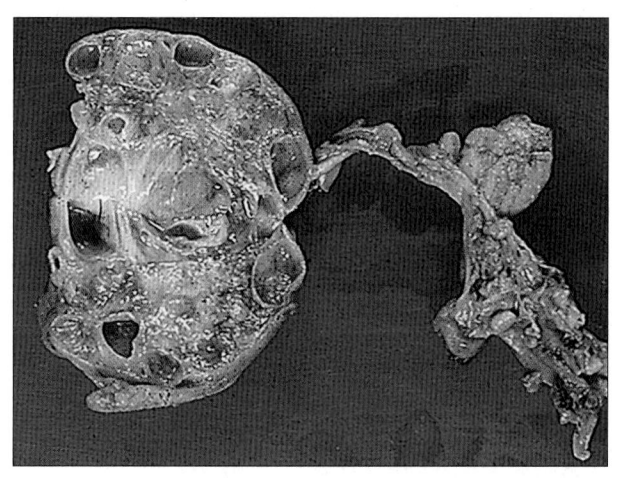

Figure 4-13. Congenitally dysplastic kidney. Gross cross-section of a dysplastic kidney from a perinatal autopsy showing cysts and absence of normal corticomedullary architecture.

Intrauterine Growth Retardation

Intrauterine growth retardation (IUGR), defined as lower than expected fetal size as measured by ultrasound in utero and/or lower than expected birth weight for gestational age, can result from abnormalities of the fetus (usually genetic or chromosomal abnormalities), the placenta, or maternal factors.

ANATOMY

Placental Structure and Function

The normal, term placenta measures approximately 18 cm in diameter and weighs approximately 500 g. It is composed of an umbilical cord, membranes, and trophoblastic villi that are intimately associated with maternal decidua.

The umbilical cord contains two arteries and one vein surrounded by mucopolysaccharide (Wharton's jelly), which protects these vessels from compression. The membranes consist of an inner amnion lined by a simple cuboidal epithelium that is juxtaposed with an external chorion with blood vessels in between.

The villi are composed of fibrovascular cores covered by cytotrophoblast with external syncytiotrophoblast. Villi develop from trophectoderm following blastocyst formation. Cytotrophoblast cells fuse together to form multinucleated syncytiotrophoblast cells.

Trophoblastic cells invade maternal decidua, which is composed of modified stromal cells (stimulated by progesterone). This interaction provides the functional apposition of maternal and fetal circulations that allows gas and nutrient exchange.

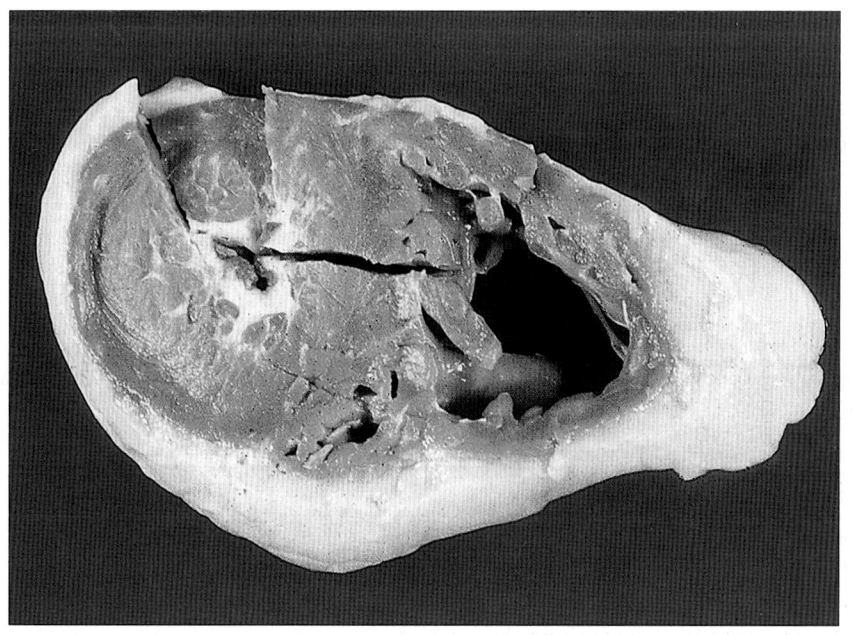

Figure 4-14. Endocardial fibroelastosis. Gross cross-section of pediatric heart showing marked fibrosis of the left ventricular endocardium (white tissue lining collapsed ventricle). This left ventricular abnormality resulted in marked compensatory hypertrophy (and ultimately failure) of the right ventricle (see Chapter 7).

Inadequate placental nutrition is a common cause of IUGR and can result from maternal hypertension (resulting in placental infarcts), toxemia of pregnancy, or maternal substance abuse.

Complications of Prematurity

Markedly premature infants (26 weeks of gestation and earlier) are at very high risk for death or severe complications involving the respiratory, nervous, and gastrointestinal systems that produce permanent dysfunction. The risk of perinatal complications diminishes progressively with gestational age in a normal pregnancy. Immature lungs cannot produce normal surfactant, resulting in high surface tension within alveolar spaces that greatly increases the work of breathing and interferes with normal oxygen transfer (neonatal respiratory distress syndrome), causing hypoxemia. Previously, infants with neonatal respiratory distress syndrome were treated with mechanical ventilation with high levels of oxygen to maintain adequate tissue oxygenation. Oxygen therapy led to multiple complications including the development of hyaline membrane disease (diffuse alveolar damage [DAD]) in which intra-alveolar exudate and cell debris form hyaline deposits around the periphery of alveoli that block gas exchange (Fig. 4-15). Hyaline membrane disease is similar to adult respiratory distress syndrome (ARDS), which can result from various insults including oxygen toxicity with free radical–mediated injury (see Chapter 8). A devastating problem, hyaline membrane disease has largely been eliminated by the availability of artificial surfactant and the induction of fetal lung maturation by a short course of corticosteroid therapy in utero.

Immaturity of vasculature in the brain can result in massive intraventricular hemorrhage in very premature infants with devastating consequences for central nervous system development (Fig. 4-16). Immaturity of the blood-brain barrier even in term infants renders the nervous system sensitive to damage from chemicals in the blood, such as bilirubin, which are excluded from the central nervous system by a mature blood-brain barrier. Extremely premature infants are also at risk for developing necrotizing enterocolitis, which is spontaneous ischemic necrosis of a large portion of the intestinal tract.

Hydrops Fetalis

Hydrops fetalis means generalized edema of the fetus or neonate and most often results from severe anemia during gestation. Anemia in this setting is often immune mediated owing to Rh incompatibility between fetus and mother (so-called immune hydrops). Other blood group antigen mismatches can also result in hemolytic disease of the newborn. The routine utilization of RhoGAM after pregnancy has greatly diminished the frequency of this complication. Nonimmune hydrops can result from other causes of fetal anemia including bone marrow failure (secondary to parvovirus infection), thalassemia (with no functional α-globin genes), and heart failure (secondary to abnormalities of the cardiovascular system).

Perinatal Tumors and Tumor-like Conditions

Hemangiomas are among the most common benign neoplasms observed in the perinatal period. Most are sporadic,

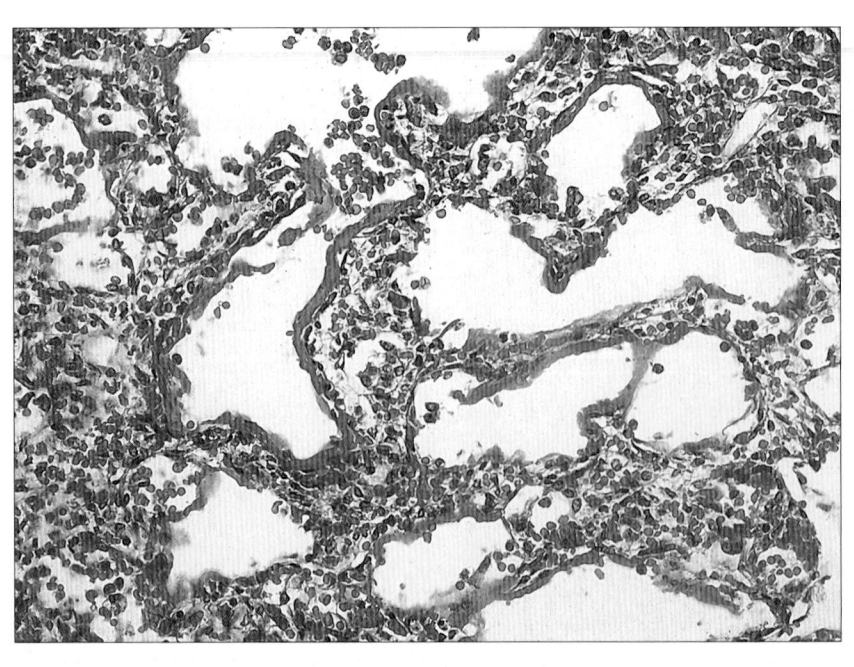

Figure 4-15. Hyaline membranes. Microscopic section of lung tissue showing fibrinoid material lining the periphery of alveolar spaces.

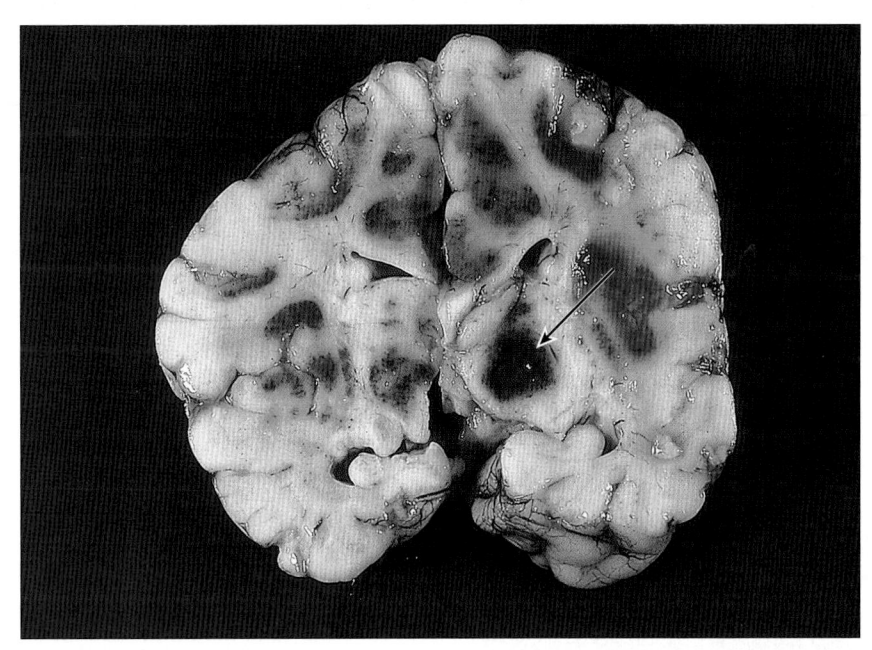

Figure 4-16. Intraventricular hemorrhage. Gross cross-section of premature infant's brain showing blood clot distending a ventricle (arrow).

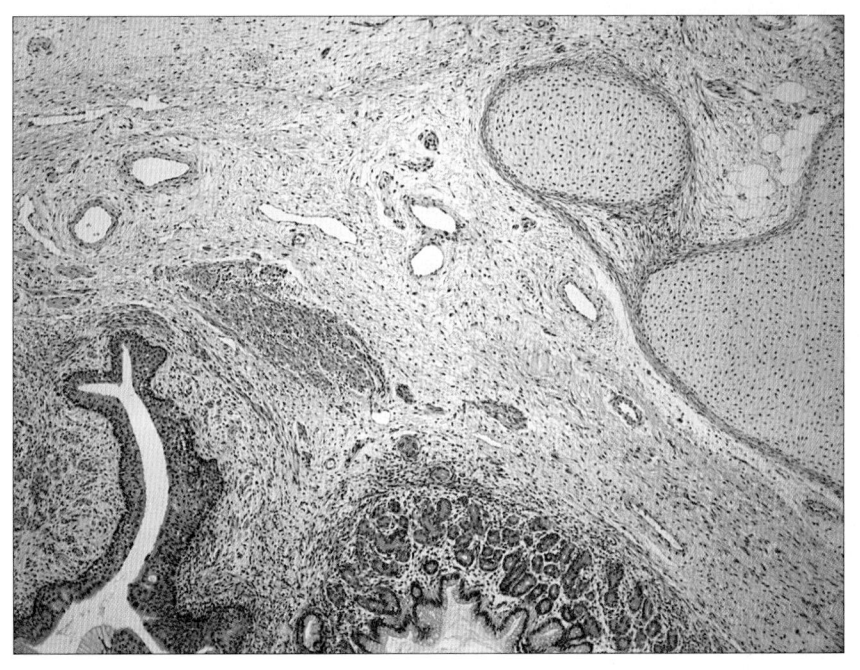

Figure 4-17. Teratoma. Mature teratoma composed of multiple mature tissues including hyaline cartilage and gastrointestinal and respiratory mucosa.

but specific types of hemangiomas are associated with different genetic syndromes and may be a clue to their diagnosis. Hemangiomas tend to grow and mature as a child ages. Some cutaneous nevi are present at birth (congenital nevi) and also develop and mature with the individual.

Heterotopia is the presence of normal tissue in an abnormal location. A common heterotopia is the presence of a small amount of gastric mucosa in the duodenum, which usually is without clinical consequence. Occasionally, heterotopic tissues can cause disease. Various diverticula and cysts can result from failure of resorption of normal embryonic structures (e.g., branchial cleft cysts or thyroglossal duct cysts in the neck). Hamartomas are abnormal benign growths composed of the normal constituents of the affected organ. Hamartomas are often present at birth, and there is diagnostic overlap between them and some benign neoplasms.

Sacrococcygeal teratomas are the most common germ cell tumors of childhood, and they may be large and deforming (Fig. 4-17). Although the majority are benign, a significant minority are malignant. Benign teratomas are composed of mature tissue of multiple different lineages (usually endodermal, mesodermal, and ectodermal structures are present). The presence of immature neural tissue or frankly malignant elements signals a poor prognosis.

A subset of malignant pediatric tumors presents in the perinatal period (Fig. 4-18). Most pediatric and perinatal tumors are associated with specific genetic alterations including specific chromosomal translocations (Fig. 4-19). Many pediatric tumors have a primitive morphologic appearance and mimic the embryologic components of the organ from which they arise. Some pediatric tumors are much more common in certain chromosomal syndromes that are associated with malformation in one or more organ systems.

Abnormalities in genes involved in the morphogenesis of these organs appear to direct tumor formation. Wilms' tumor is the most common pediatric tumor of the kidney (Fig. 4-20) and can be associated with several different genetic syndromes that result in mutations or deletions of the WT-1 or WT-2 genes (Fig. 4-21). Sporadic Wilms' tumor can also occur in genetically normal individuals and usually shows somatic mutation or deletion of the WT-1 gene. Microscopically, Wilms' tumor resembles renal blastema that is normally present early in embryogenesis but disappears after the gestational age of 26 weeks (Fig. 4-22). Other pediatric tumors including retinoblastoma and neuroblastoma are also associated with specific genetic alterations and are discussed in more detail in subsequent chapters.

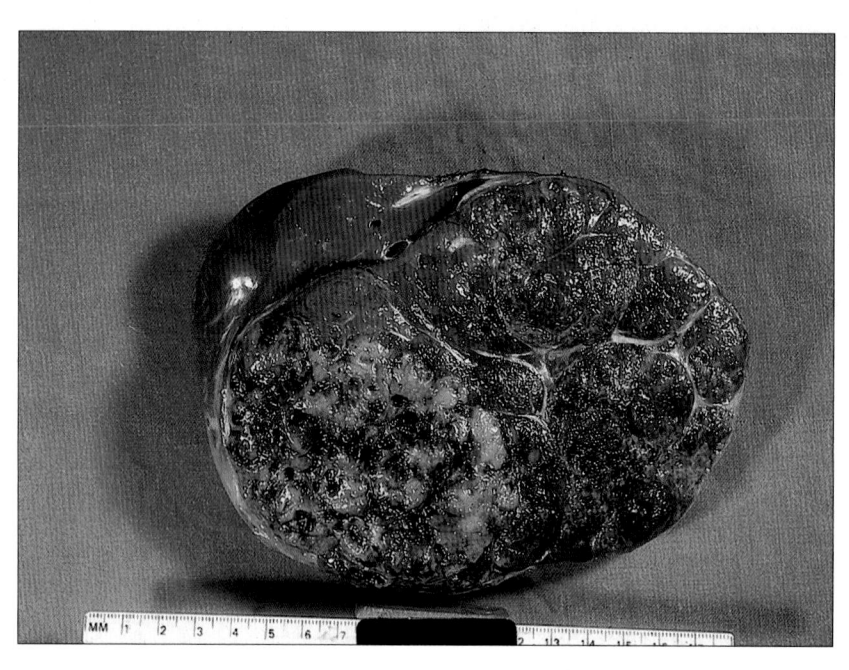

Figure 4-18. Hepatoblastoma. Gross cross-section of perinatal liver that is almost completely replaced by tumor with extensive necrosis. A small amount of residual normal liver tissue is evident in the upper right corner of the specimen.

Ewing's sarcoma
   t(11;22) t(21;22) t(7;22)
   MIC2 expression
Embroyonal rhabdomyosarcoma
   t(2;13)
   11p deletion
Wilms' tumor
   11p13 deletion/mutation
   11p15.5 deletion/mutation
   16q13 deletion
	Neuroblastoma
	   1 p deletion
	   N–myc amplification
	   Hyperdiploid
	   Neurosecretory granules
	Retinoblastoma
	   13q4 deletion/mutation
	Medulloblastoma
	   Isochromosome 17q

Figure 4-19. Common genetic alterations in pediatric tumors. Alterations associated with a good prognosis are in green and with a poor prognosis are in red.

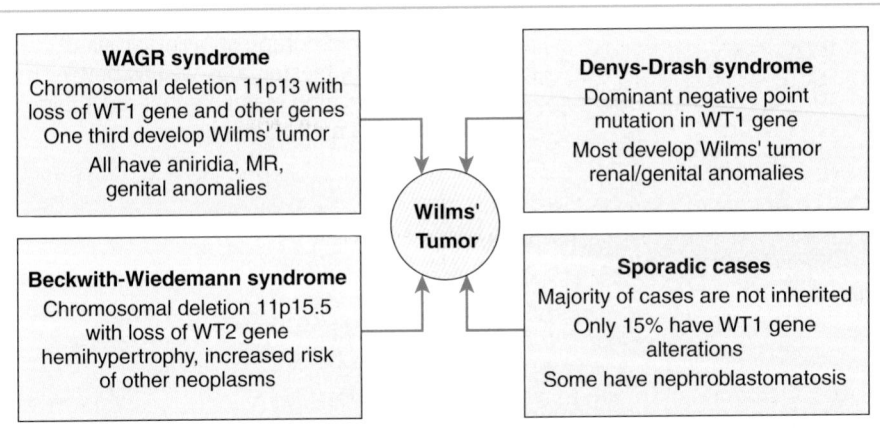

Figure 4-20. Pathways to Wilms' tumor development.

WAGR syndrome

Chromosomal deletion 11p13 with loss of WT1 gene and other genes

One third develop Wilms' tumor

All have aniridia, MR, genital anomalies

Denys-Drash syndrome

Dominant negative point mutation in WT1 gene

Most develop Wilms' tumor renal/genital anomalies

Wilms' Tumor

Beckwith-Wiedemann syndrome

Chromosomal deletion 11p15.5 with loss of WT2 gene hemihypertrophy, increased risk of other neoplasms

Sporadic cases

Majority of cases are not inherited

Only 15% have WT1 gene alterations

Some have nephroblastomatosis

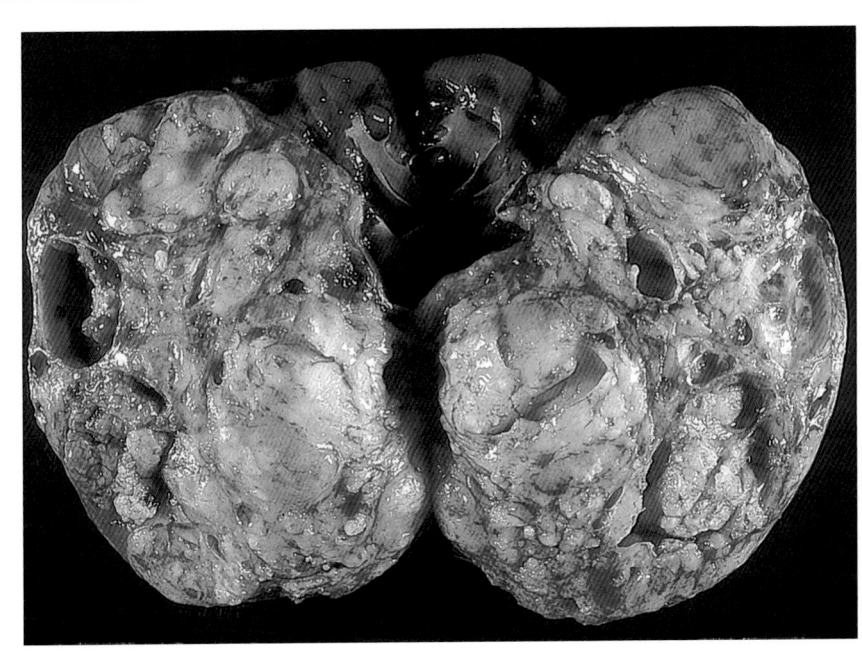

Figure 4-21. Wilms' tumor. Gross cross-section of a kidney that is almost completely replaced by Wilms' tumor. Note the fleshy appearance of the tumor with prominent areas of necrosis.

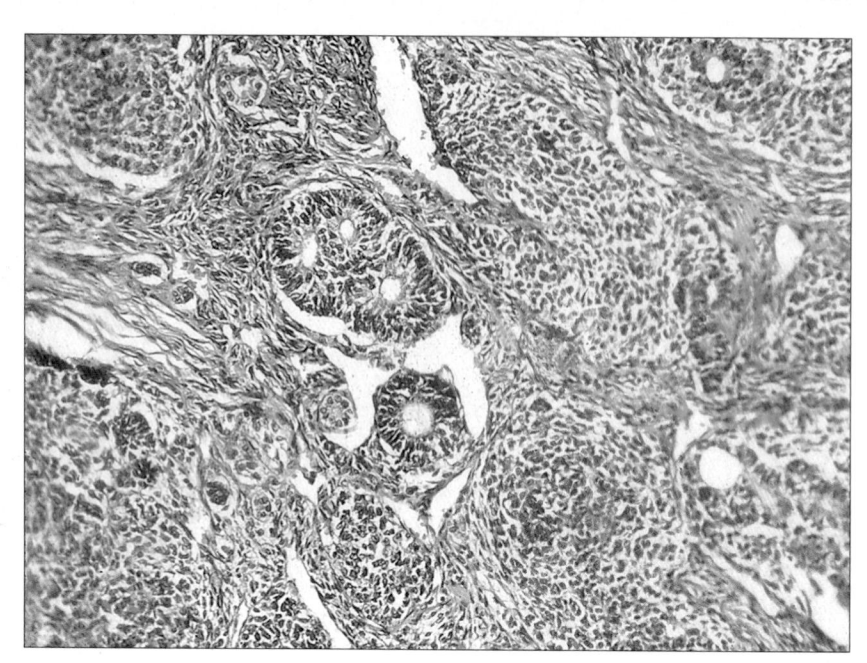

Figure 4-22. Wilms' tumor. Photomicrograph showing areas of primitive blastema as well as better differentiated elements that resemble tubules and glomeruli.

Neoplasia

5

CONTENTS

The generic term *cancer* usually implies a malignant neoplasm that has the capacity to metastasize (spread to distant location through the blood or lymphatic system) and kill its host. While this simple description is true for most forms of cancer, such as lung and breast carcinomas, it does not hold true for all types of human cancers. The word *neoplasm* means simply "new growth" and is usually interchangeable with "tumor." Cell division and growth are dysregulated in neoplasms but usually are not totally uncontrolled whether or not the tumor is malignant.

Many neoplasms tend to remain as localized growths that do not kill their host. These so-called benign neoplasms typically show more active growth than normal cells, and the increased proliferation results in the formation of a macroscopic mass lesion (i.e., a tumor). Most benign neoplasms are sharply circumscribed from surrounding tissue and often encapsulated (Fig. 5-1). Benign tumors do not invade adjacent structures or lymphatic or vascular spaces to cause metastasis.

Cancer is the second leading cause of death in the United States, and it occurs in men, women, and children but with greatly different frequencies and types of neoplasms in each group. The risk of developing almost all cancers increases dramatically in late adulthood, and this trend is enhanced by exposure to environmental carcinogens (most notably cigarette smoking for the development of many different types of cancer). Some viruses are associated with the development of specific types of cancer. The most important of these is human papillomavirus, which is the root cause of the vast majority of uterine cervical carcinomas.

Genetic factors also play an important role in cancer predisposition. There are now many well-characterized genetic syndromes that predispose to the development of some types of cancer. Although the percentage of cancers in adults that is associated with familial syndromes is quite small, these genetic diseases have been important in elucidating the genetic changes that are involved in the genesis of the more common sporadic cancers. Most of these family cancer syndromes are caused by inactivating mutations in one copy of a gene that is important for normal cell function (i.e., tumor suppressor genes; see below). Individuals with these syndromes usually inherit one defective and one normal copy of a tumor suppressor gene. Acquired genetic changes in somatic cells that result in loss or inactivation of the normal copy of this gene then cause total loss of function, which can lead to

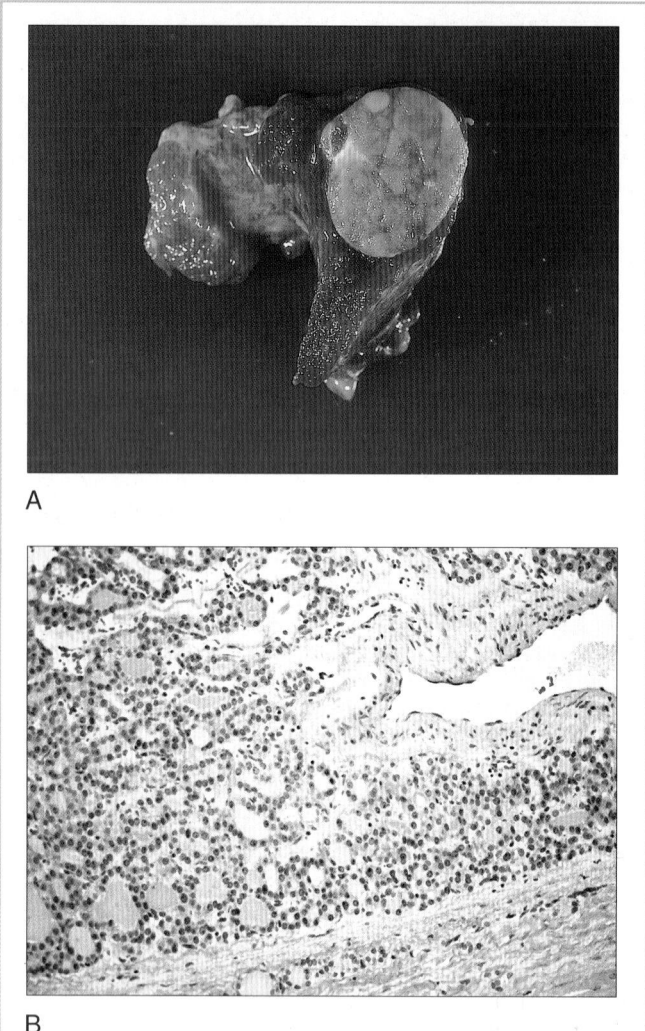

A

B

Figure 5-1. **A**, Follicular adenoma of thyroid gland. Gross cross-section of thyroid gland showing sharply circumscribed ovoid adenoma, which is distinct from surrounding red-brown thyroid tissue. **B**, Follicular adenoma of thyroid gland. Photomicrograph showing adenoma composed of monomorphous, relatively small follicles lined by bland follicular cells and surrounded by a fibrous capsule.

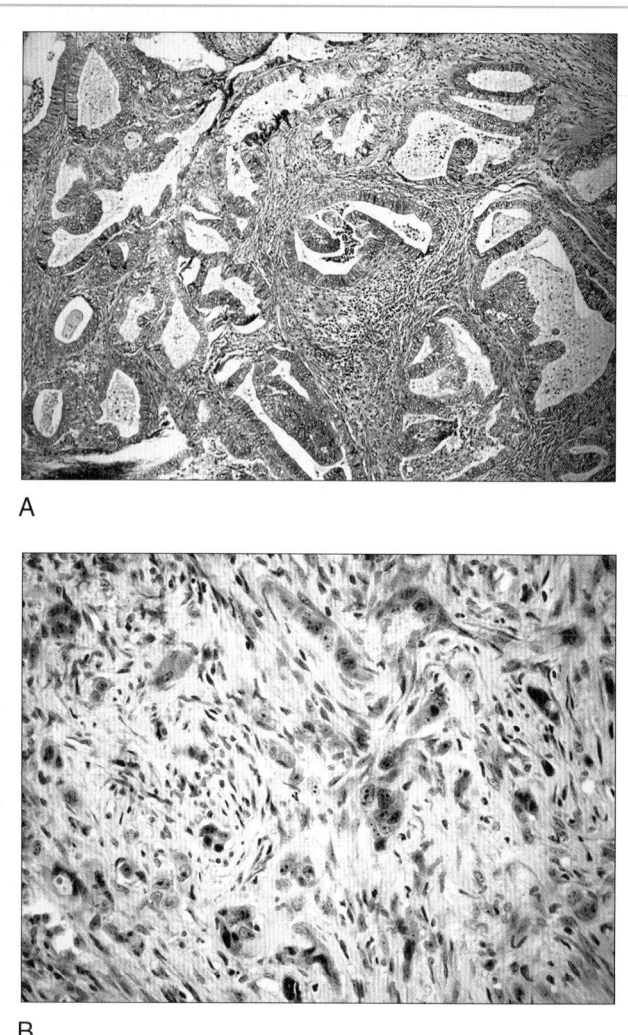

A

B

Figure 5-2. **A**, Well to moderately differentiated endometrial adenocarcinoma. Photomicrograph showing well-formed neoplastic glands lined by columnar cells with prominent nuclei. **B**, Poorly differentiated carcinoma. Photomicrograph showing scattered tumor cells with no gland formation or other differentiated features evident.

tumor formation. The normal copy of the gene may be lost by chromosomal changes that delete it or replace it with a copy of the abnormal gene. This process is referred to as loss of heterozygosity (LOH) and is an important mechanism for tumor development and progression.

More subtle forms of genetic variation are important in determining predisposition to certain kinds of cancer in many individuals. These genetic changes differ from those in family cancer syndromes because they are associated with a relatively small additional cancer risk and cancer may develop only if additional genetic lesions or environmental factors are present. Only a few of these more subtle genetic alterations have been well characterized, but the delineation of genetic variants that predispose to cancer and other serious diseases will be a major focus of molecular medicine over the next decade. The ability to identify high-risk populations offers the

opportunity to provide more intensive screening for individuals at high risk for specific cancers and to modify their lifestyle or environment to avoid factors that may further increase their cancer risk.

The clinical behavior of different malignant neoplasms is determined in large part by their level of differentiation and their cell of origin. The epigenetic programming of different types of cells in different tissues and organs provides a framework for gene expression and can be modified by genetic and epigenetic changes as tumors develop and progress (Fig. 5-2A). Poorly differentiated neoplasms retain few of the differentiated features of their cell of origin and tend to spread widely and aggressively (see Fig. 5-2B). Better differentiated neoplasms that retain most features of their cell of origin tend to grow and spread more slowly and to behave in a relatively predictable manner.

The ability of tumor cells to invade normal tissues and organs and to invade vascular spaces and metastasize is determined by the expression of many different cellular proteins. The type of tumor and its level of differentiation predict which of these abilities a given tumor may have or acquire. The cancer stage is a systematic classification of the extent of tumor spread at its site of origin and throughout the body by metastasis. The cell of origin of a tumor (i.e., the tumor type) and its pathologic stage are the most important determinants of its clinical behavior. Tumor grade (i.e., the degree of tumor cell differentiation or anaplasia; usually described as "well differentiated," "moderately differentiated," or "poorly differentiated") is also important but is almost always subordinate to tumor stage. Exceptions to these general principles occur, and in a number of pediatric malignancies, tumor grade and patient age can be much more important indicators of clinical behavior than tumor stage (e.g., neuroblastoma).

It has become clear over the past 20 years that most benign neoplasms contain genetic abnormalities (somatic mutations), some of which are similar or identical to those present in malignant neoplasms (Fig. 5-3). Genetic abnormalities in benign neoplasms are usually limited in scope and often correspond to a point mutation in a single gene. Genetic abnormalities in benign tumors tend to cause abnormal growth but usually do not result in genetic instability. Most benign neoplasms remain benign and do not progress to malignancy although a small minority eventually undergo malignant transformation.

●●● EPIDEMIOLOGY

Malignant neoplasms can develop in most human organs and tissues, but the frequency of tumor development varies greatly among different tissues. In adults, solid tumors are much more common than sarcomas or hematopoietic neoplasms (lymphomas and leukemias). Breast and prostate carcinoma each account for approximately one third of newly diagnosed cancers in women and men (respectively) in the United States.

Carcinomas of the lung follow next in incidence for both men and women (Fig. 5-4). Together these neoplasms account for more than 50% of cancers diagnosed in adults in the United States. The incidence of lung cancer grew strikingly in women after 1960 because of changes in smoking behavior (an eightfold increase in cancer death rate over 40 years). Since smoking is a major risk factor for many other types of

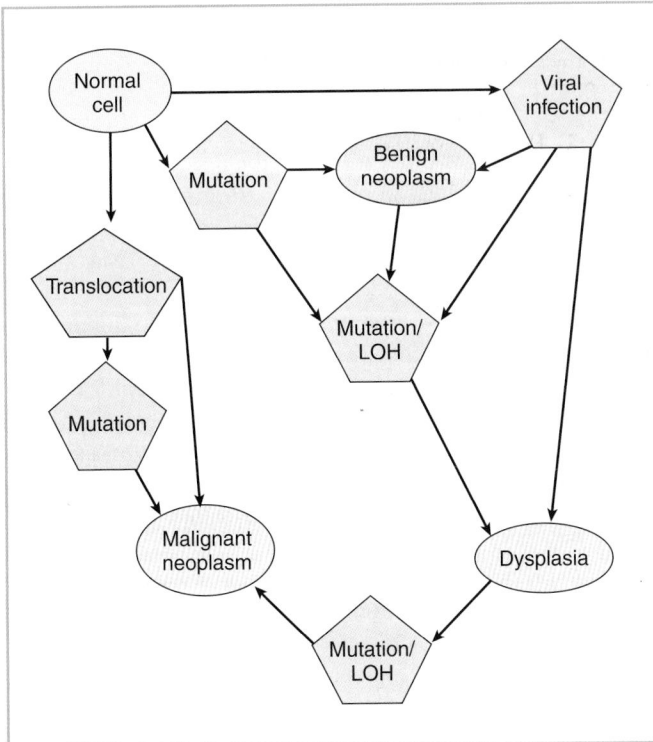

Figure 5-3. Pathways to tumor development.

CLINICAL MEDICINE

Cancer Epidemiology

The overall cancer death rate in the United States is 175 per 100,000. Cancer death and incidence rates for aggressive, incurable cancers (e.g., lung cancer) tend to be nearly identical, but there are significant differences in incidence and death rates for less aggressive cancers or cancers for which effective treatment is available. Survival with cancer for many years is typical in many cases of breast and prostate cancers. For this reason, although prostate and breast cancers are the most prevalent malignant tumors in men and women, respectively, they are each surpassed by lung cancer in terms of the number of cancer deaths per year.

Lung cancer accounts for approximately one third of cancer deaths in men and one quarter of cancer deaths in women. Conversely, prostate cancer accounts for only 10% of cancer deaths in men and breast cancer for 15% of cancer deaths in women.

Primary Site/ Tumor Type	New Cases/ 100,000	Deaths/ 100,000
Prostate	129	24
Gastrointestinal	117	61
Breast	112	28
Lung	87	77
Hematopoietic	47	26
Gynecologic	46	15
Renal/urinary	40	11
Melanoma	16	3
Oral	15	4
CNS	9	6
Endocrine	7	1
Sarcoma	4	2

Primary Site	5-Year Survival
Lung	13%
Oral	53%
Gastrointestinal	58%
Prostate	77%
Breast	79%

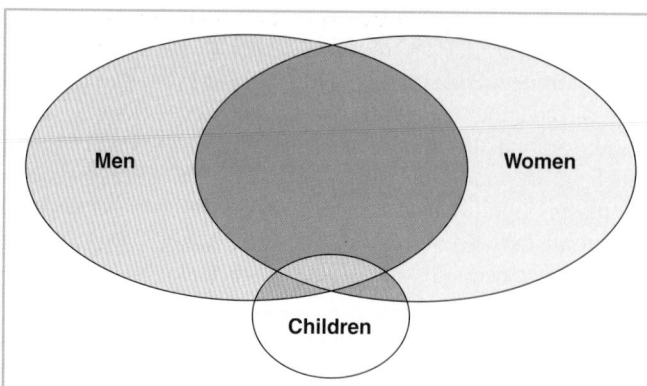

Figure 5-4. Distribution of cancer in men, women, and children.

malignant neoplasms, these behavioral changes have also shifted the incidence rates for other types of adult tumors.

Pediatric cancers are much less common than those in adults, and most childhood tumors have substantially different biology and genetics than adult tumors.

There are marked geographic differences in the incidence of some types of malignant tumors. Some of these differences reflect genetic differences in populations, but environmental influences are important as well. The incidence of breast cancer is much higher in the United States than in Japan, but native Japanese women who immigrate to the United States eventually acquire a risk for developing breast cancer similar to that in American women. Conversely, the rate of gastric adenocarcinoma is much higher in Japan than in the United States, and Japanese immigrants to the United States typically lower their risk for gastric adenocarcinoma.

Socioeconomic factors are also important in determining cancer incidence. Exposure to carcinogenic substances in the environment can be much higher in industrial areas than in rural locations. The prevalence of smoking and heavy alcohol consumption in social groups is an important determinant of cancer risk as well. In addition, viruses are important in the development of some tumors, and the venereal spread of human papillomavirus is the most important risk factor for the development of cervical carcinoma.

●●● CLONALITY OF NEOPLASMS

Neoplasms almost invariably develop from the clonal expansion of one cell (i.e., they are monoclonal rather than polyclonal) (Fig. 5-5). The conversion of a clonal cell population to a malignant neoplasm is usually a multistep process in which progeny of preneoplastic cells sequentially acquire additional genetic abnormalities. Eventually some clonally expanded cells acquire a fully malignant phenotype to produce an invasive tumor. This type of clonal selection (evolution) continues in established malignancies so that not all cells in an adult neoplasm are genetically identical and individual subclones may be identifiable (e.g., different growth patterns, different protein expression patterns, and different genotypes). Selection for different tumor cell prop-

Cancer Survival Rates and Clinical Trials

Survival rate is a statistical measure that summarizes the likelihood of different outcomes for a group of patients at a particular point in time. A survival curve is a graph of survival rates over time that is often adjusted for the age of the patient (to correct for deaths expected in individuals of this age that are not specifically related to cancer).

Since different patients in a study are usually observed for different time intervals, a mathematical model must be employed to calculate survival rates based on observable data. The most commonly employed model is the Kaplan-Meier method, which creates a life table in which the percentage of surviving patients is plotted versus time from the patient's date of cancer diagnosis or the date they were enrolled in the study. Individual patient death or disease recurrence is plotted as a data point. This method allows statistical comparison of treatment and control groups and is commonly used to compare the results of different therapies.

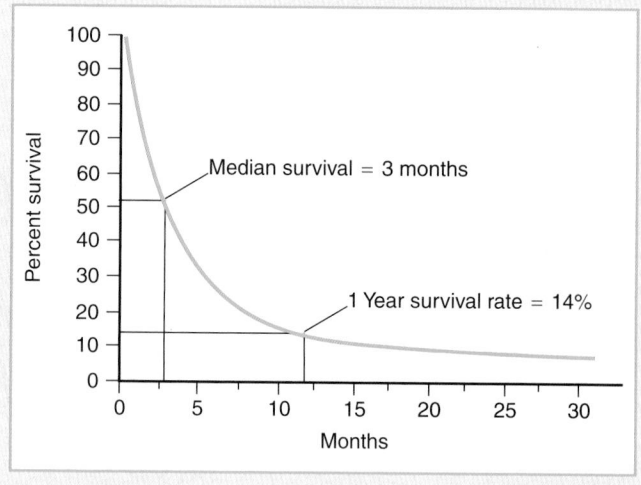

erties or capabilities often results in the development of more clinically aggressive neoplasms. Similarly, therapeutic maneuvers such as radiation therapy and chemotherapy may select for tumor subclones that are resistant to these treatments.

In addition to monoclonal tumor cells, all solid tumors contain stromal components that provide a supporting extracellular matrix and blood vessels that are essential for tumor cell growth beyond microscopic size. These stromal components are stimulated to grow by the cytokines and growth factors secreted by tumor cells and usually have a characteristic microscopic appearance called tumor desmoplasia (Fig. 5-6). Different neoplasms may be more or less adept at producing supporting vasculature and as a result may be associated with more or less ischemic necrosis.

While the stromal and vascular cells in tumors are not derived directly from tumor cells in most cases, they are usually abnormal in their configuration and in their relationship with tumor cells. Tumor-associated vasculature may express proteins not typically present on normal endothelial

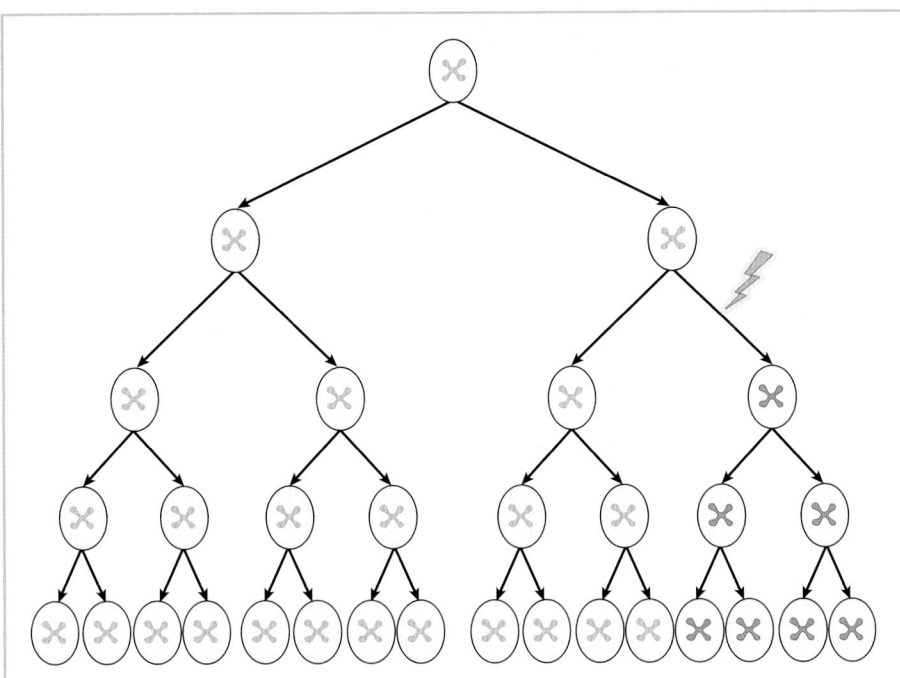

Figure 5-5. Clonal evolution of neoplasms.

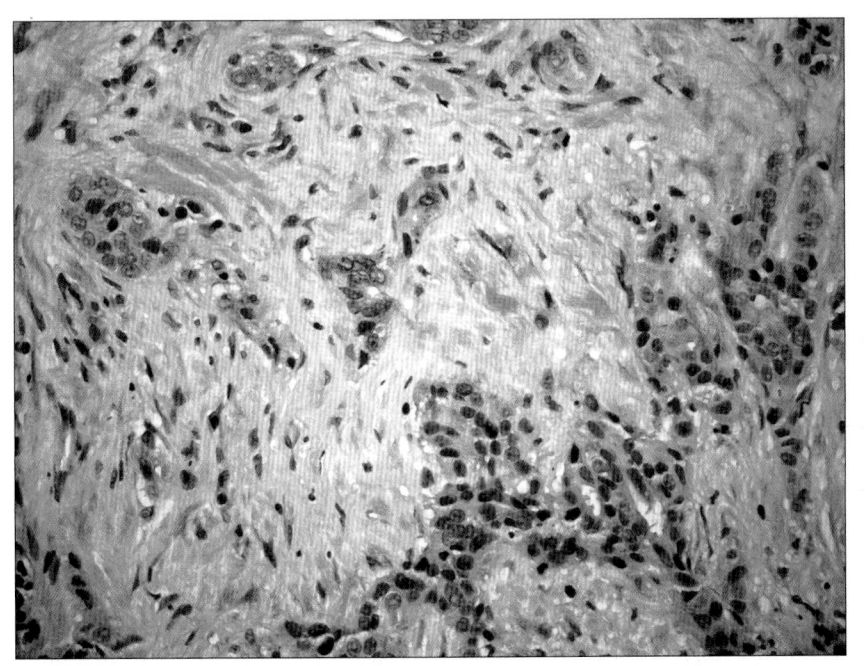

Figure 5-6. Desmoplastic stromal reaction. Section of breast carcinoma with marked stromal desmoplasia (slightly bluish [myxoid] appearance of tumor stroma similar to granulation tissue). This type of stromal reaction is a characteristic feature of most invasive carcinomas.

cells. In some situations, these different properties of tumor vasculature may provide useful therapeutic targets (e.g., blocking tumor angiogenesis or specifically attacking tumor vasculature).

●●● MOLECULAR GENETICS

The intense scientific study of cancer over the last 50 years has greatly advanced our understanding of molecular biology and molecular genetics in normal physiology. Conversely, the current level of understanding of molecular genetics permits a much more precise delineation of the changes that occur in normal cells that eventually convert them to malignant neoplasms. The study of genetic abnormalities in families with a high frequency of specific kinds of cancer has allowed the identification of specific genetic lesions in the germline and in tumors. Although these familial cancer syndromes comprise only a tiny percentage of adult cancers, many of the genetic lesions in these syndromes are causally involved in the development of sporadic cancers.

Cell Cycle Control and Genetic Instability

Abnormal proliferation is a critical feature of most malignant neoplasms. For this reason, the proteins and systems that control DNA replication and cell division are central to the development of most types of neoplasia. Normal cells (except for germ cells) have a limited ability to replicate. For most somatic cells, this replicative ability is quite limited, and growth arrest supervenes after a predetermined number of cell replications. This replication block is controlled by the activity of the enzyme telomerase, which maintains the length of telomere repeats ($TTAGGG_n$) at the ends of chromosomes. Telomerase activity in non–germ cells diminishes with each cell division, resulting in a progressive decrease in the length of telomeres in daughter cells. As telomere length diminishes, chromosome fusion and other abnormalities can occur that either trigger apoptosis (in normal cells) or result in mutations in daughter cells. Somatic stem cells have diminished telomerase activity and replicative capacity compared with embryonic stem cells, and telomerase expression is down-regulated as their progeny undergo terminal differentiation. Most tumor cells reactivate telomerase activity during tumorigenesis to overcome this potential replication block. Neoplastic transformation of the stem cells can result in tumors with nearly unlimited replicative capacity without up-regulation of telomerase expression.

Many of the first family cancer syndromes identified involved genes that control cell replication. Abnormalities of these genes can lead to major abnormalities in the control of cell division that result in genetic instability and a high incidence of cancer development. Retinoblastoma is a rare tumor of the retina of eye. A high percentage of retinoblastoma cases are heritable (autosomal dominant predisposition), resulting from defects in the retinoblastoma gene that inactivate one normal allele. The retinoblastoma protein (Rb) is central to the control of cell cycle progression at the G_1S checkpoint (see Chapter 3 and below). Therefore, it is easy to see why abnormalities of this protein can cause abnormal cell proliferation and tumor development. Tumor suppressor genes are cellular proteins that normally function to prevent tumor development, and retinoblastoma typifies the behavior of a classical tumor suppressor gene.

The G_1S cell cycle checkpoint is critical in controlling the rate of proliferation of cells and in preventing cells with genetic abnormalities from undergoing replication. Signals from growth factors stimulate cells to move from the inactive G_0 stage to G_1 and ultimately to S phase, where DNA synthesis is initiated. Stimulation of growth factor receptors is required to initiate cell division in normal cells. Many growth factors bind to receptor tyrosine kinases (RTKs), which can activate several types of signaling pathways to promote cell cycle entry (Fig. 5-7). Many of these RTKs and proteins involved in downstream signaling are targets for mutation and can contribute to the formation or progression of both benign and malignant neoplasms. Constitutive activation of these pathways in tumor cells often results in increased cell cycle entry and proliferation.

Binding of an RTK to its cognate receptor can result in activation of RAS proteins by binding GTP, which can in turn activate RAF proteins that activate MAP kinase to phosphorylate a number of specific target proteins. Protein phosphorylation causes changes in gene transcription that promote cell cycle progression in sensitive cells. Activated RAS can be inactivated by the tumor suppressor gene NF-1, which is associated with some forms of hereditary neurofibromatosis. Ligand binding by some RTKs can result in activation of PI3 kinase, which phosphorylates and activates the protein Akt. Like MAP kinase, Akt can promote cell progression by modifying gene expression. Akt activation can also indirectly inhibit apoptosis by interfering with the function of the proapoptotic protein BAD. BAD normally inhibits the antiapoptotic mitochondrial protein BCL-2 so that the ultimate effect of Akt activation is up-regulation of BCL-2 and relative protection from apoptosis. Another tumor suppressor gene PTEN (phosphatase and tensin analog deleted from chromosome 10; germline mutations cause Cowden's disease) normally functions to activate BAD, favoring apoptosis. Blockage of apoptosis can allow cells with DNA damage to escape programmed cell death at G_1S and cause mutations in daughter cells that may result in tumorigenesis or tumor progression.

Cyclin-dependent kinases are key mediators of cell cycle progression that are activated by elevated cellular levels of cyclin proteins. A major consequence of RTK stimulation is an increase in cyclin D expression, which activates cyclin-dependent kinase 4 (CDK-4) to phosphorylate the retinoblastoma tumor suppressor gene product (Rb). Rb normally binds to and sequesters the E2F transcription factor, but phosphorylation of Rb results in the dissociation of this complex and the release of E2F. E2F can then bind to transcriptional targets, resulting in the final activation of DNA synthesis and cell cycle progression. The balance of these progrowth and antigrowth activities is critical in maintaining the genetic stability of cells during and after DNA replication.

Specific molecular pathways are active at G_1S in normal cells to detect and repair genetic lesions prior to the initiation of DNA synthesis (the most important of these is the p53 tumor suppressor gene product). Activation of p53 at G_1S results in the inhibition of cell cycle progression by the direct inhibition of CDK-4.

If DNA damage is corrected, some cells may progress to DNA replication. If the genetic abnormalities are not corrected, p53 may activate apoptotic pathways, resulting in programmed cell death. While p53 occupies a central role in blocking DNA synthesis and triggering apoptosis at G_1S, other cellular proteins are important in controlling this transition as well and many of these genes are targeted in different tumors (Fig. 5-8).

The p16 gene product is an important inhibitor of CDK-4 that can be activated through the TGF-β signaling pathway. The p16 gene locus is complex, and TGF-β signaling also results in the formation of a second protein (P14ARF), which down-regulates the MDM-2 protein and prevents it from inhibiting p53.

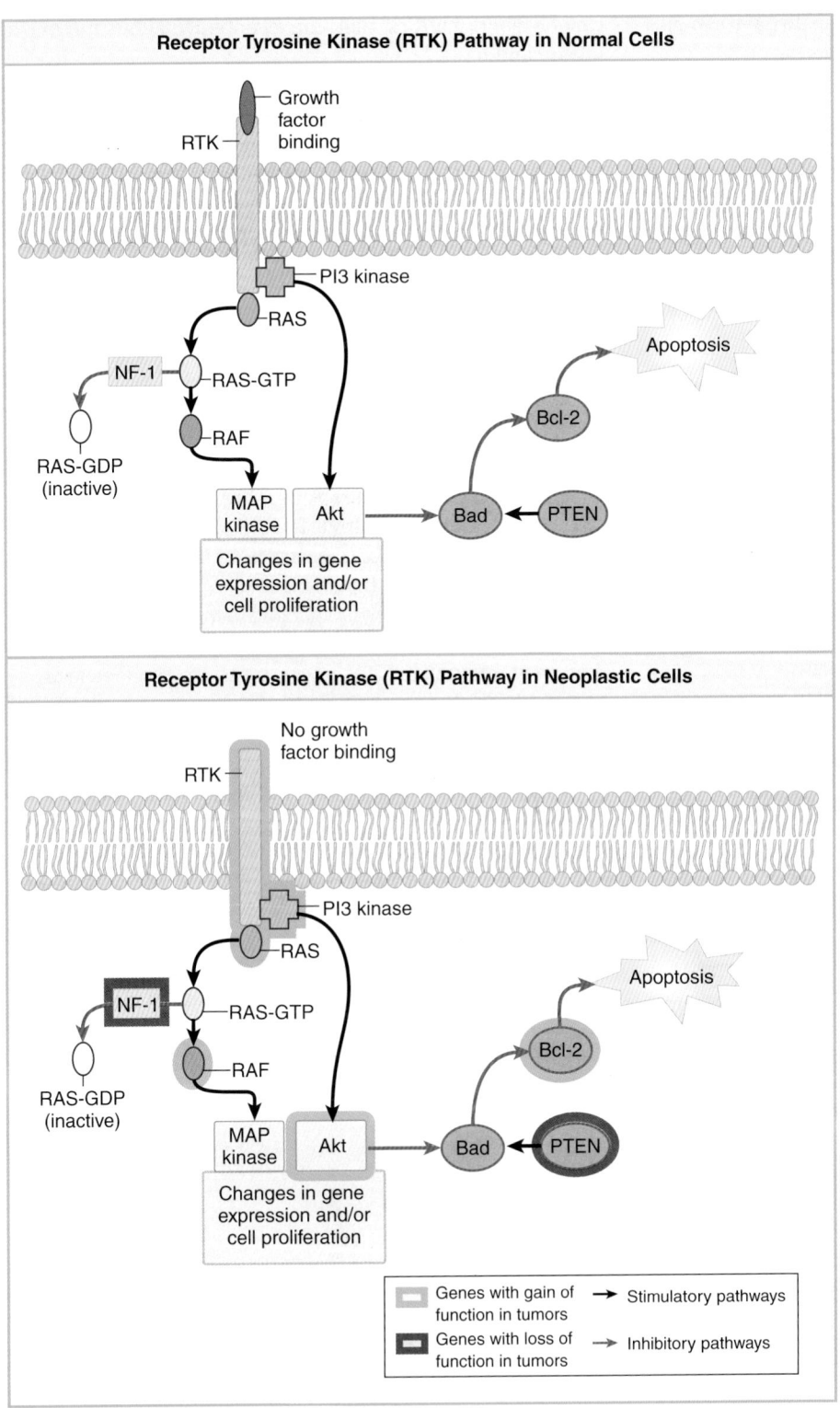

Figure 5-7. Receptor tyrosine kinase signaling in normal cells and in tumor cells.

This two-pronged affect results in enhanced p53 function and diminished CDK-4 activity. TGF-β signaling also results in up-regulation of other CDK inhibitors, such as p27, which can further inhibit cells cycle progression in sensitive cells. Loss of function of one or more of these pathways in tumor cells can result in a high level of genetic instability and resistance to apoptosis that characterizes most malignant neoplasms. This phenotype results in rapid tumor growth and enhanced selection of more biologically aggressive tumor cell variants. The G_1S cell cycle checkpoint is not the only mechanism for detecting genetic abnormalities during DNA replication. Similar checkpoints are active at the G_2M transition, but these pathways are less well characterized. The ability of tumor cells to initiate apoptosis at G_1S or at G_2M (or both) is critical for the activity of many chemotherapeutic agents and ionizing radiation that are used to treat malignant neoplasms. Defects in these key pathways can also result in profound resistance to these therapies.

Oncogenes and Proto-oncogenes

Viral oncogenes were first discovered in animal tumor viruses and correspond to mammalian genes that have been incorporated into the viral genome through genetic recombination.

Alterations in the coding sequence of these genes result in constitutively active proteins that are expressed as viral oncogenes. Most viral oncogenes are involved in signal transduction, and their expression in infected cells results in constitutive activation of critical pathways that tend to push these cells into the cell cycle. Increased and abnormal proliferation favor the acquisition of additional genetic changes in transformed cells to produce a malignant neoplasm. These changes often result in genetic instability that sets the stage for the acquisition of many additional

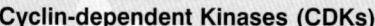

BIOCHEMISTRY

Cyclin-dependent Kinases (CDKs)

CDKs are a family of related proteins that bind to specific cyclin proteins to form active complexes that can phosphorylate specific target molecules. CDKs play a critical role in cell replication, and different CDKs are sequentially activated and inactivated during G_1, S, and M phases of the cell cycle.
- CDK4 binds cyclin D at the G_1S transition to activate it to phosphorylate the retinoblastoma protein (Rb).
- CDK2 binds cyclin E late in G_1 and with cyclin A in S phase to mediate the G_2M transition.
- CDK1 binds cyclin B in G_2M.

---

genetic abnormalities that can eventually allow tumors to invade and metastasize.

Based on information derived from the study of viral oncogenes, it became clear that many normal human genes can act as proto-oncogenes (i.e., mutations in these genes can create a constitutively active protein that may initiate tumor formation). In most cases, only very specific point mutations in proto-oncogenes result in their constitutive activation (e.g., most gain of function mutations in K-ras are restricted to specific amino acid substitutions in codons 12 or 13). Most RTK pathways include multiple proto-oncogenes, and activating mutations in the receptor tyrosine kinase itself or in downstream signaling molecules such as RAS, RAF, or PI3 kinase can result in constitutive signaling. Inactivation of some tumor suppressor genes, NF-1, or PTEN can also up-regulate these signaling pathways in normal cells or potentiate the effects of activating mutations in other oncogenes.

The effects of constitutive RTK signaling are different in cells of different types. Activation of these pathways can substitute for growth factor signals to promote cell replication, or they may result in more complex transcriptional changes that allow tumor cells to acquire new phenotypes that may be needed for local invasion, angiogenesis, or metastasis. Mutation of single proto-oncogenes such as RAS and RAF are often involved in the formation of benign neoplasms, such as intestinal polyps, which show abnormal proliferation but usually do not necessarily progress to malignant neoplasms.

Tumor Suppressor Genes

Tumor suppressor genes usually function in a manner that prevents or diminishes the likelihood of malignant transformation. Loss of function of a tumor suppressor gene

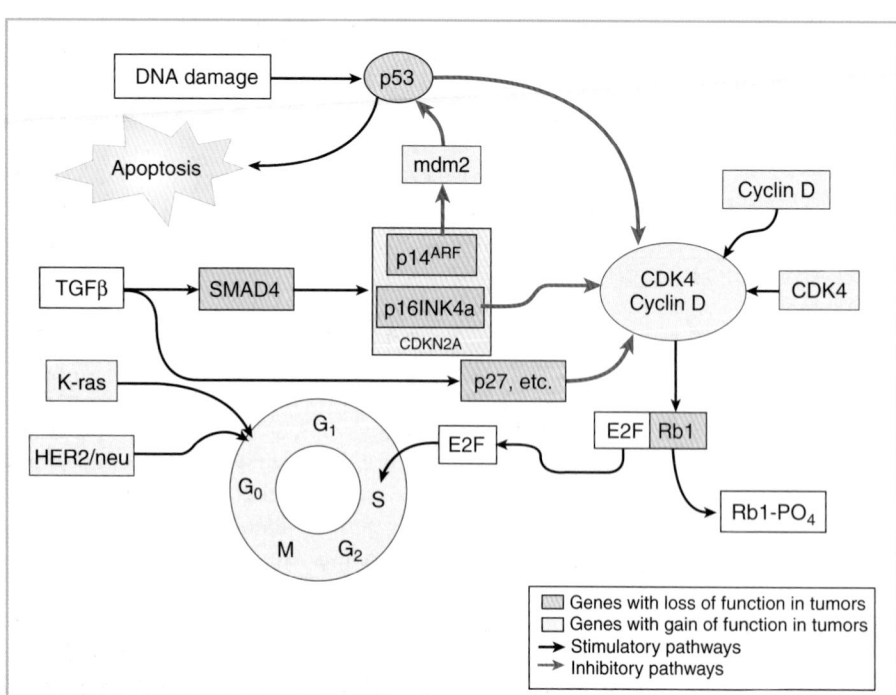

Figure 5-8. G_1S cell cycle checkpoint in tumor cells.

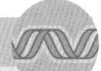

GENETICS

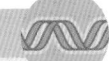

p16 Gene Organization

The CDKN2A locus (also known as INK4a/ARF) consists of four exons (1α, 1β, 2, and 3) that encode the P16P16^{INK4a} and P14^{ARF} proteins. The P16^{INK4a} protein is produced by transcripts that include exons 1α, 2, and 3 and functions as an inducible inhibitor of CDK4 and CDK6, blocking their ability to phosphorylate the retinoblastoma protein RB. Phosphorylated RB (pRB) is required to activate cell cycle progression. P16^{INK4a} contains four ankyrin domains, the second and third of which interact with CDK4/6 and are targeted by point mutation in tumors.

P14^{ARF} protein is produced by transcripts that include exons 1β, 2, and 3 but utilizes an alternative reading frame in exons 2 and 3 and so has a protein sequence that is not homologous with P16^{INK4a}. The purpose of this unusual gene organization is not known. P14^{ARF} inhibits MDM2, which normally targets the P53 protein for ubiquitination and subsequent destruction in the proteosome.

Mutations or deletions of the CDKN2A locus can thereby result in loss of both P16^{INK4a} and P14^{ARF} function to disrupt both P53 and CDK4-RB pathways at G$_1$S. It is not surprising that this dual inactivation event can result in substantial genetic instability and act as a pathway to malignancy. The evolutionary purpose of the unusual genetic organization of this locus (encoding two important tumor suppressors) is not known.

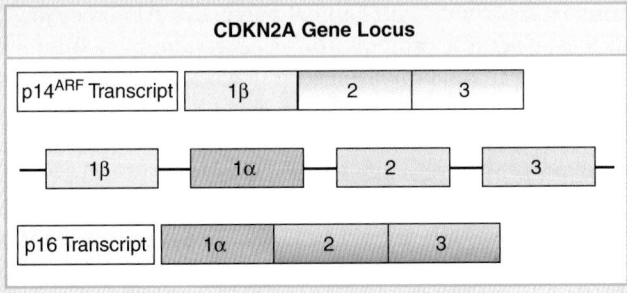

CDKN2A Gene Locus

GENETICS

Oncogenes

Oncogenes are mutated or overexpressed cellular genes (proto-oncogenes) that are normally involved in cell growth and differentiation. Mutations that result in gain of function for a proto-oncogene can produce a dominant neoplastic phenotype if only one copy of the gene is affected. (In contrast, inactivation of both copies of most tumor suppressor genes is required to produce a neoplastic phenotype.) Oncogenes typically belong to one of five classes of molecules:

- Growth factors that are overexpressed (e.g., PDGF, FGF, TGF, and HGF)
- Growth factor receptors with mutations that result in their constitutive activation (e.g., RET and c-kit)
- Growth factor receptors that are overexpressed (e.g., HER2/neu, EGFR, PDGF-R)
- Signal transduction proteins with mutations that result in their constitutive activation (RAS, ABL, BRAF)
- Transcription factors that are overexpressed (c-myc, N-myc, and L-myc)
- Cell cycle regulatory proteins that are overexpressed (cyclin D, cyclin E, and CDK4)

retinoblastoma protein in cell cycle control, abnormalities of this single gene are sufficient to produce a malignant tumor in susceptible cells. Patients with familial retinoblastoma are also at increased risk for osteosarcoma but surprisingly are not at markedly increased risk for many other common cancers.

Germline genetic alterations in the p53 and p16 tumor suppressor genes also occur and predispose to the development of different tumors. p16 gene mutations typically can cause familial melanoma, with a substantially increased risk for development of this highly malignant tumor. p53 gene mutations produce the Li-Fraumeni syndrome, in which patients are at substantially increased risk for many types of solid tumors. Presentation with a sarcoma at a young age or with multiple primary solid tumors is typical. Mutant p53 often acts somewhat differently from a classic tumor suppressor gene. Because normal p53 protein functions as a homodimer, the abnormal p53 protein can bind to and functionally inactivate normal copies of p53, resulting in a dominant-negative phenotype. Abnormal p53 proteins are often more stable than normal p53 so that sequestration of normal p53 in nonfunctional heterodimers can result in the near total loss of p53 function in cells with a point mutation in only one allele. In this way, some p53 gene mutations genetically mimic proto-oncogene–activating mutations. This prominent dominant-negative phenotype is unusual; alterations in most other tumor suppressor genes result in a simple loss of function without dominant-negative effects.

Microsatellite Instability

Abnormalities of mutation repair pathways can result in the accumulation of mutations in many different genes in affected cells. In particular, cells with defective mismatch repair tend

---

predisposes a cell to neoplastic transformation. Many tumor suppressor genes are involved in cell cycle control (e.g., p53, p16, Rb). Heritable alterations in these genes can markedly increase the risk for tumor development in many different cell types. Patients with familial retinoblastoma develop normally with one defective copy (and one normal copy) of the retinoblastoma gene (Fig. 5-9). Somatic mutation (ultraviolet radiation) or loss of the normal copy of the retinoblastoma gene (LOH) in retinal cells triggers tumor formation. In normal individuals who carry two functional copies of the retinoblastoma gene, two independent somatic mutations in a retinal cell are required for tumor development. This "one-hit" versus "two-hit" model for tumor development was originally suggested by Knudson and underlies the genetics of classic tumor suppressor genes. Mutations in tumor suppressor genes are usually inherited as autosomal dominant genetic diseases (i.e., the predisposition for tumor development is inherited in a dominant manner) (see Fig. 5-9). Because of the central importance of the

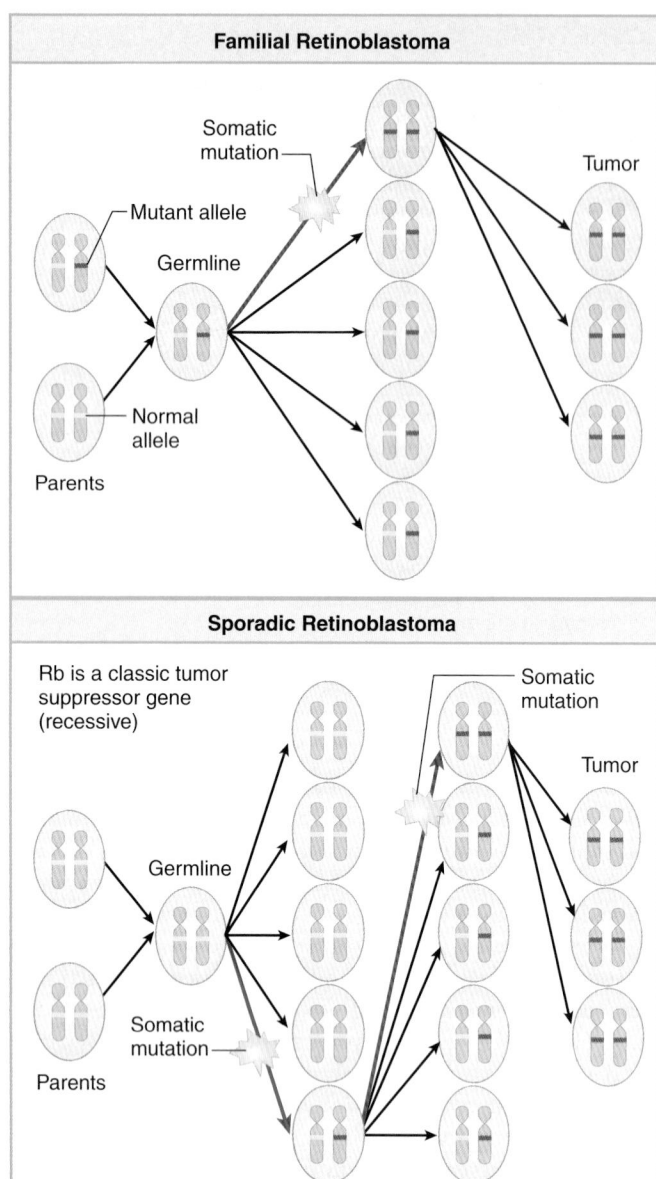

Figure 5-9. Genetics of familial and sporadic retinoblastoma.

to show great variability in the number of short nucleotide repeats in specific genes. These size differences can be detected by PCR analysis of affected loci and this type of assay defines the microsatellite instability (MSI) phenotype (Fig. 5-10A). Addition or subtraction of repeats can result in inactivation of susceptible genes so that high-MSI tumors (i.e., tumors with detectable microsatellites in two or more loci) have a high mutation rate.

Heritable deficiency of one mismatch repair gene (usually MLH-1 or MSH-2) causes the familial syndrome of hereditary nonpolyposis colorectal cancer (HNPCC; also called Lynch syndrome). This is an autosomal dominant disease in which loss of expression of the normal mismatch repair allele in tumors impairs the ability to repair acquired point mutations (see Fig. 5-10B). This syndrome frequently results in the development of colon cancer at a young age as well as tumors

in other organs (e.g., increased risk for endometrial carcinoma). Most tumors arising in HNPCC patients are high-MSI tumors that have a distinctive phenotype with abundant mucin production (mucinous tumors) and heavy infiltration by T lymphocytes. These tumors have a better prognosis (stage for stage) than do MSI-negative tumors. High-MSI tumors can also occur in individuals who inherit normal mismatch repair genes. In these sporadic MSI tumors, hypermethylation of the promotor region of one or more mismatch repair genes greatly reduces gene expression, resulting in functional inactivation of the gene (epigenetic gene silencing).

Other Pathways Involved in Cancer

Alterations in cell cycle control genes and in RTK signaling pathways are important in most human neoplasms, whereas genetic alterations in several other types of signaling pathways are important in some specific types of tumors.

Wnt Signaling Pathway

The Wnt signaling pathway operates by modulation levels of β-catenin in the nucleus and cytoplasm (Fig. 5-11A). Most β-catenin is bound to the integral membrane protein E-cadherin, and free β-catenin is rapidly inactivated through the activity of the APC protein (i.e., the product of the adenomatous polyposis coli gene, which is mutated in the germline of patients with familial polyposis). APC specifically attaches ubiquitin proteins to lysine residues on β-catenin that target it to the proteasome for degradation. This degradative pathway normally prevents β-catenin from translocating to the nucleus, where it can induce c-myc and cyclin D1 expression to promote cell cycle entry and progression. Binding of the WNT ligand to a specific GPCR promotes the dissociation of β-catenin from the E-cadherin, facilitating the translocation of β-catenin to the nucleus. WNT signaling also inhibits the APC protein, which would otherwise target free β-catenin to the proteasome. In this manner, cytoplasmic and nuclear levels of β-catenin are elevated and the affected cell is stimulated to enter the cell cycle. Inactivating mutations of the APC gene result in constitutive WNT signaling, which is a key event in the formation of sporadic and heritable adenomatous colon polyps. Abnormalities in β-catenin and E-cadherin can also result in constitutive activation of WNT signaling and increased cell cycle entry. E-cadherin is an essential component of the tight junctions (desmosomes) between cells, and loss of functional E-cadherin in tumors results in poorly cohesive tumor cells.

Adenocarcinomas with defective E-cadherin expression have constitutively active WNT signaling and tend to infiltrate as single cells (i.e., they do not form architectural structures such as glands). Diffusely infiltrating adenocarcinomas often have an E-cadherin–negative phenotype and tend to be clinically aggressive (see Figs. 5-11B and C).

TGF-β Signaling Pathway

TGF-β is an important inhibitor of cell cycle entry or progression in some cells types and may act to prevent tumor

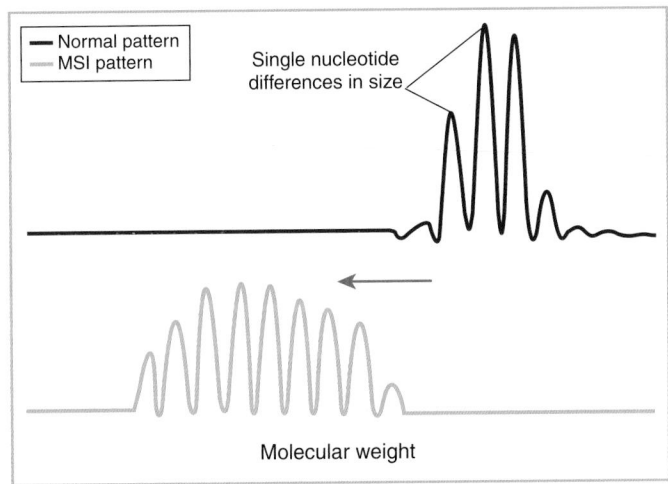

Figure 5-10. A, Microsatellite instability (MSI). Capillary electrophoresis pattern of PCR products generated from a normal cell (*top*) or from a high-MSI tumor (*bottom*). There is increased size variability and a shift in the average length of PCR products with the high-level MSI phenotype. **B**, MSI and hereditary nonpolyposis coli (HNPCC).

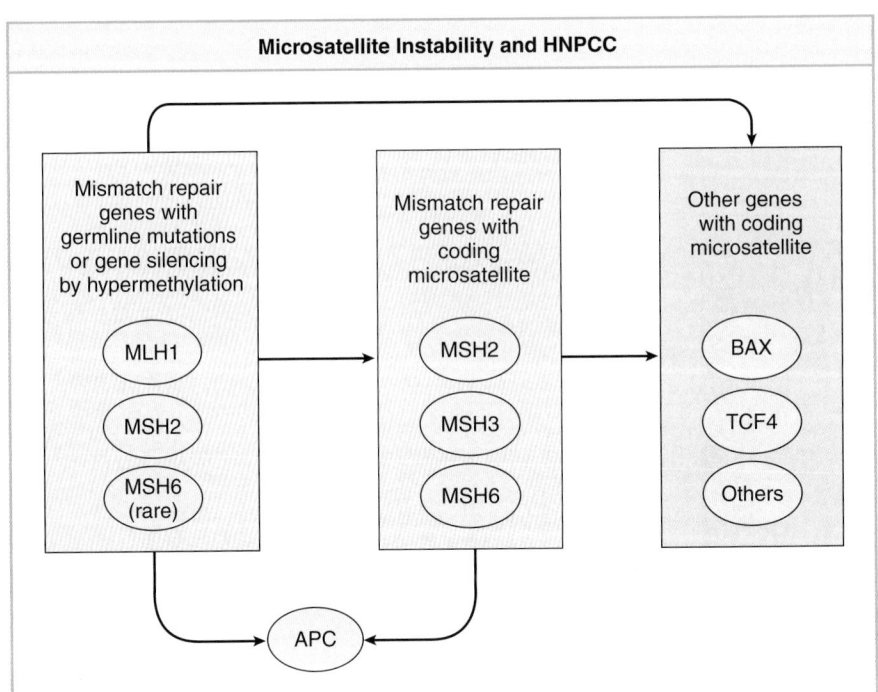

Von Hippel–Lindau (VHL) Gene and Angiogenesis

development. TGF-β signals through a membrane receptor that signals by phosphorylation of SMAD2 protein, which in turn activates SMAD4. SMAD4 can then activate multiple specific inhibitors of cell cycle progression at G_1S including p16 (and p14ARF) and p27 (Fig. 5-12). Together, these proteins directly inhibit CDK-4 or up-regulate p53 (to indirectly inhibit CDK-4 and promote apoptosis). These effects help maintain genetic stability in TGF-β–responsive cells. SMAD2 and SMAD4 as well as the TGF-β receptor itself can be inactivated in tumor cells. The MEN1 protein (which enhances the activation of SMAD4 by activated SMAD2) is altered in a heritable syndrome that results in the development of multiple endocrine tumors as well as several other specific tumors in other organs.

Von Hippel–Lindau (VHL) disease is an autosomal dominant genetic disease in which patients inherit a defective copy of the VHL tumor suppressor gene that is involved in the regulation of angiogenesis induced by hypoxia. This important pathway controls the production of the angiogenic cytokines (VEGF and PDGF) and epidermal growth factor receptor (EGFR). The VHL protein normally down-regulates expression of oxidized HIF-1 (hypoxia-inducible factor 1) by targeting it to the proteasome for destruction (by attaching ubiquitin to lysine residues on the HIF-1 protein) (Fig. 5-13A). HIF-1 normally acts as a metabolic sensor for oxygen levels, and inactivation of VHL results in increased intracellular concentrations of HIF-1 that cause enhanced

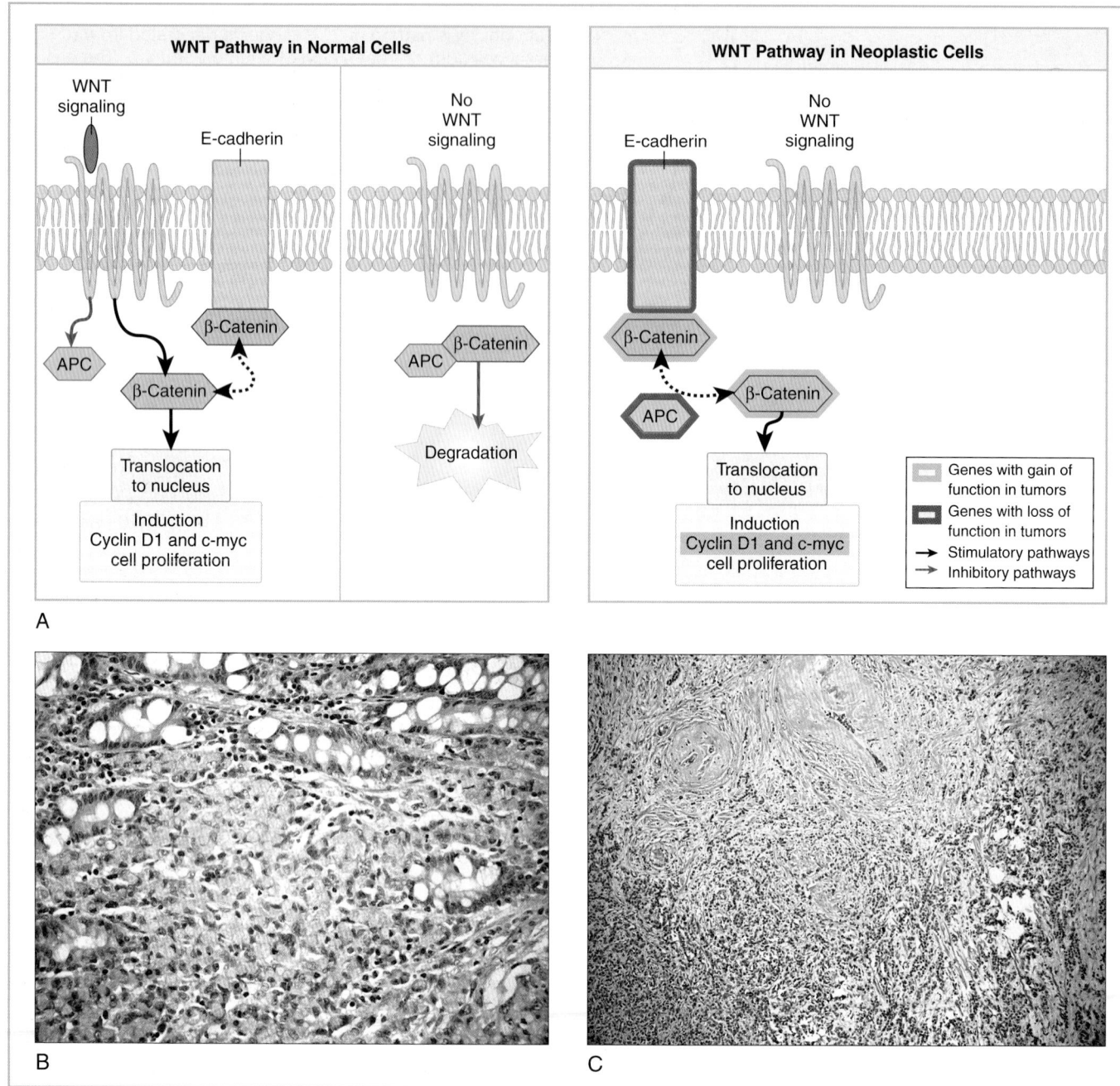

Figure 5-11. A, WNT signaling pathway in normal cells and in tumor cells. **B**, Signet ring cell adenocarcinoma. Photomicrograph of a poorly differentiated colon cancer with prominent signet ring cells and lack of cellular cohesion resulting from loss of E-cadherin expression. **C**, Lobular carcinoma of the breast. Photomicrograph of invasive lobular breast cancer showing single tumor cells infiltrating stroma associated with loss of E-cadherin expression.

transcription of proangiogenic cytokines and EGFR. Patients with VHL disease develop multiple specific types of benign tumors at characteristic locations (e.g., cerebellar hemangioblastoma, a largely vascular tumor) (see Fig. 5-13B) and also are at increased risk for clear-cell carcinoma of the kidney (a highly vascular malignant tumor) (see Fig. 5-13C). Sporadic clear-cell carcinoma of the kidney is also associated with very prominent vascular proliferation, and almost all these tumors have targeted disruption of the VHL gene on chromosome 3p in addition to other genetic changes.

Gene Amplification

Gene amplification means the abnormal presence of more than two copies of a gene in a nondividing cell (a few genes are normally present in more than one copy per diploid genome, e.g., α-globin). Gene amplification usually results in enhanced expression of the amplified gene and amplification of some proto-oncogenes is an important mechanism in the progression of some types of tumors. It is unclear why amplification characteristically develops in some types of tumors

HISTOLOGY

Desmosomes

Desmosomes are junctional complexes (adhering junctions) between the membranes of adjacent cells. Hemidesmosomes form between epithelial cells and their underlying basement membrane.

Desmosomes are composed of desmoplakin and other proteins, which form an electron-dense plaque immediately beneath the plasma membrane. Tonofilaments and the cytoplasmic portion of some transmembrane proteins insert into the plaque. Cadherins (calcium-dependent adherence proteins) also are associated with desmosomes and penetrate the cell membrane to interact with cognate proteins on adjacent cells. Cadherins function to hold the cells in contact with one another across desmosomes. Since cadherin binding is calcium dependent, these cell junctions are also calcium dependent. Cadherins also connect to actin in the cytoskeleton through α- and β-catenins. β-Catenin also plays a key role in Wnt signal transduction.

In routine histologic sections, the presence of desmosomes can be inferred by the scalloping of cell membranes between desmosomes that result from retraction artifact (tissue shrinkage during formalin fixation).

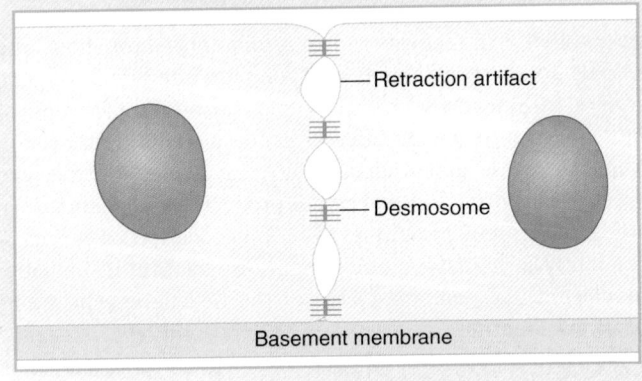

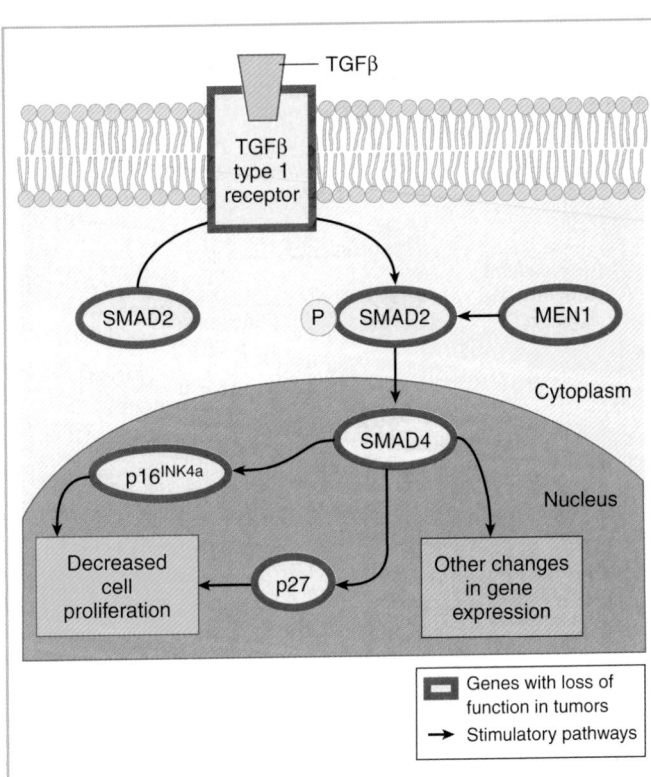

Figure 5-12. TGF-β/SMAD signaling pathway.

and not in others. Gene amplification can occur in situ, forming a so-called homogeneously staining region (HSR) in the normal chromosomal location of the gene (many copies of the gene are present as tandem repeats) or as so-called double minute chromosomes (extra chromosomal fragments of DNA containing multiple copies of the amplified gene). Gene amplification is much more likely to occur in tumor cells that have already acquired genetic instability through alterations in cell cycle checkpoint pathways. Gene amplification can also occur as an artifact when tumor cells are cultured in vitro.

Amplification of the N-myc gene in neuroblastoma is an adverse prognostic factor for neuroblastoma that is correlated with decreased survival and was one of the first clinical applications of a molecular biologic assay. HER2/neu proto-oncogene amplification occurs in a subset of clinically aggressive breast cancers that can be detected by fluorescence in situ hybridization.

High-level expression of HER2/neu results in increased HER2/neu protein expression and signaling for proliferation through this RTK (Fig. 5-14). HER2/neu gene amplification is important also because it provides a specific biologic target for a humanized monoclonal antibody (trastuzumab), which binds to the overexpressed receptor protein. Antibody binding to the HER2/neu protein can induce apoptosis in some tumor cells. As expected, trastuzumab is more effective in treating tumors that strongly overexpress HER2/neu, and so protein overexpression and gene amplification are important predictive markers for response to trastuzumab. The success of this targeted therapy (trastuzumab) has become an important paradigm in oncology, and many other biologic therapies are currently under development.

Chromosomal Translocation

Specific chromosomal translocations can serve as useful diagnostic markers for some types of neoplasms. For instance, translocation of a portion of the bcl-2 proto-oncogene to the immunoglobulin heavy chain gene locus is common in follicular non-Hodgkin's lymphoma (NHL) and is a clinically useful genetic marker for this neoplasm. This translocation results in the overexpression of BCL-2 protein to inhibit apoptosis in tumor cells.

Chromosome translocations can also result in the actual fusion of two different genes to produce a novel chimeric protein (fusion protein) that is not normally present in human cells. Chimeric proteins often have new and abnormal functions (Fig. 5-15). Many fusion proteins act as transcription

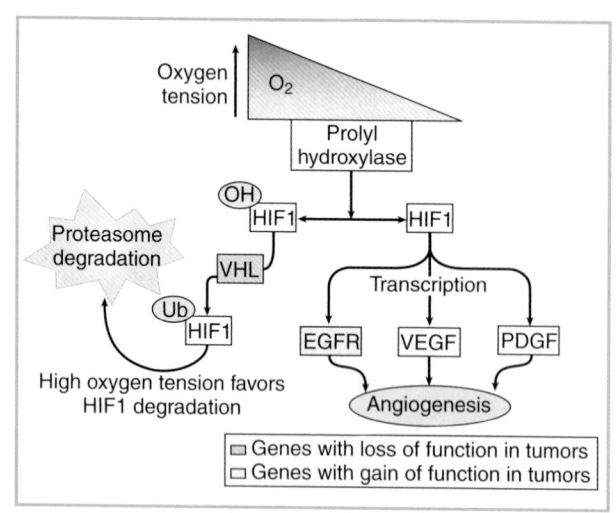

A

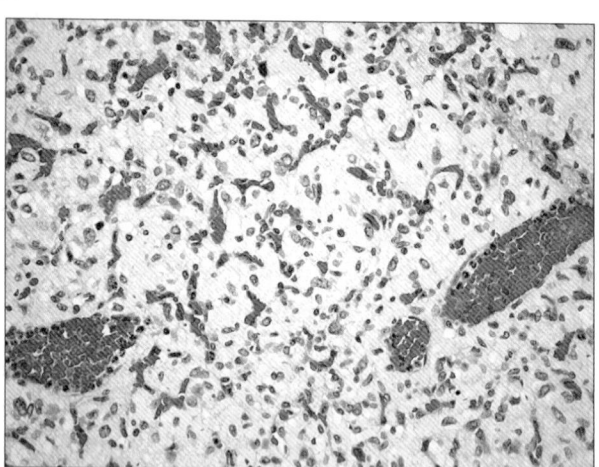

B

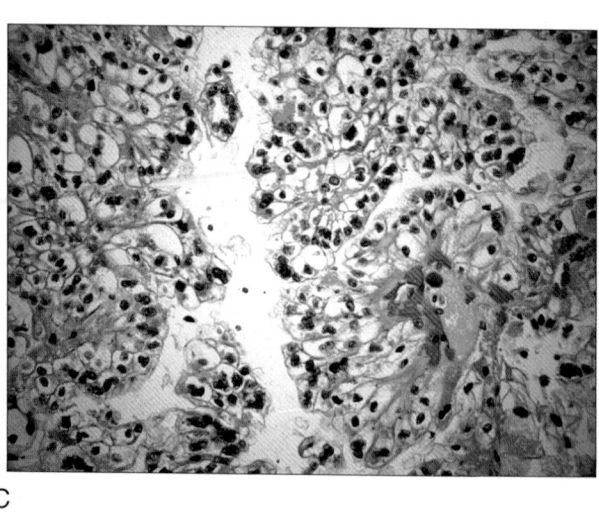

C

Figure 5-13. A, Control of angiogenesis. **B**, Hemangioblastoma. Photomicrograph of benign, highly vascular brain tumor, which frequently develops in patients with VHL disease. **C**, Renal clear-cell carcinoma. Photomicrograph of a highly vascular, malignant clear-cell carcinoma of the kidney, which is almost always associated with somatic deletion of the VHL gene.

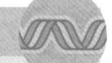

GENETICS

Fluorescence in Situ Hybridization (FISH)

FISH is an in vitro assay that uses a fluorescent reporter attached to a DNA probe to detect the presence of specific DNA sequences in chromosomes by molecular hybridization. Although FISH can be used to help identify individual metaphase chromosomes in classical cytogenetics (e.g., chromosome painting), it has a wider clinical application in interphase cytogenetics that can be performed on routine histologic sections (i.e., metaphase chromosomes are not required).

During interphase, chromosomes are distributed throughout the nucleus, but the number of hybridization signals in a cell's nucleus (as enumerated by fluorescence microscopy) can provide information about gene copy number (e.g., the presence of gene deletion or gene amplification). The use of two different colored probes specific for each gene involved in the translocation can allow identification of the translocation. Translocation results in the colocalization of the two hybridization probes to produce a fused color signal (e.g., gene fusion converts separate red and green signals to a single, fused yellow signal).

factors that can activate novel promoters throughout the genome to cause extensive and complex alterations in gene expression. Since these hybrid proteins can activate (or repress) the expression of many different genes, a single translocation event can cause global changes in gene expression that can directly transform a normal cell to produce a malignancy.

Fusion proteins resulting from translocation occur most frequently in hematopoietic neoplasms, a subset of pediatric neoplasms, and sarcomas. One of the first neoplastic translocations identified is a marker chromosome (the so-called Philadelphia chromosome) in patients with chronic leukemia. Tumors that express chimeric proteins are often defined diagnostically by the presence of these specific translocation events. For example, the pathologic diagnosis of acute promyelocytic leukemia (a variant of myeloid leukemia) now rests on the demonstration of a translocation between the retinoic acid receptor (RAR) protein gene and the PML gene. Treatment of patients who have leukemias expressing this fusion protein with all-*trans*-retinoic acid can induce clinical remission in a high percentage. Malignant neoplasms resulting from single translocation events tend to retain intact apoptotic pathways and are often more responsive to cancer treatment than are many carcinomas. Since most carcinomas develop by the sequential accumulation of numerous genetic alterations, they often have defective apoptotic pathways and are resistant to many forms of therapy.

Epigenetic Change

While the study of mutations and translocations has dominated cancer research to date, it is now clear that epigenetic changes in tumor cells (which are at least partially heritable) are also important in the development of many human

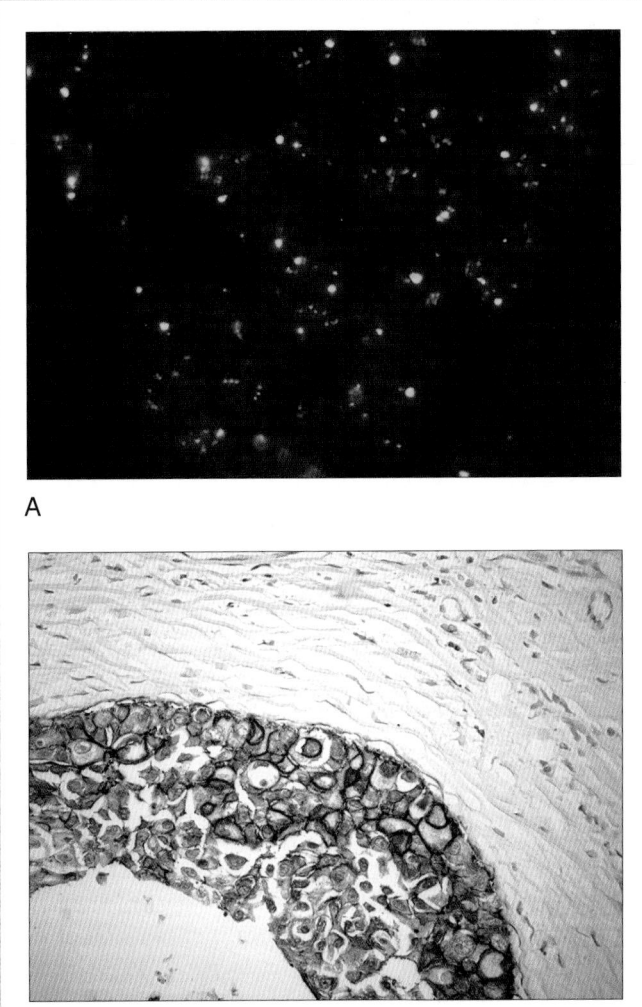

A

B

Figure 5-14. A, Fluorescence in situ hybridization (FISH) showing high-level HER2/neu gene amplification in breast cancer cells. The HER2/neu gene probe appears as orange dots. A control centromeric probe for chromosome 17 (*green*) is also visible. Nuclear envelopes are visible as faint staining above the black background of the photomicrograph. On average, two control probes are present per nucleus, whereas numerous HER2/neu probes (*orange*) are present, consistent with high-level gene amplification. **B,** Immunohistochemical staining for HER2/neu protein in intraductal breast cancer. Photomicrograph of breast cancer stained for HER2/neu protein. The brown cytoplasmic membrane staining corresponds to abundant HER2/neu protein expressed by these tumor cells.

tumors. Epigenetic changes often result in gene silencing through hypermethylation of promoter regions in tumor suppressor genes. This is the most common mechanism whereby mismatch repair genes are silenced in sporadic MSI tumors (see above). DNA methylation pattern is passed on to daughter cells as a relatively stable phenotype that does not depend on changes in DNA sequence. Epigenetic programming of normal differentiated cells is responsible for many of their phenotypic features (Fig. 5-16A). These differentiated

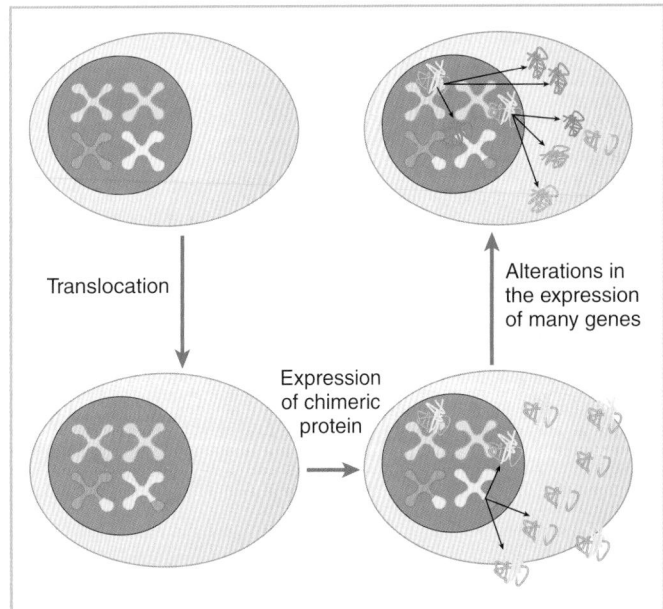

Figure 5-15. Chromosomal translocations in tumorigenesis.

features dominate the current classification of most adult tumors (e.g., squamous cell carcinoma, adenocarcinoma) and provide highly accurate information about their likely clinical behavior (see Fig. 5-16B). The loss of such differentiated features in tumor progression is likely due in part to the abrogation of epigenetic programming. Epigenetic changes are considerably more difficult to measure experimentally than are DNA sequence changes, and the true importance of epigenetic changes in the development and progression of cancer may be substantially underestimated because of these technical limitations.

●●● CARCINOGENESIS

Carcinogenesis is the process by which normal cells are converted to tumor cells. Carcinogenesis progresses by substantially different mechanisms in different tissue types and may be initiated by environmental exposure to carcinogens (chemicals, ionizing radiation, etc.) or infectious agents. While carcinogenesis may result from a single chromosomal translocation event (see above), this mechanism is unusual in the most common adult solid tumors. Carcinogenesis in most carcinomas occurs as a stepwise process in which normal cells are incrementally converted to tumor cells by the acquisition of multiple genetic and epigenetic alterations that ultimately cause genetic instability (Fig. 5-17). The genetic and epigenetic alterations that accumulate during carcinogenesis tend to target the seven critical cellular pathways/systems (proliferation, receptor tyrosine kinase, WNT, mutation repair, apoptosis, TGFB, and angiogenesis) discussed in detail above, which have important interconnections (Fig. 5-18). These pathways are consistently targeted in different types of tumors. In some cases (best demonstrated in colon cancer development), the acquisition of these genetic alterations appears to follow a relatively stereotyped order or pathway.

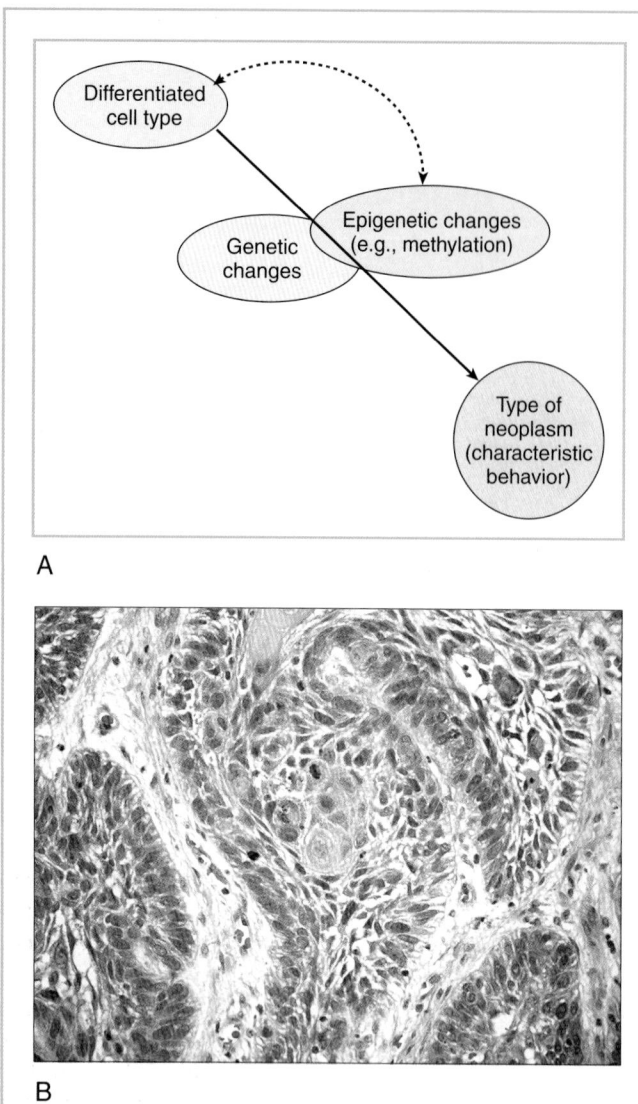

A

B

Figure 5-16. A, Factors determining tumor phenotype. **B,** Squamous cell carcinoma. Photomicrograph showing a moderately differentiated squamous cell carcinoma with prominent foci of keratinization.

This progression usually involves morphologic alterations (visible microscopically) that can be recognized as dysplasia or carcinoma in situ (see below) as well as genetic changes.

Irradiation

Ionizing radiation can be a potent carcinogen and acts predominantly by creating free radicals that can damage DNA and result in heritable genetic changes. High levels of ionizing radiation can result in double-strand DNA breaks. Ultraviolet (UV) radiation from the sun results in dimerization of thymidine residues in DNA, and defective repair of these dimers leads to mutation. Skin pigmentation (melanin) can absorb UV radiation to protect DNA, so dark-skinned individuals are much less susceptible to UV carcinogenesis. Hereditary deficiency of specific DNA repair enzymes (e.g., ataxia-telangiectasia) results in markedly increased sensitivity to DNA damage by irradiation.

Chemical

Chemical carcinogens are prevalent in the environment both as natural products and as synthetic compounds. Most mutagens are potential carcinogens although some mutagens are more potent than others. The route of exposure and dose of carcinogens are important in determining their effectiveness. Many carcinogens are ingested as inactive agents that must be activated by cellular enzymes such as liver cytochrome P-450 enzymes. Genetic variations in these enzymes can either enhance or diminish the conversion of substances to active carcinogens. Similarly, genetic differences in DNA repair machinery may either predispose or protect cells from various types of carcinogens.

Viral

Tumor viruses are the dominant cause of both leukemia and solid tumors in many lower animal species (Fig. 5-19). Surprisingly, tumor viruses are a much less prevalent cause of human cancer in the United States.

Hepatitis Viruses

Worldwide, hepatocellular carcinoma (related to chronic hepatitis B virus infection) is a major cause of cancer death. Hepatitis B virus infection and hepatocellular carcinoma are highly prevalent in Asia, where vertical transmission of virus (from mother to fetus) is common. Hepatitis B infection is also a risk factor for hepatocellular carcinoma in the United States, but the prevalence of chronic hepatitis B virus infection is relatively low and hepatocellular carcinoma is uncommon. Hepatitis B is a DNA virus that can integrate into the host genome, where it expresses transactivating genes that can alter cell cycle control in infected hepatocytes. These genetic alterations, as well as damage mediated by a chronic immune response to the virus, probably drive carcinogenesis in association with other environmental factors. Chronic hepatitis C virus infection is more prevalent in the United States and is a numerically more important risk factor for hepatocellular carcinoma than is hepatitis B. Hepatitis C virus appears to cause tumors indirectly by inciting a strong, chronic inflammatory response that drives cell proliferation (to replace damaged or destroyed cells) and generates free radicals (which damage DNA and proteins; see below).

Lymphotrophic Viruses

Human T-cell lymphotrophic virus type 1 (HTLV-1) is a retrovirus that is the cause of an unusual type of human T-cell leukemia/lymphoma. HTLV-1–associated leukemia and lymphoma are rare in the United States but more common in the Caribbean and in Japan, where viral infection is endemic. Epstein-Barr virus can act as a tumor promoter in some situations and is associated with the development of Burkitt's lymphoma in Africa and nasopharyngeal carcinoma in Asia.

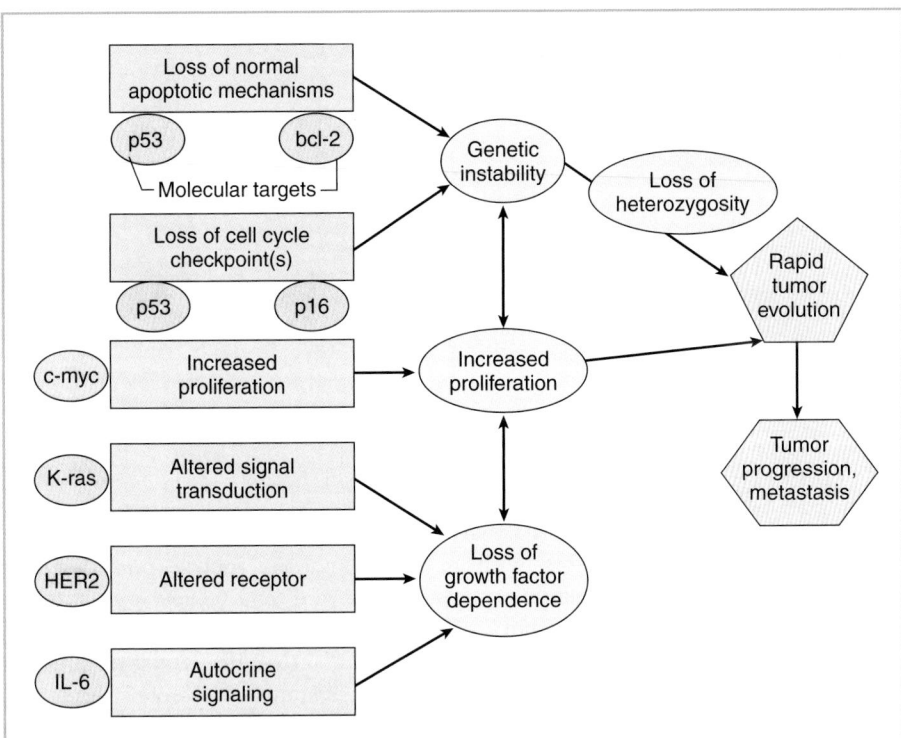

Figure 5-17. Tumor evolution.

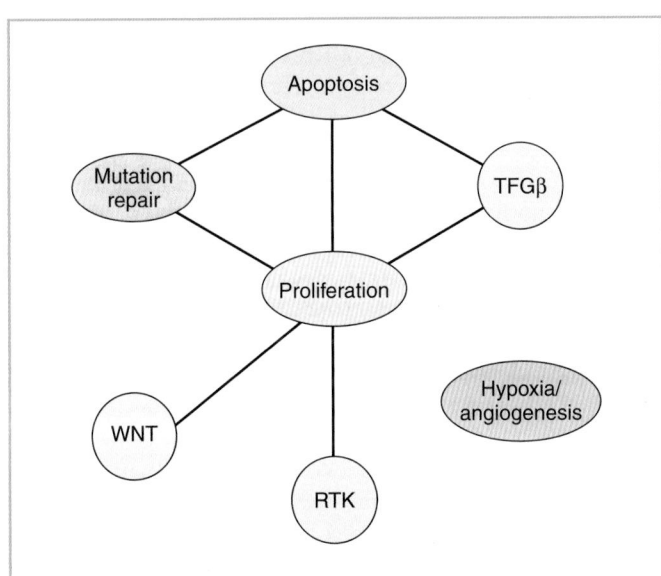

Figure 5-18. Relationships between key pathways in tumorigenesis.

Human Papillomavirus

Cancer of the uterine cervix caused by chronic infection with some strains of human papillomavirus (HPV) occurs world-wide. Although cancer screening by Papanicolaou (Pap) smear has greatly reduced the incidence of cervical cancer in developed countries, cervical cancer remains a significant cause of mortality in the developing world. HPV infects cervical epithelial cells, resulting in cytologic changes in these cells that can be detected by Pap smear. Integration of the

virus into the cellular genome is usually required for car-cinogenesis and activates expression of virus-transactivating proteins E6 and E7. Both these viral products have potent effects on the G_1S cell cycle checkpoint. E6 binds to the p53 protein, resulting in loss of normal p53 function. E7 binds directly to the Rb protein and liberates E2F from Rb to initiate DNA synthesis. The expression of both these viral proteins can result in increased cell proliferation and genetic instability with loss of p53-dependent apoptosis (Fig. 5-20A). These changes in cell cycle control and gene regulation produce many of the morphologic changes of dysplasia in association with HPV infection (see Fig. 5-20B) and facilitate the acquisition of additional genetic alterations that lead to invasive cancer. Other specific HPV serotypes are associated with the development of squamous cell carcinoma of the larynx and oral cavity although their importance for carcinogenesis at these sites is probably much less than that of tobacco and alcohol exposure. Few other viruses are known to have a direct role in human carcinogenesis.

Inflammatory

Inflammation results in the formation of free radicals that can damage DNA and cause mutations. Although free radical damage is usually repaired and genetically defective cells are eliminated by apoptosis, persistent chronic inflammation can predispose to cancer (e.g., chronic hepatitis C virus infection of the liver can increase the risk of developing hepatocellular carcinoma by many fold). Inflammation resulting in cell death increases cell division by progenitor and stem cells, and increased cell proliferation may also contribute to carcino-genesis in some situations. The production of growth factors

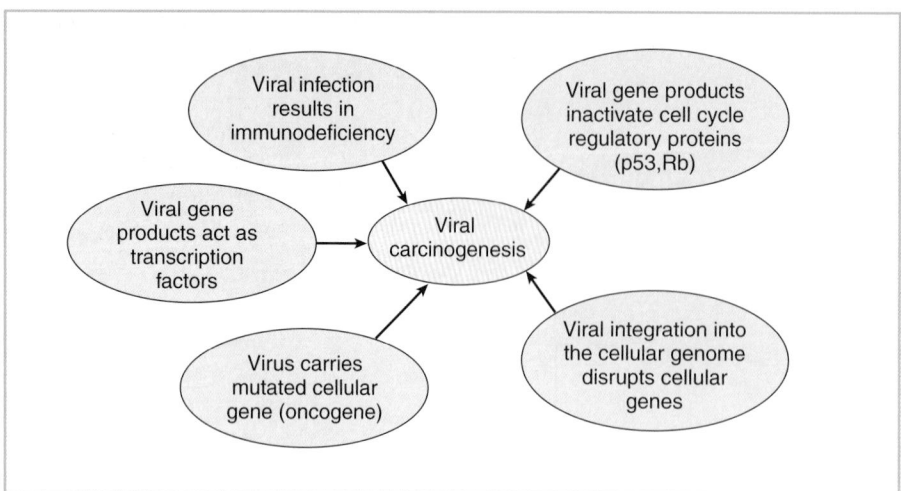

Figure 5-19. Viral carcinogenesis.

and cytokines at sites of inflammation is potentially important and may also support the growth of abnormal cells.

Chronic immune stimulation appears can also produce tumors of inflammatory cells (e.g., B lymphocytes in MALT lymphoma) by persistently driving their proliferation. Acquired genetic changes in proliferating lymphocytes can result in the emergence of clones that grow independently of antigen stimulation and may progress to aggressive lymphomas. The combination of chronic inflammation with environmental carcinogens may act synergistically to produce tumors in some situations.

Genetic

The identification of familial cancer syndromes has been important in defining many key genes involved in sporadic cancers. Rare genetic disorders in which patients inherit one defective copy of the p53 or retinoblastoma gene (Li-Fraumeni and familial retinoblastoma) are discussed above. These and other family cancer syndromes are also important because individuals with these syndromes usually require enhanced screening and may benefit from prophylactic removal of certain targeted organs (e.g., removal of both ovaries in individuals with BRCA1 mutations who have a high likelihood of developing ovarian carcinoma during their lifetime). In some cases, tumors that develop in patients with these genetic syndromes are also qualitatively different from sporadic cancers.

Heritable alterations in the DNA repair genes BRCA1 and BRCA2 result in a markedly increased predisposition to breast and ovarian cancer or ovarian cancer, respectively (Fig. 5-21). Both these gene products are involved in the detection and repair of DNA damage and cooperate with other proteins (p53, CHK2, and ATM) to accomplish this function. Unlike most other family cancer syndromes, BRCA1 and BRCA2 are not prominently targeted in sporadic breast and ovarian cancers. Individuals with homozygous defects of the ATM gene have ataxia-telangiectasia and have marked sensitivity to mutations induced by irradiation as well as a high rate of leukemia.

Patients with neurofibromatosis inherit one defective NF-1 tumor suppressor gene and tend to develop numerous benign tumors of nerves (neurofibromas). Neurofibromas develop in the skin as well as in deeper structures and can cause severe deformity and dysfunction. A small percentage of these neurofibromas may undergo malignant transformation to aggressive sarcomas. The NF-1 protein is involved in the modulation (down-regulation) of the RAS signaling pathway, where it converts activated RAS bound to GTP to an inactive form of RAS (bound to GDP). Patients with neurofibromatosis are at increased risk for the development of other malignant neoplasms including carcinomas of the kidney.

Some forms of MEN are caused by mutations in the MEN gene that normally enhances signaling through the TGF-β pathway to decrease cell proliferation and enhance p53 function. Affected patients develop hyperplasia of the parenchymal cells of multiple endocrine organs, some of which progress to malignant tumors.

Familial adenomatous polyposis (FAP) is an autosomal dominant disease that results from mutations in the adenomatous polyposis coli (APC) tumor suppressor gene, which is involved in modulating the WNT signaling pathway (see above). Somatic loss of function of the remaining normal APC allele in FAP patients results in constitutive Wnt signaling that drives cell proliferation. Patients with FAP can have innumerable colonic adenomatous polyps (as well as polyps in other parts of the gastrointestinal tract), and colon cancer develops at a young age.

●●● CARCINOMA VERSUS SARCOMA VERSUS HEMIC NEOPLASMS

The cells of origin for most human tumors can be categorized in terms of their derivation from the three embryonic layers: ectoderm, mesoderm, and endoderm. Embryonic derivation implies some relatively specific features about a neoplasm that are useful diagnostically and in predicting tumor behavior (see below) (Fig. 5-22). Almost all carcinomas are malignant neoplasms of epithelial cells (ectoderm and

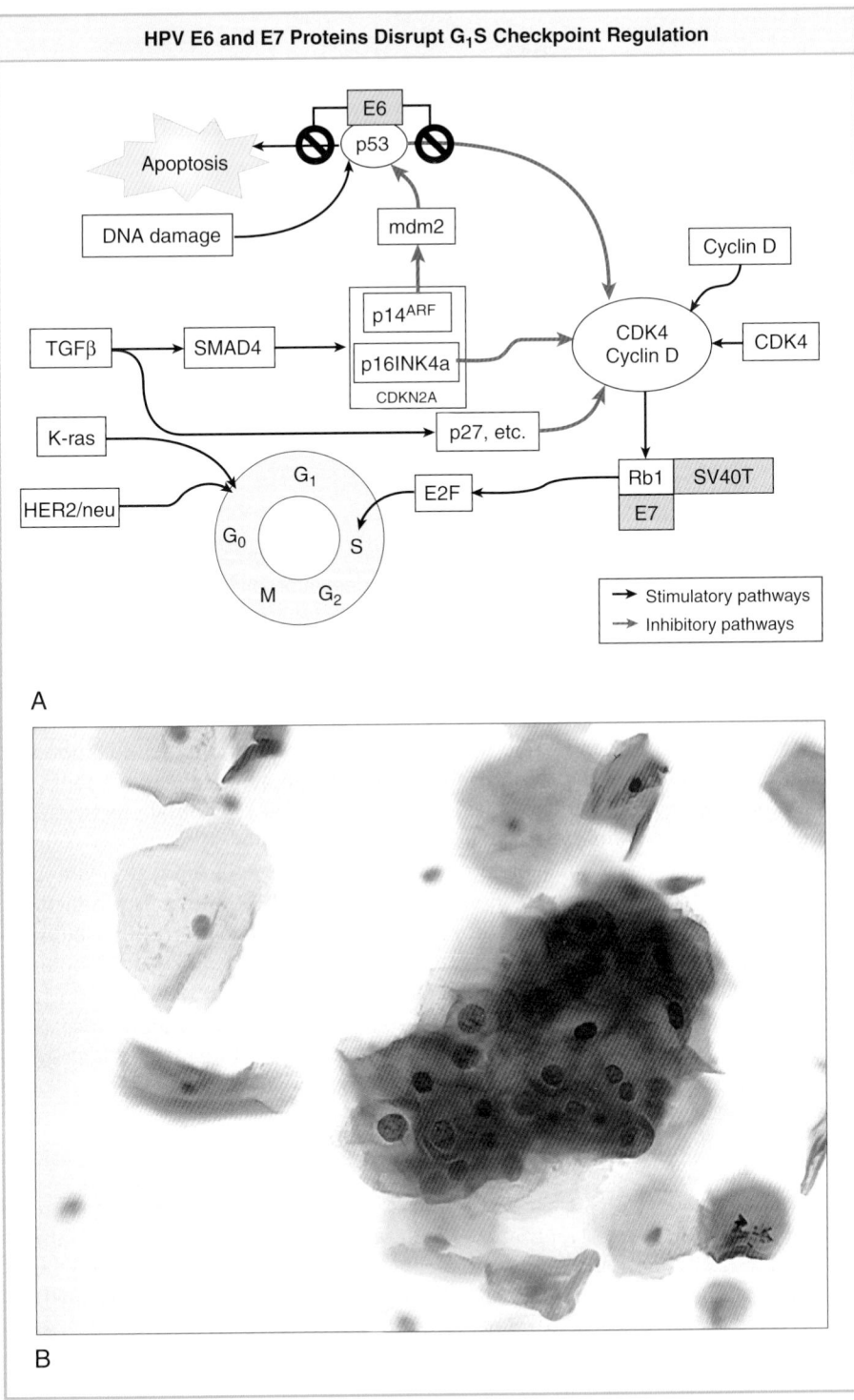

Figure 5-20. A, Interactions between human papillomavirus (HPV) proteins and components of the G₁S cell cycle checkpoint. **B**, Dysplastic cervical squamous cells in a Papanicolaou smear. Cluster of HPV-infected squamous cells with nuclear enlargement, binucleation, and perinuclear clearing (koilocytosis). Normal squamous cells are visible at the periphery.

endoderm) (Fig. 5-23A), whereas sarcomas are malignant neoplasms of mesenchymal cells (mesoderm) (see Fig. 5-23B). In humans, carcinomas vastly outnumber sarcomas in incidence, whereas sarcomas predominate in some laboratory animals. Some unusual human tumors combine features of carcinoma and sarcoma and are termed carcinosarcomas (most of these rare neoplasms are now thought to be carcinomas that have undergone metaplastic change to resemble mesenchymal cells).

Carcinomas

Most carcinomas in adults develop through a multistep process of dysplasia involving sequential genetic alterations affecting multiple different cellular pathways. Carcinoma in situ can sometimes be recognized before malignant cells invade through the basement membrane and form a tumor mass. Carcinomas tend to invade locally and to metastasize via the lymphatic system, giving rise to lymph node metastases. In

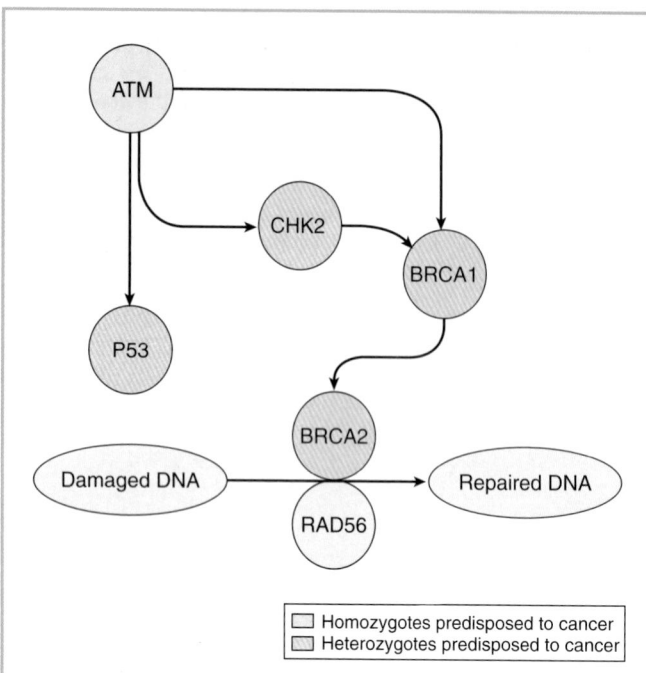

Figure 5-21. Abnormalities of DNA repair pathways that predispose to cancer.

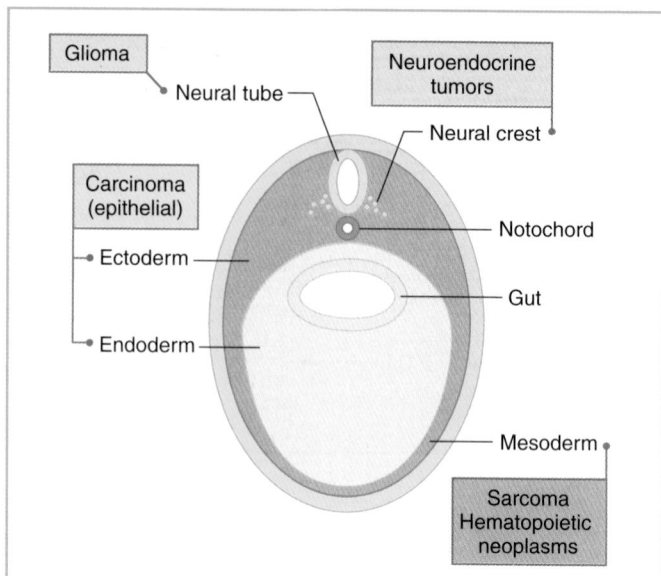

Figure 5-22. Embryonic derivation of different types of neoplasms.

most carcinomas, lymphatic metastases precede hematogenous metastases. Some carcinomas preferentially invade vascular spaces and give rise to hematogenous metastases early in their clinical course. Most carcinomas have relatively well-developed junctions between tumor cells, whereas these junctions are much less well developed in sarcomas.

Sarcomas

Most sarcomas arise in deep soft tissue, and all sarcomas are locally invasive, since their progenitors are not delimited by basement membranes (as are epithelial cells). Morphologically, sarcomas tend to be composed of spindle cells, whereas most carcinomas retain an epithelial appearance. A growing percentage of adult sarcomas are known to have specific chromosomal translocations that create unique fusion proteins. The acquisition of these specific translocations may be sufficient to initiate tumor formation in some cases. Local growth of sarcomas may result in death by compromise of vital structures. Most sarcomas metastasize hematogenously, and lymph node metastases from sarcomas are unusual.

Neuroendocrine Tumors

Tumors of neuroendocrine cells can arise in nearly any organ and form a morphologically and clinically distinct group of neoplasms. Neuroendocrine cells derive from neural crest cells (see Fig. 5-23C), which can differentiate into a number of different lineages including melanocytes.

Neuroendocrine tumors vary from low grade (e.g., carcinoid tumors) to highly malignant small-cell undifferentiated carci-

nomas that are often widely metastatic at the time of initial diagnosis. Most neuroendocrine tumors contain specific neuroendocrine markers such as chromogranin A (a component of dense core neurosecretory granules) and synaptophysin. Melanomas have morphologic and phenotypic features that are intermediate between carcinoma and sarcoma (spindle cell and epithelioid morphology). Most melanomas retain some features of normal melanocytes (e.g., melanin production), from which they arise. Tumors arising from neuroectoderm (brain tumors) tend to have very different properties from carcinomas and only rarely give rise to metastases (see Fig. 5-23D). Most neuroectodermal tumors arise from glial cells in the central nervous system, and high-grade tumors can be rapidly fatal owing to mass effect.

Pediatric Tumors

Most malignant tumors developing in young children recapitulate primitive embryonic tissues and share many morphologic features with one another (so-called small blue round-cell tumors). Many of these tumors are called blastomas (e.g., neuroblastoma, nephroblastoma), and they have primitive nuclei with finely divided chromatin (i.e., most genes capable of expression) and a high nuclear cytoplasmic ratio (see Fig. 5-23E). Most have relatively primitive cell junctions and tend to form primitive tubules of different types (e.g., rosettes). Many of these tumors result from specific chromosomal translocations that result in novel fusion proteins.

Hematopoietic Neoplasms

Normal hematopoietic cells express cell surface receptors that allow them to migrate from place to place using the vasculature as a conduit with specialized receptors that recognize endothelial cells in specialized lymphoid organs. Many

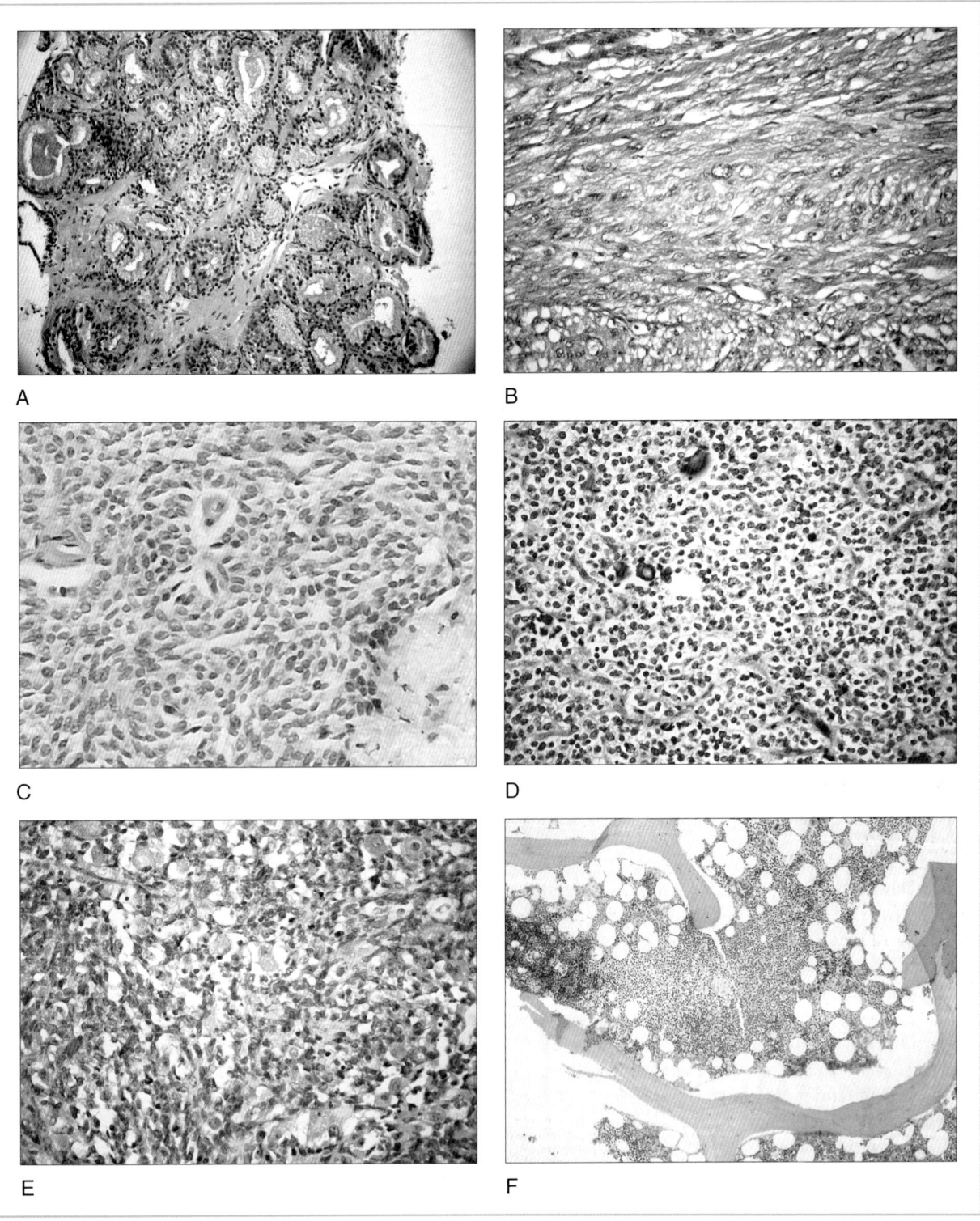

Figure 5-23. A, Prostatic adenocarcinoma. Photomicrograph showing an adenocarcinoma composed of well-formed glandular structures. **B**, Leiomyosarcoma. Photomicrograph showing an intermediate-grade sarcoma composed of spindle cells, which morphologically resemble smooth muscle cells. **C**, Carcinoid tumor. Photomicrograph showing tumor cells with nuclei containing finely divided chromatin characteristic of neuroendocrine cells. Well-differentiated neuroendocrine tumors, such as this pulmonary carcinoid tumor, typically show a trabecular growth pattern. **D**, Oligodendroglioma. Photomicrograph showing a well-differentiated brain tumor recapitulating some morphologic features of normal oligodendroglial cells ("fried egg" appearance). **E**, Embryonal rhabdomyosarcoma. Photomicrograph showing a high-grade sarcoma composed of cells with primitive (blastic) nuclei alternating with more differentiated cells with eosinophilic cytoplasm resembling skeletal muscle. **F**, Follicular lymphoma. Photomicrograph showing bone marrow with paratrabecular aggregates (adjacent to bony trabeculae) of small, angulated lymphocytes, which is characteristic of involvement by follicular lymphoma.

EMBRYOLOGY

Neural Crest

Neural crest cells are sometimes called the fourth germ cell layer and derive from a group of specialized cells that reside adjacent to the crest of the neural ridge during neurulation. Neural crest cells then migrate extensively into the cranium, trunk, vagal and sacral regions, and heart. Their migration is associated with down-regulation of N-cadherin expression. Differentiation of neural crest cells is largely controlled by environmental stimuli, including paracrine signaling:

- BMP2 (bone morphogenetic protein) → cholinergic neurons
- Glial growth factor → Schwann cells
- Endothelin-3 → melanocytes and adrenergic neurons
  Neural crest cells also give rise to a wide variety of other mature cell types including neurons in the peripheral nervous system, melanocytes in the skin, epinephrine-producing cells in the adrenal medulla, and connective tissue cells in the head and neck. Many neural crest cell derivatives retain some differentiated features typical of neuroendocrine cells.

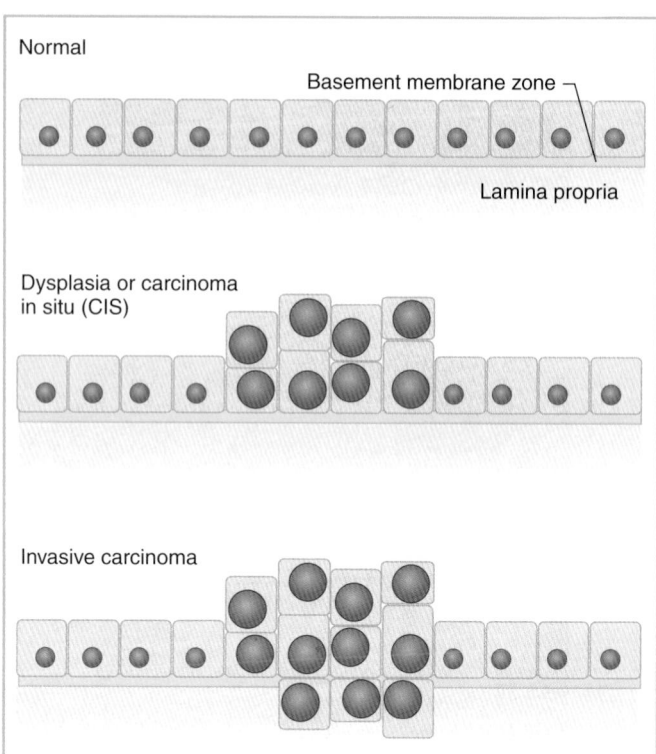

Figure 5-24. Invasive and in situ carcinoma.

hematopoietic neoplasms traffic extensively through the vascular or lymphatic systems (or both), since they retain these specialized receptors (see Fig. 5-23F). Hematopoietic cells also have cytoskeletons that permit them to undergo diapedesis and transmigrate endothelial surfaces into tissue. Because of these intrinsic properties, the spread of most hematopoietic neoplasms through the body is not referred to as metastasis, and many hematopoietic neoplasms (e.g., leukemia) are widely disseminated at the time of diagnosis. In contrast, most carcinomas and sarcomas must acquire new abilities before they can metastasize.

Other characteristics of hematopoietic neoplasms differentiate tumorigenesis in these cells from tumorigenesis in epithelial cells. Leukemias tend to develop from committed stem cells or progenitor cells that have substantial replicative capacity. Because of this, disruption of fewer cellular pathways may be required for tumorigenesis in hematopoietic cells. Many leukemias, lymphomas, sarcomas, and pediatric neoplasms develop as a consequence of specific translocation events that form chimeric proteins with novel functions (see above). These specific translocations are now used to diagnose and classify many of these neoplasms. In some circumstances, myelodysplasia (similar to epithelial dysplasia) can develop in hematopoietic lineages with the stepwise accumulation of genetic abnormalities. Leukemias that arise in the setting of myelodysplasia are usually phenotypically and clinically distinct from those resulting from specific chromosomal translocations and typically are refractory to treatment.

●●● IN SITU CARCINOMA AND OTHER PRECURSOR LESIONS

Most carcinomas arise from precursor lesions referred to as in situ carcinoma that develop in the setting of progressive epithelial dysplasia. Neoplastic polyps share some features with carcinoma in situ and are the predominant precursor lesion of carcinoma in some organs (e.g., colonic adenocarcinoma).

Carcinoma in situ corresponds to high-grade dysplasia without evidence of invasion of tumor cells through the epithelial basement membrane (Fig. 5-24). In most anatomic locations, high-grade dysplasia and in situ carcinoma are viewed as equivalent (and morphologically indistinguishable) processes that are associated with multiple genetic abnormalities in the involved cells. Dysplasia (or carcinoma in situ) does not typically result in the formation of a mass lesion although morphologic changes in a flat epithelium (usually epithelial thickening) may be visible (e.g., leukoplakia or white patches in the oral mucosa produced by squamous cell dysplasia).

In situ carcinoma is viewed as a direct precursor to invasive carcinoma in some organs, but in others the relationship between in situ and invasive lesions is less clear. For example, invasive prostatic adenocarcinoma and high-grade dysplasia (high-grade prostatic intraepithelial neoplasia, HGPIN) frequently coexist; however, a direct precursor-product relationship has not been clearly demonstrated between them. Nonetheless, it is generally accepted that dysplasia precedes the development of overt invasive or in situ carcinoma in most adult carcinomas.

Dysplasia

Most human carcinomas arise through the stepwise acquisition of multiple genetic abnormalities (Fig. 5-25). It is possi-

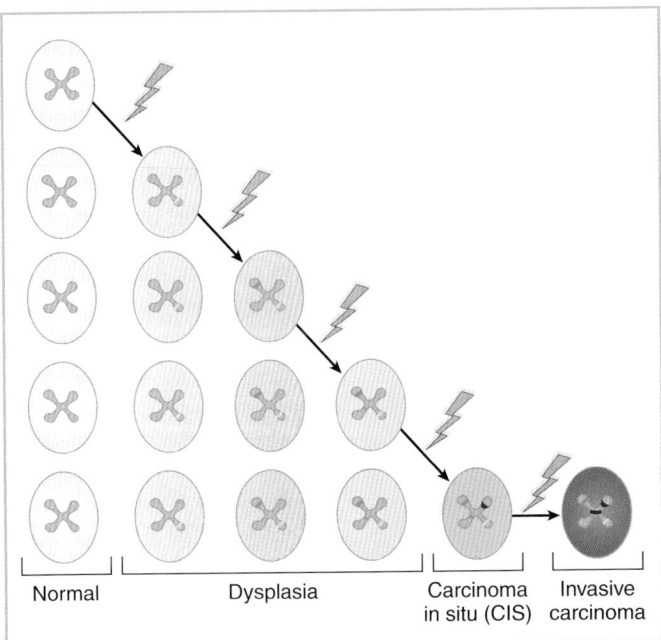

Figure 5-25. Dysplasia and carcinoma development.

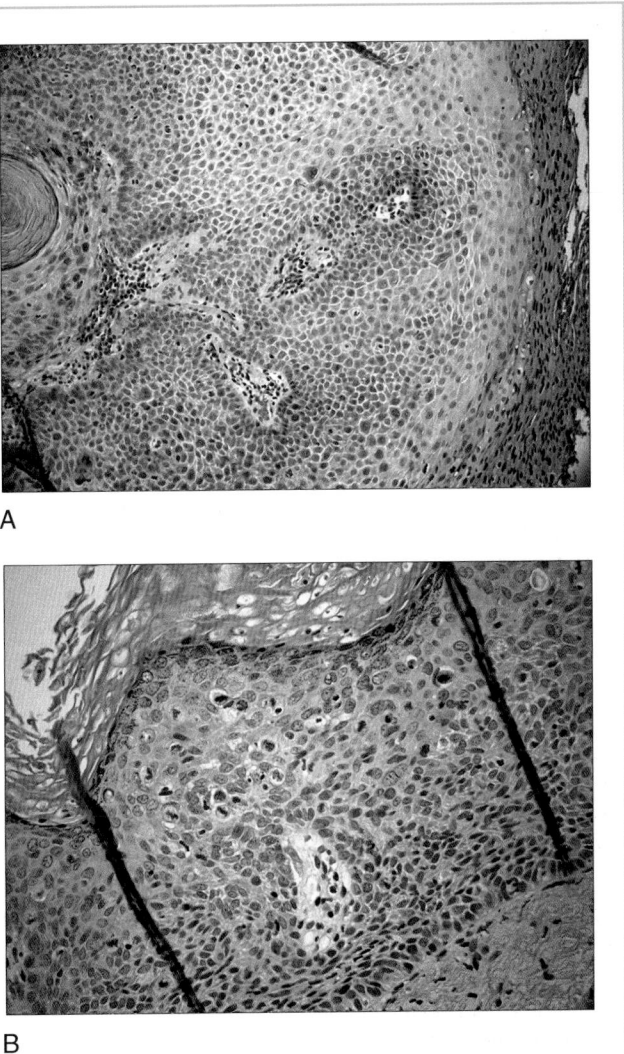

Figure 5-26. A, Low-grade squamous dysplasia. Photomicrograph showing cervical squamous mucosa composed of cells with nuclear hyperchromasia and increased size, demonstrating disordered maturation (partial loss of nuclear polarity and orientation). **B,** High-grade squamous dysplasia. Photomicrograph showing thickened squamous mucosa with marked variation in nuclear size and complete loss of orderly maturation. Scattered abnormal mitotic figures are present at all levels of the epithelium.

ble to sample the at-risk cell population and measure abnormalities to assess the risk of tumor development at some anatomic sites (e.g., the uterine cervix), but it is much more difficult in many other locations (e.g., the pancreas). Progression from dysplasia to carcinoma has been fully demonstrated in the uterine cervix, where Pap smears can detect cytologic changes in premalignant cells that are likely to progress to fully malignant cells and ultimately invasive carcinoma. In the uterine cervix, these morphologic changes are largely induced by human papillomavirus infection. Integration of the virus into the genome causes targeted disruption of p53 and Rb protein function, which directly results in increased proliferation and diminished apoptosis. These genetically unstable cells are then at substantially increased risk for acquiring additional genetic lesions that may convert them to fully malignant tumors. The fact that this stepwise acquisition of genetic changes results in measurable morphologic changes makes it possible to stratify risk in individual patients by cytologic screening of Pap smears (Fig. 5-26). While the stepwise progression from dysplasia to carcinoma has been well documented in the uterine cervix, this progression has not been as convincingly demonstrated in other anatomic sites (because of difficulty in reliably sampling these areas).

Dysmyelopoietic syndromes precede some leukemias and share some features with epithelial dysplasia. Preneoplastic lesions of lymphoid cells are rarely observed, however. This may reflect technical difficulties in identifying abnormal populations and intrinsic differences between hematopoietic cells (which have intrinsic ability to migrate through the vascular system and often develop as a consequence of specific translocations) and epithelial cells. Similarly, dysplastic lesions in soft tissue are only rarely identified.

Neoplastic Polyps

Polyps are defined as exophytic growths from the skin or mucous membranes and are a heterogeneous group of lesions, some of which constitute true neoplasms while others are purely reactive or inflammatory processes. Adenomatous polyps of the colon are neoplastic lesions that can progress to invasive adenocarcinomas. Most adenomatous polyps develop as a result of mutations in the APC gene (see above) and are composed of benign stromal components and neoplastic epithelium. Adenomatous polyps can grow in a villous (papillary) or tubular (similar to normal colonic crypts) con-

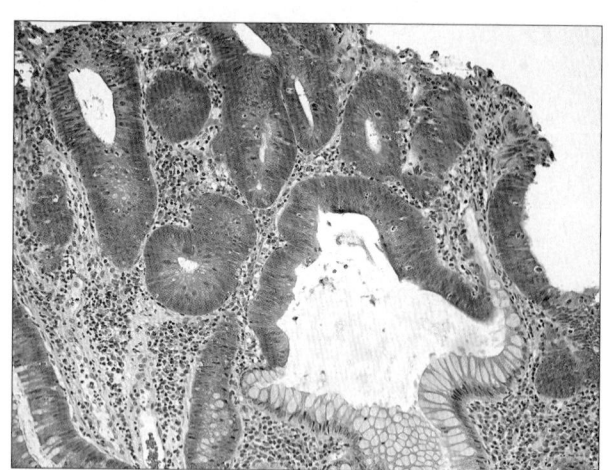

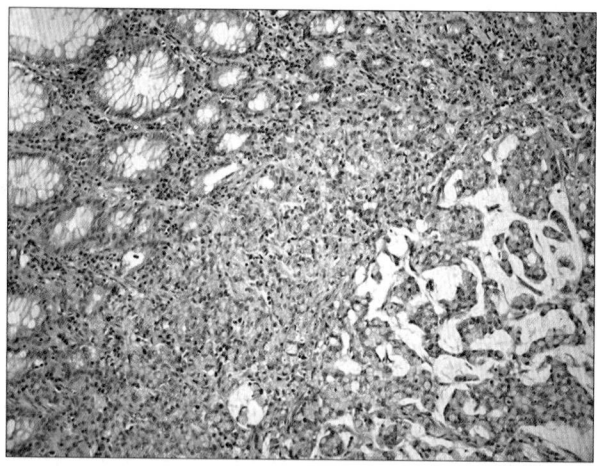

Figure 5-27. A, Adenomatous polyp of the colon. Photomicrograph showing increased nuclear size and hyperchromasia in adenomatous epithelium. There is also increased nuclear stratification and mucin depletion as compared with normal epithelium (*bottom right*). **B,** Signet ring cell adenocarcinoma of the colon.

figuration (Fig. 5-27A). All adenomatous polyps form mass lesions that may be relatively flat (sessile) or pedunculated (stalked) relative to surrounding mucosa. By definition, adenomatous polyps lack metastatic potential but unlike most other benign neoplasms, have a significant likelihood of transforming into invasive adenocarcinomas (see Fig. 5-27B). Adenomatous polyps are best viewed as dysplastic lesions in that they have a significant potential for progression to invasive carcinoma, although they differ from flat epithelial dysplasias that do not form mass lesions. As adenomatous polyps enlarge, they often acquire additional genetic changes (e.g., RAS, SMAD, and p53 mutations) that accelerate their growth or cause them to invade beyond the basement membrane (i.e., become an invasive adenocarcinoma).

TUMOR INVASION

In epithelial neoplasms, invasion implies the ability of tumor cells to digest through the underlying basement membrane and migrate downward into underlying submucosal tissue. Invasive tumors must also be capable of inducing angiogenesis as they invade to form a tumor mass. Invasion is a complex phenotype that involves the expression of multiple enzymes and pathways (Fig. 5-28). Metalloproteinases are important for digesting through the basement membrane zone, but tumor cells must also acquire the ability to rearrange their exoskeleton to actively move through gaps created in basement membranes.

Tumor cells must express integrins and other adhesion molecules on their surface so that they can interact with extracellular matrix components, such as laminin and fibronectin. Finally, if tumors are able to successfully invade and grow, they must generate a de novo blood supply to provide oxygen and nutrition for a rapidly increasing number of tumor cells.

Different types of epithelial tumors are more or less efficient in inducing angiogenesis.

In some tumors, loss of normal VHL tumor suppressor gene function results in aberrant expression of angiogenic factors (see Von Hippel–Lindau (VHL) Gene and Angiogenesis, above). Other tumor cells may retain a normal capacity to respond to hypoxic conditions through the HIF1 pathway with the elaboration VEGF and PDGF. The underlying phenotype of the cells that gave rise to the tumor often influence a tumor's ability to establish effective angiogenesis.

The meaning of invasion for sarcomas is less clear than for carcinomas in that their cells of origin are not separated from surrounding tissues by basement membrane. For this reason, it is usually not possible to define in situ sarcomas. Different types of sarcomas are more or less effective in inducing angiogenesis as judged by the amount of associated tumor necrosis. Invasion is not a relevant concept for hematopoietic tumors, since they can move through the vasculature by virtue of specific integrins on the surface.

TUMOR METASTASIS

Like tumor invasion, metastasis is a complex process involving the expression of multiple gene products. To metastasize, tumor cells must be able to gain access to vascular spaces (either lymphatic or vascular), travel to new locations, and establish effective tumor growth at these sites. Metastatic tumor cells must also have cytoskeletal properties that allow them to migrate into and out of vascular spaces. Tumors that give rise to metastases have usually acquired all these capabilities. Some metastatic tumors express cell surface proteins that allow their specific adhesion to endothelial cells and facilitate their transmigration into target tissues. More commonly, clusters of tumor cells that gain access to the vasculature mechanically embolize in small blood vessels (lung and liver provide effective vascular filters) (Fig. 5-29). In other cases, the tumor vasculature is partially lined by

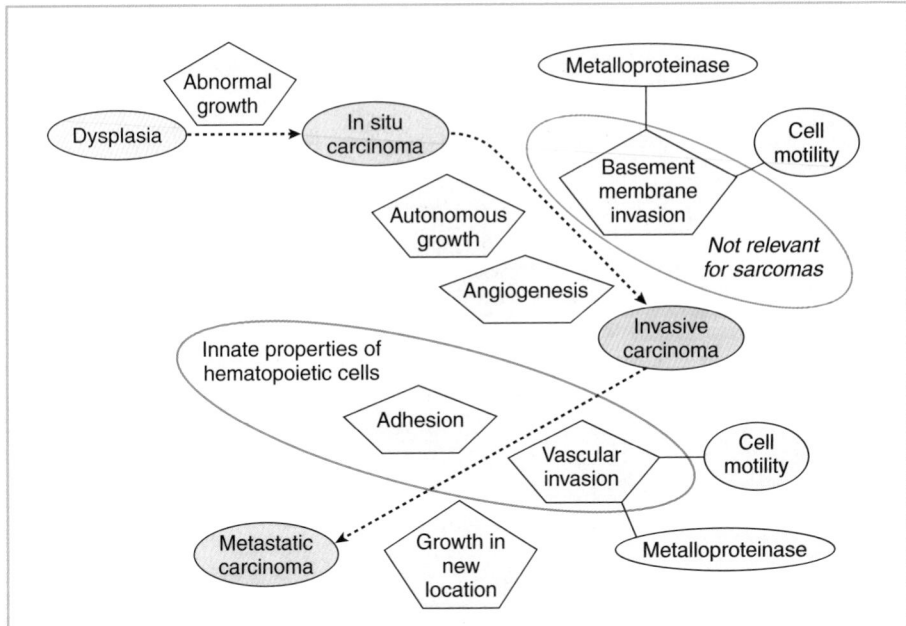

Figure 5-28. Mechanisms of tumor invasion and metastasis.

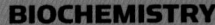

BIOCHEMISTRY

Matrix Metalloproteinases

Matrix metalloproteinases (MMPs) are a family of closely related Zn^{++}-dependent endopeptidases that are involved in remodeling the extracellular matrix in normal physiology and in disease. All protein components of the extracellular matrix can be cleaved by at least one MMP. MMPs are produced as inactive zymogens by many cell types and can be secreted or remain bound to the plasma membrane.

MMP zymogens can be activated by plasmin, and their production is frequently regulated by cytokines. MMPs are inhibited by TIMPs (tissue inhibitors of metalloproteinases), which are often secreted by the same cells that produce MMPs. Three groups of MMPs are distinguished:

- Type IV collagenases (gelatinase), including MMP-2 and MMP-9, which can digest basement membrane components
- Stromelysins (MMP-3)
- Interstitial collagenase (MMP-1)

MMPs also are essential for angiogenesis and are expressed on endothelial cells and vascular smooth muscle cells. MMP expression is up-regulated in some tumors and is thought to be important in tumor metastasis and invasion.

BIOCHEMISTRY

Tumor Angiogenesis

The microvasculature of most tumors is qualitatively different from that of normal blood vessels. The endothelial cell layer in tumor capillaries is often discontinuous, and in some cases, these vascular spaces are lined by a mosaic of endothelial cells and tumor cells. As a result, tumor microvasculature tends to be leaky (larger proteins tend to diffuse out of the vasculature, resulting in tumor edema) and is prone to hemorrhage and thrombosis. Most tumor blood vessels are induced to sprout from normal vessels by VEGF and other angiogenic factors produced by tumor cells.

VEGF-A is a heparin-binding glycoprotein with at least four different splice variants that can bind to VEGFR1 and VEGFR2 receptor tyrosine kinases on endothelial cells.

Angiopoietins Ang1 and Ang2 also are important in initiating new blood vessel formation, with Ang2 favoring vessel sprouting and Ang1 stabilizing normal vessels and favoring the formation of nonleaky vascular networks.

PDGF and bFGF also are needed to recruit perivascular-supporting cells for new blood vessels.

VEGF-C and VEGF-D bind to VEGFR3 and direct the formation of tumor lymphatic vessels.

tumor cells that form a mosaic pattern with endothelial cells. Some tumors show extensive vascular space invasion within or adjacent to the primary tumor, and these neoplasms are more likely to be associated with metastatic disease.

Once tumor cells have arrived at a new location, they must be able to egress from the vascular space and establish growth in the new environment. If tumor cells are able to grow in the environment where they lodge, they form small metastatic deposits that may grow if angiogenesis is induced. Not all tumor cells are clonogenic, and so-called tumor stem cells may be required for effective metastasis. Most tumor cells are at least partially dependent on hormonal or cytokine stimulation for continued growth and viability, and secondary tumor deposits in other tissues and organs may not find a suitable growth environment. Metastatic disease may be restricted to more favorable geographic environments, or

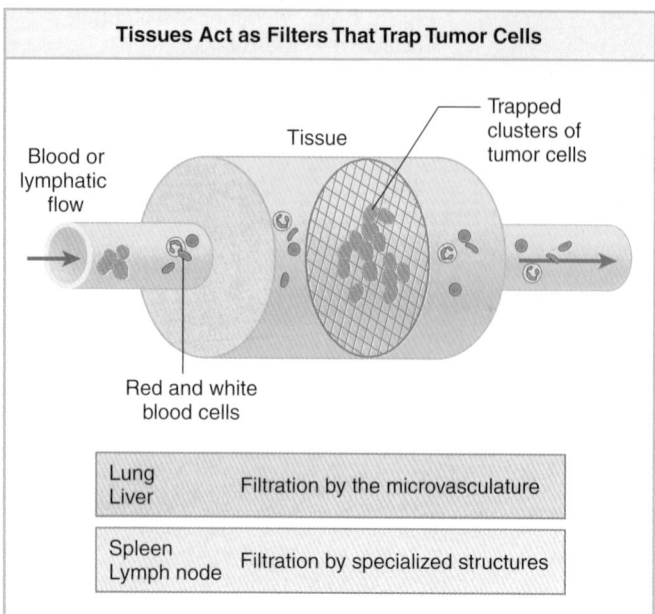

Figure 5-29. Different types of metastatic spread.

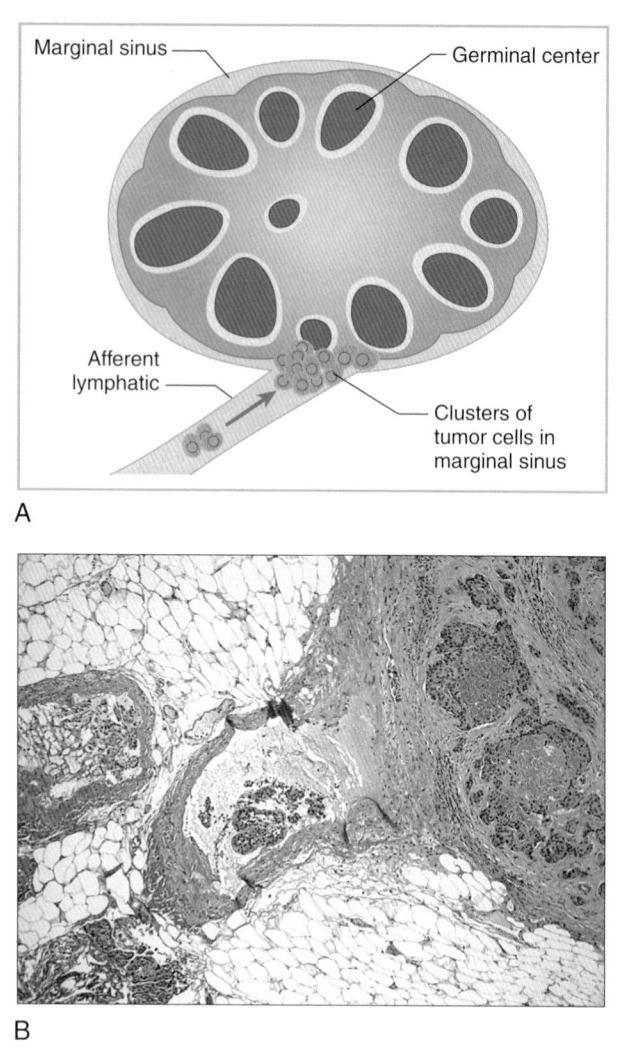

Figure 5-30. A, Lymph node metastasis. **B,** Photomicrograph showing a dilated afferent lymphatic vessel (containing breast cancer cells) connecting with a draining lymph node (*at right*) that is partially replaced by metastatic tumor.

metastasis may not be possible for some tumors unless they become independent of stimulatory or inhibitory factors and develop completely autocrine growth.

Some anatomic sites usually are resistant to tumor cell metastasis because of normally hypoxic conditions or other factors. For example, normal cartilage is a relatively hypoxic tissue that is resistant to both contiguous tumor invasion and tumor metastasis. Some tumors show marked tropism for particular metastatic sites. This is true for prostate cancer, which preferentially metastasizes to bone and gives rise to characteristic blastic (bone-forming) metastases. This type of tropism is less clear for most other types of metastatic tumors, and their anatomic relationship to draining lymph nodes is a significant factor in determining their pattern of metastatic spread.

Tumors can invade perineural spaces and travel across anatomic boundaries within nerves. Perineural invasion is a characteristic feature of some tumors, including adenocarcinoma of the prostate and adenoid cystic carcinoma of the salivary gland. Some tumors preferentially spread along the surfaces of organs (e.g., serous ovarian carcinoma) or may grow in liquid suspension in malignant pleural or peritoneal effusions. Tumor cells that gain access to lymphatic vessels tend to be filtered and trapped in the subcapsular sinus of draining lymph nodes, where most early lymph node metastases are observed (Fig. 5-30).

The advent of sentinel lymph node biopsy (in which the primary draining lymph node is identified by means of a radioactive probe after a radioactive tracer has been instilled in the primary tumor bed) has permitted more accurate staging of tumors with limited lymph node dissection. Patients with negative sentinel lymph nodes have a very low risk of occult metastases in other draining lymph nodes. Most carcinomas develop detectable lymph node metastases before systemic hematogenous metastases are discovered, so lymph node sampling provides important pathologic information.

Metastatic tumor deposits are usually spherical and often multiple. These two features are helpful in distinguishing primary tumors (usually solitary and irregular in shape) from metastatic tumor deposits (Fig. 5-31). Metastatic lesions may ultimately grow to replace organs or lymph nodes and are the ultimate cause of death in many cancer patients.

● ● ● PARANEOPLASTIC SYNDROMES

Some tumors give rise to characteristic syndromes that are not related to tumor mass effect, loss of normal parenchyma, or metastatic disease. Some of these syndromes appear to be hormonal and are related to the abnormal production of cytokines, growth factors, and hormones by tumor cells or tumor stroma. Some tumors characteristically produce

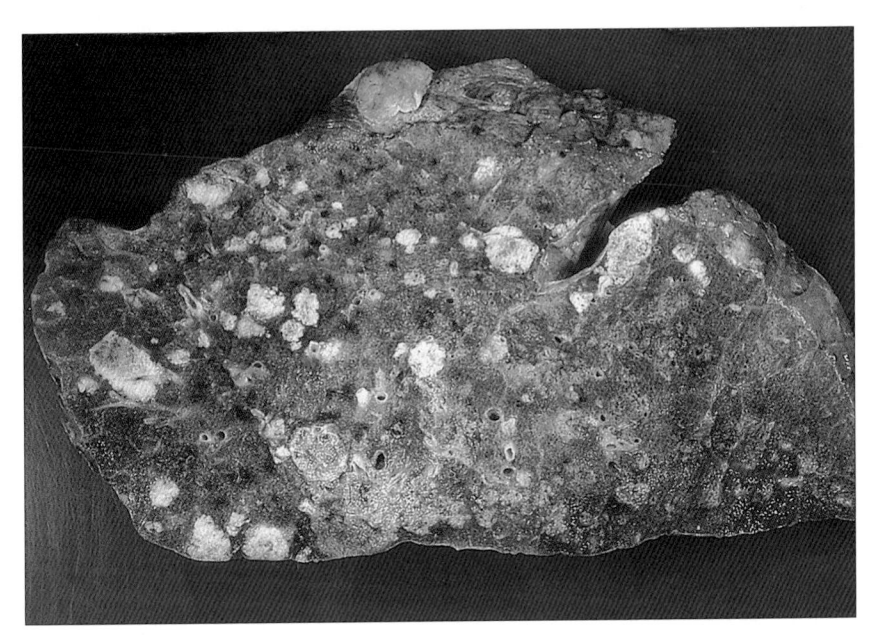

Figure 5-31. Multifocal metastatic carcinoma in lung tissue.

ectopic hormones or secrete novel peptides that have hormonal activities. A relatively common syndrome associated with small-cell undifferentiated carcinomas of the lung is the ectopic production of parathyroid hormone–like peptides, which activate osteoclasts to induce bone resorption, causing tumor-associated hypercalcemia. Some paraneoplastic syndromes are clearly related to the production of cytokines by tumor cells (e.g., TNF-α), whereas others may result from autoimmune phenomena triggered by tumor cells. The pathogenesis of some paraneoplastic syndromes remains entirely unexplained.

Cachexia (lack of appetite and muscle wasting) frequently develops in patients with advanced malignancy. Tumor cachexia is directly related to the production of TNF-α, interferon γ, or IL-6 by tumor cells. These cytokines have direct effects on the nervous system and skeletal muscle. Together, these cytokines specifically inhibit the synthesis of muscle contractile proteins and enhance their degradation, resulting in marked muscle wasting (Fig. 5-32). Other systemic effects of TNF-α include appetite depression and more complex central nervous system effects.

TUMOR STAGING

Clinical and pathologic staging of tumors is the most important prognostic factor for most adult neoplasms once the tumor type has been established. The extent of local spread of a tumor (its T stage), the presence and/or extent of lymph node metastases (the N stage), and the presence or absence of systemic metastases (the M stage) provide this critical staging information that helps guide therapy. For example, if a tumor has given rise to distant metastases, therapy targeted only at the primary tumor cannot be curative. Therapeutic trials in clinical and surgical oncology have defined the optimal

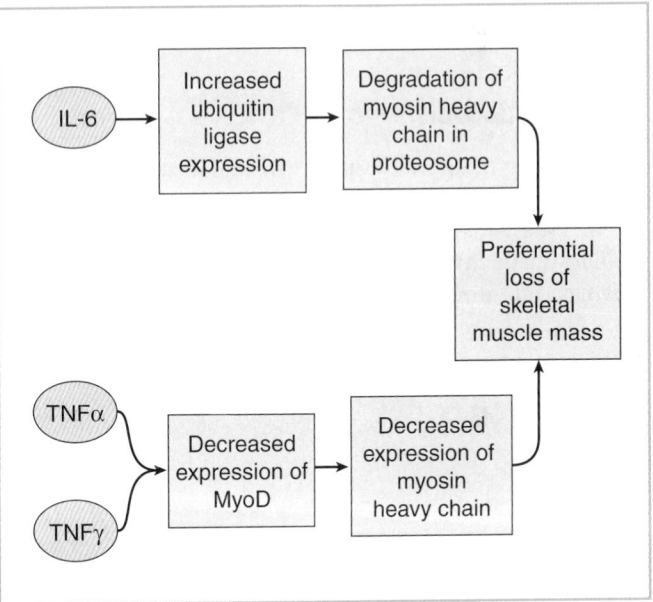

Figure 5-32. Tumor-induced cachexia.

therapeutic interventions for many tumors at various pathologic stages, and the accurate assessment of tumor stage is paramount in determining the most effective and useful therapy as well as for assessing the prognosis.

Although radiographic imaging allows the detection of metastatic disease with increasing accuracy and sensitivity, pathologic staging is still the gold standard for most human solid tumors. This is accomplished through the therapeutic excision of the involved organ, usually in continuity with the draining lymph nodes. Careful pathologic analysis of the primary tumor and lymph nodes is essential for accurate staging. The precise staging criteria for different neoplasms at various anatomic sites are complex but are closely related to the size of the primary tumor and the number of lymph node metastases. The TNM stage is combined into an overall AJCC (American Joint Committee on Cancer) stage for each neoplasm, which usually implies a specific form of therapy or combination of therapies (surgery, irradiation, and chemotherapy).

●●● TUMOR MARKERS

Tumor markers are biomarkers that may be useful in the early detection of tumors, assessment of the extent of tumor growth or spread, and identification of tumor recurrence. Most tumor biomarkers in clinical use correspond to proteins or peptide fragments (although nucleic acids, lipids, etc., may also serve as biomarkers) that are made by tumor cells. Many tumor biomarkers may be shed in the blood or other bodily fluids (e.g., urine) as tumor cells undergo necrosis or apoptosis. Tumor biomarkers are rarely unique to tumor cells (i.e., true tumor-specific antigens) and more often correspond to normal proteins that are aberrantly expressed by tumor cells or to reactivation of expression of fetal proteins (e.g., α-fetoprotein). True tumor-specific antigens are usually restricted to neoplastic B and T cells that have rearranged antigen receptor genes with unique protein sequences.

Immunohistochemical Markers

Identification of specific proteins in tumor cells can provide therapeutically important information about the cell of origin for that tumor. Many tumor markers correspond to intermediate filaments (e.g., cytokeratins expressed in most carcinomas) and differentiation antigens (e.g., CD20 expressed on most B-cell lymphomas) that can be detected by immunohistochemical methods (binding of specific labeled antibodies to antigens in tissue sections).

Immunohistochemistry is used in routine pathologic diagnosis of many different types of tumors, and the ability to detect specific antigens is particularly important in unusual, metastatic, and poorly differentiated neoplasms. Although the expression of one protein may be aberrant in some tumors, evaluation with a panel of different antibodies usually allows unambiguous characterization of tumor lineage.

Serum Biomarkers

Most tumor markers are tumor cell products resulting from abnormal expression of particular molecules. They may correspond to the ectopic expression of normal proteins by tumor cells or the reactivation of expression of proteins normally restricted to embryogenesis or fetal life (e.g., the production of α-fetoprotein by malignant hepatocytes of hepatocellular carcinoma). The amount of biomarkers in the serum is usually a rough index of the bulk of tumor in the patient. Serum tumor markers are usually detected by enzyme-linked immunoadsorption assay (ELISA) of serum. Specific antibodies coated on microtiter plates bind antigen if present in serum samples, and bound antibody is detected by immunohistochemical techniques. Serum biomarkers can be used to screen individuals who may be at risk for tumors and to monitor for recurrent disease.

There is great interest in identifying new screening biomarkers in serum or urine that are capable of detecting tumors at an early stage of development when they are curable by conventional therapy. For a biomarker to be useful

---

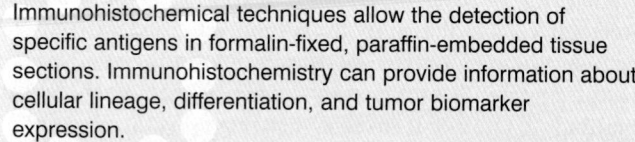

CLINICAL MEDICINE

AJCC Tumor Staging

AJCC tumor stage is assigned based on a combination of individual parameters that measure local tumor growth (T stage), regional lymph node metastasis (N stage), and distant metastasis (M stage). Although tumor-specific staging criteria differ, small tumors confined to their organ of origin are usually AJCC stage I while tumors of any size with distant metastases are usually classified as AJCC stage IV. In a few tumor types, serum tumor markers or other features play a direct role in the staging system (e.g., testicular germ cell tumors).

For example, a 2.1-cm breast carcinoma with negative lymph nodes and no evidence of distant metastasis is AJCC stage I (pT2, pN0, pM0). The "p" prefix indicates that staging is based on pathologic rather than clinical or radiographic data. A similar carcinoma with one lymph node metastasis would be AJCC stage II (pT2, pN1, pMX) while four lymph node metastases would up-stage the tumor to AJCC stage III (pT2, pN2, pMX). A liver biopsy showing metastatic carcinoma would be stage IV (pT2, pN2, pM1).

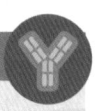

IMMUNOLOGY

Immunohistochemistry (IHC)

Immunohistochemical techniques allow the detection of specific antigens in formalin-fixed, paraffin-embedded tissue sections. Immunohistochemistry can provide information about cellular lineage, differentiation, and tumor biomarker expression.

Usually, an indirect immunoperoxidase technique is employed by applying a primary antibody (usually a monoclonal antibody raised in mice against a specific human protein) to a tissue section on a glass slide. After incubation, unbound primary antibody is washed away and a secondary antibody (frequently antimouse immunoglobulin covalently linked to biotin) is applied. After incubation and washing, an avidin-biotin-peroxidase detection system is applied. Avidin has multiple binding sites for biotin and forms a bridge between the peroxidase and the antibody. After washing, a chromogenic substrate is applied, which is converted to a colored precipitate by the peroxidase. This chromogen is visible by routine light microscopy in areas where the primary antibody has bound. The specificity and sensitivity of the technique must be verified with control tissues of known reactivity.

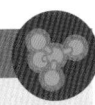

BIOCHEMISTRY

Tumor Markers

Tumor biomarkers can be characterized as markers of cancer risk, tumor-host interaction, tumor burden, or functional tumor markers.

Most cancer risk biomarkers are genetic (e.g., tumor suppressor gene mutations or SNPs and polymorphisms that are statistically associated with increased risk).

Markers that reflect tumor-host interaction relate to organ system dysfunction (e.g., increased liver enzymes in patients with liver metastases) or to features of the host immune response to tumors.

Biomarkers of tumor burden usually correspond to substances produced by tumors, such as prostate-specific antigen (PSA), α-fetoprotein (AFP), and carcinoembryonic antigen (CEA). Most of these biomarkers are not exclusively produced by tumor cells, so their diagnostic specificity is limited. In patients with known malignancies, serum levels of these biomarkers can be useful measures of tumor burden.

Functional tumor markers correspond to the expression or alteration of particular genes or pathways that influence tumor cell behavior (e.g., angiogenesis induced by VEGF or metastasis). Many of these markers may be predictive biomarkers that allow selection of optimal therapies for individual cancer patients.

for tumor screening in a low-risk population, it must have high specificity (very few false-positive results) as well as high sensitivity (very few false-negative results) if it is to be used effectively. If a biomarker with low specificity is applied to a low-risk population, the ratio of false-positive to true-positive results will be high, and many individuals will be subjected to unnecessary additional testing (i.e., the test will have a low positive predictive value). Conversely, if a biomarker with low sensitivity is applied to a low-risk population, many individuals with disease may be missed because of false-negative assay results. Tumor markers with lower specificity may still be useful in high-risk populations (such as patients with genetic cancer syndromes) because the high prevalence of disease in this population greatly increases the positive predictive value of the assay.

Prostate-specific antigen (PSA), which is expressed only by prostatic epithelial cells, has proved to be a useful screening marker for prostate cancer. While PSA is present in the serum of all normal men, patients with prostate cancer usually have increased serum PSA levels. Although a significant elevation of PSA is not diagnostic of prostate cancer (elevation may result from inflammation of the prostate gland), it does identify a group of men who are at increased risk for prostate cancer who may benefit from more intensive evaluation (e.g., prostate needle biopsy). Patients with prostate cancer who are treated surgically by radical prostatectomy theoretically have all prostate tissue removed. As a result, their serum PSA levels are expected to be undetectable, and serum PSA is an ideal means of monitoring for tumor recurrence in these patients.

Human chorionic gonadotropin (hCG) is an excellent serum tumor marker for some testicular tumors because of its high specificity. Most other currently employed tumor markers have more limited specificity that significantly limits their clinical utility. CA125 is usually elevated in patients with ovarian carcinoma but may also be elevated in patients with any inflammatory process of the peritoneal cavity. Because ovarian cancer is a rare disease and because the specificity of CA125 is relatively low, it is not a practical marker for population screening for ovarian carcinoma. Rising levels of CA125 are usually indicative of tumor recurrence or progression in ovarian cancer patients, however.

Emerging Tumor Biomarkers

Recently, mass spectroscopy has been used to identify peptides in patient serum or urine that may allow detection of tumors very early in their clinical course (e.g., ovarian carcinoma), but it remains to be seen whether these results will translate into clinically useful biomarkers. Some tumors cause the generation of antibodies to tumor cells or autoantibodies to normal cellular components. These antibodies are potential biomarkers, but they have not been demonstrated to be of great clinical utility to date. Genetic changes in tumor cells are used clinically as biomarkers and are considered in the following section.

●●● MOLECULAR DIAGNOSTICS

Molecular genetic changes underlie the genesis of most human neoplasms. Because of this, all human neoplasms contain genetic changes that are potentially useful for their diagnosis. To date, molecular diagnostics has been used most extensively in hematopoietic diseases to assess clonality and the presence of specific chromosomal translocations. PCR technology has been extensively employed in hematopathology and allows the sensitive and specific detection of monoclonal lymphoid populations as well as individual translocation events. Molecular diagnostics has also been an important tool for characterizing and diagnosing pediatric neoplasms that are associated with specific translocations or specific gene amplification events (e.g., N-myc amplification in neuroblastoma).

Molecular diagnostics has played a much smaller role in the diagnosis of adult solid tumors, in which heterogeneous mutations in multiple different genes involving cell signaling, proliferation, and apoptosis pathways are common. Because many of these pathways are targeted in adult human tumors, demonstration of individual genetic lesions has relatively little specificity for particular tumor types. Conversely, many different genes would have to be evaluated to exclude the presence of genetic abnormalities in a given tumor sample. Mutations in some oncogenes (RAS and RAF) occur in benign neoplasms (hyperplastic colon polyps) so that the detection of these mutations is not always indicative of malignancy or dysplasia.

Unique antigen receptor gene rearrangements occur in the precursor cells of most NHLs. These DNA rearrangements are usually conserved in daughter tumor cells and can serve as unique clonal markers for these neoplasms. PCR analysis provides a clinically useful assay for clonal antigen receptor gene rearrangement, since the size (and DNA sequence) of PCR products produced using primers that span the complementarity-determining regions (CDRs) of the antigen receptor genes is a marker of each unique rearrangement event (Fig. 5-33A). Polyclonal lymphoid populations produce a smear pattern of PCR products on gel electrophoresis in this type of assay, whereas a discrete band can be produced from a monoclonal lymphoid population (see Fig. 5-33B). The assessment of small biopsies of lymph nodes for the presence of monoclonality can thus be a sensitive and specific test for the presence of NHL and lymphoid leukemia. The assessment of a particular translocation, such as the bcl-2 to immunoglobulin heavy chain gene translocation, by PCR can also be useful in the diagnosis and categorization of NHLs, such as follicular lymphoma.

More recently, gene expression profiling using RNA isolated from tumor cells has been used as a tool to discover new biomarkers that are prognostically useful or may help direct therapy in individual patients.

While this type of assay allows interrogation of the expression of thousands of genes, it is sensitive to tumor cell preservation (mRNA is highly labile) and has been clinically validated in only a few studies.

Minimal Residual Disease

Depending on the type of primary tumor, different assessment modalities (e.g., palpation, CT scan, PET scan) may have widely varying sensitivity for the detection of residual tumor after cancer treatment. Minimal residual disease means that a treated patient has residual tumor that is not detectable by clinical, radiographic, or pathologic examination. Minimal residual disease means the presence of residual tumor (either as tumor cell nests or as single tumor cells) in treated patients. Pathologic staging is the main modality used to evaluate residual disease after surgery, but it is usually not capable of detecting single tumor cells. Target amplification techniques such as PCR offer the possibility of detecting even single tumor cells if unique markers can be exploited. Molecular evaluation of minimal residual disease is most meaningful in hematopoietic tumors, which are often represented in blood or other body fluids (e.g., CSF) that can be sampled relatively easily. Since somatic genetic changes in lymphoid cells tend to be relatively stable over time, they can be used to assess minimal residual disease after therapy.

Minimal residual disease in children with acute lymphoblastic leukemia often takes the form of residual central nervous system involvement. Cytologic evaluation of CSF may show unequivocal evidence of residual or recurrent disease, but a fairly large number of tumor cells must be present for them to be differentiated unambiguously from cytologic atypia resulting from chemotherapy effects.

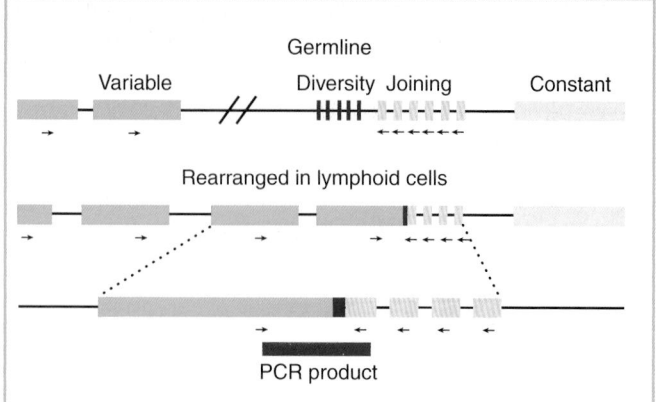

A

B

Figure 5-33. **A**, PCR detection of antigen receptor gene rearrangement in T and B lymphocytes. The germline arrangement of antigen receptor genes is shown at the top of the figure with the normal pattern of somatic rearrangement in lymphoid cells shown below. The small arrows indicate the positions and directions of PCR primers. No PCR product is generated from the germline configuration. PCR products ranging from 80 to 200 nucleotides in length are produced from rearranged IgH genes in B cells. **B**, Gel electrophoresis of PCR products. PCR products appear as bright bands against a black background in this acrylamide gel stained with ethidium bromide. Monoclonal rearrangement produces a discrete band while polyclonal rearrangement produces many different sized products visualized as a smear on gel electrophoresis.

Detection of clonal antigen receptor rearrangements can be a sensitive marker for tumor persistence or recurrence in this situation. Since not all tumor cells are clonogenic, care must be taken in assessing the significance of very small numbers of tumor cells.

DNA Microarrays

DNA microarrays provide a means of assessing the level of expression of many different genes at one time by hybridizing labeled cellular RNA to the array. A DNA microarray is a collection of microscopic deposits of specific DNA sequences on a solid support medium (usually glass). The position of a spot in the array determines the DNA sequence represented. Early arrays used predominantly cDNA and had hundreds to thousands of spots per array. Most modern arrays use synthetic oligonucleotides and more than 10,000 sequences can be represented on one array.

RNA isolated from cells is labeled by making a cRNA copy using fluorescently labeled nucleotides. Sometimes mRNA must be amplified before labeling to produce sufficient signal. If RNA is isolated from paraffin blocks using laser capture microdissection (see Laser Capture Microdissection box), the small amounts obtained always require RNA amplification prior to labeling, which can significantly skew the final results. Labeled RNA is hybridized to the array under high stringency conditions and the fluorescence intensity of individual spots is read by means of a specialized scanner.

The intensity of fluorescence is a measure of relative gene expression. The signal from housekeeping genes serves as a standard for the amount of input RNA and allows comparison between different samples.

Since many thousands of data points are produced by one experiment, computer analysis is essential to analyze the data and permits clustering of genes with up- and down-regulation (so-called hierarchical clustering). Genes can also be grouped into functional classes for comparison of expression in normal and diseased tissue.

 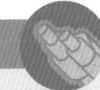

Laser Capture Microdissection (LCM)

LCM permits the isolation of small fragments of tissue from a histologic section using a specialized microscope to select the areas for excision. A clear plastic cap is placed directly on a stained tissue section (frozen or fixed), and the operator triggers a pulse from a laser beam that melts a small area of the plastic cap to fuse the cap to selected areas in the tissue, forming a spot weld. When the cap is removed, adherent cells at the spot weld are specifically removed and can be used to purify nucleic acid or protein.

The diameter of the laser beam can be adjusted so that single cells can be isolated under optimal conditions. LCM is a straightforward technique for the collection of DNA from cells selected visually or by immunohistochemical staining. Usually several hundred individual laser pulses are required to produce enough DNA for multiple PCR assays.

RNA isolation is more difficult because of the lability of RNA (RNA degradation occurs in situ during microdissection at room temperature). Many thousands of laser pulses may be required to obtain a useful amount of RNA for PCR analysis. RNA amplification is required for microarray applications because of the small amount of RNA obtained by LCM.

Detection of clonality in nonlymphoid tumors is more problematic because predictable genetic markers such as antigen receptor gene rearrangement or specific translocations are rarely present in these tumors. In some situations, measurement of expressed genes by RT-PCR has been used to identify small numbers of tumor cells, but the specificity of many of these assays is limited.

Prognostic Markers

Accurate definition of the likely clinical outcome for a cancer patient is an important clinical goal. Tumor staging currently provides the most important prognostic information, but the variation in prognosis within a tumor stage is usually significant, and additional, accurate prognostic markers would be beneficial. The presence of a few specific molecular genetic changes are associated with adverse prognosis in some neoplasms (e.g., p53 gene mutations in NHL are associated with shorter survival). Most adult solid tumors are quite genetically heterogeneous, however, with diverse alterations in many of the same genetic pathways. As a result, the identification of single genetic changes has not been of clear prognostic value in most neoplasms. Although comprehensive characterization of tumor genotype might yield more useful prognostic information, this type of analysis is beyond the scope of current technology.

Global evaluation of mRNA expression (i.e., gene expression profiling of thousands of individual genes by DNA microarray analysis) can define subgroups of NHL and leukemia that have significantly different prognoses. Evaluation of expression of a set of 20 genes selected by microarray analysis in breast cancer is now available commercially as a clinical prognostic assay. It is not clear whether this paradigm will be extended to other neoplasms or whether the value of these novel approaches will be confirmed by subsequent studies. These types of molecular assays critically depend on the isolation of pure populations of tumor cells for DNA and RNA analysis. Contamination of tumor nucleic acids with material from normal cells or necrotic tumor can potentially skew results, leading to false-positive or false-negative findings. Laser capture microdissection has emerged as a useful technique that allows precise sampling of tumor tissue under direct microscopic examination.

It is unclear whether the effort and expense associated with all these methodologies will be justified by the prognostic information obtained.

Predictive Markers

Predictive tumor markers differ from prognostic tumor markers in that their presence implies an enhanced (or diminished) response of a particular tumor to a specific therapeutic intervention. A simple example is the demonstration of HER2/neu gene amplification/overexpression in breast cancer. Patients who overexpress HER2/neu are much more likely to respond to a monoclonal antibody targeted against this receptor protein, and in this sense; HER2/neu overexpression is a predictive tumor marker.

IMMUNOLOGY & PHARMACOLOGY

Trastuzumab

Trastuzumab (Herceptin) is a humanized mouse monoclonal antibody that binds to the extracellular domain of the human epidermal growth factor receptor HER2/neu. Trastuzumab binding can induce apoptosis in many breast cancers that overexpress HER2/neu and can be very effective in combination with other forms of chemotherapy (particularly doxorubicin-containing regimens). Trastuzumab does not carry a toxin or irradiation, and its antitumor mechanism is not completely understood. Fc receptors on NK cells can bind trastuzumab, and antibody-mediated cytotoxicity (ADCC) by these cells may play a role in tumor cell killing in some circumstances.

The overexpressed HER2/neu receptor is not mutated and is thought to function normally. High receptor density in the membrane favors receptor dimerization, leading to autoactivation. Trastuzumab can trigger internalization of the HER2/neu receptor and decrease receptor density on the surface of tumor cells, but it is difficult to understand how this triggers apoptosis in sensitive cells.

HER2/neu is expressed at lower levels on some normal cells including cardiac myocytes, and trastuzumab therapy can damage these cells, particularly in combination with other cardiotoxic drugs. Recent data suggest that breast cancer patients who are successfully treated with trastuzumab have decreased rates of local tumor recurrence compared to those treated with standard chemotherapy protocols.

As more biologic therapies are developed, it seems clear that additional predictive markers will come into clinical practice. The development of imatinib, which was designed to target the chimeric receptor tyrosine kinase produced by bcr-abl gene translocation in chronic myelogenous leukemia (Fig. 5-34), is a recent example.

Leukemias that lack this translocation cannot respond to imatinib, making its genetic evaluation an essential prerequisite for treatment.

●●● TUMOR IMMUNITY

Tumor immunity refers to the generation of an immune response against a malignant neoplasm. Tumor immunity may be cell mediated or humoral although humoral responses are

PHARMACOLOGY

Imatinib

Imatinib mesylate is a potent inhibitor of a small number of structurally related tyrosine kinases including the bcr-abl fusion protein that is present in most cases of chronic myelogenous leukemia (CML). Imatinib can induce hematologic and cytogenetic remission in a significant percentage of patients with CML although resistance can develop in tumors via new mutations in their bcr-abl fusion protein.

Imatinib's activity against the c-kit receptor has been employed in gastrointestinal stromal tumors (GISTs). These low- to intermediate-grade sarcomas frequently have activating mutations in their c-kit receptor gene that make it constitutively active and stimulate tumor cell growth. These mutations also make the receptor sensitive to inhibition by imatinib. This type of molecularly designed therapy serves as an important paradigm for the development of other kinase inhibitors as cancer therapeutics.

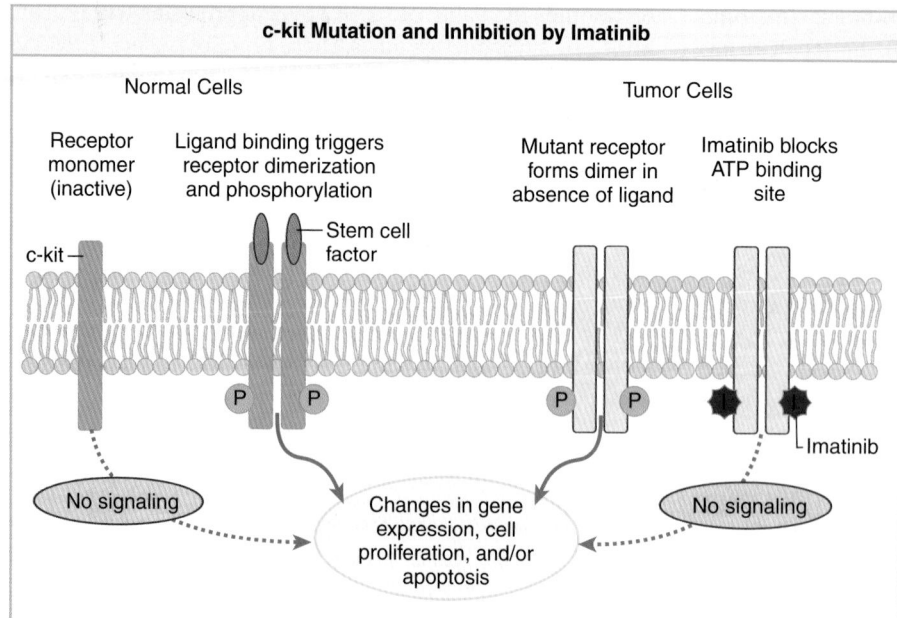

Figure 5-34. c-kit Mutations and gastrointestinal stromal tumors.

probably not effective in controlling tumors. Natural killer cells (innate immunity) are probably important in the early response to some neoplasms, and tumor-infiltrating lymphocytes (predominantly T cells) can be demonstrated in most malignant tumors. T cell–mediated responses are clearly important in some specific types of neoplasms. In cutaneous melanoma and some types of B-cell NHL, the presence of abundant tumor-infiltrating lymphocytes obviously is a positive prognostic indicator.

It is also clear that host immune response is insufficient to eradicate established malignant neoplasms in most situations. Although modulation of the immune system of cancer patients with cytokines and tumor vaccines has had occasional encouraging results, it is unlikely that this will become first- or second-line anticancer therapy. Nonetheless, in combination with chemotherapy, surgery, and/or irradiation, host immunity may be essential to eliminate residual microscopic foci of disease. In patients treated with bone marrow transplantation for myelogenous leukemia, it is apparent that limited graft-versus-host disease (in part directed against residual tumor cells) is a functionally important part of the therapeutic effect. It is also clear that patients with severe immunosuppression, either iatrogenic or due to HIV infection, are at substantially increased risk for the development of tumors (both typical adult neoplasms and unusual neoplasms that occur only in the context of immunosuppression). All these observations are consistent with the idea that immunosurveillance is important in the prevention and early destruction of different types of neoplasms and in the eradication of microscopic residual disease after cytotoxic therapy.

Host immunity can play a somewhat different role in preventing neoplasms that are induced by viral infection. Immunization against HPV has shown encouraging early results as a mechanism to prevent persistent viral infection that can lead to cervical dysplasia and ultimately cervical cancer. Similarly, prevention of persistent HBV infection by immunization protects individuals from potential hepatocarcinogenesis.

Skin and Musculoskeletal Pathology

6

●●● SKIN

Skin is largest organ of the body, and diffuse involvement of the skin by inflammation or injury can result in a massive fluid loss as well as a portal of entry for infectious agents. In addition to this mechanical barrier function, the skin is an important immune organ with numerous resident antigen-presenting cells. Solar and ultraviolet radiation are the major risk factors for the development of skin cancer, with fair-skinned individuals being most susceptible. Skin cancer is numerically the most common form of adult cancer, but most cases are cured by local excision although field effect changes in sun-exposed skin can lead to multiple primary tumors.

Dermatitis

Dermatitis means an inflammatory condition of the skin. Different forms of dermatitis may involve predominantly the epidermis, dermis, or both. The nature of the inflammatory infiltrate and the pattern of inflammation are key features in establishing a histologic diagnosis. For instance, most diseases that result in blister formation are clinically and pathologically distinct from most other types of dermatitis. In many cases, the gross appearance of the skin lesions, their pattern, and time course of evolution are critical factors in arriving at a specific pathologic diagnosis.

Eczema

Acute spongiotic dermatitis (also called call *eczematous dermatitis*) is an inflammatory condition that primarily involves the epidermis and results in intercellular edema (spongiosis), which produces visible separations between keratinocytes (Fig. 6-1). Edema may be so extensive that it results in the formation of fluid-filled cysts (bullae) that may rupture. The nature of the inflammatory infiltrate associated with edema may be useful in establishing the class of dermatitis (e.g., eosinophils are often prominent in allergic reactions). Many clinicopathologic subtypes of spongiotic dermatitis are recognized and differ in terms of their clinical features as well as specific morphologic features. A common cause of spongiotic dermatitis is the delayed-type hypersensitivity reaction such as occurs with exposure to poison ivy. In this case, sensitized T cells react with proteins in the skin that have been modified by haptens derived from poison ivy. These activated T cells release cytokines that attract other inflammatory cells and result in epidermal inflammation.

Erythema Multiforme

Erythema multiforme can result from hypersensitivity reactions to various drugs or be associated with infections (e.g., mycoplasmal pneumonia), malignancy, or collagen vas-

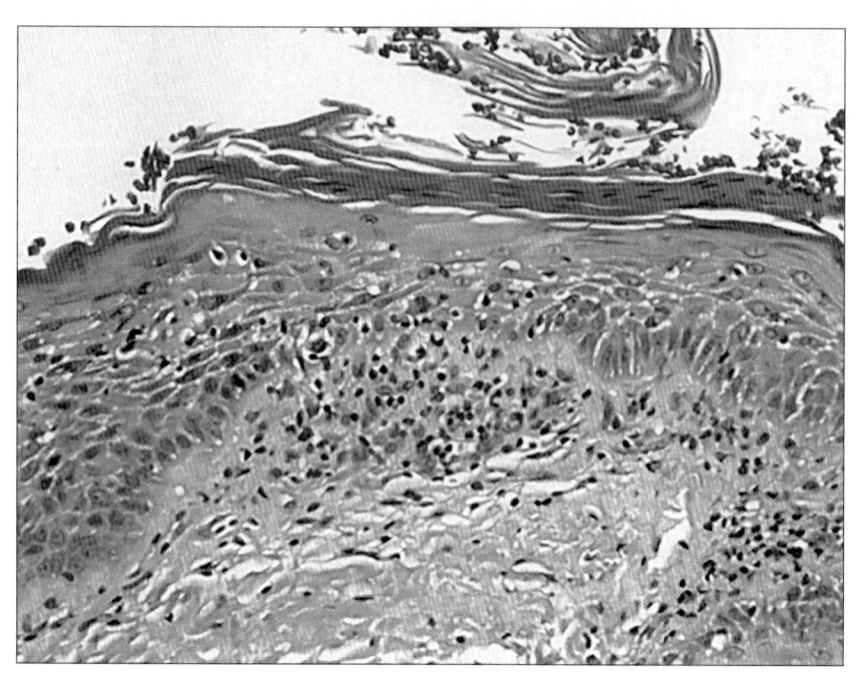

Figure 6-1. Spongiotic dermatitis. Microscopic section of skin showing a focal chronic inflammatory cell infiltrate in the superficial dermis and edema in the epidermis as evidenced by separations between keratinocytes (spongiosis). Mild hyperkeratosis is also present.

cular disease. Patients usually have numerous lesions of variable appearance consisting of macules, papules, and vesicles. These lesions tend to ulcerate, resulting in erosions (shallow ulcers). Histologically, there is a moderate to marked neutrophilic infiltrate. Eosinophils are often prominent in cases resulting from hypersensitivity reactions. Like other forms of spongiotic dermatitis, the primary cause of erythema multiforme likely is sensitized cytotoxic T cells. The most severe form of erythema multiforme is the so-called Stevens-Johnson syndrome in which the skin and mucous membranes are diffusely inflamed and ulcerated.

Lichen Planus

Lichen planus is a chronic inflammatory lesion of skin that results in papules with flattened surfaces that may coalesce to a confluent area of involvement. The biopsy specimen demonstrates a dense chronic inflammatory cell infiltrate that closely approximates the dermal-epidermal junction (Fig. 6-2). This is usually associated with thickening of the epidermis, hyperkeratosis, and liquefactive degeneration of the basal cell layer of the epidermis. Civatte bodies (round eosinophilic globules that are formed from necrotic keratinocytes) are frequently present in the epidermis. The morphologic pattern of lichen planus is often sufficiently characteristic to permit a specific pathologic diagnosis. Lichen planus is mediated by cytotoxic T cells, but its pathogenesis is not understood in detail.

Systemic Lupus Erythematosus

Systemic lupus erythematosus (SLE) and discoid lupus can produce morphologically identical skin lesions. In discoid lupus, the autoimmune process is limited to the skin and predominantly affects the scalp, often resulting in alopecia. In systemic lupus, a malar rash ("butterfly rash" over the cheek bones) is typical, but any area of the skin may be involved. Histologically, there is a marked chronic inflammatory cell infiltrate in the superficial dermis associated with hyperkeratosis (Fig. 6-3) as well as marked follicular plugging of hair shafts in discoid lupus. Immunofluorescence stains show granular deposition of immunocomplexes along the basement membrane zone in lesional skin (type III hypersensitivity). In patients with SLE, immunocomplexes are also observed in morphologically normal skin, whereas in discoid lupus, immunocomplexes are limited to skin lesions.

Psoriasis

Psoriasis is relatively common chronic inflammatory dermatitis that results in persistent scaling (desquamation of the stratum corneum) and may involve large areas of the body. The nails may also be affected. Histologically, there is marked thickening of the epidermis (acanthosis) with elongation of rete ridges. Neutrophils tend to form small microabscesses in the stratum corneum (Fig. 6-4). Many different subtypes of psoriasis are distinguished clinically and pathologically. The pathogenesis of psoriasis remains unclear but is thought to be related to T-cell infiltration.

Blistering Disorders

Blistering disorders can result from autoimmune disease or genetic abnormalities of components of the basement membrane zone.

Pemphigus is an uncommon autoimmune disease (type II hypersensitivity) that results in the formation of numerous blisters that wax and wane over time. Pemphigus is caused by binding of autoantibodies to the junctions between

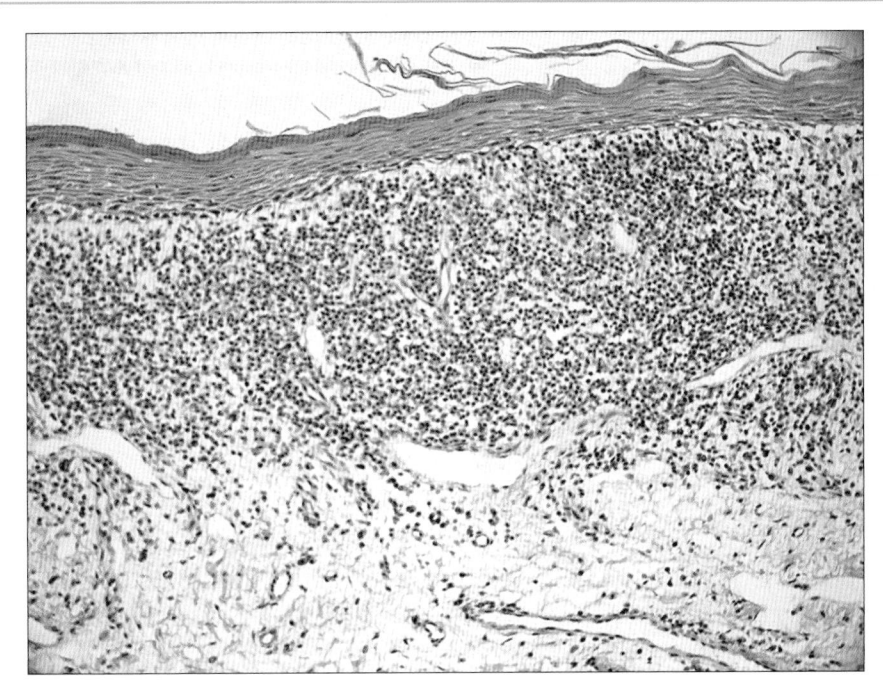

Figure 6-2. Lichen planus. Microscopic section of skin showing a prominent band-like chronic inflammatory cell infiltrate that closely approximates the dermal-epidermal junction. Basal keratinocytes show liquefactive degeneration. There is mild hyperkeratosis.

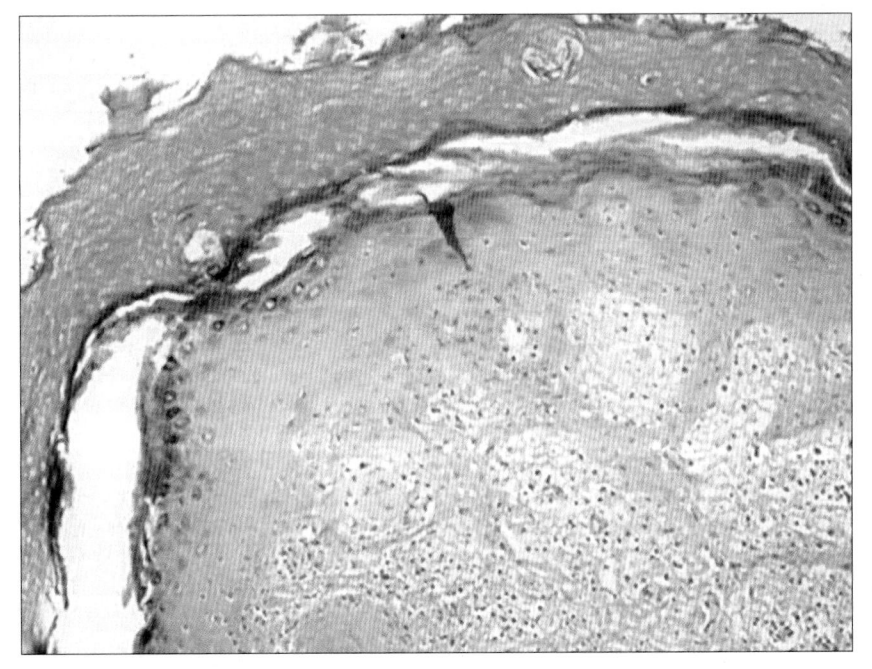

Figure 6-3. Systemic lupus erythematosus. Microscopic section of skin showing prominent hyperkeratosis and parakeratosis with a dense chronic inflammatory cell infiltrate in the dermis. Liquefactive degeneration of the basal cell layer of the epidermis is prominent. Immunofluorescence stains would show granular deposition of immunocomplexes along the dermal-epidermal junction.

keratinocytes, causing the separation of epidermal cells from one another (so-called acantholysis). Acantholysis can be observed in histologic sections and ultimately results in the formation of suprabasal blisters (Fig. 6-5). Immunofluorescence stains can demonstrate antibody deposition at the junctions between keratinocytes; this finding is important for establishing the diagnosis. Multiple clinical subtypes are distinguished.

Bullous pemphigoid also is a type II hypersensitivity disorder in which binding of autoantibodies to basement membrane zone components creates a cleft between the basal layer of the epidermis and the basement membrane, resulting in a subepidermal blister. Immunofluorescence stains show deposition of antibodies in the basement membrane zone.

Dermatitis herpetiformis is rare autoimmune disease caused by deposition of IgA at the tips of dermal papillae

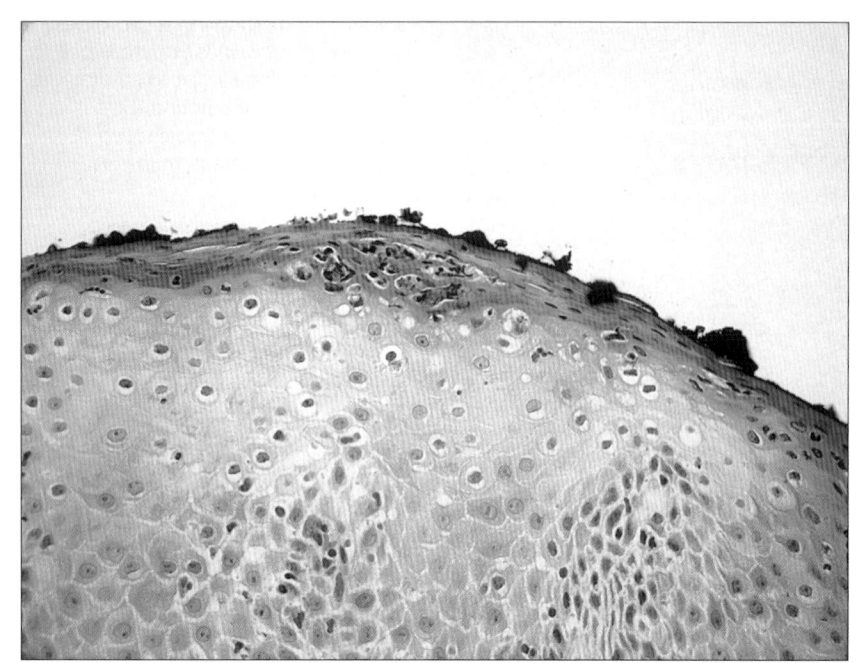

Figure 6-4. Psoriasis. Microscopic section of skin showing a Munro microabscess in the corneal layer of the epidermis.

IMMUNOLOGY

Psoriasis

Psoriasis affects approximately 2% of the population, and genetic predisposition to psoriasis shows a pattern consistent with multifactorial inheritance. Psoriasis shows a strong association with some MHC alleles, particularly HLA Cw6.

Environmental factors play a role, and infection of susceptible individuals with appropriate bacterial strains (e.g., those producing bacterial superantigens) may initiate a T-cell immune response that drives persistent skin inflammation and hyperproliferation of keratinocytes. T cells in the epidermis of patients show an activated phenotype, and T_H1 cells predominate. T cells are recruited to the skin by chemokines including TARC (thymus and activation regulated chemokine, which binds chemokine receptor CCR4) and CTACK (cutaneous T cell–attracting chemokine, which binds CCR10).

Replication in basal keratinocytes may increase by up to 50 times the normal rate, resulting in thickening of the epidermis to form plaques. Persistent inflammation in the epidermis results in expression of intercellular adhesion molecule–1 (ICAM-1) and MHC class II molecules by many cells, resulting in enhanced T-cell activation. This inflammatory milieu also primes endothelial cells for angiogenesis.

Immune-mediated arthritis (psoriatic arthritis) also develops in up to 20% of patients.

HISTOLOGY

Blistering Disorders

The level at which blisters form in the epidermis is critical in the differential diagnosis of all of blistering disorders. Subcorneal blisters form in the region just below the keratinized layer of the epidermis. Suprabasal blisters form between the basal layer (stratum basale) and upper layers of the epidermis. Subepidermal blisters form between the basement membrane zone and the basal cell layer of the epidermis.

Histologic evaluation of blisters is best performed while they are actively forming because secondary infection and repair processes can rapidly obscure the primary pathology. Biopsy specimens should be taken at the margin of a blister.

Chapter 9), possibly by cross-reacting with proteins in the basement membrane zone.

Infectious Skin Diseases

Systemic infections can result in transient skin changes that may be helpful in establishing the clinical diagnosis (e.g., viral exanthems such as measles). In viral infections such as smallpox and varicella zoster virus (VZV), skin lesions dominate the clinical presentation in some patients and can result in significant morbidity and mortality.

Bacterial Infections

Bacterial infections of skin can be caused by many different organisms and may serve as the portal of entry for deeper (e.g., fasciitis) or systemic infection. Streptococci can produce

resulting in an inflammatory reaction that tends to form sub-epidermal blisters. Some cases of dermatitis herpetiformis are associated with celiac disease, suggesting that the immune response to gluten-associated antigens in the intestine may contribute to IgA-mediated disease in the skin (see

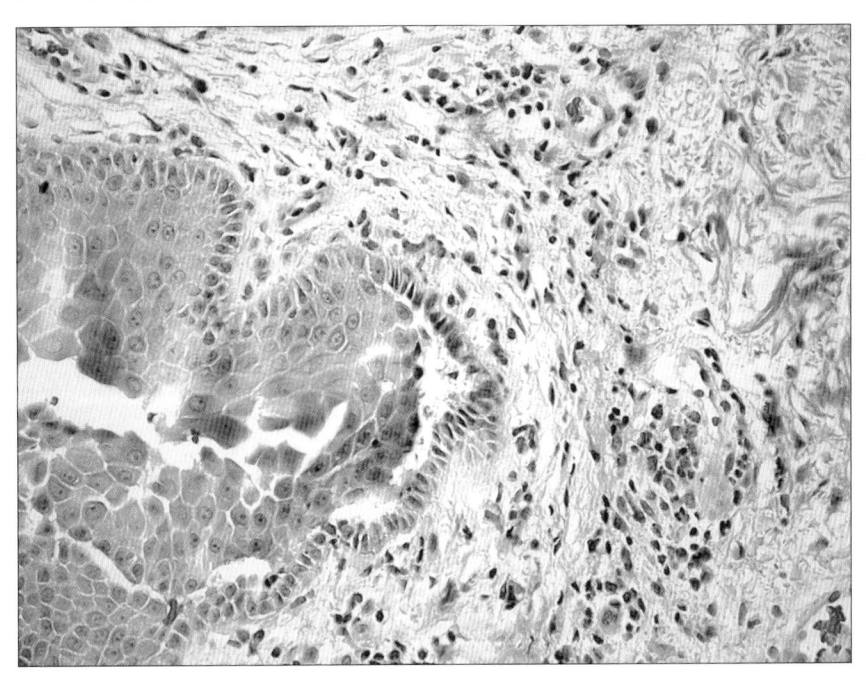

Figure 6-5. Pemphigus vulgaris. Microscopic section of skin showing a mild chronic inflammatory cell infiltrate in the superficial dermis. Acantholysis (separation of keratinocytes from each other) is prominent and has resulted in the formation of a small suprabasal bulla. Immunofluorescence stains would show immunoglobulin deposition around acantholytic keratinocytes.

the clinical syndrome of erysipelas with erythema of the skin that spreads in a wave-like pattern. Staphylococci usually result in a more localized infection with abscess formation.

Warts

Cutaneous warts (verrucae) are caused by infection with human papillomavirus (HPV). Viral serotypes have tropisms for different types of skin and mucous membranes. The morphologic features of verrucae vary with location, but most cutaneous warts show papillomatosis (papillary extension of rete ridges) in association with prominent hyperkeratosis (thickening of the stratum corneum), parakeratosis (presence of nucleated squames in the stratum corneum), and hypergranulosis (prominence of the granular cell layer of the epidermis with large keratohyaline granules) (Fig. 6-6). Cutaneous warts are not associated with an increased risk for the development of squamous cell carcinoma, but infection of the cervix or oropharynx with certain subtypes of human papillomavirus is an important risk factor for tumor development.

Herpesviruses

Many human herpesviruses cause cutaneous or mucosal eruptions at the site of infection or produce generalized skin eruptions. In most cases, these lesions are associated with relatively characteristic viral cytopathic changes. Herpes simplex virus (type 1, cold sores; and type 2, venereal spread) tends to produce ulcerating papules that show nuclear clearing and multinucleation of infected cells. Cytomegalovirus (CMV) more commonly involves mucous membranes and produces large intranuclear eosinophilic inclusions in infected cells and, less commonly, cytoplasmic inclusions. VZV produces crops of vesicles during the acute phase of chickenpox with

associated viral cytopathic effects evident on the Tzanck test. Most herpesviruses produce lifelong latent infection that can reactivate during periods of stress or immunosuppression. VZV typically localizes to dorsal root ganglia, and reactivation produces a skin eruption (similar to chickenpox) in areas supplied by that nerve.

Tumors and Tumor-like Conditions

Most tumors and premalignant lesions of skin can be identified by gross visual inspection, and most primary skin tumors grow to large size before metastatic disease develops. The major exception to this rule is malignant melanoma, which may metastasize very early in its course. Small squamous cell carcinomas occasionally metastasize, but this is much more common in larger, neglected tumors. Most other common skin tumors are benign and have little or no metastatic potential.

Seborrheic Keratosis

Seborrheic keratoses are common benign lesions that usually appear as hyperpigmented papules (slightly raised, dome-shaped lesions). Morphologically, they are composed of a thickened and usually hyperkeratotic epidermis with typical pseudohorn cysts (rounded concentric foci of keratinization within the epidermis). Different subtypes of seborrheic keratosis show variations on this general architectural scheme. Seborrheic keratoses may become inflamed but almost never undergo malignant degeneration.

Actinic Keratosis and Squamous Cell Carcinoma

Actinic keratosis is preneoplastic dysplasia of epidermal keratinocytes that is associated with significant sun or UV light

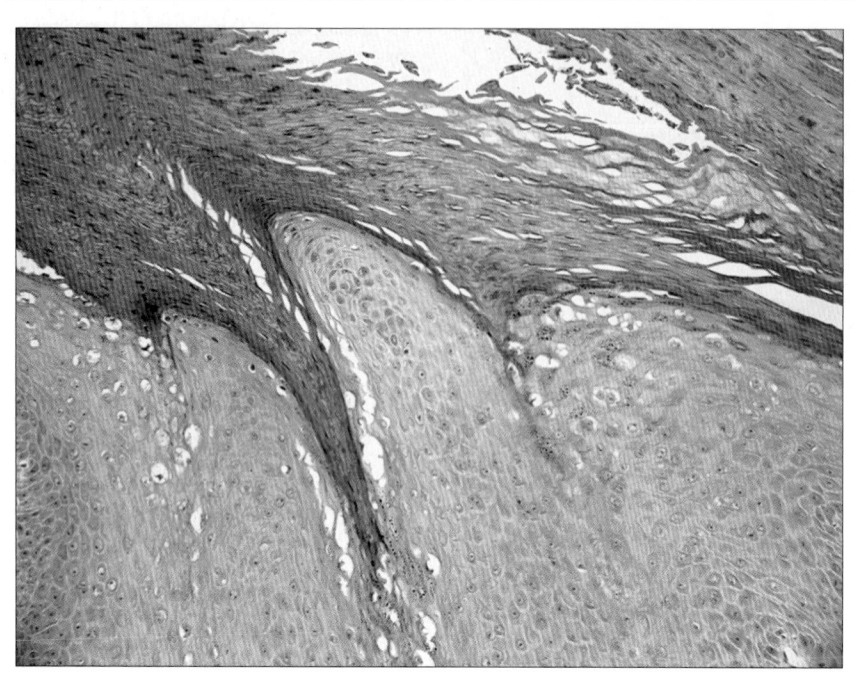

Figure 6-6. Verruca vulgaris. Microscopic section of skin showing marked thickening of the epidermis (acanthosis) with prominent papillomatosis. Prominent parakeratosis is also present with marked prominence of the granular cell layer, which contains large keratohyaline granules. Some infected keratinocytes show binucleation.

exposure. Actinic keratoses often show thickening of the epidermis (acanthosis) with cytologic atypia of keratinocytes demonstrating disorderly maturation. Mitotic figures are often abnormally present above the basal cell layer. Some lesions show marked hyperkeratosis forming a so-called keratin horn that may project outward for a centimeter or more. Underlying dermal collagen also shows evidence of sun damage with basophilic staining and fragmentation of collagen fibers (so-called solar elastosis) and a variable chronic inflammatory cell reaction.

The dysplastic keratinocytes in actinic keratoses are confined by the basement membrane, and progression to squamous cell carcinoma is signaled by the extension of neoplastic cells through the basement membrane into the dermis with an associated desmoplastic reaction (Fig. 6-7). Squamous cell carcinomas occasionally result in lymph node metastases early in their course. Various subtypes and grades of squamous cell carcinoma have differing biologic aggressiveness and metastatic potential.

Basal Cell Carcinoma

Basal cell carcinoma is a common tumor of the epidermis that is strongly associated with sun exposure. Tumor cells resemble basal cells of the epidermis and invade the dermis as nests and cord-like extensions. Connection of these nests to the overlying epidermis is usually maintained, and they show prominent peripheral palisading of tumor cell nuclei (the long axis of nuclei is oriented perpendicular to the edge of the tumor cell nests), which is a characteristic feature of this tumor (Fig. 6-8). Numerous subtypes of basal cell carcinoma are recognized, and some are associated with specific genetic syndromes. Basal cell carcinoma can be locally aggressive, but

metastasis almost never occurs even with very large primary tumors.

Skin Appendage Tumors

Most tumors of skin appendages (hair shafts, sweat glands, and apocrine glands) have characteristic morphologic features that mimic their cell of origin (e.g., hair shaft, eccrine gland). The vast majority of these tumors behave in a benign (or at most locally aggressive) fashion, and metastasis is exceptionally rare.

Melanocytic Nevi and Malignant Melanoma

Melanocytic nevi are common lesions that may be present at birth (so-called congenital nevi) or develop during life (acquired nevi). Nevi tend to go through a cycle of maturation in which they begin as nests of nevus cells along the dermal-epidermal junction (a so-called junctional nevus). Over time nevus cells migrate downward into the dermis with conversion of the junctional nevus to an intradermal nevus. Intermediate stages of this process are described as compound melanocytic nevi (Fig. 6-9). Normal nevus cells become smaller as they penetrate deeper into the epidermis (so called vertical maturation) and remain in an organized, relatively circumscript configuration. Most nevi in adults have completed their maturation and are pure intradermal nevi.

Some nevi have atypical morphologic features (so-called dysplastic nevi) and are precursors of malignant melanoma. Dysplastic nevi often show predominance of the junctional over the epidermal component and less well formed nests of nevus cells along the dermal-epidermal junction. Of even more concern is the development of cytologically atypical nevus cells and the presence of lamellar fibrosis in the dermis

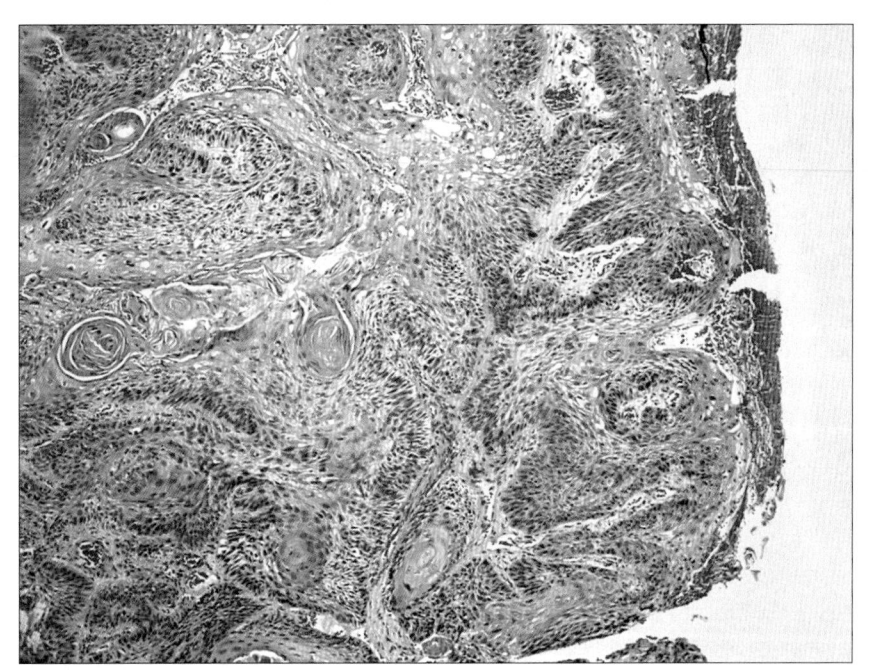

Figure 6-7. Squamous cell carcinoma. Microscopic section of skin showing a deeply invasive, moderately differentiated tumor with irregular masses of neoplastic squamous cells invading deep into the dermis. There is prominent keratinization of invasive tumor cell nests.

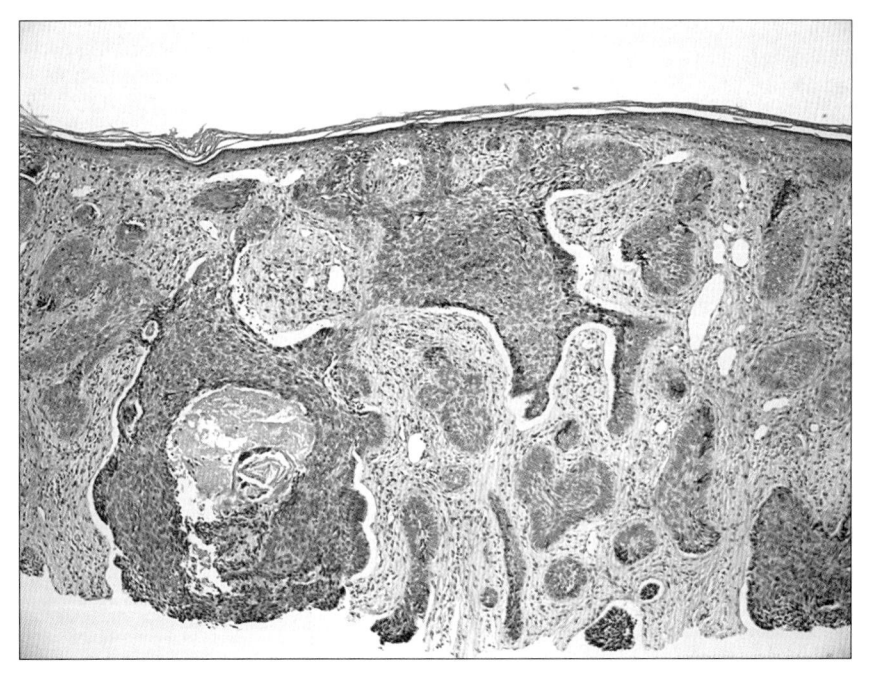

Figure 6-8. Basal cell carcinoma. Microscopic section of skin showing connection of tumor cell nests to the basal cell layer of the epidermis. There is prominent palisading (parallel alignment) of tumor cells at the periphery of tumor nests.

beneath the nevus. Transformation to malignant melanoma is often heralded by extension of nevus cells into the epidermis (so-called epidermotropism), where they interdigitate between keratinocytes.

Malignant melanomas can also arise de novo (i.e., with no precursor nevus), and some dermatopathologists think that all melanomas arise de novo. Melanoma in situ corresponds to the presence of cytologically malignant melanocytes along the dermal-epidermal junction with associated epider-

motropism. Melanomas may spread laterally (so-called radial growth phase) before they invade the dermis (so called vertical growth phase) (Fig. 6-10). A number of different morphologic variants of in situ melanoma are recognized and some of these (so-called minimal deviation melanoma) may be difficult to differentiate from benign or atypical nevi.

The development of melanoma is strongly associated with sun exposure. This is particularly true in light-skinned individuals, in whom UV radiation easily penetrates the epider-

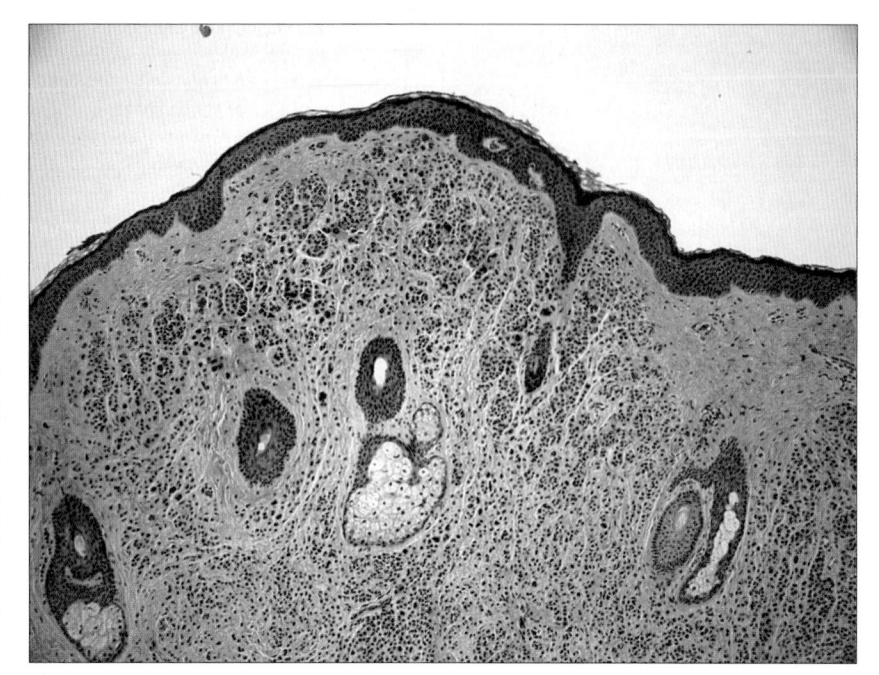

Figure 6-9. Melanocytic nevus. Microscopic section of skin showing nevus cells extending downward into the dermis, demonstrating vertical maturation. No epidermal component remains in this mature (intradermal) nevus.

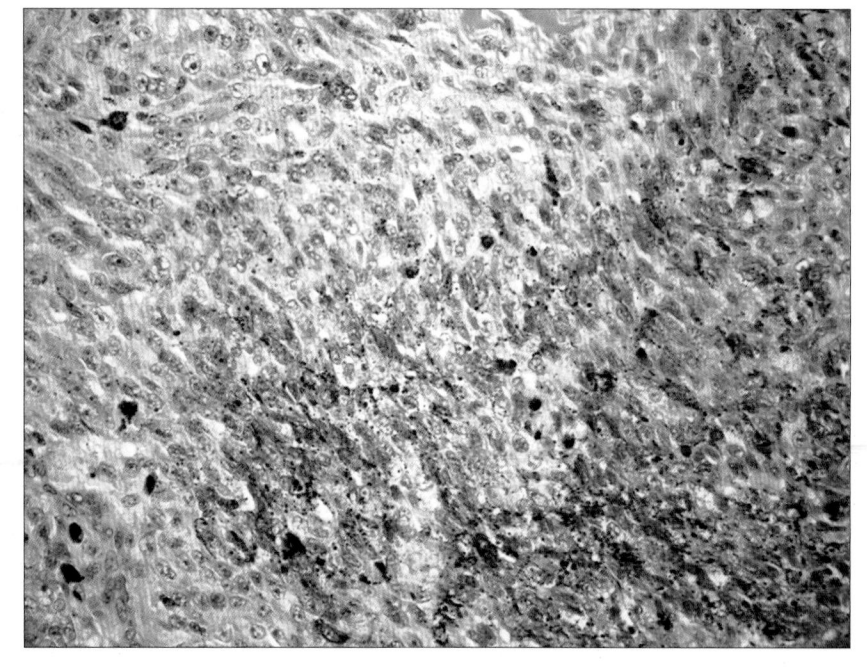

Figure 6-10. Malignant melanoma. Microscopic section of skin showing a high-grade malignant melanoma composed predominantly of spindle cells with prominent melanin pigment.

mis. A history of moderate to severe sunburns during childhood is a significant risk factor. Heritable genetic abnormalities in the p16 tumor suppressor gene can result in a high frequency of melanoma in some families (i.e., familial melanoma). p16 and PTEN gene alterations are common in sporadic melanomas.

Clinically, melanomas may present as a color or shape change in a preexisting nevus or as a new pigmented lesion.

A high index of suspicion is required to identify these lesions early in their preinvasive stage when surgical excision is curative. As melanomas begin to invade the dermis, there is often a host immune response to the invading tumor cells, and the intensity of this lymphocytic infiltrate is an important prognostic factor. The depth of invasion is the most important prognostic feature in invasive melanomas. Depth can be characterized by Clark level (a descriptive staging system based

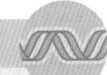

Familial and Hereditary Melanoma

Approximately 10% of patients with melanoma report a positive family history of melanoma, and a family history of melanoma is associated with a twofold increased risk that is largely the result of polygenic and environmental factors (e.g., light skin and sun exposure).

Hereditary melanoma is an uncommon syndrome (probably less than 1% of all melanomas) in which one genetic alteration results in a marked predisposition to melanoma. Mutations in the p16 gene and in cyclin-dependent kinase 4 (CDK4) can each cause hereditary melanoma. CDK4 mutations tend to cluster in the region of the protein that normally interacts with p16, suggesting a convergence of oncogenic mechanisms at this control point. Both mutations can result in uncontrolled cell cycle progression at G_1S that causes genetic instability. Most p16 gene mutations in hereditary melanoma are in exons 1α and 2.

Although p16 gene mutations predispose to melanoma, it is not clear that that p16 is involved in the dysplastic nevus syndrome in which patients develop numerous dysplastic nevi that may progress to melanoma. Other genetic lesions may cause this syndrome.

on penetration of the superficial to deep dermis) and Breslow depth (a measurement in millimeters from the granular cell layer of the epidermis to the deepest point of invasion by melanoma cells). The Breslow depth is a strong predictor of clinical outcome, with lesions greater than 0.5 mm bearing a significant risk for metastasis. Patients with moderately to deeply invasive melanomas are typically managed by complete excision of the lesion and sentinel lymph node biopsy (see Chapter 13). Other features may affect the likelihood of metastasis including mitotic activity and expression of CD10 (a membrane-bound metalloproteinase).

Although most melanomas arise in the skin in association with sun exposure, they can arise primarily in some visceral sites (e.g., in the distal rectum). Some patients have metastatic melanoma with no evidence of a primary tumor, and in these cases, a strong host immune response may have caused complete regression of the primary tumor. Most melanomas are associated with the production of melanin pigment although this may be lost in metastases and in more poorly differentiated tumors (so-called amelanotic melanomas). Some melanomas may mimic carcinomas or sarcomas (e.g., desmoplastic melanoma). Melanocytes derived from the neural crest and most melanomas stain negatively for cytokeratins and express S100 protein and Mart-1, and these immunohistochemical markers are quite useful diagnostically.

●●● JOINTS

Degeneration of joint surfaces is responsible for significant physical impairment in many older individuals, whereas inflammatory diseases of joints are more common in younger people. Tumors and tumor-like conditions of joints are rare.

Osteoarthritis

Osteoarthritis is a degenerative condition that is almost universally present in older individuals. Osteoarthritis is thought to result from age-related changes and repetitive minor joint trauma. Abnormal skeletal structure, trauma, or excessive weight bearing (obesity) can greatly accelerate this degenerative process. Pathologically, osteoarthritis corresponds to thinning and erosion of articular cartilage. In more severe cases, subchondral cysts form in articular bone because synovial fluid is forced (under pressure) through defects in cartilage into bony tissue (Fig. 6-11). This results in additional deformity of the bone and increasing dysfunction of the joint. Over time, microfractures develop in articular bone, resulting in more extreme deformity and associated pain.

Rheumatoid Arthritis

Rheumatoid arthritis is an autoimmune disease that typically presents in young to middle-aged adults. Women are much more frequently affected than men are. Morphologically, joints are inflamed, with a prominent lymphoplasmacytic cellular infiltrate (Fig. 6-12A). The synovial membranes are hyperplastic and are converted from their normal linear architecture into masses of hyperplastic papillary membranes filled with chronic inflammatory cells. Untreated, rheumatoid arthritis results in marked damage to the articular cartilage and can result in the formation of granulation tissue (pannus), which replaces the articular cartilage and can result in bony fusion across joint spaces (ankylosis) with complete loss of joint mobility. Rheumatoid arthritis characteristically involves the small joints of the hands and feet but may also involve larger joints. Hand involvement typically results in ulnar deviation of the fingers and, in severe cases, the "swan neck" deformity (see Fig. 6-12B).

Most evidence favors cell-mediated immunity as the major driver of inflammation in joints. Macrophages are key players in this inflammatory reaction and provide cytokines that are critically involved in the pathogenesis of this disease. TNF is particularly important in promoting inflammatory activity and probably underlies many of the systemic effects of this disease. T_H1 helper T cells likely stimulate macrophages in joints to produce TNF-α. Although rheumatoid arthritis is thought to be a T cell–mediated disease, recent studies have shown efficacy of monoclonal antibody therapy directed against mature B cells, suggesting that B cells and/or plasma cells play a key role in pathophysiology.

Simple categorization of rheumatoid arthritis as a cell-mediated or humoral disease is not possible. Many patients with rheumatoid arthritis have an autoantibody (so-called rheumatoid factor) that reacts with the Fc receptors of other immunoglobulins. Rheumatoid factor can also be present in individuals with other types of autoimmune disease who do not have arthritis.

Rheumatoid arthritis usually causes severe joint pain, and although anti-inflammatory analgesic drugs such as aspirin and nonsteroidal anti-inflammatory agents may provide some

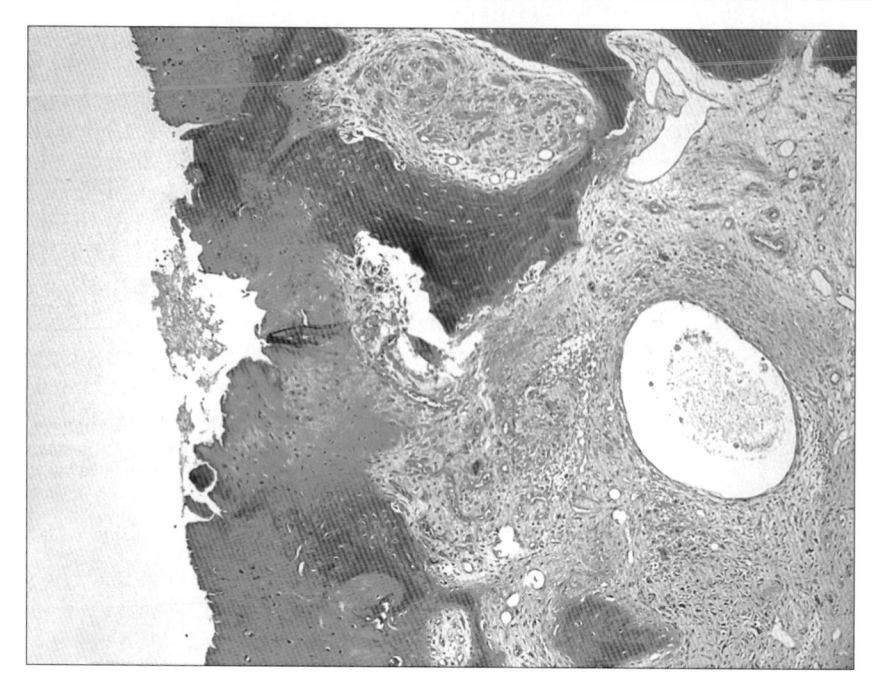

Figure 6-11. Osteoarthritis. Microscopic section of a hip joint showing marked degeneration and erosion of articular cartilage and the formation of small subchondral cysts.

symptomatic pain relief, they do not modify the clinical course of arthritis. Agents such as corticosteroids and methotrexate can slow the progression of joint destruction and are now referred to as DMARDs (disease-modifying anti-rheumatic drugs). Monoclonal antibody therapy targeted at TNF-α is effective in relieving symptoms and slowing joint destruction. While these therapies can be effective in arresting disease progression, all produce significant immunosuppression and increased risk for opportunistic infection and immunodeficiency-associated lymphoproliferative disorder.

Patients with rheumatoid arthritis frequently develop extra-articular manifestations of autoimmune disease. Rheumatoid nodules are subcutaneous foci of necrobiosis of collagen that are surrounded by palisading histiocytes (see Fig. 6-12C). Rheumatoid nodules typically occur along extensor surfaces (e.g., elbow) and must be distinguished from opportunistic infections, which may produce similar morphologic features in immunocompromised patients. More serious but less common extra-articular manifestations of rheumatoid arthritis include interstitial pulmonary fibrosis, which may lead to significant pulmonary dysfunction.

Crystalline Arthritis

The accumulation of crystals in joint spaces incites a severe inflammatory reaction (e.g., uric acid crystals in gout and calcium pyrophosphate crystals in pseudogout). Crystals ingested by inflammatory cells tend to cause membrane rupture with release of proteolytic enzymes and cytokines. These changes result in pain and inflammation in joints with swelling and joint effusions. Microscopic examination of joint fluid under polarized light can show characteristic

crystal morphology and is usually diagnostic. One joint is often involved in a single attack (monoarticular), but multiple joints are typically involved over time. Peripheral joints are affected most frequently owing to the decreased temperature, which facilitates crystal formation. Repeated cycles of inflammation can result in significant joint deformity. Gout can also result in the formation of tophi (solid masses of uric acid crystals in a proteinaceous matrix with associated giant cell inflammatory response).

Infectious Arthritis

Transient arthritis (arthralgias) is associated with many types of viral infection and results from immune mechanisms rather than direct infection of joints in most cases. Many different types of bacteria can cause infection if they are directly inoculated into joints, but several organisms characteristically localize to joints during systemic infection.

Lyme Disease

Lyme disease is caused by infection with a spirochete (*Borrelia burgdorferi*) that is transmitted by tick bite (usually deer ticks). Infection produces a skin lesion at the site of inoculation (erythema marginatum) with a "bull's-eye" pattern of erythema.

The joints are often affected in subacute and chronic disease, and organisms can be demonstrated in joint tissue by sensitive techniques (e.g., PCR). Immune-mediated injury and persistent infection may both play a role in chronic Lyme disease. Serologic testing for Lyme disease is not fully reliable (many equivocal or false-positive tests), making definitive diagnosis difficult.

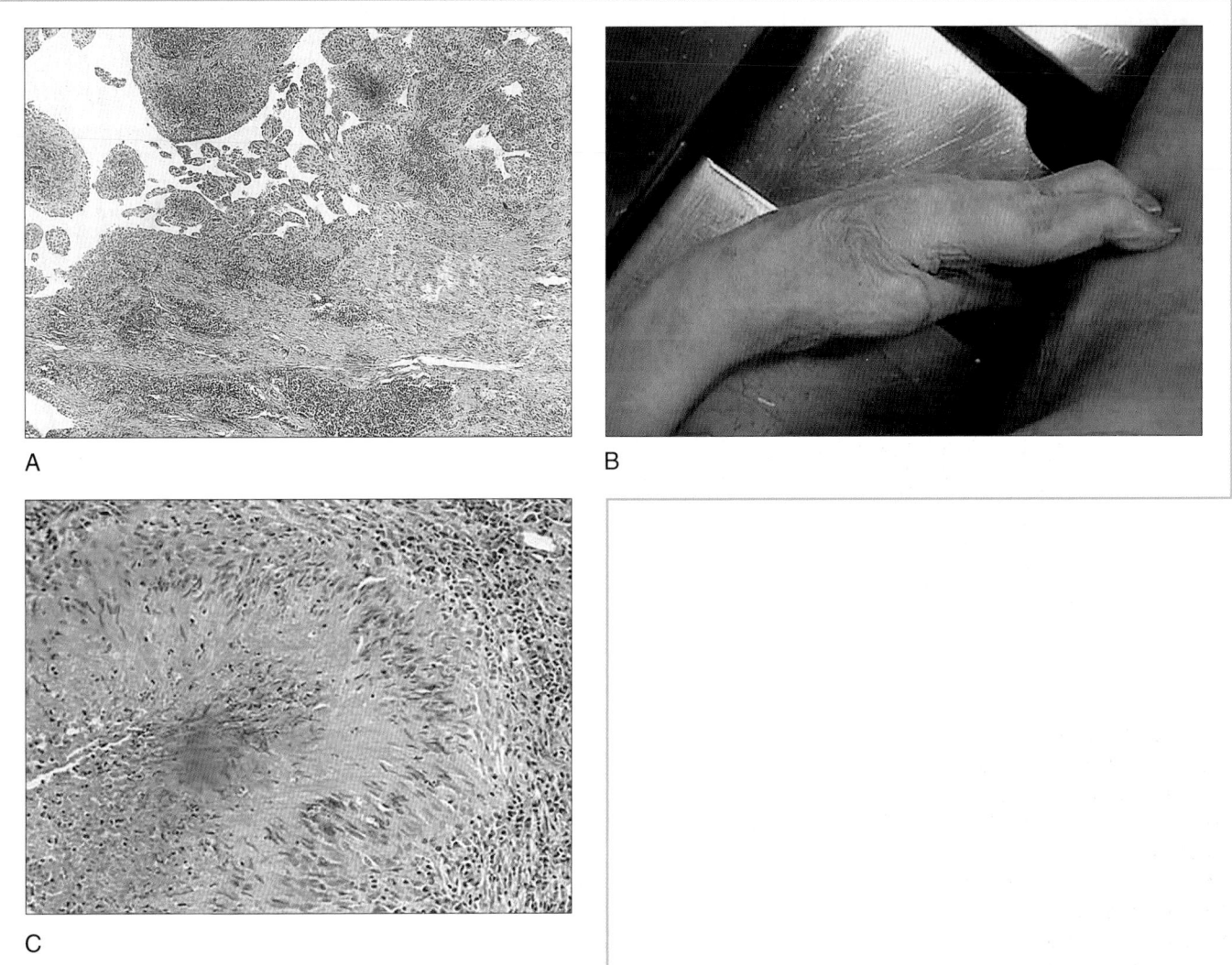

Figure 6-12. **A,** Inflamed synovium in rheumatoid arthritis. Microscopic section showing papillary proliferation of the synovial membrane, which is infiltrated by lymphocytes and plasma cells. **B,** Rheumatoid arthritis with joint subluxation. **C,** Rheumatoid nodule. Microscopic section showing central necrobiosis surrounded by palisading histiocytes (oriented histiocytes that assume an architectural pattern reminiscent of columnar epithelium).

Neisseria gonorrhoeae

Systemic infection with *Neisseria gonorrhoeae* (after venereal transmission) can result in a painful, pyogenic arthritis that can be monoarticular or polyarticular. Joint aspiration demonstrates intracellular gram-negative cocci in neutrophils and is diagnostic. The joint tropism of this organism is not well explained.

●●● BONE

Bones provide mechanical integrity for the skeleton but are also critical endocrine organs involved in maintaining calcium homeostasis as well as providing an appropriate environment for hematopoiesis. Cortical bone provides most of the mechanical strength in the skeleton while trabecular bone (with a much larger surface area) subserves endocrine functions (Fig. 6-13).

Genetic Bone Disease

Most genetic diseases affecting bone present in infancy or early childhood with abnormal bone growth and remodeling with or without decreased skeletal integrity.

Achondroplasia

Achondroplasia results from mutations in the fibroblast growth factor receptor 3 (FGF-R3) gene that produces a constitutively active receptor. Abnormal signaling disrupts cartilage formation, thereby preventing endochondral ossification.

Since all long bones are formed by endochondral ossification, patients have short stature and deformity of most long bones (achondroplastic dwarfs).

Osteogenesis Imperfecta

Osteogenesis imperfecta (so-called brittle bone disease) is a family of diseases that result from abnormalities in type I

PHARMACOLOGY

Monoclonal Antibody (MAb) Therapy

MAbs were first developed in 1975, and they offer the possibility of crafting highly specific effectors to attack disease targets. Most MAbs are produced in mice although therapeutic mouse antibodies are often "humanized" by replacing the mouse Fc sequences with human sequences. These changes may decrease the antigenicity of the antibody in humans (still a problem with repeated injections) and allow binding of MAbs to host cells with Fc receptors. If host immunity develops, therapeutic MAbs are rapidly cleared from the circulation, decreasing or eliminating their therapeutic benefit. More recently, advanced molecular biology techniques permit construction of fully human MAbs in mice.

MAbs can be directed against cellular or protein/glycoprotein targets to effect the removal of circulating cells (e.g., B lymphocytes, anti-CD20) and inflammatory mediators (e.g., TNF-α) by the spleen. MAbs can also be conjugated with toxins (e.g., diphtheria toxin or ricin have been used in cancer therapy) that are activated only if the antibody binds to a cell and is internalized. MAbs conjugated with radioactive isotopes have also been used in cancer chemotherapy. The short half-life of isotopes makes these MAbs inconvenient and costly, but some radioactive MAbs have shown impressive anticancer activity in small trials.

MICROBIOLOGY

Borrelia burgdorferi

B. burgdorferi is a spirochete that uses axial filaments (endoflagella) for locomotion. Organisms are 20 to 30 μm in length but only 0.2 μm in width, making them visible by dark-field but not by bright-field microscopy. *B. burgdorferi* has an outer membrane composed of LPS-like material similar to gram-negative bacteria. *B. burgdorferi* expresses a number of surface proteins that are thought to be involved in virulence.

The natural host and reservoir for *B. burgdorferi* is thought to be the white-footed mouse. *B. burgdorferi* can be transferred from the mouse to humans and deer via a tick vector (usually the deer tick *Ixodes*) that is much smaller (<2 mm) than the common dog tick.

Human infection initially produces a rash at the site of a tick bite (erythema marginatum) that forms an expanding red ring-like lesion. Spirochetes can be cultured from erythema marginatum lesions, which usually persist for 3 to 4 weeks. Dissemination of spirochetes though blood can occur within days to weeks of initial infection and is associated with systemic symptoms including fever, fatigue, headache, and arthralgias. Signs of persistent infection usually develop months to years after infection, with intermittent joint pain and neurologic symptoms. Treatment with doxycycline usually is effective at all stages of disease. Infected individuals develop antibodies, but serologic tests are often inconclusive.

collagen (a major component of normal osteoid and bone). Both autosomal dominant and recessive forms of disease can result in bones with very low tensile strength that are easily fractured. Children often die in infancy as a result of multiple fractures.

Osteopetrosis

Osteopetrosis (so-called marble bone disease) is caused by alterations in the macrophage colony-stimulating factor (MCSF) gene, which is essential for normal osteoclast differentiation from monocyte precursors in the bone marrow. Affected patients have few osteoclasts and cannot normally resorb bone. As a consequence, unopposed osteoblastic activity fills the marrow space with bone. Excess bone eventually impinges on cranial and spinal nerve roots and disrupts normal hematopoiesis.

Bone Fractures

Fractures usually result from skeletal trauma that is sufficient to break normal bones. Fractures of normal bone heal with the formation of the callus, composed of reactive bone formation (woven bone) around the fracture (Fig. 6-14). If the fracture is not complicated by infection (e.g., an open fracture) and is properly aligned, healing results in the remodeling of the callus to mature lamellar bone (i.e., restoration of normal function).

Fractures caused by very mild trauma or by normal wear and tear are called pathologic fractures, meaning that they result from an underlying abnormality of the bone. Pathologic fractures can result from intrinsic abnormalities of bone including osteopenia (e.g., abnormally low bone density), osteomalacia (e.g., abnormal, deficient mineralization of bone), tumors (primary or metastatic), and tumor-like conditions of bone.

Osteomyelitis

Osteomyelitis means a direct bacterial infection of bone that can occur as a complication of an open fracture or by hematogenous seeding of microorganisms. If necrotic bone is present at an infected fracture site (so-called sequestrum), usually it is not possible to resolve the infection without surgical removal of the necrotic tissue (Fig. 6-15). Osteomyelitis is often difficult to cure with antibiotics and may require prolonged therapy with intravenous antibiotics. Osteomyelitis can complicate systemic infection with *Mycobacterium tuberculosis*, which typically localizes to the vertebral bodies (Pott's disease).

Sickle Cell Anemia

Sickle cell anemia causes small and large bone infarcts (pain crisis) that put these patients at markedly increased risk for developing osteomyelitis, frequently caused by *Salmonella* spread hematogenously from the gastrointestinal tract. The basis of this tropism is not well understood.

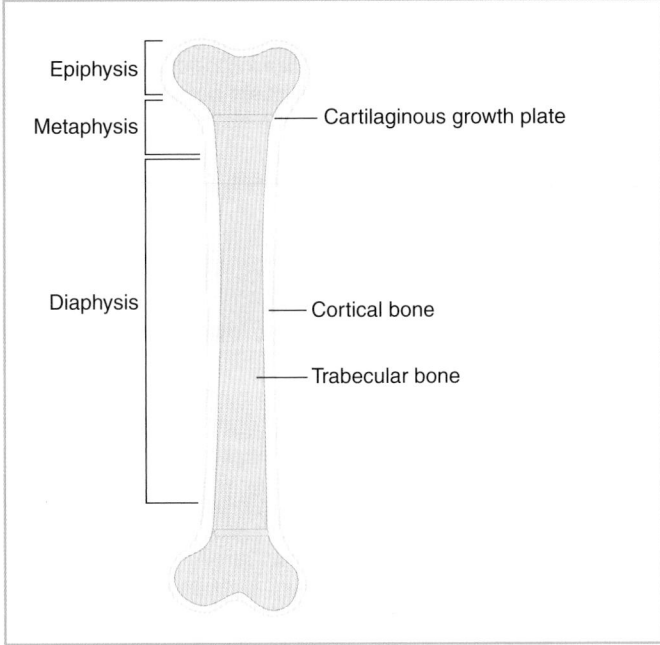

Figure 6-13. Schematic diagram of a long bone.

Epiphysis
Metaphysis
Diaphysis
Cartilaginous growth plate
Cortical bone
Trabecular bone

Endochondral Ossification

Endochondral ossification is the normal process that forms all long bones. After a cartilaginous framework of a bone is formed, endochondral ossification results in the sequential conversion and resorption of calcified cartilage and its replacement by bone. Osteoblasts migrate to the ossification front and synthesize bone matrix. Endochondral ossification is a well-ordered process that has definite polarity with residual cartilage on one edge and newly formed osteoid on the other. Trailing osteoid is mineralized in an orderly fashion to form new mineralized bone.

In long bones, ossification begins in the diaphysis during embryonic development, whereas ossification of the epiphysis does not start until after birth. In neonates, the ossification fronts move toward each other until only the growth plates (epiphyseal plates) remain between the metaphysis and epiphysis. Continued endochondral ossification at the growth plates permits a linear increase in bone length until closure of the epiphyses in late adolescence or early adulthood.

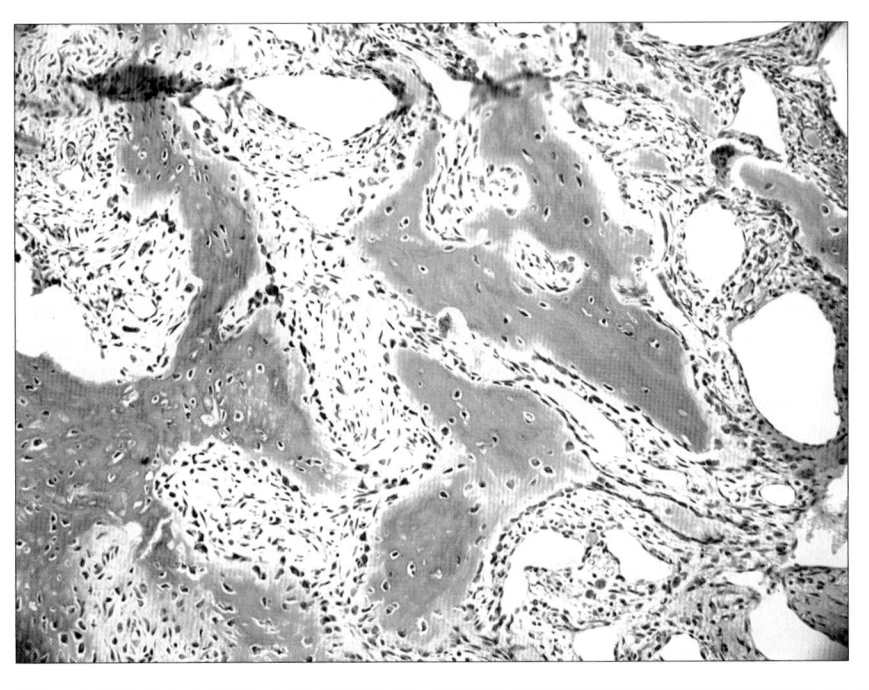

Figure 6-14. Woven bone. Microscopic section showing newly formed bone in a fracture callus. The collagen in the irregular bony trabeculae is poorly aligned, and numerous osteoblasts and osteoclasts are present about newly formed trabeculae.

Metabolic Bone Disease

Metabolic bone disease includes a variety of abnormalities in the endocrine function of the bone in calcium homeostasis as well as abnormalities of mineral deposition in newly formed or remodeled bone. Since bony remodeling is a constant process throughout life, even minor persistent abnormalities in bone mineralization can eventually result in marked changes in bone structure or loss of mineralized bone. Abnormalities of mineralization in growing children cause different clinical features with prominent deformity of long bones.

Osteoporosis

Osteoporosis is an extremely common disease in United States and tends to be most severe in postmenopausal women. Progressive bone loss after menopause sets the stage for pathologic fractures in multiple bones. Normally, skeletal

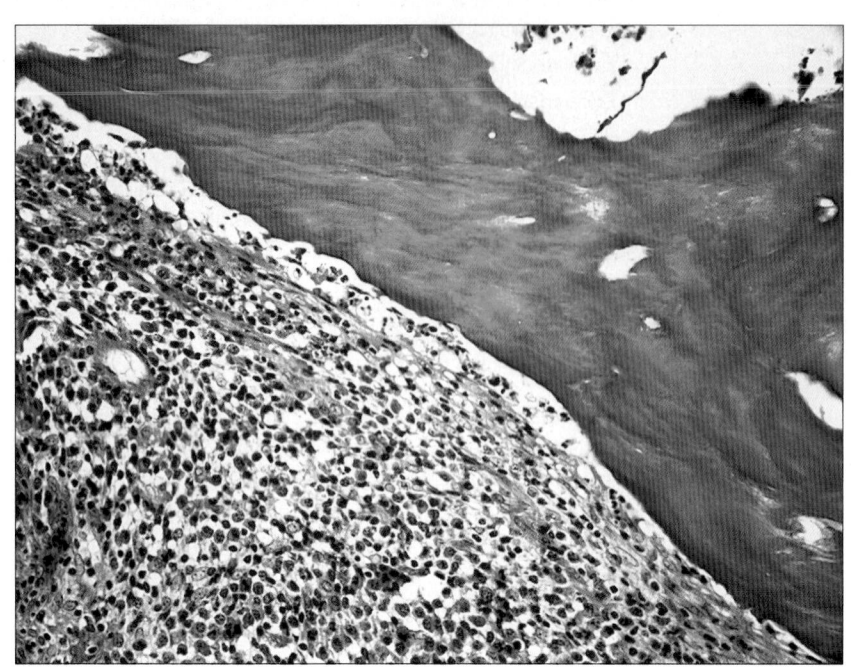

Figure 6-15. Acute osteomyelitis. Microscopic section showing a dense inflammatory cell infiltrate in the marrow space. The adjacent bony trabeculae are necrotic (note the absence of osteocytes in lacunae).

density increases during childhood and reaches a peak in young adulthood in all individuals, with men having greater bone density than women. There is a slow, progressive loss of bone mineral after young adulthood, and this loss can be accelerated by inactivity (mechanical stimulation is necessary to maintain bone mass), nutritional deficiency, and other factors. The extent of peak mineralization and the rate of bone mineral loss are the key determinants of when (and whether) individuals will develop symptomatic osteoporosis during their lifetime (and be at risk for pathologic fractures).

Most patients with osteoporosis appear to have an unequal balance between osteoblastic and osteoclastic activity. Over time, bony remodeling (in response to changing mechanical stress) accelerates age-dependent loss of bone mineral. It is now thought that the predominant defect in most patients with osteoporosis is decreased new bone formation. Osteoporosis affects bones with a large percentage of trabecular bone (metabolically active bone that modulates calcium homeostasis) most severely. For this reason, compression fractures of the vertebrae are very common in osteoporosis, and patients may experience decreasing height and nerve root compression as initial symptoms.

At menopause, there is a marked increase in bone mineral loss that is probably related to differences in cytokine secretion in bony tissue. For instance, increased TNF-α production by macrophages favors the differentiation of macrophages to osteoclasts and can enhance bone resorption. Estrogen replacement and calcium supplementation may be helpful in some patients but usually are not sufficient to reverse bone loss. Known genetic risk factors for osteoporosis include polymorphisms in the vitamin D receptor.

Hyperparathyroidism

Increased secretion of parathyroid hormone by the parathyroid glands results in increased osteoclastic activity in bone with increased resorption and release of free calcium into the circulation (Fig. 6-16). Hyperparathyroidism is characterized as primary if the abnormality resides in the parathyroid glands themselves (as a result of either hyperplasia or a functional adenoma). Secondary hyperparathyroidism results from abnormalities in free calcium and phosphorus levels in plasma that cause compensatory hyperplasia of the parathyroid glands, which then secrete large amounts of parathyroid hormone. This condition is common in patients with end-stage renal disease and contributes to the bony abnormalities in renal osteodystrophy (see below). Severe, prolonged hyperparathyroidism can result in the formation of so-called brown tumors, which are solid aggregates of osteoclasts stimulated by parathyroid hormone. Brown tumors are not true neoplasms, and removal of parathyroid hormone results in their regression. Hypercalcemia and bone mineral loss can also occur as a paraneoplastic syndrome, which may be mediated by parathyroid hormone–like peptides or osteoclast activating factor (OAF).

Osteomalacia

Osteomalacia means defective mineralization of newly formed osteoid. Osteomalacia can result from a deficiency of vitamin D (as occurs in rickets) or from resistance to vitamin D (e.g., abnormalities of the vitamin D receptor). In growing children, abnormal bone mineralization results in weakened long bones that tend to bow and curve, resulting in the characteristic skeletal deformities of rickets. Osteomalacia can also result from abnormal serum concentrations of calcium

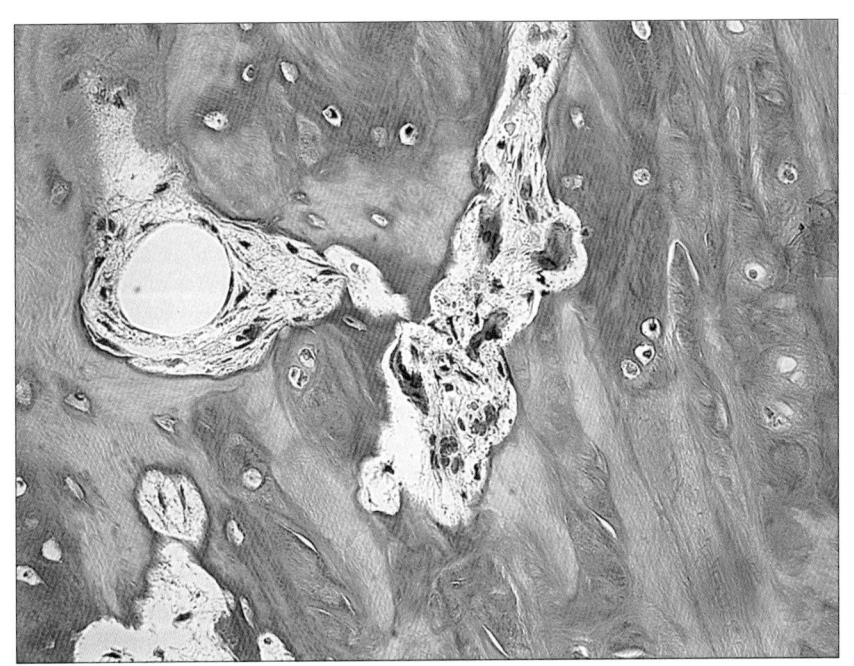

Figure 6-16. Bone resorption. Microscopic section of bone showing prominent osteoclastic activity with large resorption bays formed in trabecular bone.

and phosphorus in patients with end-stage renal disease (so-called renal osteodystrophy) that prevent normal formation of hydroxyapatite.

Bone Tumors and Tumor-like Conditions

Tumors and tumor-like conditions of bone often present as pathologic fractures. The inherent difficulties in obtaining samples of mineralized bone and of preparing histologic sections from calcified bony tissue make evaluation of most bone lesions problematic. There is also significant histologic overlap among different bone lesions so that their location, radiographic appearance, and the age of the patient are all important factors in establishing a correct diagnosis. Some bone lesions may present as tumors but are better characterized as developmental abnormalities (e.g., osteomas of the skull are regions of increased bone density). Slowly growing bone lesions tend to produce a sclerotic rim of reactive bone that is visible radiographically, and this feature is usually associated with a benign process. Conversely, lesions that grow quickly are not associated with a sclerotic bonyrim. Malignant bone tumors may penetrate the cortex of the bone, resulting in Codman's triangle.

Bone Cysts

Bone cysts typically occur during childhood and adolescence and may be unilocular or multiloculated. Aneurysmal bone cysts are cystic lesions that are usually related to trauma and show evidence of prior hemorrhage (hemosiderin pigment) and contain multinucleated giant cells. Bone cysts usually enlarge over time and cause pressure resorption of cortical bone, which may result in a pathologic fracture. In patients

HISTOLOGY

Codman's Triangle

Elevation of the periosteum (i.e., pulling the periosteum off the surface of cortical bone) by tumor penetrating the bone cortex initiates new reactive bone formation in the periosteum. Ossified or calcified periosteal tissue is visible in plain film radiographs, and its separation from cortical bone produces a pattern that is known as Codman's triangle. This triangle pattern on radiography is usually a feature of malignant bone tumors (often osteosarcoma), which can perforate the cortex, and is distinct from the reactive osteosclerosis that usually forms around benign bone tumors or lesions.

with pathologic fractures associated with benign cysts, reactive bone formation may simulate malignant bone tumors such as osteosarcoma. Careful attention to the organization of the repair process and the bland cytology of bone-forming cells usually allows clear distinction between these two processes.

Osseous Tumors

Different bone-forming tumors tend to involve characteristic locations within affected bones (e.g., metaphysis, diaphysis, or epiphysis).

Osteoid Osteoma and Osteoblastoma

Osteoid osteomas usually occur in adolescents and involve the cortex of long bones. These lesions are often painful, and the pain may be relieved by aspirin. Morphologically, a sclerotic band of reactive bone formation surrounds a small central nidus of active bone formation. The osteoblasts that rim newly formed bone do not have malignant cytologic features, and the overall organization of the lesion confirms its benign nature, and osteoid osteomas are cured by local excision. The nidus of bone formation in an osteoid osteoma has similar morphologic features to osteoblastomas, which typically occur in vertebral bodies and lack a sclerotic rim. Osteoblastomas may expand and erode cortex and cause compression fractures.

Osteochondroma

Osteochondromas form as an abnormal outgrowth from the surface of different bones (e.g., ribs and long bones) and recapitulate normal endochondral ossification (i.e., osteochondromas result from normal endochondral ossification in an abnormal location). Osteochondromas typically have a thick cartilaginous cap at their leading edge that is remodeled into normal bone (Fig. 6-17A). The normal organization and polarity of the ossification process demonstrates that this is a benign lesion. Rarely, chondrosarcoma can develop in the cartilaginous cap of an osteochondroma, and increased thickness of this cap is a risk factor for malignant degeneration.

Osteosarcoma

Osteosarcoma is a malignant neoplasm of osteoblasts that usually occurs in childhood or adolescence in the metaphysis of long bones. The demonstration of osteoid formation by tumor cells is required to establish a diagnosis of osteosarcoma. Osteosarcomas may also produce cartilage and thus may mimic cartilaginous tumors (see Fig. 6-17B). Extensive sampling of tumor tissue is important to establish the correct diagnosis to direct therapy. Osteosarcomas may perforate bone cortex (resulting in Codman's triangle) and may eventually penetrate the epiphyseal growth plate to extend through joint spaces to involve adjacent bones. Osteosarcomas often metastasize early in their course (pulmonary metastases are typical). Treatment typically involves amputation or en bloc resection of the affected bone, followed by adjuvant chemotherapy.

Many osteosarcomas demonstrate mutations in the p53 gene, and patients with hereditary abnormalities in either p53 (Li-Fraumeni syndrome) or Rb (hereditary retinoblastoma) genes are at markedly increased risk for the development of osteosarcoma as well as other tumors. Osteosarcomas can also arise in the setting of Paget's disease of bone, and these tumors develop in elderly individuals with radiographic evidence of Paget's disease (see Paget's Disease of Bone section).

Cartilaginous Tumors

Enchondroma

Enchondromas are small masses of mature cartilage that typically form in the small bones of the hands and feet. In this setting, they are invariably benign, even if cytologic atypia is present.

Chondrosarcoma

Chondrosarcomas are malignant tumors of cartilage that usually develop in large joints, with the hip being the most common location. Chondrosarcomas are tumors of older individuals, and most show extensive cartilage formation. Tumors vary from well-differentiated (consisting of nearly normal appearing hyaline cartilage) to high-grade neoplasms with minimal cartilaginous differentiation. The combination of a tumor mass in a large joint with variable degrees of cytologic atypia in chondrocytes allows a confident diagnosis of malignancy even in very well-differentiated chondrosarcomas (see Fig. 6-17C). Chondrosarcomas typically appear as large, soft tissue masses with "popcorn" calcifications on x-ray. Chondrosarcomas tend to cause predominantly localized tissue destruction with metastasis occurring late in their course. Mesenchymal chondrosarcoma occurs in younger patients and may present as a bone tumor but is often extraskeletal. It is composed of foci of neoplastic cartilage alternating with small, undifferentiated cells. If the undifferentiated cells predominate, it may be confused with one of the small blue round-cell tumors of childhood (e.g., Ewing's sarcoma).

Metastatic Tumors to Bone

Metastatic tumors to bone greatly outnumber primary bone tumors in adults. Some tumors have a marked propensity to metastasize to bone, including prostate cancer, clear-cell carcinoma of the kidney, and hepatocellular carcinoma. Breast and lung cancer also give rise to skeletal metastases that can result in pathologic fractures (see Fig. 6-17D). Most metastatic tumors result in mixed lytic and blastic lesions that show both bone resorption and new bone formation. Prostate cancer causes characteristic osteoblastic (bone-forming) metastases, and bone pain rather than pathologic fractures characterizes its clinical course. Focal involvement of the bone marrow by plasma cell myeloma tends to result in purely lytic bone lesions that are radiographically characteristic (so-called punched-out lesions with a sharp margin between residual bone and the lytic lesion).

Other Lesions

A variety of different bone tumors and tumor-like conditions as well as neoplasms of other constituents of bone (e.g., nerves, blood vessels, etc.) can occur. Most of these are quite rare, and only the more frequently encountered lesions are described here.

Giant Cell Tumor of Bone

Giant cell tumor of bone tends to involve the epiphysis of growing long bones in adolescents and young adults. It is a locally destructive tumor that can result in a pathologic fracture. Uncomplicated giant cell tumor is not thought to have metastatic potential, but giant cell tumors recurring after inadequate therapy may ultimately give rise to metastases. Giant cell tumors have relatively characteristic biphasic morphology with spindled stromal cells merging

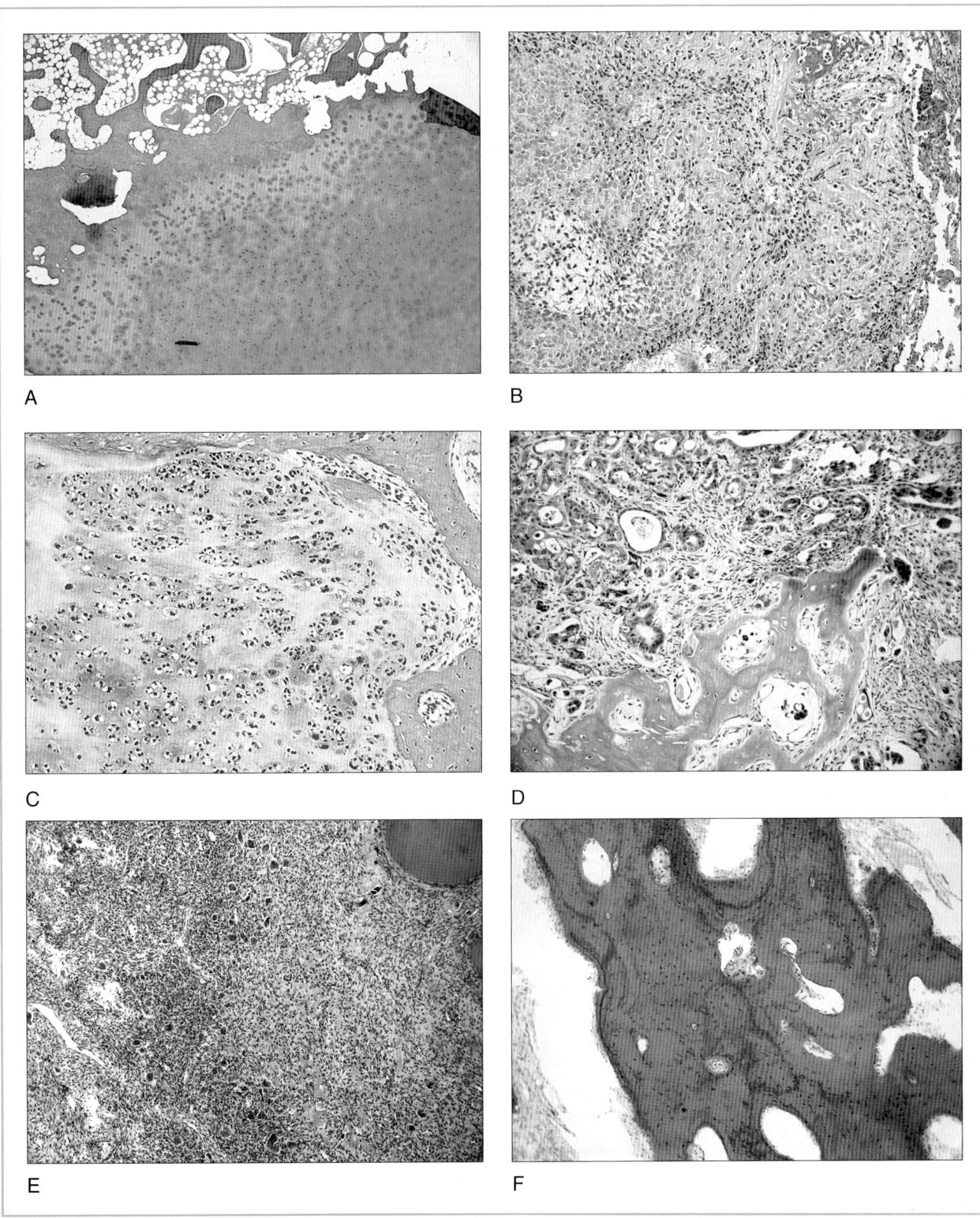

Figure 6-17. **A**, Osteochondroma. Microscopic section showing normal endochondral ossification adjacent to a thick cartilaginous cap. **B**, Osteosarcoma. Microscopic section showing pleomorphic malignant cells forming osteoid. This finding is pathognomonic of osteosarcoma. **C**, Chondrosarcoma. Microscopic section showing hypercellular hyaline cartilage with prominent atypia of chondrocytes. Benign reactive bone formation is evident at right. **D**, Bone metastasis. Microscopic section showing malignant glands infiltrating bony tissue. Reactive bone formation is evident in the lower portion of this figure. **E**, Giant cell tumor of bone. Microscopic section showing prominent tumor giant cells that merge with the spindle cell component of this neoplasm. **F**, Paget's disease of bone. Microscopic section showing thickened bony trabeculae with prominent cement lines that form a mosaic pattern.

with multinucleated giant cells (see Fig. 6-17E). The nuclei in both cell types have similar morphology. Giant cell tumors must be distinguished from osteosarcomas, which may also contain abundant multinucleated giant cells. Similarly, the osteoclastic lesions (brown tumors) associated with hyperparathyroidism sometimes mimic the giant cell tumor.

Fibrous Dysplasia

Fibrous dysplasia is a tumor-like condition that may involve a single bone (monostotic) or multiple bones (polyostotic). Fibrous dysplasia corresponds to a focus of trabecular bone composed of bony trabeculae with complex shapes often described as a "Chinese letter" configuration. Osteoblasts are scant or absent in fibrous dysplasia. Lesions can grow, causing resorption of normal lamellar bone or teeth (the jaws are a common location), which can result in fracture and tooth loss.

Paget's Disease of Bone

Paget's disease of bone is an abnormality of bony remodeling which begins with a lytic phase that results in extensive resorption of normal bone. The lytic phase transitions to a sclerotic phase in which extensive new bone formation results in increased bone density. Most of the new bone formed is woven bone, which is not normally converted to lamellar bone. In most patients with Paget's disease, the sclerotic phase ultimately dominates, resulting in dense, calcified masses of abnormal bone. Histologically, the presence of mosaic cement lines (shaped like jigsaw puzzle pieces) is highly suggestive of Paget's disease (see Fig. 6-17F). Patients with active Paget's disease tend to have increased levels of serum alkaline phosphatase as a result of increased bone remodeling and are at increased risk for the development of osteosarcoma. The pathogenesis of Paget's disease remains unclear; although viral infection has been suspected for many years, proof is still lacking.

●●● MUSCLE

In addition to the biomechanical function of skeletal muscle, it is also critical for maintaining glucose homeostasis under the influence of insulin and other metabolic hormones. Muscle fibers require frequent contraction to maintain normal trophic hormones, and loss of normal stretch stimulation due to inactivity or denervation results in profound atrophy with resorption of contractile proteins. Skeletal muscle can undergo marked physiologic hypertrophy in response to exercise but has no (or very limited) capacity for hyperplasia and regeneration if muscle fibers are irreversibly injured.

Myositis

Myositis is an inflammatory condition of muscle that can develop in the setting of collagen vascular disease or as a paraneoplastic syndrome. Patients with dermatomyositis have a combination of skin lesions and inflammatory myopathy. Muscle biopsy can be helpful in clarifying the etiology of myositis by virtue of the types of fibers involved and the chronicity of the changes observed (Fig. 6-18). Some genetic diseases result in inclusion bodies in muscle fibers, which can be identified by electron microscopy.

Bacterial infection of muscle is uncommon; however, fasciitis (infection of connective tissue) can secondarily involve muscle, resulting in a rapidly progressive infection

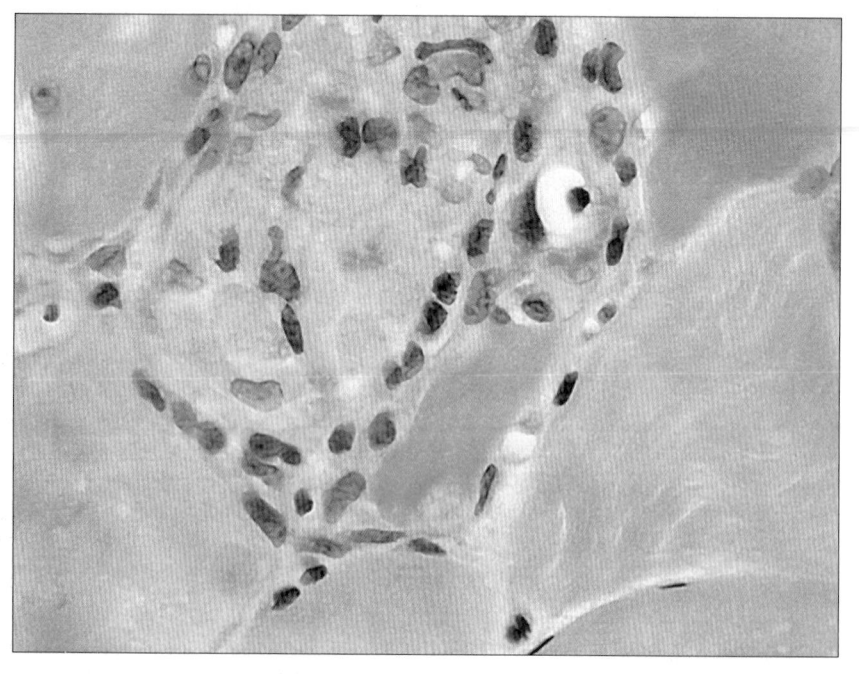

Figure 6-18. Myositis. Microscopic section showing skeletal muscle fibers surrounded by T lymphocytes. Cytopathic effects are evident is some muscle cells.

(e.g., necrotizing fasciitis). Parasitic myositis can result from ingestion of undercooked pork when *Trichinella spiralis* encysts in muscle tissue. Rhabdomyolysis is rupture of muscle cells, which can be caused by trauma or electrolyte abnormalities. If rhabdomyolysis is extensive, myoglobin released into the circulation can produce acute renal failure.

Muscular Dystrophy

Duchenne's muscular dystrophy results from genetic alterations in the dystrophin gene that cause chronic injury to muscle cells and ultimately results in their replacement by adipose and fibrous tissue. Duchenne's dystrophy is discussed in more detail in Chapter 4.

Myasthenia Gravis

Myasthenia gravis results from autoantibodies directed against the acetylcholine receptor on skeletal muscle fibers. Antibodies bound to this receptor block neuronal stimulation of muscle contraction, producing episodic weakness that is characteristic. In some patients, myasthenia gravis is progressive, but in most it follows a relapsing and remitting course. A fraction of patients with myasthenia gravis have thymic tumors (thymomas), and surgical removal of thymomas may induce remission of muscle disease. Severe symptoms can be managed with plasmapheresis to remove the offending autoantibody.

Tumors

Tumors of skeletal muscle are quite rare, whereas tumors of smooth muscle are very common (e.g., uterine leiomyomas). Rhabdomyomas are usually benign tumors of skeletal or cardiac muscle that often arise in patients with tuberous sclerosis. These unusual lesions are composed of bizarre-appearing muscle cells with prominent glycogen accumulations having a spider-like morphology.

Rhabdomyosarcoma

Rhabdomyosarcoma is usually a tumor of childhood and is one of the so-called small blue round-cell tumors of childhood. It can present as undifferentiated, but most rhabdomyosarcomas retain some evidence of skeletal muscle differentiation (e.g., expression of desmin and actin proteins), which can be detected by immunohistochemistry. Better differentiated rhabdomyosarcomas contain spindle cells with rudimentary sarcomeres that produce cross-striations on light microscopy (so-called strap cells) (Fig. 6-19A).

Two different forms of rhabdomyosarcoma have relatively characteristic clinical and morphologic features. Embryonal rhabdomyosarcoma is composed of small spindle cells that tend to cluster beneath mucosal surfaces, forming a so-called cambium layer. These tumors can present as botryoid sarcomas (i.e., they form grape-like masses that can fill the urinary bladder or vagina). Alveolar rhabdomyosarcoma usually involves the extremities and is associated with a specific

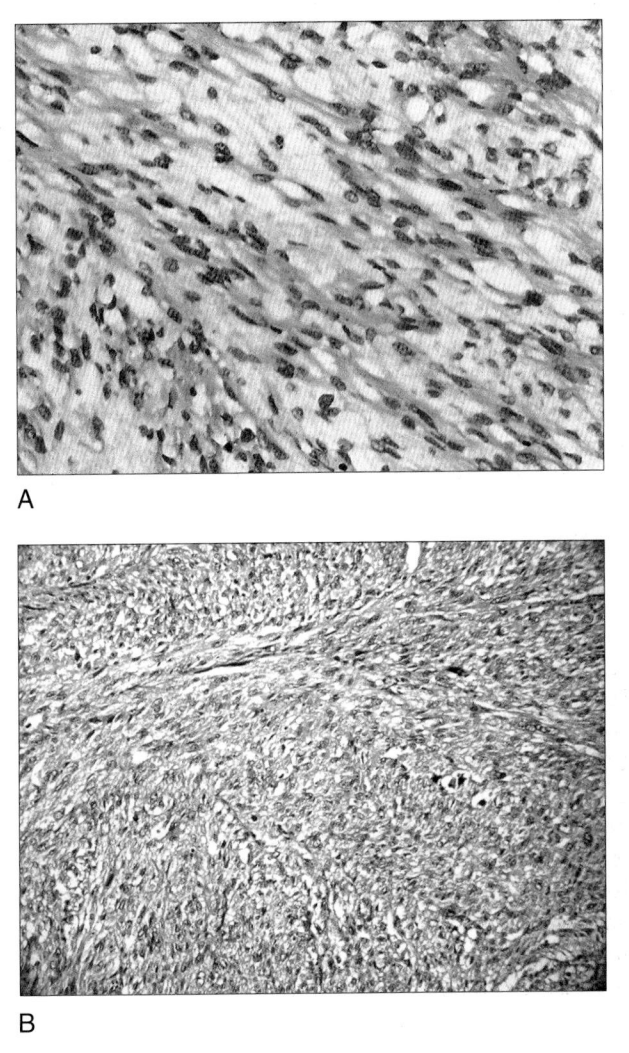

Figure 6-19. A, Rhabdomyosarcoma. Microscopic section showing elongated tumor spindle cells with eosinophilic cytoplasm and occasional cross-striations indicative of skeletal muscle differentiation. **B**, Leiomyosarcoma. Microscopic section showing plump tumor spindle cells that resemble normal smooth muscle cells.

chromosomal translocation between the PAX3 gene and the FLI1 gene.

Leiomyoma and Leiomyosarcoma

Leiomyomas are benign tumors of smooth muscle. They can arise in almost any site in the body in which smooth muscle is present. Since vascular smooth muscle is present in all organs, essentially all sites are at risk. Leiomyomas tend to be sharply circumscribed from surrounding tissues and are composed of bland-appearing spindle cells with elongated, cigar-shaped nuclei. They are extremely common in the uterine myometrium and can cause symptoms related to mass effect.

Leiomyosarcomas are the malignant counterparts of leiomyomas (see Fig. 6-19B) and vary from borderline lesions to highly malignant sarcomas. Leiomyosarcomas are probably most common in the uterine myometrium, where most are thought to arise from malignant transformation of common benign leiomyomas. Mitotic activity and tumor necrosis are the best predictors of biologic aggressiveness.

●●● ADIPOSE TISSUE

Adipose tissue is highly vascular and contains a significant number of macrophages, which are important in modulating hormonal and cytokine signaling. Adipose tissue is a dynamic tissue that undergoes continuous self-renewal through the differentiation of preadipocytes from committed stem cells residing in adipose and from macrophages that can differentiate into adipocytes. Adipose tissue performs several critical functions. (1) It provides a mechanical cushion to protect internal organs. (2) It provides effective thermal insulation as well as a large store of nutrients. (3) It also controls glucose and lipid homeostasis in response to the secretion of insulin and other trophic hormones. Brown fat has an important role in heat generation in some species but is only minimally present in human adults and probably does not have an important physiologic role.

There is accumulating evidence that different types of adipose tissue (e.g., subcutaneous, mesenteric, omental) have a different composition (differing ratio of adipocytes to macrophages) and respond differentially to hormonal signaling. The composition and properties of various fat deposits can be markedly altered in obesity. Steroid hormones including glucocorticoids and estrogens can trigger redistribution of adipose tissue from one location to another. Some drugs can also result in the redistribution of adipose tissue between different storage sites and may produce lipodystrophy (loss of adipose tissue) in some critical areas.

Inflammatory Lesions

Inflammatory lesions of adipose tissue include fat necrosis, which can result from mechanical trauma, inflammation, or release of activated pancreatic enzymes. Fat necrosis can take on multiple morphologic forms that may lead to confusion with certain neoplasms. Dystrophic calcification in fat necrosis can cause dystrophic calcifications in breast tissue and other sites.

Panniculitis is an inflammatory condition that specifically targets adipose tissue. In septal panniculitis, chronic inflammation is centered on fibrous septae dividing lobules of adipose tissue, and this pattern is frequently associated with autoimmune disease (Fig. 6-20). Erythema nodosum is a localized inflammatory lesion that forms nodules within adipose tissue and is sometimes associated with autoimmune disease, although many cases are idiopathic.

Diabetes Mellitus

Adipocytes and macrophages both express insulin receptors, and there is significant cross-talk between these two cell types in adipose tissue. Insulin stimulates adipocytes to take up lipoproteins from plasma, which are processed and stored as lipid vacuoles that can be mobilized by β-oxidation. Insulin signaling also stimulates glucose uptake by adipocytes. Insulin-mediated cross-talk between adipose tissue and adjacent skeletal muscle helps activate glucose uptake by myocytes. Skeletal muscle accounts for the bulk of rapid glucose uptake in response to insulin. Increased adipose tissue in obesity is associated with a greater number of macrophages in adipose tissue and an increased number of insulin receptors, forcing insulin to occupy a much larger number

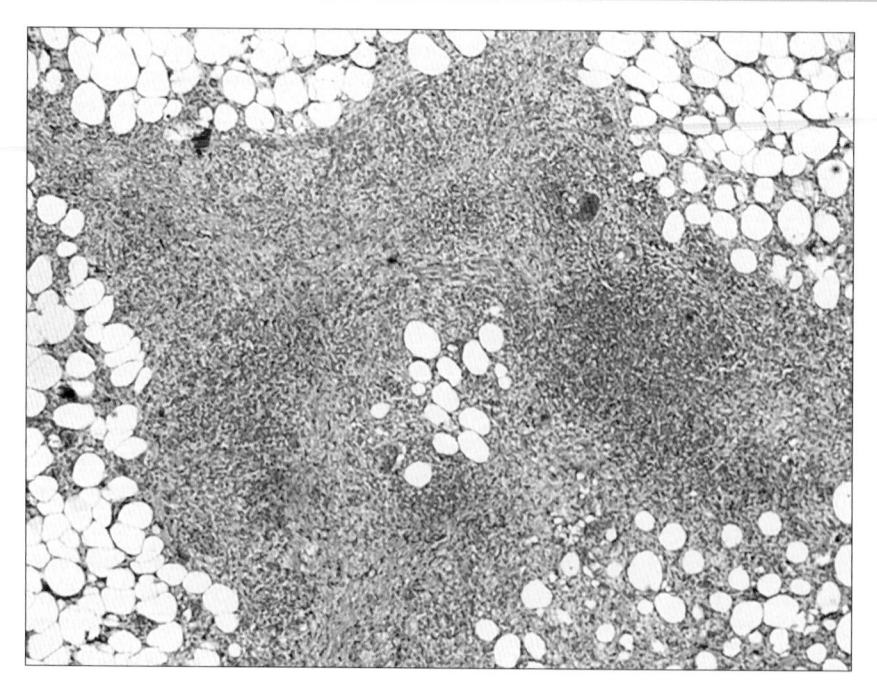

Figure 6-20. Panniculitis. Microscopic section showing subcutaneous adipose tissue with a prominent septal chronic inflammatory cell infiltrate and associated fibrosis.

of receptors to achieve the same physiologic response (i.e., insulin resistance). Increased synthesis of TNF-α by macrophages in adipose tissue further inhibits the effects of insulin. Expression of resistin by adipocytes additionally contributes to insulin resistance (see Chapter 10). These alterations in adipose tissue contribute to the development of the metabolic syndrome that is strongly associated with obesity and contributes to the high incidence of diabetes mellitus and heart disease in the United States.

Tumors

Lipoma

Lipomas are benign tumors of adipocytes, which usually are superficial in location and sharply circumscribed from surrounding tissue. The adipocytes that make up these tumors are morphologically identical to normal mature adipocytes.

Liposarcoma

Liposarcoma is a rare malignant tumor of varying biologic potential that usually arises in deep adipose tissue (below the fascial layer). These tumors have multiple morphologic forms (e.g., myxoid, round cell, pleomorphic, and well differentiated), which may intermingle. Most liposarcomas are locally aggressive neoplasms that rarely metastasize. Because many of these tumors arise in the retroperitoneum, complete surgical excision usually is not technically feasible, and many patients ultimately succumb to local effects of tumor growth. Adipocytes are subject to high oxidative stress from fatty acid oxidation, which may contribute to carcinogenesis in this tissue. Many liposarcomas are associated with specific chromosomal translocations that produce unique fusion proteins.

●●● SOFT TISSUE TUMORS AND TUMOR-LIKE CONDITIONS

Tumors and tumor-like conditions of soft tissue often show mixed features of fibroblastic, histiocytic, and myoid differentiation. In some cases, it is not possible to assign a definite cell of origin for tumors arising in soft tissue. Most malignant soft tissue tumors share common clinical features because of their tendency to arise in deep soft tissue and because of other inherent properties of mesenchymal cells.

Some sarcomas are associated with unique chromosomal translocations, which may define the neoplasm and dictate a specific pathologic diagnosis. Morphologic distinction between some reactive conditions of soft tissue and sarcomas can occasionally be difficult.

Nodular Fasciitis

Nodular fasciitis is an uncommon response to injury in soft tissue. It consists of a localized proliferation of fibroblast-like cells in fascia that grows rapidly and then spontaneously involutes over the course of weeks. A history of prior trauma

---

 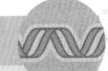

and the rapid growth of a soft tissue mass in a young person are typical clinical features that help distinguish nodular fasciitis from sarcomas and other lesions. Morphologic distinction of nodular fasciitis from sarcoma can occasionally be difficult, and it depends on subtle architectural features (feathery growth pattern) in a mitotically active lesion.

Fibromatosis

Fibromatoses are uncommon, slow-growing proliferations of fibroblast-like cells that are associated with extensive collagen production (Fig. 6-21). Fibromatoses can occur at multiple sites throughout the body and tend to have a relatively distinct biologic behavior at different sites. For instance, palmar fibromatoses (so-called Dupuytren's contracture) is a fibrotic lesion of the fascia of the palm of the hand or sole of the foot that can result in dysfunction of digits. This type of fibromatosis is hypocellular and does not behave like a soft tissue neoplasm.

In contrast, abdominal fibromatoses (so-called desmoid tumors) present as a slow-growing soft tissue mass in the abdomen and may ultimately kill the patient by local extension. Despite this potentially aggressive biologic behavior, abdominal fibromatoses are sparsely cellular and cytologically bland with almost no demonstrable mitotic activity. Desmoid tumors are more common in women and may be associated with pregnancy and prior abdominal surgery. These tumors are very poorly defined grossly and tend to have markedly infiltrative borders. Tumor cells may extend centimeters beyond the apparent limit of the tissue mass, making complete excision difficult or impractical. Many desmoid tumors express estrogen receptors, and hormonal therapy may be beneficial in some patients. Desmoid tumors

develop preferentially in a subset of patients (Gardner's syndrome) with germline mutations in the adenomatous polyposis coli (APC) gene that causes familial polyposis.

Other forms of localized fibromatoses of intermediate biologic aggressiveness occur at various sites. Fibromatoses arising in infancy usually have a benign clinical course and a characteristic clinical presentation.

Fibrohistiocytic Tumors

Fibrohistiocytic tumors are classified on the basis of expression of both fibroblastic and histiocytic markers in tumor cells. Some of these lesions are poorly differentiated sarcomas with little tendency toward any specific form of differentiation (e.g., malignant fibrous histiocytoma [MFH]) and probably constitute a heterogeneous group of neoplasms. The tumors described below are relatively well-defined clinicopathologic entities, some of which are associated with specific chromosomal translocations.

Dermatofibrosarcoma Protuberans

Dermatofibrosarcoma protuberans (DFSP) is a distinctive sarcoma of the dermis that can grow to large size but only rarely metastasizes. It is composed of fibroblast-like cells that expand and infiltrate the dermis, producing an elevated mass (protuberans) in the skin, most frequently in the head and neck region.

Fibrosarcoma

Pure fibrosarcoma is a rare malignant neoplasm of fibroblast-like cells having a distinctive architectural pattern of growth that produces an interlacing "herringbone" pattern in histologic sections.

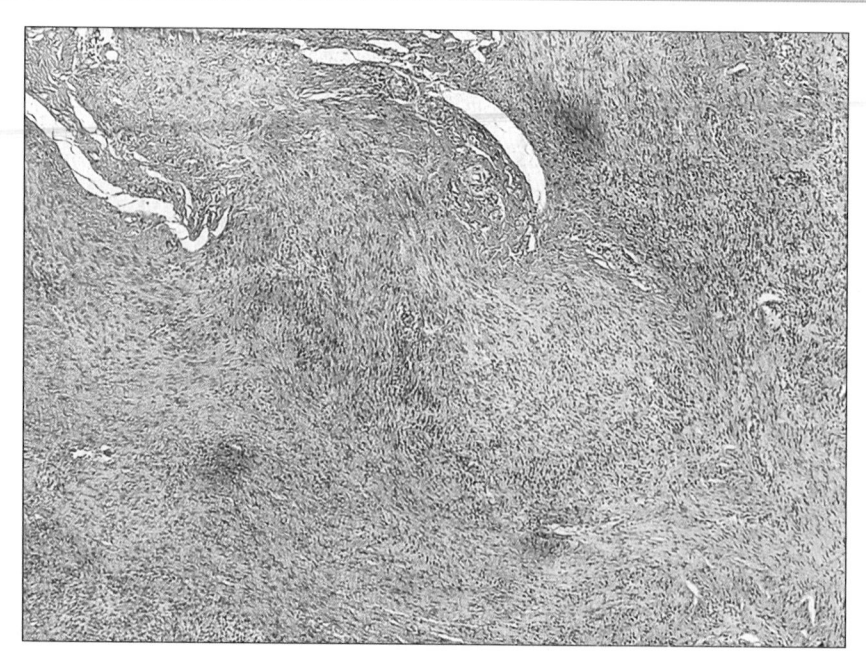

Figure 6-21. Palmar fibromatosis. Microscopic section showing a cytologically bland proliferation of fibroblast-like cells with no necrosis or demonstrable mitotic activity.

Solitary Fibrous Tumor

Solitary fibrous tumor is a neoplasm of intermediate biologic potential that can occur at many sites throughout the body. Tumors are relatively circumscript and are composed of spindle cells with inconsistent orientation (so-called pattern-less pattern). These tumors express CD34 but do not express the more specific angiogenic marker CD31 (PECAM). The consistent expression of CD34 in these tumors has allowed the regrouping of several different tumor types (e.g., hemangiopericytoma and solitary fibrous tumor of pleura) into a single diagnostic category. Some solitary fibrous tumors behave as benign neoplasms, whereas others are locally aggressive and may even result in metastasis. Their biologic behavior is partially predicted by their histologic features (e.g., extent of mitotic activity and presence of tumor necrosis).

Synovial Sarcoma

Synovial sarcoma is a distinctive malignant neoplasm of soft tissue that often occurs in the vicinity of joints but is not limited to this location. The most characteristic form of synovial sarcoma is biphasic with alternating areas of spindle cells and epithelial differentiation (gland-like structures or nests). Most synovial sarcomas have a specific chromosomal translocation t(X;18) between the SYT and the SSX1 or SSX2 genes. Synovial sarcoma is a malignant tumor that can give rise to both lymph node and hematogenous metastases.

Peripheral Neuroectodermal Tumor and Ewing's Sarcoma

Peripheral neuroectodermal tumors (PNETs) include Ewing's sarcoma and similar primitive neoplasms of childhood, which can occur at many different anatomic sites throughout the body. All PNETs fall under the differential diagnostic entity of "small blue round-cell tumors of childhood." Ewing's sarcoma is an undifferentiated tumor (usually arising in bone) that is composed of small cells with blastic chromatin and often containing abundant cytoplasmic glycogen. PNETs occurring in the pleura and other sites may be morphologically indistinguishable from Ewing's sarcoma (Fig. 6-22). These tumors typically metastasize at an early stage and are usually treated with systemic chemotherapy. PNETs typically have translocations between the FLI-1 and Ewing's sarcoma (EWS) genes, but other translocation partners are utilized in some tumors.

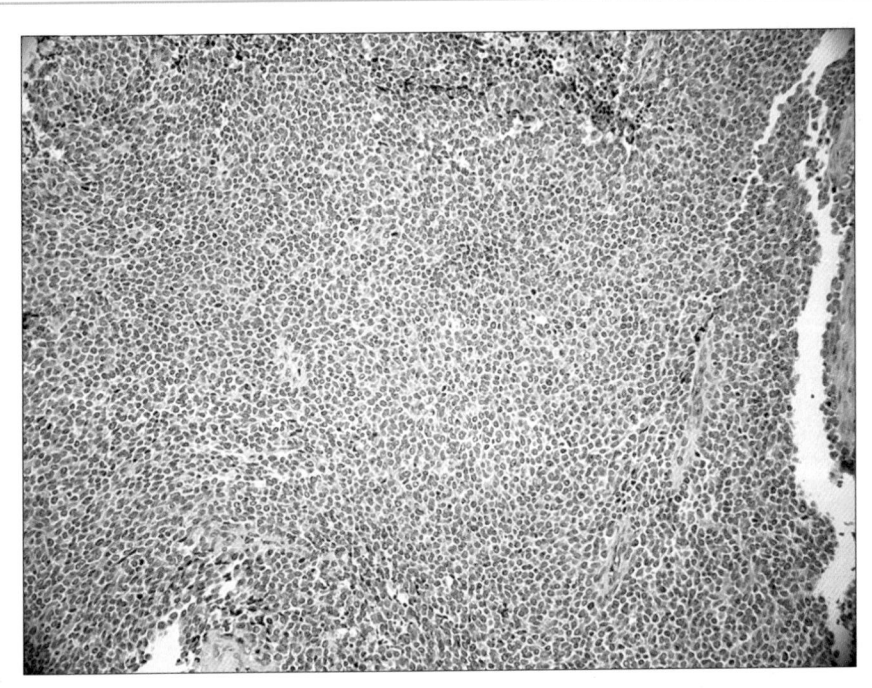

Figure 6-22. Peripheral neuroectodermal tumor (PNET). Microscopic section showing undifferentiated tumor cells, which demonstrate occasional rosette formation.

GENETICS

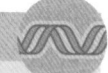

Ewing's Sarcoma (EWS) and FLI1 Genes

The native EWS gene is a nuclear protein that functions as a transcription factor. It serves as a translocation partner for a number of different genes (many are members of the ETS family of transcription factors) in Ewing's sarcoma.

- The most common translocation in Ewing's sarcoma (90% to 95%)—t(11;22)(q24;q12)—involves EWS and FLI1 genes. FLI1 is a transcription factor named for Friend leukemia virus integration site 1 (the animal heterolog of this gene is targeted for retroviral integration). FLI1 expression is important for hematopoiesis and early vascular development.
- A translocation between EWS and ERG (another transcription factor)—t(21;22)(q22;q12)—occurs in 5% to 10% of cases of Ewing's sarcoma.
- Variant translocations involving EWS are seen in less than 1% of Ewing's sarcoma cases and involve fusion of EWS with ETS family transcription factors (ETV1, E1AF, FEV, and ZSG).
- EWS is the translocation partner of other genes in neoplasms other than Ewing's sarcoma.

Translocation	Fusion Protein	Disease
t(11;22)	EWS-FLI1	Ewing's sarcoma
t(21;22)	EWS-ERG	Ewing's sarcoma
f(17;22)	EWS-E1AF	Ewing's sarcoma
t(7;22)	EWS-ETV1	Ewing's sarcoma
t(9;22)	EWS-?	Extraskeletal myxoid chondrosarcoma
t(11;22)	EWS-WT1	Desmoplastic small round-cell tumor
t(12;22)	EWS-?	Clear-cell sarcoma

Cardiovascular Pathology 7

CONTENTS

The heart and the vasculature make up a cardiovascular system that is a functionally closed loop. Because of this, pathology at any level of the cardiovascular system can result in abnormalities and compensatory changes at other levels. By the time patients have cardiovascular symptoms (or resected organs come to pathologic evaluation), these secondary changes may overshadow the primary pathology. For example, the backflow of blood into the left atrium that results from moderate mitral valve regurgitation is usually asymptomatic, but over time results in right ventricular hypertrophy and pulmonary vascular remodeling. Such patients often come in for medical attention (with pulmonary hemorrhage and right heart failure) at a time when massive right ventricular hypertrophy may overshadow the inciting abnormalities in the mitral valve. To pinpoint the root cause of a pathologic lesion, it is essential to understand the functional link between all components of the cardiovascular system and the secondary and tertiary pathologic consequences of any abnormality.

●●● FUNCTIONAL CARDIOVASCULAR ANATOMY

Blood vessels have three layers: intima, media, and adventitia.

HISTOLOGY

Blood Vessel Structure

The intima, media, and adventitia form the three functional layers of blood vessels. Elastin fibers in the media provide elastic recoil and are much more prominent in larger "elastic arteries" such as the aorta. The media is separated from the other layers by an elastic lamina composed of elastin fibers. The internal and external elastic laminae are best developed in larger muscular arteries.

There is dynamic interaction between endothelial cells in the intima and the smooth muscle cells in the media to maintain vascular tone and respond to injury or changing metabolic demands. Medium-sized and larger arteries have blood vessels of their own known as vasa vasorum that penetrate the tunica adventitia and tunica media of the parent blood vessels and provide essential nutrition for the media.

The intima is composed of a thin layer of connective tissue with a basement membrane covered by endothelial cells, and it is separated from the media by an internal elastic lamina that is made up of an organized band of elastin fibers (Fig. 7-1). The internal elastic lamina is clearly visible in muscular arteries but becomes much less prominent in smaller arteries and arterioles. The media is composed of smooth muscle cells with a predominantly circular orientation. Again, this layer is best developed in muscular arteries that are functional resistance blood vessels. In the largest arteries, elastic fibers are prominent in the media and provide a cushioning effect that smoothes blood pressure during the cardiac cycle. The adventitia is composed of loose connective tissue with small blood vessels (vasa vasorum) that penetrate the larger arteries to provide nutrition to the media. Most of these elements become inconspicuous as the vasculature diminishes in size; at the level of capillaries, only endothelium with a small amount of supporting connective tissue is visible. Medium-sized veins include one-way valves that are functionally important in assisting return flow. Flow through the vasculature is almost exclusively laminar.

This arrangement with the slowest flow rate adjacent to the blood vessel wall minimizes shear stress on the endothelial lining.

The heart is an embryologically modified blood vessel that is also composed of three layers: an endocardium similar to the intima of blood vessels, a muscular wall made up of cardiac myocytes, and an epicardium consisting of adipose tissue covered by mesothelium containing coronary arteries and veins (Fig. 7-2). Because the arteries penetrate the myocardium from the outside of the heart (epicardium), the subendocardium (i.e., the myocardium just beneath the

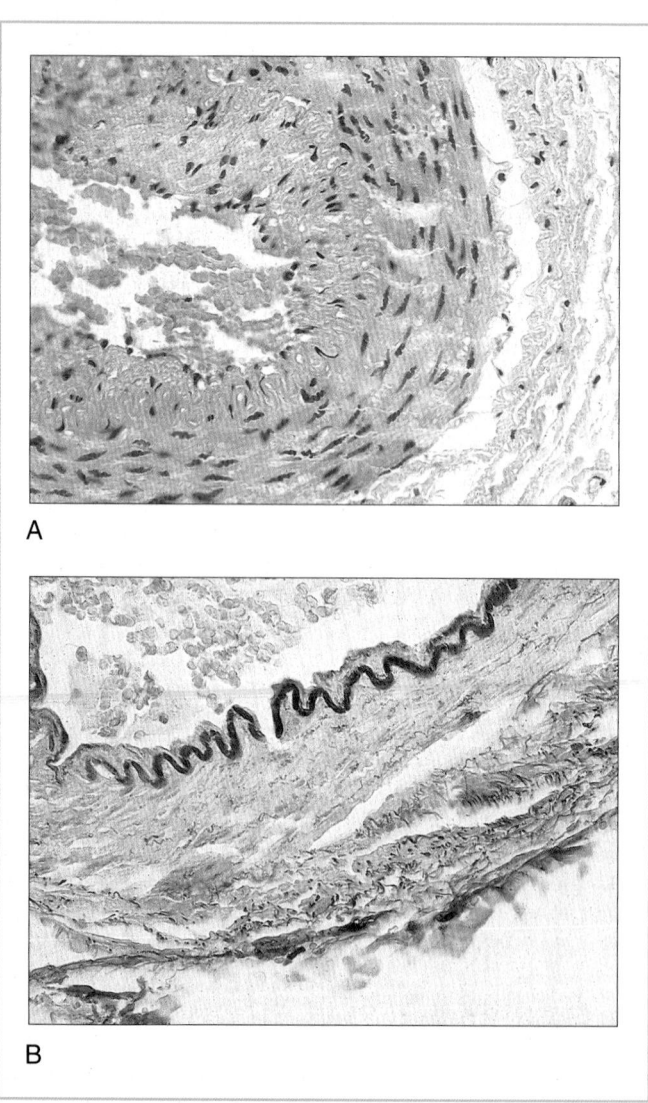

A

B

Figure 7-1. A, Normal artery. Microscopic section showing a small muscular artery. The internal elastic lamina is barely visible beneath the thin intimal layer. **B**, Normal artery. Microscopic section showing a silver stain of a small muscular artery highlighting the internal elastic lamina (black).

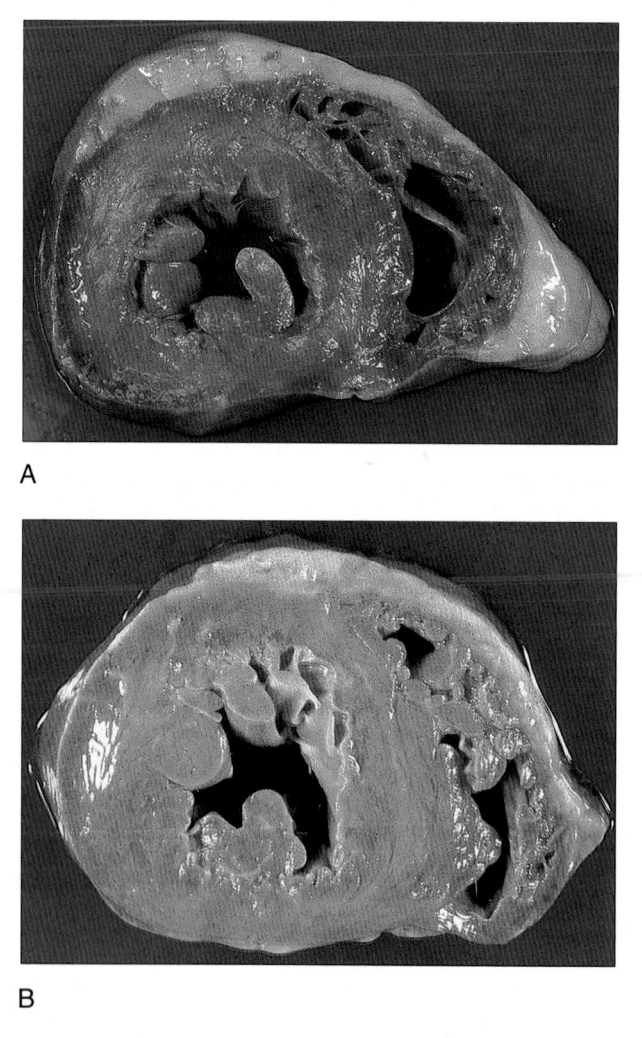

A

B

Figure 7-2. A, Normal heart. Gross cross-section of a normal heart. **B**, Left ventricular hypertrophy. Gross cross-section of a heart with marked left ventricular hypertrophy secondary to systemic hypertension.

endocardium) is the most vulnerable to low flow states (i.e., "watershed area"). Adult cardiac myocytes can respond to increased demand by hypertrophy, but their capacity for self-renewal (hyperplasia) is limited or absent.

The cardiac valves are simple structures composed of a fibrous annulus to which are attached valve leaflets made up of a core of collagen covered by endothelium. No blood vessels or lymphatics are normally present in cardiac valves, and they derive nutrition exclusively from luminal blood and have a limited ability to repair damage or respond to infection.

●●● ARTERIOSCLEROSIS

Arteriosclerosis literally means hardening of the arteries and corresponds to three separate pathologic entities: atherosclerosis, Mönckeberg's medial calcific sclerosis, and arteriolosclerosis. *Mönckeberg's sclerosis* is dystrophic calcification of the media of muscular arteries, which frequently occurs in older individuals. Since this calcification does not result in significant luminal narrowing, it is usually without significant functional consequence. *Arteriolosclerosis* refers to the thickening of small arteries and arterioles in which even small changes in wall thickness result in significant luminal compromise. This process is age dependent but is markedly accelerated in individuals with hypertension or diabetes mellitus. Two forms of arteriolosclerosis are recognized. *Hyaline arteriolosclerosis* is typical of diabetes and consists of the thickening of arterial walls by amorphous protein deposits that apparently result from leakage of plasma proteins into the blood vessel wall (Fig. 7-3A). *Hyperplastic arteriolosclerosis* is characterized by hypertrophy/hyperplasia of smooth muscle cells in the media of small arteries, resulting in concentric muscle layers with an "onionskin" appearance (see Fig. 7-3B). This process is typically observed in the kidneys in the setting of severe (malignant) hypertension. It may be associated with the fibrinoid necrosis of the blood vessel wall in its most severe form.

Atherosclerosis

Atherosclerosis is the most common and clinically important variety of arteriosclerosis. Atherosclerosis is almost universally present in the larger arteries of the Western population because of frequent genetic and environmental risk factors (Table 7-1). Atherosclerosis is characterized by the progressive accumulation of lipid, inflammatory cells, smooth muscle cells, and connective tissue within the intima of large- and medium-sized arteries. Incremental accumulation of these materials results in progressive luminal narrowing and predisposition to thrombosis, which ultimately results in end-organ ischemia and infarction. The essential lesion of atherosclerosis is the atheroma (atherosclerotic plaque), which develops as an eccentric thickening of the arterial intima (see below). Atheromas are composed of cellular, lipid, and extracellular matrix components (Table 7-2).

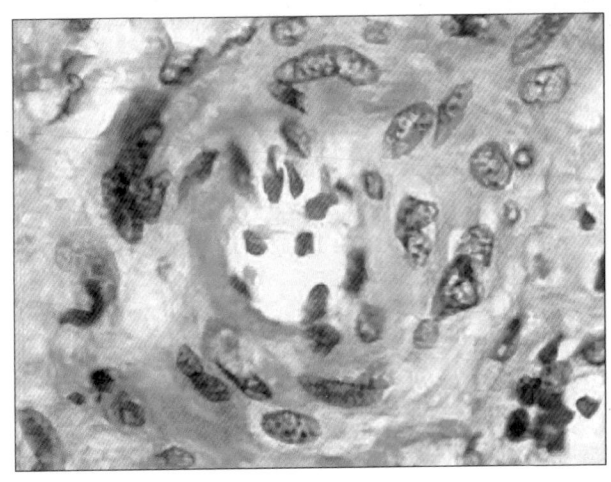

A

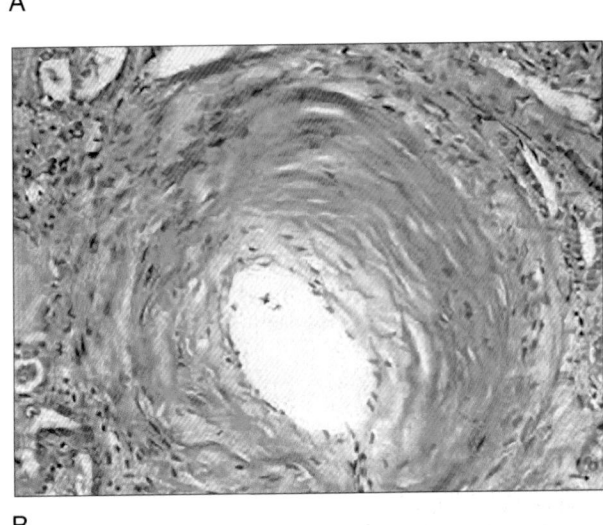

B

Figure 7-3. A, Hyaline arteriolosclerosis. Microscopic section showing the accumulation of amorphous material in the wall of an arteriole. **B,** Hyperplastic arteriolosclerosis. Microscopic section showing concentric rings of fibrous tissue around an arteriole.

Pathogenesis of Atherosclerosis

Although some controversy remains regarding the pathogenesis of atherosclerosis, the reaction to injury hypothesis is strongly favored by current evidence. Alternative theories that describe atherosclerosis as a primary proliferative abnormality of smooth muscle cells and or as a consequence of chronic infection by microorganisms have limited support at this time. The reaction to injury model proposes that atherosclerosis develops as a result of a chronic inflammatory response to subtle vascular (endothelial) injury occurring over a long period of time. According to this hypothesis, the interaction of multiple cell types with each other and with chemical and inflammatory mediators drives the incremental growth of atherosclerotic plaques. As plaques enlarge, additional changes develop that increase the risk of complications (thrombosis and acute vascular occlusion).

TABLE 7-1. Risk Factors for Atherosclerosis

Major Risk Factors		Minor Risk Factors
Modifiable	**Nonmodifiable**	**Minor Risk Factors**
Hyperlipidemia	Increasing age	Obesity
Hypertension	Male gender	Stress (type A personality)
Cigarette smoking	Family history	Factors affecting thrombosis
Diabetes mellitus	Genetic abnormalities: LDL-R, ApoB, ApoE, 5'-lipoxygenase	High carbohydrate intake
		Homocysteinemia

TABLE 7-2. Components of Atherosclerosis

Cellular	Extracellular Matrix	Lipid
Endothelial cells	Collagen	Cholesterol esters
Smooth muscle cells	Elastin	
Macrophages	Proteoglycans	
Other inflammatory cells		

The accumulation of macrophages with lipid droplets in their cytoplasm (foam cells) is the first step in atherogenesis (Fig. 7-4). Initially these accumulations form barely perceptible whitish yellow, nonraised longitudinal streaks on the endothelial surface of arteries, which are called "fatty streaks." Fatty streaks are almost universally present in the Western population, even in children. While they appear to be precursors of atheromatous plaques, the development of a fatty streak into an atheroma is not inevitable, since not all areas with fatty streaks develop plaques. Plaques tend to develop at specific anatomic locations, suggesting that other cofactors (probably chronic endothelial injury related to turbulent blood flow) are important. The development of fatty streaks is closely correlated with some of the major risk factors for atherosclerosis, particularly hyperlipidemia and the genetic syndrome of familial hypercholesterolemia that results from homozygous deficiency of the LDL receptor.

Even though most of the pathophysiologic events in atherosclerosis take place beneath the endothelial layer, endothelial cells are key players in this process and produce many of the mediators that direct plaque formation and attract or recruit key inflammatory cells and platelets from the blood. Endothelium is an active tissue that maintains hemostasis, regulates vascular tone (nitric oxide), and modulates leukocyte and platelet adhesion. Endothelial injury can result from mechanical shear stress (e.g., turbulent flow at arterial bifurcations), hyperlipidemia, free radicals, and hyperhomocysteinemia. These insults can cause endothelial cell activation and dysfunction, which ultimately result in increased vascular wall permeability and changes in gene expression that enhance leukocyte adherence (increased ICAM-1 and VCAM-1 expression). Some or all of these factors may be important in the development of atheromas in different individuals.

Hyperlipidemia and increased endothelial permeability favor the accumulation of LDL and very-low-density lipoprotein (VLDL) in the arterial intima.

Uptake of LDL by macrophages and endothelial cells results in intracellular oxidation of LDL. Alternatively, free radicals generated by the auto-oxidation of homocysteine (favored in individuals with high serum levels of homocysteine) can also oxidize extracellular LDL. The production of oxidized LDL in early plaques appears to be a key event driving atherosclerosis. Oxidized LDL is preferentially taken up by the scavenger receptor on macrophages, resulting in formation of foam cells. Oxidized LDL is also toxic to endothelial cells and promotes proinflammatory cytokine release, which further stimulates atherogenesis by recruiting additional inflammatory cells. Oxidized LDL is also a direct chemoattractant for macrophages/monocytes as well as smooth muscle cells (see below).

Many cell types are recruited into the developing plaque. These include inflammatory cells such as monocytes/macrophages (as discussed above) as well as T and B lymphocytes, which can be activated by cytokines, such as IL-1 and TNF-α, and oxidized LDL. Neutrophils may also play a role in atherosclerosis, since polymorphisms in the 5'-lipoxygenase pathway (predominantly expressed in neutrophils) have been genetically implicated as a risk factor for atherosclerosis. The presence of all these cell types in the developing plaque results in an environment in which both autocrine and paracrine stimulation of these cells favors the generation of additional oxidized LDL and proinflammatory cytokines. These positive feedback loops (Table 7-3) are the engine that drives plaque formation forward. In some cases, inflammatory mediators synthesized by one cell type are taken up by other cells and chemically modified to produce additional mediators.

Small plaques enlarge incrementally through the accumulation of additional inflammatory cells and extracellular lipid material (cholesterol clefts). Oxidized LDL and other chemotactic factors eventually stimulate the migration of smooth muscle cells from the arterial media across the internal elastic lamina into the intima. These smooth muscle cells are not normally present in the vascular intima, and in the setting of a developing plaque they also ingest lipids, converting themselves to foam cells. PDGF (platelet-derived growth factor), FGF (fibroblast growth factor), and TGF-α stimulate these cells to produce collagen, elastin, and proteoglycans to form a "fibrous cap" over the lipid core of the mature atheroma (see Fig. 7-4).

As atheromas increase in size, hypoxia at their center results in the release of proangiogenic factors that cause

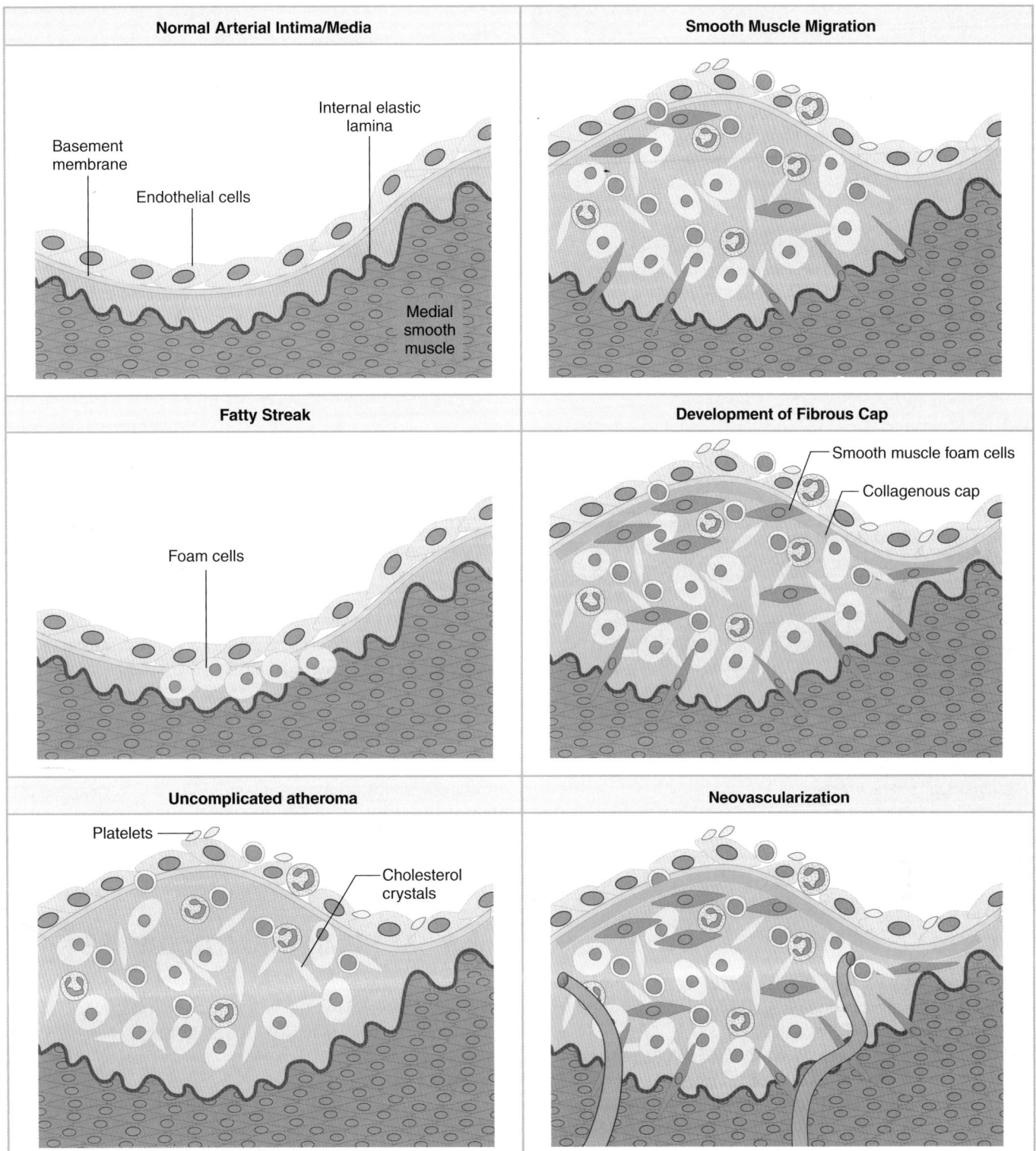

Figure 7-4. Schematic illustration of the development of an atheroma from a normal artery to mature plaque.

neovascularization (new blood vessel formation) at the periphery of the plaque. These small blood vessels are not normally present in the intima, and they predispose to hemorrhage within the plaque. Episodes of hemorrhage contribute hemosiderin (derived from the metabolism of hemoglobin) to the plaque core as well as additional lipid material and cholesterol (derived from erythrocyte membranes). All these factors cooperate to cause incremental growth of the plaque and predispose to plaque rupture/thrombosis. Enlargement of the plaque eventually results in significant obstruction to vascular flow, with resultant end-organ ischemia. In addition, altered flow around irregular

BIOCHEMISTRY

Low-density Lipoprotein (LDL)

LDL is composed of microparticles that include specific lipoproteins and cholesterol derived primarily from the digestion of food material and reprocessing of other lipoprotein particles (VLDL and IDL) by the liver. The amount of LDL cholesterol in the plasma is controlled by interaction of dietary and genetic factors.

Polymorphisms in genes coding for some lipoproteins can alter the structure and function of LDL. Deficiency of LDL receptors results in increased hepatic cholesterol synthesis and very high blood levels of LDL that facilitate its uptake by scavenger receptors on macrophages and histiocytes to contribute to atherosclerosis.

Table 7-4. Complications of Atherosclerosis

Pathophysiologic Event	Complication
Acute arterial occlusion secondary to plaque rupture/thrombosis	End-organ infarction
Progressive luminal narrowing	Chronic ischemic heart disease
Erosion/replacement of the arterial media by plaque with loss of tensile strength	Aneurysm formation
Dislodgment of a plaque thrombus and/or release of the highly thrombogenic components of the plaque core	Thromboembolism, atheroembolism

TABLE 7-3. Interactions of Cell and Inflammatory Mediators in the Development of Atherosclerosis*

Causes	Endothelial injury/dysfunction	Mononuclear cell recruitment	Lipid accumulation	Oxidized LDL	Myocyte recruitment	Fibrosis
Hyperlipidemia	×		×	×		
Endothelial injury/dysfunction	×	×	×	×		×
Mononuclear cell recruitment	×		×	×	×	×
Lipid accumulation	×			×		
Oxidized LDL	×	×			×	×
Myocyte recruitment	×	×				×

*An × indicates facilitating interactions that drive the development of atherosclerotic plaques.

atheromas causes turbulence resulting in injury or dysfunction in adjacent endothelial cells, which may result in linear propagation of the plaque.

Over time, some atheromas are completely replaced by collagen deposition to form a fibrous plaque (scar). Others develop dystrophic calcification at their core or enlarge to impinge on and cause atrophy of the arterial media. Such complicated atheromas are of greater clinical significance and may contain foci of dystrophic calcification or internal hemorrhage. All these factors are associated with an increased risk of thrombosis.

Complications of Atherosclerosis

Atherosclerosis accounts for more deaths and serious morbidity in the Western world than any other disease. The major complications of atherosclerosis, including ischemic heart disease, myocardial infarction, stroke, and gangrene of the extremities, account for more than half of the annual mortality in the United States. Most of these complications are related to plaque rupture/thrombosis (Table 7-4). The endothelium overlying atheromas is maintained in an activated state by diffusion of inflammatory mediators from the core of the plaque. This activation results in enhanced platelet adherence and an increased risk of thrombosis. Abnormal flow over the eccentric atheroma also favors endothelial injury or erosion and exposure of thrombogenic subendothelial collagen. Mechanical disruption of an atherosclerotic plaque can also be induced by vasospasm, hypertension, or hemorrhage of abnormal small blood vessels within the plaque. The formation of small platelet and fibrin thrombi on the surface of atheromas can initiate occlusive thrombosis or release microthrombi, which embolize into cardiac circulation, causing microinfarcts. Plaque rupture exposes highly thrombogenic components of the lipid core, stimulating the production of an occlusive thrombosis or release of atheroemboli (cholesterol crystals) into the coronary circulation.

●●● ISCHEMIC HEART DISEASE

Ischemic heart disease is a constellation of disorders in which myocardial ischemia is the common pathophysiologic mechanism. In the vast majority of cases, this ischemia results from obstruction of coronary artery blood flow by atherosclerosis, but its severity and consequences are affected by other factors that affect myocardial oxygen demand (e.g., concurrent valvular disease, chronic hypertension, blood oxygenation, microvascular disease [arteriolosclerosis is most important in diabetes mellitus]). There is a large functional reserve in normal coronary arteries so that coronary atherosclerosis typically becomes symptomatic only when the luminal cross-sectional area is reduced by more than 75% (i.e., a 50% decrease in luminal diameter). Atheromas typically involve the proximal portions of the left anterior descending and left coronary arteries and the entire right coronary artery (Fig. 7-5A). Plaques can progressively occlude flow (severe, fixed coronary obstruction), resulting in a slow diminution of blood flow. Alternatively,

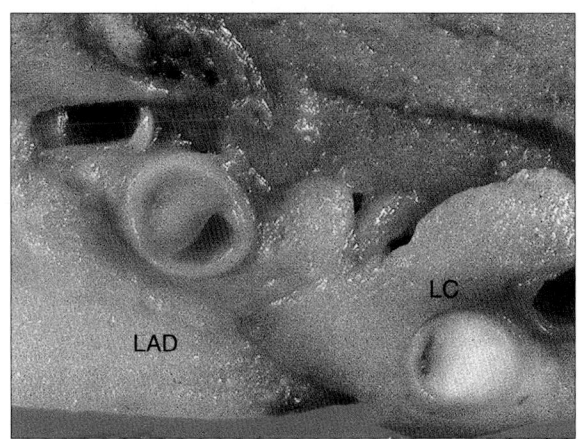

A

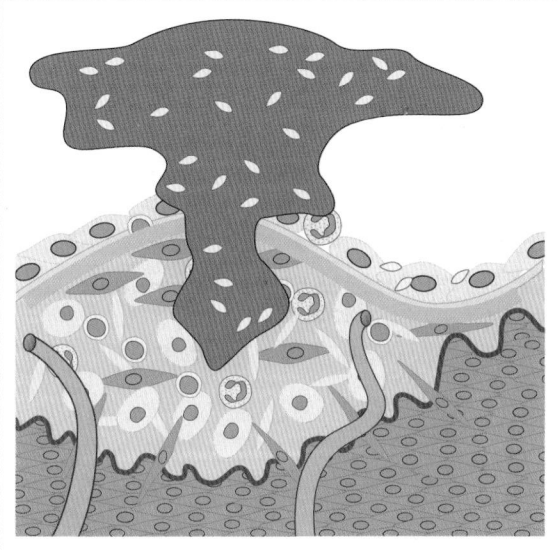

B

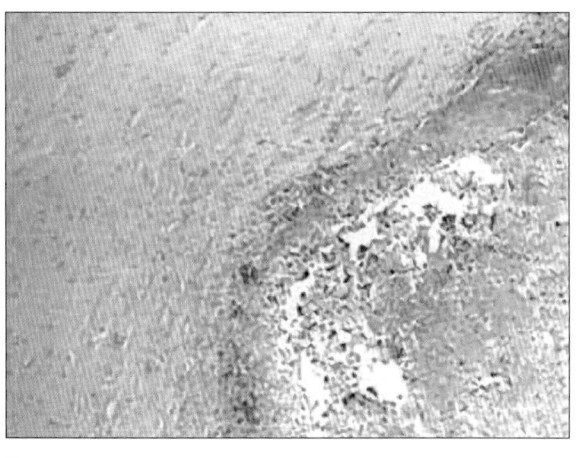

C

Figure 7-5. **A**, Coronary atherosclerosis. Gross cross-section of left coronary (LC) and left anterior descending (LAD) arteries in situ showing severe fixed lesions (>95% and 85% stenosis, respectively). **B**, Diagram showing plaque rupture and resulting thrombosis in a complicated atheroma. **C**, Coronary artery thrombosis. Microscopic section showing an acute thrombus filling an atherosclerotic coronary artery.

acute plaque change (hemorrhage, rupture, erosion) can result in catastrophic occlusion of blood flow or embolization to the distal coronary vasculature with microinfarction (see Figs. 7-5B and C). These lesions contribute to the four clinical syndromes of ischemic heart disease: angina pectoris, myocardial infarction, chronic ischemic heart disease, and sudden cardiac death.

Angina Pectoris

Angina pectoris is a symptom complex characterized by recurrent attacks of crushing substernal chest pain, which often radiates to the left arm and jaw. Three variants are recognized, but they have overlapping features.

Stable (Typical) Angina

Stable (typical) angina is characterized by chest pain and shortness of breath precipitated by exertion and relieved by rest or nitroglycerin. Pathologically stable angina usually corresponds to a fixed coronary obstruction.

Unstable (Crescendo) Angina

Unstable (crescendo) angina is characterized by chest pain and shortness of breath that occur either at rest, with progressively less exertion, or with increasing frequency. Pathologically, unstable angina is associated with acute plaque change and often with microscopic foci of infarction secondary to embolization of microthrombi. Unstable angina is associated with a significant risk of acute transmural myocardial infarction and may not be clinically distinguishable from a small transmural infarct (see Acute Coronary Syndrome section).

Prinzmetal's (Variant) Angina

Prinzmetal's (variant) angina is uncommon, with pain occurring at rest as a result of primary coronary vasospasm (contraction of medial smooth muscle resulting in luminal narrowing). This syndrome typically responds to calcium channel blockers, distinguishing it from other forms of angina. Vasospasm may also contribute to acute plaque change and myocardial infarction but is superimposed on atherosclerosis in this setting.

Acute Coronary Syndrome

Acute coronary syndrome (ACS) is a clinical symptom complex that corresponds to unstable angina and acute MI. These two conditions cannot be reliably distinguished in all cases, and patients with ACS have been shown to benefit from aggressive clinical management, including angioplasty and/or thrombolysis. In most cases, the clinical diagnosis of ACS corresponds pathologically to acute changes in a coronary atheroma with associated platelet microthrombi (Fig. 7-6). Embolization of these microthrombi can produce micro-infarcts that may not be clinically distinguishable from small transmural infarcts (e.g., changes in troponin levels, C-reactive protein, ECG).

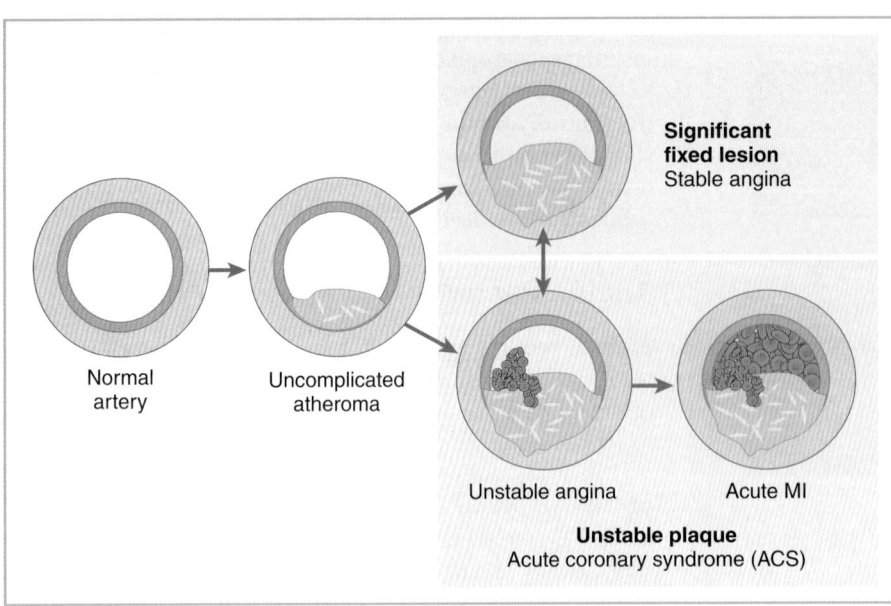

Figure 7-6. Relationship of coronary artery pathology to acute coronary syndrome (ACS).

TABLE 7-5. Chronology of Complications Following Myocardial Infarction

Complication	Time of Occurrence After Infarction
Cardiogenic shock	Variable; risk is dependent on baseline myocardial function and volume of infarct, may improve with recovery of function by "stunned" myocardium
Arrhythmia	Anytime; ventricular fibrillation occurs most often in first 12 hours postinfarct
Mural thrombus formation	Anytime
Papillary muscle rupture resulting in mitral valve incompetence	3–6 days postinfarct
Myocardial rupture with cardiac tamponade	3–6 days postinfarct
Ventricular aneurysm	Weeks to months postinfarct
Chronic ischemic heart disease	Months to years postinfarct

Myocardial Infarction

Myocardial infarction is a discrete focus of ischemic necrosis (coagulation necrosis) in the heart that occurs when myocardial ischemia is prolonged for more than 20 or 30 minutes. Transmural (full wall thickness) and subendocardial (limited to the subendocardial watershed area) infarcts are usually clinically and pathologically distinct processes although they sometimes overlap.

Transmural Infarction

Ninety percent of transmural infarcts are caused by an occlusive intracoronary thrombus, usually associated with an ulcerated atheromatous plaque. Thrombosis results in an area of infarction in the territory supplied by that artery. Right ventricular infarction may occur in conjunction with left ventricular and septal infarcts, but isolated right ventricular infarction is quite rare. Infarction begins in the subendocardium (watershed) and propagates outward toward the epicardium. Ischemia first results in myocyte dysfunction secondary to ATP depletion. ATP levels drop very rapidly, and such "stunned" myocytes at the periphery of an infarct may regain function over time if their vascular supply improves. Over the course of 20 to 30 minutes, ischemia produces irreversible cell injury, with membrane disruption and coagulative necrosis. Morphologic changes in acute infarcts develop on a relatively well-defined time scale that allows pathologic dating of many infarcts (Table 7-5). Light microscopic changes are subtle (wavy fiber change) for up to 12 hours postinfarct while ultrastructural evidence of necrosis is well developed by 1 hour. Necrotic myofibers induce chemotaxis of neutrophils (clearly evident by 24 hours and maximal at 48 hours) (Figs. 7-7A and 7-7B).

Gross pathologic changes in an acute transmural myocardial infarct become visible after approximately 4 hours as a discrete, dark, mottled area in the myocardium. Over the next 3 days, the infarct becomes more clearly defined with an increasingly pale center (see Figs. 7-7C and D). Over the next

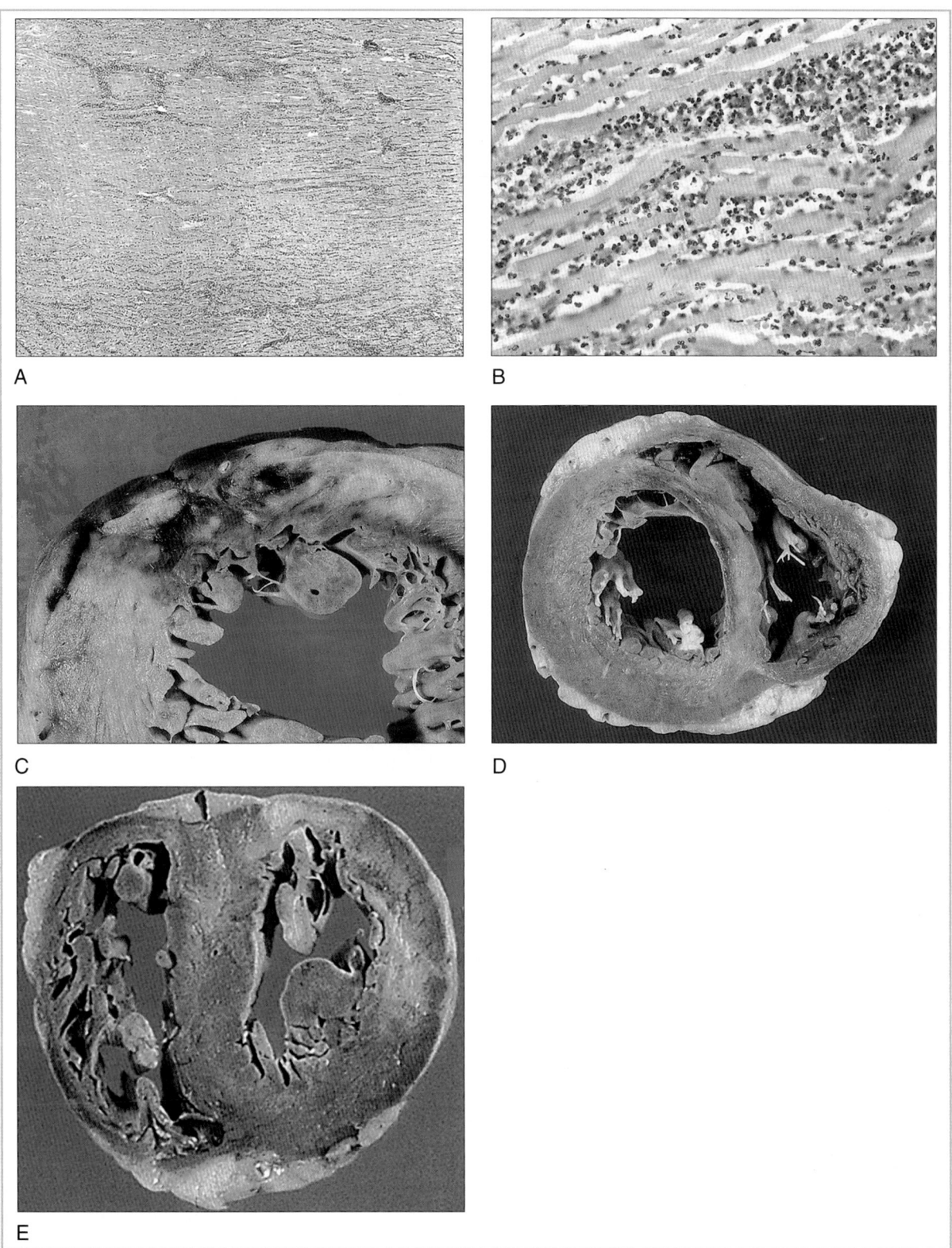

A

B

C

D

E

Figure 7-7. Acute myocardial infarction. Microscopic section of an acute myocardial infarct at 48 hours showing coagulation necrosis and maximal neutrophilic infiltrate at low power (**A**) and high power (**B**). **C**, Acute myocardial infarct. Gross cross-section of a left ventricle showing an acute myocardial infarct at 3 days complicated by ventricular rupture through the infarct. **D**, Subacute myocardial infarct. Gross cross-section of a septal myocardial infarct showing volume loss (thinning) and fibrosis of the intraventricular septum with compensatory right ventricular hypertrophy as a result of congestive heart failure. **E**, Healed myocardial infarct. Gross cross-section showing healed infarcts in the posterior and lateral walls free walls with prominent fibrosis (white tissue).

week, the infarct is sharply outlined with a central pale yellowish center (coagulation necrosis and neutrophilic infiltrate) bordered by a hyperemic zone composed of granulation tissue. Over the course of months, the infarcted region progresses to an organized gray-white scar, and necrotic tissue is removed by histiocytes and replaced with collagen from proliferating fibroblasts (see Fig. 7-7E).

The size of the infarct and whether or not vascular flow is restored to the affected area (reperfusion) affect the precise time scale for these changes. Large infarcts in which reperfusion does not occur tend to progress more slowly, since inflammatory cells must travel a relatively longer distance through extravascular tissue to reach the infarct's center. Conversely, early reperfusion can accelerate this process as well as predispose to hemorrhage from damaged blood vessels.

Clinical Findings in Transmural Infarcts

The clinical diagnosis of transmural myocardial infarction is critically dependent on electrophysiologic changes as well as serum biomarkers (Fig. 7-8).

Elevation of these cardiac biomarkers results from release of cytoplasmic proteins into the bloodstream by necrotic myocytes. The time course of appearance and disappearance of these biomarkers varies pending on the size and nature of the proteins and the volume of infarcted tissue. These parameters affect the clinical usefulness (sensitivity, specificity, time course) of these assays for detecting myocardial infarction.

Revascularization After Infarction

The development of transmural infarcts can be modified by rapid revascularization of the affected myocardium. Revascularization is usually a result of medical intervention through angioplasty (with or without stent placement) or treatment with thrombolytic agents (streptokinase, tissue plasminogen activator). If revascularization is achieved soon after infarction, myocytes at the periphery of the infarct that are damaged but have not undergone irreversible injury may recover and regain function. Similarly, these interventions may prevent propagation of thrombosis and infarct extension.

Revascularization also causes irreversibly damaged myocytes to develop contraction band necrosis. Contraction bands are visible by light microscopy as linear densities (perpendicular to the long axis of myocytes) that result from regeneration of ATP in myocytes with calcium leakage (hypercontraction of sarcomeres in this setting causes them to override their normal contraction positions). Although reperfusion is often associated with hemorrhage, this is not usually associated with adverse consequences and has been shown to improve long-term survival of the patient.

Acute and Subacute Sequelae of Transmural Infarcts

The consequences of myocardial infarction depend on size and location of the infarct as well as on therapeutic inter-

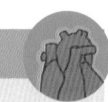

PHYSIOLOGY

Cardiac Electrophysiology

In a 12-lead electrocardiogram (ECG), leads II, III, and aVF reflect activity from the inferior wall while leads I, aVL, V5, and V6 monitor the lateral wall. Leads V1–V6 represent the anterior wall. Changes in the axis of the ECG can indicate right ventricular hypertrophy or a conduction block. Increased amplitude of electrical impulses is indicative of cardiac hypertrophy.

- P waves result from atrial contraction, and the QRS complex is produced by septal conduction and ventricular contraction. T waves are caused by repolarization of the ventricles.
- ST-segment elevations on ECG are indicative of acute cardiac ischemia that may or may not result in infarction.
- Q waves are usually indicative of transmural myocardial infarcts.
- Non–Q wave infarcts are usually subendocardial.

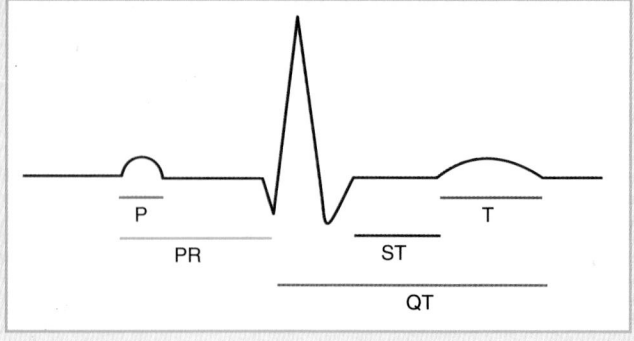

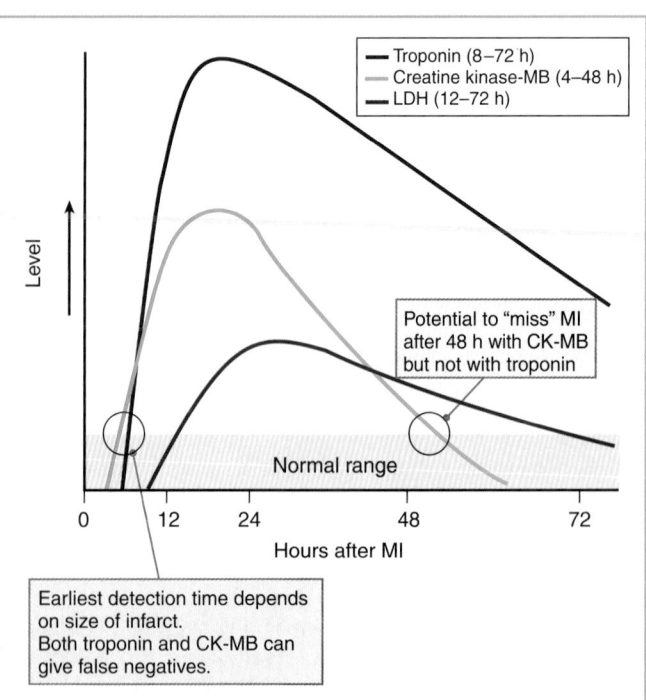

Figure 7-8. Serum cardiac biomarker changes following acute myocardial infarction.

ventions such as thrombolysis (Table 7-6). Cardiogenic shock results when an infarct affects a large percentage of the left ventricular myocardium or when myocardial reserve has been diminished by prior episodes of infarction/chronic ischemia. In either case, shock is the result of inadequate systemic perfusion to meet tissue demands. The hypotension associated with shock may further compromise myocardial blood flow, resulting in extension of an infarct. Conversely, successful reperfusion may allow recovery of stunned myocardium at the periphery of the infarct, with functional improvement.

Arrhythmias are serious complications of myocardial infarction that may result from abnormal conduction through the area of infarct with reentrant circuits or from direct interruption of the conduction system by the infarct. Arrhythmias can occur at any time postinfarct although ventricular fibrillation is most often observed within the first 12 hours. Mural thrombi may form at any time after infarction because diminished or abnormal wall motion can result in blood stasis in the ventricles and atria. Anticoagulation and antiplatelet agents may reduce the risk of thrombus formation, which can lead to catastrophic systemic thromboemboli. Papillary muscle rupture and ventricular wall rupture (free wall or septum) through an infarct usually occur between 3 and 6 days postinfarct at a time when neutrophilic infiltrate and tissue lysis are maximal but before significant fibrosis has developed. Papillary muscle rupture results in severe mitral regurgitation, requiring emergent surgical correction if clinically feasible. Ventricular free wall rupture is usually fatal with the rapid development of cardiac tamponade from intrapericardial hemorrhage that prevents diastolic filling. Septal rupture produces a ventricular septal defect with a left-to-right shunt that usually requires surgical closure. Ventricular aneurysm is typically a late complication of myocardial infarction. In this case, fibrous scar formation does not provide sufficient tensile strength and undergoes progressive dilatation secondary to luminal blood pressure. Such aneurysms diminish ejection fraction and predispose to mural thrombi. Repeated episodes of myocardial infarction result in chronic ischemic heart disease.

Subendocardial Myocardial Infarcts

Subendocardial myocardial infarcts are usually not caused by acute coronary thrombosis. The subendocardial region is a "watershed area" that is more susceptible to ischemic damage, since it is far from its vascular supply (i.e., the coronary arteries). Most patients with subendocardial infarcts have diffuse stenosis of all coronary arteries without evidence of plaque rupture or thrombosis. Subendocardial ischemia/infarction results from diminished blood flow to this watershed secondary to systemic hypotension and/or hypoxia (diminished pulmonary function, anemia, and carbon monoxide from smoking). The areas of subendocardial infarction usually extend outside the territory of a single coronary artery and may be circumferential. In patients with severe fixed coronary obstruction, the subendocardium is typically fibrotic, and residual myocytes show dystrophic changes, including vacuolization (myocytolysis), which result

TABLE 7-6. Microscopic Characteristics of Evolving Myocardial Infarcts

Time	Pathologic Findings	Clinical Correlation
1.5–4 hours	Wavy fiber change	Chest pain/shortness of breath; cardiogenic shock may occur if myocardial reserve is inadequate; mural thrombi can form early and embolize
4–12 hours	Hypereosinophilia of myofiber, edema, hemorrhage	CK and CK-MB elevated after 4–48 hours; troponin I elevated after 8–72 hours; ventricular fibrillation usually occurs in first 12 hours
12–24 hours	Early coagulation necrosis with pyknosis and hypereosinophilia, contraction band necrosis, early infiltration by neutrophils	Arrhythmias can occur at any time
1–3 days	Karyolysis of myocyte nuclei; neutrophilic infiltrate peaks at 48 hours	Pericardial friction rub may occur
3–7 days	Early disintegration of necrotic myofibers, macrophages, minimal blood vessel proliferation at periphery of infarct	Greatest risk of ventricular or papillary muscle rupture
7–10 days	Proliferation of blood vessels, numerous macrophages with extensive phagocytosis	
10–14 days	Granulation tissue peak, fibroblasts, few collagen fibers	
2–8 weeks	Increased collagen and decreased cellularity	Ventricular aneurysm
>2 months	Dense scar	Chronic ischemic heart disease

in diminished contractile function. This slow, progressive loss of cardiac myocytes in the subendocardium is an important component of chronic ischemic heart disease.

Chronic Ischemic Heart Disease

Chronic ischemic heart disease typically occurs in elderly patients with a previous history of myocardial ischemia/infarction who have progressive congestive heart failure (sometimes called ischemic cardiomyopathy). Marked subendocardial fibrosis secondary to severe fixed coronary obstruction is almost always present, with focal discrete scars corresponding to prior acute transmural infarcts. Myocytolysis (hydropic degeneration) is typically present throughout the subendocardium. Some patients with predominantly microvascular disease and/or severe fixed coronary lesions have only diffuse fibrosis and myocyte loss without discrete healed infarcts. There is usually moderate to marked left ventricular hypertrophy and dilatation. Histologically, there is myocardial hypertrophy and interstitial fibrosis resulting from loss of individual myofibers.

Myocardial Hypertrophy

The heart and cardiovascular system respond to changes in short- and long-term alterations in demand for blood supply using different mechanisms. Short-term changes are accommodated by changes in heart rate and vascular resistance. Long-term changes initiate adaptive responses that typically involve actual remodeling of the heart and vasculature. Dilatation of the ventricles can increase stroke volume.

Myocardial hypertrophy results in increased myocardial mass with an increase in both the size of myocytes and the amount of interstitial connective tissue present in the myocardium. Myocardial hypertrophy is a complex process involving changes not only at the gross and microscopic levels but also at the molecular level because of alterations in the pattern of gene expression.

It is important to recognize that some of these compensatory changes in response to preload and afterload stress can lead to significant dysfunction. Hypertrophy causes wall thickening that results in decreased compliance and always produces a degree of diastolic dysfunction. In extreme hypertrophy, this diastolic dysfunction may overwhelm any contractile advantage achieved. Similarly, dilatation of the left ventricle in an attempt to increase stroke volume can cause dilatation of the mitral valve ring, with valvular insufficiency and decreased functional cardiac output.

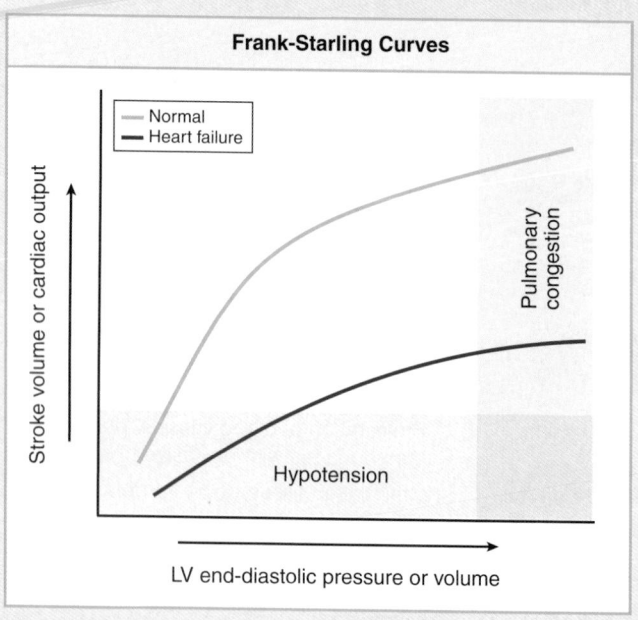

Frank-Starling Curves

Normal
Heart failure

Stroke volume or cardiac output

Pulmonary congestion

Hypotension

LV end-diastolic pressure or volume

Although some aspects of hypertrophy are adaptive (increasing contractile force to produce higher blood pressure or to replace the contractile function of dead myocytes), other aspects of myocyte function are abnormal and predispose to complications including arrhythmias. Additional complex changes in gene expression occur as congestive heart failure supervenes when compensatory mechanisms are overwhelmed.

Congestive Heart Failure

Heart failure is a physiologic state in which the heart is unable to maintain sufficient output for the metabolic requirements of organs and tissues. When heart failure is accompanied by significant edema in end organs, it is called congestive heart failure. Congestive heart failure (CHF) has marked effects on the lungs, liver, and kidneys as well as producing dependent edema in subcutaneous tissues. End-organ dysfunction is a consequence of both inadequate blood flow and abnormal fluid accumulation. Heart failure can result from either systolic or diastolic dysfunction or more commonly a combination of the two.

Diastolic dysfunction means ineffective filling of the ventricles during diastole. Since this is a low-pressure event, relatively small changes in the compliance (stiffness, rigidity) of the ventricles can result in significant dysfunction. Decreased compliance results in backup of pressure into the pulmonary and venous circulation as well as diminished cardiac output. Systolic dysfunction reflects a loss of myocardial contractility resulting from loss of muscle fibers (prior infarction) and/or increased intracellular connective tissue (increased resistance to contraction). There are also specific changes in gene expression in CHF that result in decreased β-adrenergic receptor density on cardiac myocytes and induction of brain natriuretic peptide (BNP). BNP synthesis is triggered by volume or pressure overload, and the serum level of BNP is a useful biomarker for clinically significant CHF. Myocyte apoptosis also is increased in CHF and may exacerbate failure.

Diastolic dysfunction in CHF results in increased pulmonary vascular pressure, producing pulmonary congestion and pulmonary edema. Pulmonary edema directly decreases oxygenation and decreases lung compliance, increasing the work of breathing. This edema fluid is a transudate that is exacerbated by sodium retention, hypoproteinemia, or both. Transudate can also accumulate in the pleural spaces, further decreasing functional lung volume. Right ventricular diastolic dysfunction results in increased systemic venous pressures, which increases pressure in hepatic central veins, causing dysfunction or necrosis of centrilobular hepatocytes.

Systolic dysfunction leads to hypoperfusion of the kidneys, which decreases glomerular filtration rate (GFR) with retention of sodium (further exacerbating tissue and organ edema) or acute tubular necrosis with renal failure. CHF can thereby produce a vicious cycle that results in worsening edema and increased myocardial demand that ultimately results in decompensation.

Hypertensive Heart Disease

Hypertensive heart disease is defined as left ventricular hypertrophy in the absence of cardiovascular causes other than hypertension (although this process almost always coexists with chronic ischemic heart disease).

BIOCHEMISTRY

B-Type Natriuretic Peptide (BNP)

BNP is a member of a family of three known natriuretic peptides (also including ANP and CNP) that share a common ring structure made up of 17 amino acids linked by a disulfide bond. BNP is produced predominantly in ventricular cardiac myocytes as a pro-protein (BNP-108) that is processed to the functional 32-nucleotide hormone BNP (BNP-32, composed of amino acids 72 to 108 of pro-BNP).

Most BNP exists in myocytes as BNP-32 and it is secreted in patients who develop heart failure, renal failure, some forms of secondary hypertension, and liver disease. BNP elicits diuretic, natriuretic, and hypotensive effects that tend to protect against fluid overload and increased blood pressure. BNP binds to the type A receptor that also binds ANP and signals by elevating cytoplasmic cyclic GMP (target tissues include kidney, adrenal glomerulosa cells that produce aldosterone, and vascular smooth muscle cells).

BNP is a clinically useful cardiac biomarker. Increased BNP levels in serum are a better marker of heart failure than pro-ANP levels. There is interest in pro-BNP as a biomarker of heart failure but it is not clear that it is superior to BNP. BNP has been used as a therapeutic agent in the treatment of heart failure and can improve hemodynamic parameters in the short term, but its use is controversial because of its high cost and possible increased death rate in treated patients.

PHYSIOLOGY

Hypertension and Blood Pressure Control

Hypertension is defined as sustained diastolic blood pressure greater than 90 mm Hg or sustained systolic blood pressure greater than 140 mm Hg.

Primary (essential) hypertension is hypertension of unknown cause that is not secondary to an identified disease (e.g., renal artery stenosis with excess renin production by the kidney). Approximately 95% of hypertensive patients have essential hypertension. Essential hypertension often shows polygenic inheritance with genetic variations in pathways that up-regulate or down-regulate various components of the cardiovascular system (e.g., vascular tone, natruresis, kaluresis, and ventricular contraction). The mechanisms controlling these aspects of cardiovascular and renal physiology are diverse (neural, endocrine, paracrine), and a combination of multiple factors is responsible for essential hypertension in most patients.

Sustained hypertension accelerates atherosclerosis, causes direct end-organ damage (kidney and heart), and increases the risk of cerebral infarction.

This hypertrophy is a compensatory mechanism to accommodate the increased afterload present in systemic hypertension. The left ventricle is thickened, and the overall weight of the heart is increased, exceeding 375 g in men and 350 g in women. Microscopically, the myocardial cells appear hypertrophic with enlarged nuclei secondary to duplication of nuclear DNA (polyploid), and they demonstrate the specific alterations in gene expression discussed above.

Cor Pulmonale

Cor pulmonale is right ventricular failure (usually with both hypertrophy and dilatation) generally secondary to pulmonary hypertension, which may be primary or secondary to left ventricular dysfunction or valvular heart disease.

Sudden Death

Sudden death is defined as unexpected death from cardiac causes (lethal arrhythmia) within 1 hour of the onset of symptoms and frequently is the first manifestation of underlying coronary atherosclerosis (often severe lesions with plaque disruption or occlusive thrombus). Less commonly the cause can be nonatherosclerotic (e.g., primary cardiomyopathy; see below).

●●● VASCULITIS

Vasculitis (angiitis) is the destructive inflammation of blood vessel walls. Vascular inflammation is present in all ulcers and infarcts as a secondary process, but the term *vasculitis* is typically reserved for primary inflammation of the vasculature that is usually immune mediated. Primary vasculitis is quite rare in the general population with the exception of giant cell arteritis that occurs with some frequency in older individuals. Vasculitis can affect any blood vessel from the aorta to capillaries to veins. Microscopically, it is characterized by the presence of inflammatory cells within the vessel wall and varying degrees of endothelial and medial injury. The sizes of the involved blood vessels and the nature of the inflammatory reaction are critical features in the differential diagnosis of different forms of vasculitis.

Although almost all cases of vasculitis are immune mediated, the precise mechanisms involved are clearly understood for only a few entities. For example, Goodpasture's syndrome results from an autoantibody that is specific for basement membrane components in the kidney and lungs (type II hypersensitivity)

Similarly, immunocomplex deposition (type III hypersensitivity reaction) is clearly the cause of some types of vasculitis (leukocytoclastic vasculitis resulting from a hypersensitivity reaction to a drug; i.e., serum sickness). However, immunocomplexes are not readily demonstrable in most clinical specimens with vasculitis (pauci-immune vasculitis). Many patients with vasculitis have autoimmune diseases, but others develop vasculitis as a paraneoplastic syndrome.

Some specific types of vasculitis are used as eponyms to describe a number of separate clinicopathologic syndromes (mainly rheumatologic diseases) that affect specific organ systems. Although some of these disorders fit into well-defined clinical categories (e.g., giant cell arteritis), a significant percentage show overlapping features, complicating their classification. Serum antineutrophil cytoplasmic antibodies (ANCAs) are a useful adjunct to histologic examination in the diagnosis of some forms of vasculitis.

While the pathologic diagnosis of vasculitis is important in terms of treatment decisions, it is often complicated by the

---

IMMUNOLOGY

Hypersensitivity Reactions

Type II hypersensitivity results from the binding of high-affinity antibodies directly to specific target molecules. Bound antibodies may fix complement or act as opsonins to promote phagocytosis.

Type III hypersensitivity results from the deposition of preformed antigen-antibody complexes at different sites in the body (usually in the vasculature). These complexes initiate an inflammatory reaction by activating complement. The ensuing inflammatory reaction may lead to necrosis, thrombosis, and hemorrhage. Accumulation of antigen-antibody complexes in glomerular capillaries can ultimately result in blockage of ultrafiltration and renal failure.

IMMUNOLOGY

Antineutrophil Cytoplasmic Antibody (ANCA)

ANCAs are autoantibodies that develop in some patients with vasculitis. They were first identified by incubating patient sera with normal neutrophils and staining with labeled antihuman immunoglobulin antibodies. Sera from a subset of patients with vasculitis produced a pattern of either cytoplasmic (c-ANCA) or perinuclear staining (p-ANCA).

Subsequently, it has been shown that most c-ANCA antibodies recognize proteinase III while most p-ANCA antibodies recognize myeloperoxidase. ANCA titers correlate with disease activity and response to therapy in some patients with vasculitis. It remains controversial whether ANCA antibodies have a direct causal role in vascular inflammation. Antibody binding to neutrophils may trigger their activation and cause endothelial injury.

While ANCA titers are a clinically useful test, their specificity for vasculitis is limited, since these autoantibodies can be observed in other conditions that are not associated with vasculitis such as chronic inflammatory bowel disease.

Antineutrophil Cytoplasmic Antibodies (ANCA) in Vasculitis

Antigen	c-ANCA Proteinase III	p-ANCA Myeloperoxidase
Wegener's granulomatosis	+++	+
Polyarteritis nodosa (microscopic)	+	+++
Polyarteritis nodosa (classic)	−	−
Churg-Strauss angiitis	+	+++

difficulty of obtaining appropriate tissue samples. Since many forms of vasculitis are deep seated, invasive surgical procedures may be required to obtain diagnostic tissue specimens. Morphologic findings alone are often insufficient to arrive at a specific diagnosis, and demographic features relating to patient age, sex, geographic location, and HLA type as well as key serologic tests (ANCA, rheumatoid factor, ANA) are also needed to arrive at a specific diagnosis. Because of overlapping clinical and pathologic features and lack of detailed understanding of the pathophysiology of many forms of vasculitis, a provisional classification based on the size of involved blood vessels is currently in use (Fig. 7-9). In the future, clearer understanding of the underlying pathophysiology may permit a more useful classification.

Infectious arteritis refers to the direct bacterial or fungal infection of vessel walls.

Large-Vessel Vasculitis

Temporal Arteritis (Giant Cell Arteritis)

Temporal arteritis is a distinct clinical syndrome that occurs almost exclusively in older individuals and is associated with HLA-DR4 allele. Headache is typically present with pain over the temporal artery and jaw. The erythrocyte sedimentation rate (ESR; a measure of acute-phase reactants) is typically elevated in these patients. Most of the symptoms relate to vasculitis of the medium-sized arteries of the head and neck. This process can involve the ophthalmic artery, leading to blindness, so that recognition of this disease and prompt treatment with corticosteroids are critical. Morphologically, there is a destructive vasculitis of the arterial media that is often associated with multinucleated giant cells (Fig. 7-10A). There is typically fragmentation of the internal elastic membrane most easily recognized in a silver stain for elastin fibers. Giant cell arteritis can involve arteries in a focal fashion, making extensive sampling of temporal artery biopsies important in establishing the diagnosis. Disease is usually not limited to the temporal artery, but its superficial location makes it accessible to biopsy. Many patients with giant cell arteritis also develop the symptom complex of polymyalgia rheumatica, which includes arthralgias and myalgias in multiple joints and muscle groups.

Takayasu's Arteritis (Pulseless Disease)

Takayasu's arteritis is a granulomatous arteritis of the aorta and larger arteries that typically affects young women. Morphologically, there are multinucleated giant cells within the media with associated fibrosis and thickening of the media along with loss of normal elastin fibers (see Fig. 7-10B). Involvement of the aortic branches results in wall thickening and luminal narrowing, causing peripheral ischemia and the loss of pulses in the upper extremities and coronary ischemia (see Fig. 7-10C). The cause of this disease is unknown. It is rare in the United States and more common in Asia.

Small-Vessel Vasculitis

Goodpasture's syndrome is caused by autoantibodies that recognize the basement membrane (type II hypersensitivity) of the pulmonary and renal blood vessels, resulting in glomerulonephritis (see Chapter 12) and pulmonary hemorrhage. This is usually a disease of childhood.

Intermediate-Vessel Vasculitis

Classic Polyarteritis Nodosa

Classical polyarteritis nodosa (PAN) occurs predominantly in young men with vasculitis of medium-sized muscular arteries typically leading to thrombosis and end-organ ischemia or infarction. Symptoms in multiple organ systems result from

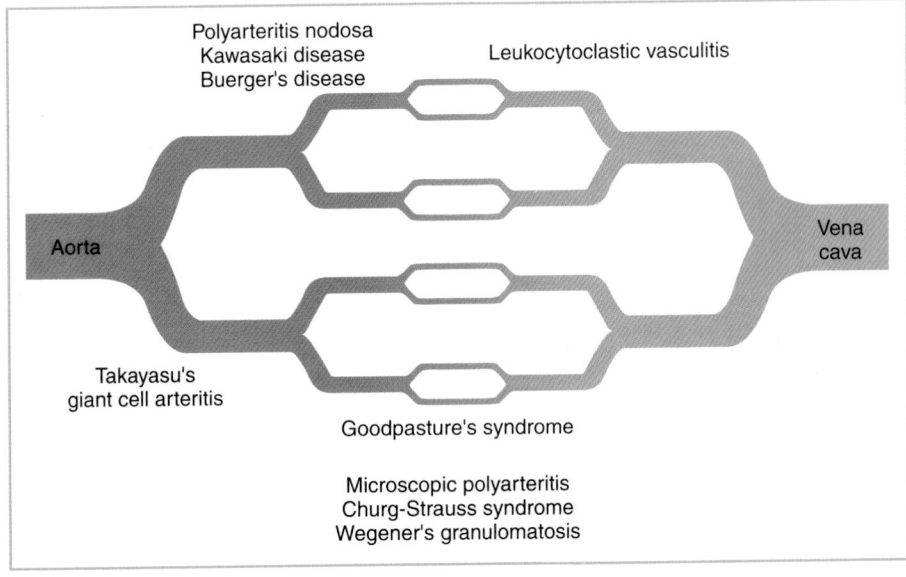

Polyarteritis nodosa
Kawasaki disease
Buerger's disease

Leukocytoclastic vasculitis

Aorta

Vena cava

Takayasu's
giant cell arteritis

Goodpasture's syndrome

Microscopic polyarteritis
Churg-Strauss syndrome
Wegener's granulomatosis

Figure 7-9. Classification of vasculitis by the size of the involved blood vessels.

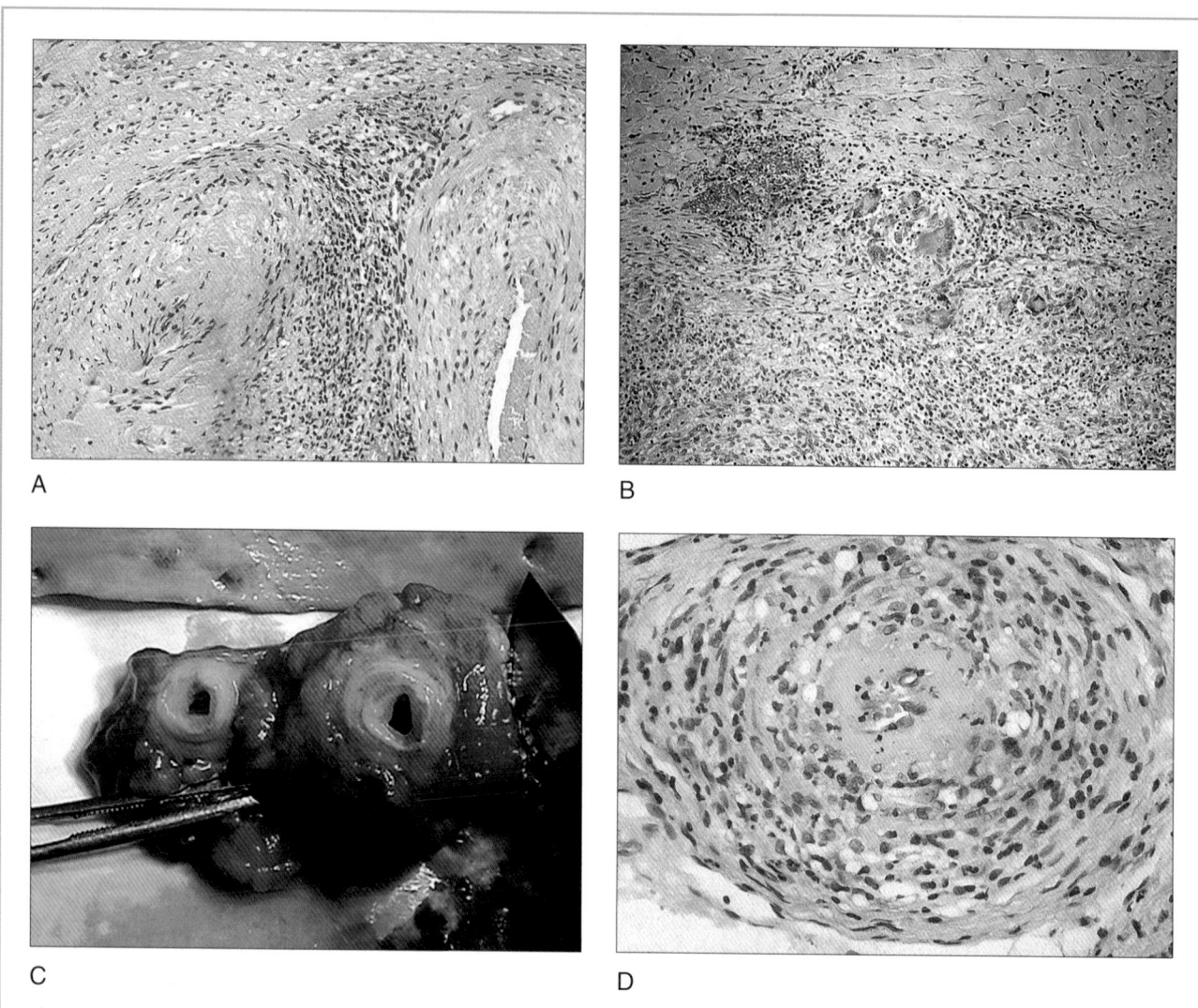

Figure 7-10. A, Giant cell arteritis, temporal artery. Microscopic section showing a prominent, lymphocytic infiltrate in the media of a temporal artery with destruction of smooth muscle cells. **B,** Takayasu's arteritis. Microscopic section showing prominent granulomatous inflammation and fibrosis in the aortic media. **C,** Takayasu's arteritis. Gross cross-section of coronary arteries showing extensive medial fibrosis and intimal narrowing that resulted in myocardial infarction. **D,** Leukocytoclastic vasculitis. Microscopic section showing prominent karyorrhectic debris in the wall of a venule in the superficial dermis associated with a mixed inflammatory cell infiltrate.

ischemia or infarction of organs by involvement of muscular arteries. Up to 30% of patients with polyarteritis nodosa have hepatitis B antigenemia, suggesting immunocomplex-mediated disease. Involvement of arteries is segmental, and healing lesions are generally present at the same time as active lesions. This temporal dissociation of lesions is important in the differential diagnosis. Morphologically, these lesions typically show fibrinoid necrosis with a mixed inflammatory cell infiltrate that often includes eosinophils. Segmental destruction of blood vessel walls can result in the formation of microaneurysms, which may be recognized radiographically. Renal involvement is typical. Patients are usually pANCA negative, and there is variable response to immunosuppressive therapy. Allergic granulomatosis and angiitis share features with classic PAN but are almost always associated with asthma and prominent eosinophilia of the peripheral blood. Involvement of the lungs and peripheral nerves is typical, and patients are usually pANCA positive.

Microscopic Polyarteritis

Microscopic polyarteritis shares some pathologic features with classic PAN but involves small arteries. pANCA is almost always positive in these patients, and immunocomplexes are usually not present (pauci-immune vasculitis). Patients frequently have other manifestations of autoimmune disease, but the pathogenesis is unclear. Many different organs and tissues can be involved.

Leukocytoclastic Vasculitis

An important subclass of microscopic polyarteritis, which usually is self-limited, is leukocytoclastic vasculitis. Leukocytoclastic vasculitis is usually pANCA negative and presents clinically with purpura (hemorrhage into the skin or mucous membranes). Hemorrhage results from involvement of venules, and in contrast with classic PAN, lesions are synchronous. In the majority of cases, immuno-complex deposition secondary to a hypersensitivity reaction to a drug is implicated, and eosinophils are often prominent. Morphologically, there is prominent inflammation within the wall of venules, with fragments of nuclear material (karyorrhectic debris) resulting from apoptosis (see Fig. 7-10D). This morphologic pattern can also be observed as a paraneoplastic syndrome, a component of essential mixed cryoglobulinemia, and with Henoch-Schönlein purpura.

Wegener's Granulomatosis

Wegener's granulomatosis is typically a disease of older individuals with a significant male predominance. The upper respiratory tract and kidney may be involved together or individually, and most patients are positive for cANCA. Patients may have necrotizing granulomas of the upper airways or respiratory tract that produce geographic necrosis in the lungs or crescentic glomerulonephritis (rapidly progressive glomerulonephritis; see Chapter 12). Open lung biopsy may be required for diagnosis, and the necrotizing granulomatous inflammation must be distinguished from tuberculosis. Aggressive immunosuppressive therapy may be lifesaving.

Kawasaki Disease (Mucocutaneous Lymph Node Syndrome)

Kawasaki disease is a febrile illness of childhood associated with lymphadenopathy and edema and erythema of hands and feet. It is rare in the United States but relatively common in Japan. It results in necrotizing vasculitis of the coronary arteries with morphologic features similar to PAN. Surprisingly, it is almost always a self-limited process with low mortality probably because of the substantial luminal reserve in the coronary arteries of children. Patients usually make a complete recovery.

Thromboangiitis Obliterans (Buerger's Disease)

Thromboangiitis obliterans occurs exclusively in heavy smokers and consists of an acute inflammatory infiltrate in the walls of small arteries in the extremities with focal microabscess formation. This inflammation often leads to thrombosis with infarction of fingers and toes. There is an association with HLA-A9 and -B7 alleles.

●●● ANEURYSM

A true aneurysm is an arterial dilatation that is composed of all three normal components of the vessel wall. They can be cylindric, saccular, or fusiform in shape.

Atherosclerotic Aneurysm

Atherosclerotic aneurysms of the abdominal aorta are the most common and clinically significant types of athero-sclerotic aneurysms. Aneurysm formation is a direct con-sequence of erosion and replacement of the media by the growth of a complicated atheroma. The media is largely replaced by lipid material, inflammatory cells, and prominent dystrophic calcification (Fig. 7-11). Aneurysms are usually located below the renal arteries. Tension in a wall of a blood vessel is related to the product of luminal pressure and vessel diameter so that as aneurysms enlarge, the tension in their wall increases in direct proportion to their diameter. This relationship between tension and size results in a critical diameter for rupture (typically 6 cm for atherosclerotic aneurysms). Patients with aneurysms larger than 6 cm have a substantially greater risk of rupture and typically undergo elective surgical repair of the aneurysm. In addition to rupture, atherosclerotic aneurysms provide a nidus for thrombus formation that can result in embolization and infarction. Atherosclerotic aneurysms typically extend to involve tributary vessels (iliac arteries), and the resulting thickening of the wall of these smaller blood vessels results in significant luminal narrowing and diminished blood flow (i.e., peripheral vascular disease).

Luetic (Syphilitic) Aneurysm

Luetic (syphilitic) aneurysms are a complication of tertiary syphilis that affect the thoracic aorta. Treponemes are present in the small blood vessels of the adventitia (vasa vasorum) and induce a plasma cell vasculitis that eventually obliterates these vessels.

Loss of the vas vasorum results in ischemia of the aortic media with fibrous replacement of medial smooth muscle and loss of normal elasticity. These aneurysms can become large and impinge on normal mediastinal structures. Extension of the aneurysm to the aortic valve ring results in annular dilatation and aortic valvular insufficiency (regurgitation).

Dissecting Aneurysm

Dissecting aneurysms are not true aneurysms but rather hematomas within the arterial media that occur almost exclusively in the aorta. An intimal tear allows access of blood to the media, and luminal blood pressure causes propagation of the thrombus through the arterial media over the course of hours to days (Fig. 7-12). Aortic dissection can have three outcomes. (1) Blood may rupture through the adventitia, resulting in massive hemorrhage into the peri-cardium, pleura, or other structures. (2) The hematoma may reenter the aortic lumen, resulting in a double-barreled aorta. (3) The hematoma may extend down tributary blood vessels (e.g., the carotid artery). In these smaller vessels, the dissection compresses the lumen, resulting in end-organ infarction. Type A dissecting aneurysms involve the ascending aorta, putting the carotid and brachial arteries at risk for occlusion. For this reason, type A aneurysms are treated by emergent surgery. Type B aneurysms involve the descending aorta and are typically managed by lowering blood pressure.

Most patients under 40 years of age with dissecting aneurysms have Marfan syndrome or have been recently

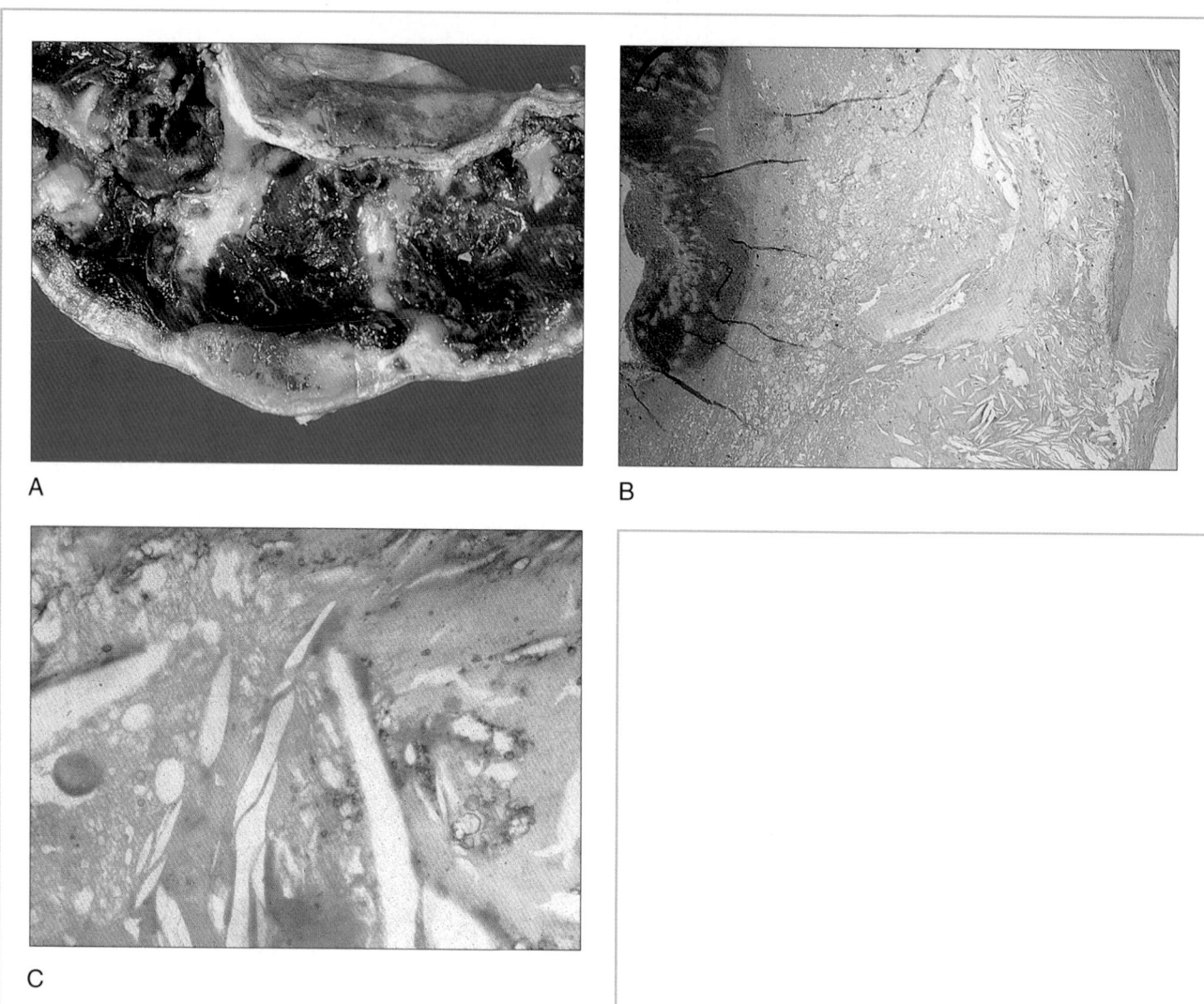

Figure 7-11. Atherosclerotic aneurysm. **A**, Gross cross-section of an abdominal atherosclerotic aneurysm showing intraluminal thrombus and yellow gray lipid material expanding the wall of the aorta. **B**, Microscopic section showing atherosclerosis replacing the aortic wall with cholesterol clefts and dystrophic calcification. **C**, High-power micrograph showing cholesterol clefts (needle-shaped spaces) and dystrophic calcifications (blue-purple deposits, right).

pregnant. Both of these conditions result in the accumulation of mucopolysaccharide ground substance within the media of the aorta, with loss and disorder of elastin fibers. In Marfan syndrome, this lesion (called cystic medial necrosis) is caused by point mutations in the fibrillin gene that prevent normal deposition of elastin in the extracellular matrix. These connective tissue abnormalities predispose patients to aortic dissection. In patients older than 40 years, typical risk factors for aortic dissection are hypertension and bicuspid aortic valve (which results in abnormal flow and endothelial injury).

False Aneurysm

False aneurysms are usually caused by trauma that results in a mechanical defect in a blood vessel wall which is then sealed by fibrosis with organization and recanalization of associated hematoma. The result is a false blood channel that is not composed of normal blood vessel wall components. A

mycotic aneurysm is one caused by an infectious agent, resulting in weakening and dilatation of an artery.

Berry Aneurysm

Berry aneurysms are outpouchings of connective tissue at the junction of arteries in the circle of Willis. These are not true aneurysms and are thought to result from congenital weakness at this site. Expansion of these lesions can impinge on cranial nerves, which may lead to the diagnosis. Rupture results in life-threatening subarachnoid hemorrhage.

●●● MYOCARDITIS

Many viral infections produce a transient myocarditis with replication of virus within cardiac myocytes that is usually subclinical (Fig. 7-13). In susceptible individuals, myocarditis may be prolonged or associated with an unusually strong host

Tertiary Syphilis

Syphilis passes through three stages of infection with a primary chancre developing at the initial site of infection. Secondary syphilis is usually asymptomatic and typically transitions to tertiary syphilis after many years.

Tertiary syphilis is an active infection in which treponemes are viable and demonstrable in diseased tissue. Most of the tissue damage results from the host's immune response to the microorganisms. Gummas are expansile, tumor-like fibrotic lesions containing treponemes that can develop at almost any site in the body and erode bone or other vital structures.

Syphilitic aneurysms of the aorta are caused by infection and inflammation of the vasa vasorum of the aorta. These small vessels are eventually obliterated, resulting in ischemia and fibrosis of the aortic media that causes loss of elasticity. Over time, the aorta dilates (predominantly the ascending and thoracic aorta are involved), resulting in secondary aortic valvular insufficiency because of dilatation of the aortic valve ring. Syphilitic aneurysms almost never rupture because of the extensive fibrosis present, but as they grow larger, they can compress and damage vital mediastinal structures.

Tabes dorsalis is myelopathy of the posterior columns of the spinal cord that results from direct infection of neural tissue by spirochetes.

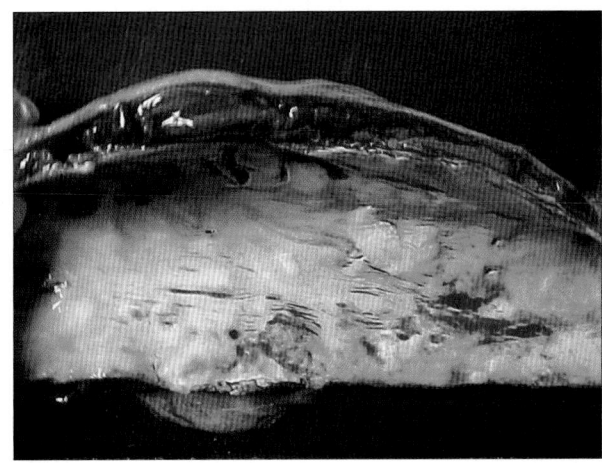

A

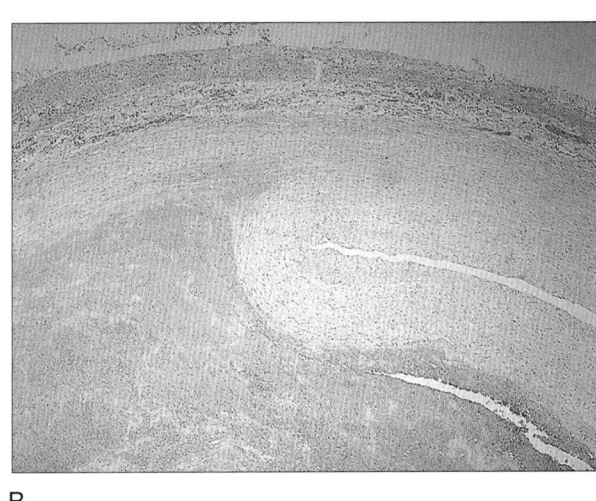

B

Figure 7-12. Aortic dissection. **A**, Gross longitudinal section of an aorta with a dissecting hematoma expanding its wall (top portion of the figure). **B**, Microscopic section showing a blood clot that forms a false channel in the aortic media that compresses the true lumen. The rate of dissection in this case was too rapid for extensive organization to occur in the hematoma.

immune response that causes symptomatic myocarditis. In a subset of these patients, the inflammatory process, which is orchestrated predominantly by activated T lymphocytes, may be sustained or progressive (Fig. 7-14A). While viral myocarditis is rare, it is probably a numerically significant cause of dilated cardiomyopathy (see below). Other forms of acute infectious myocarditis occur in the setting of protozoal disease and in some idiopathic conditions such as sarcoidosis (see Fig. 7-14B). These forms of myocarditis may interfere with the conduction system as well as directly damage cardiac myocytes.

●●● CARDIAC TRANSPLANTATION

Rejection of transplanted hearts is due to an immune response similar to that described for viral myocarditis but directed against transplantation antigens. In severe acute rejection, myocardial necrosis and heart failure may result. This type of acute rejection is generally well controlled by current immunosuppressive therapy if the HLA type of the graft and host are reasonably well matched. In contrast, chronic rejection corresponds to diffuse intimal hyperplasia of the graft coronary arteries (Fig. 7-15). This intimal hyperplasia results in significant luminal narrowing over the course of years and is not currently amenable to therapy. Chronic rejection is a major cause of long-term graft failure. This process is distinct from atherosclerosis in terms of both its histopathology and geographic distribution. The onset of myocardial ischemia in a transplant does not result in typical angina-like pain because transplanted hearts are denervated.

●●● CARDIOMYOPATHY

Cardiomyopathy is a rare condition that is typically defined as a primary disease of heart muscle. Atherosclerotic cardiovascular disease is usually not included with cardiomyopathy, since the damage to myocytes is secondary to the primary vascular lesion. In practice, it may be difficult to distinguish cardiomyopathy (rare) from ischemic heart disease (very common) during life. Cardiomyopathy is typically classified by three functional categories: hypertrophic, restrictive, and dilated (Fig. 7-16). While these three categories are useful clinically, there is usually some functional overlap at the time of diagnosis because of compensatory changes in myocardial architecture.

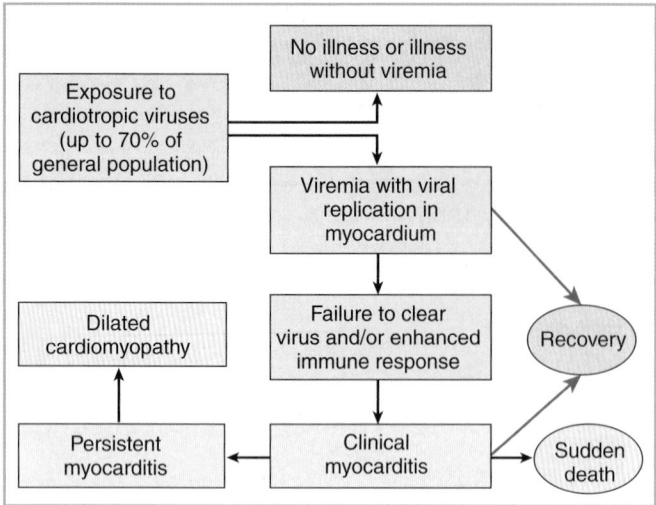

Figure 7-13. Pathogenesis of viral myocarditis.

Hypertrophic Cardiomyopathy

Hypertrophic cardiomyopathy results in thickening of the myocardial wall and is almost always inherited as an autosomal dominant trait caused by point mutations in structural proteins within the contractile apparatus of cardiac myocytes (Fig. 7-17A). The most common gene involved is the cardiac β-myosin heavy chain gene, which accounts for nearly 50% of cases. Amino acid substitutions in this gene result in defective contraction with compensatory hypertrophy of cardiac myocytes, myofiber disarray, and associated interstitial fibrosis. Different amino acid substitutions are associated with different penetrance and severity of disease. Mutations in other sarcomeric proteins account for most the other cases of hypertrophic cardiomyopathy. Patients typically are young or middle-aged adults with enlarged hearts and evidence of congestive heart failure without significant coronary artery disease. The age and severity of presentation can be strongly influenced by environmental factors such as alcohol consumption and exercise training, which may accelerate the development of symptomatic disease. Left ventricular hypertrophy of any cause is associated with an increased risk of sudden death (probably secondary to arrhythmia) and hypertrophic cardiomyopathy is commonly found in young athletes with sudden death. Most cases of hypertrophic cardiomyopathy are associated with disproportionate septal hypertrophy, which results in aortic outflow obstruction, further exacerbating hypertrophy. Ventricular thickening decreases myocardial compliance and causes defective diastolic filling (a prominent feature of restrictive cardiomyopathy; see below).

Dilated Cardiomyopathy

Dilated cardiomyopathy results from primary systolic dysfunction with massive dilatation of the left ventricle and a markedly diminished ejection fraction (see Fig. 7-17B). There

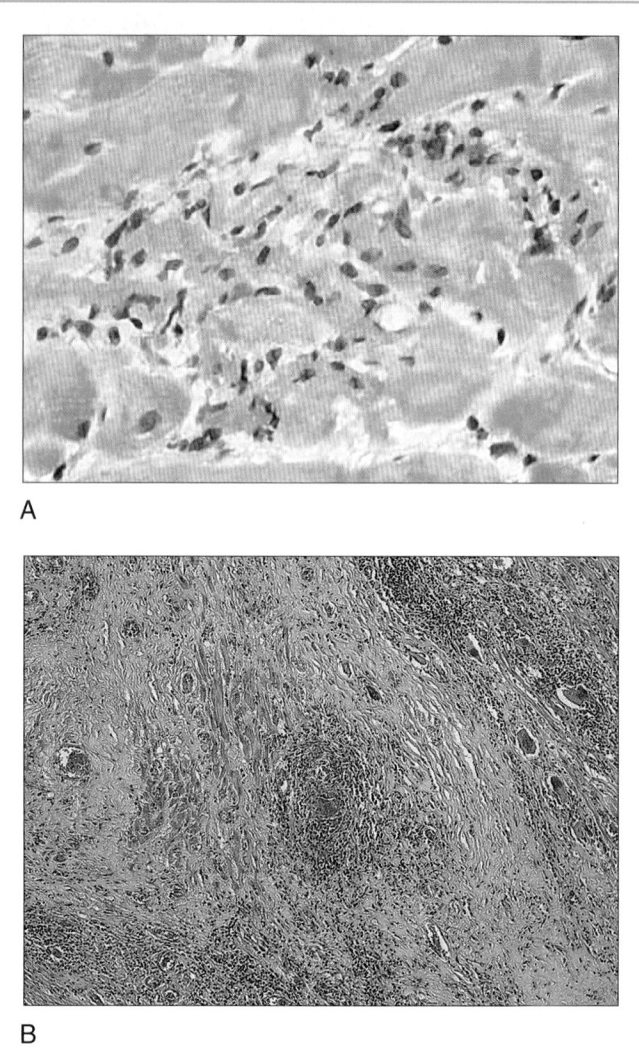

Figure 7-14. **A**, Viral myocarditis. Microscopic section showing a moderately dense infiltrate of T cells surrounding cardiac myocytes with cytopathic effects in individual myocytes. **B**, Sarcoid myocarditis. Microscopic section showing granulomatous inflammation with prominent giant cells and fibrosis that obliterates cardiac myocytes.

are multiple known genetic causes of dilated cardiomyopathy including some storage diseases (glycogen and lysosomal) as well as Duchenne's muscular dystrophy. While cardiac involvement in these diseases is an important cause of death, abnormalities in other organ systems (e.g., musculoskeletal) tend to dominate the clinical course. Some cases of dilated cardiomyopathy are clearly familial, but inheritance patterns are heterogeneous and only a few single gene defects have been implicated to date.

Genetic lesions are responsible for a relatively small percentage of patients with dilated cardiomyopathy. Undiagnosed myocarditis that has progressed to congestive heart failure probably accounts for a significant percentage of cases. The inciting virus may no longer be present when heart failure supervenes so that definitive diagnosis may not be possible.

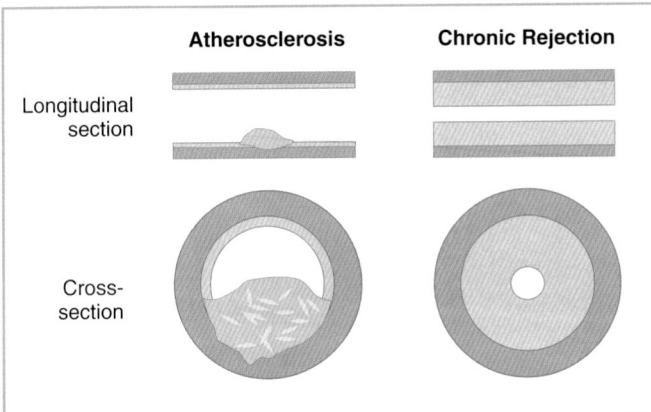

Figure 7-15. Comparison between coronary artery atherosclerosis and chronic graft rejection.

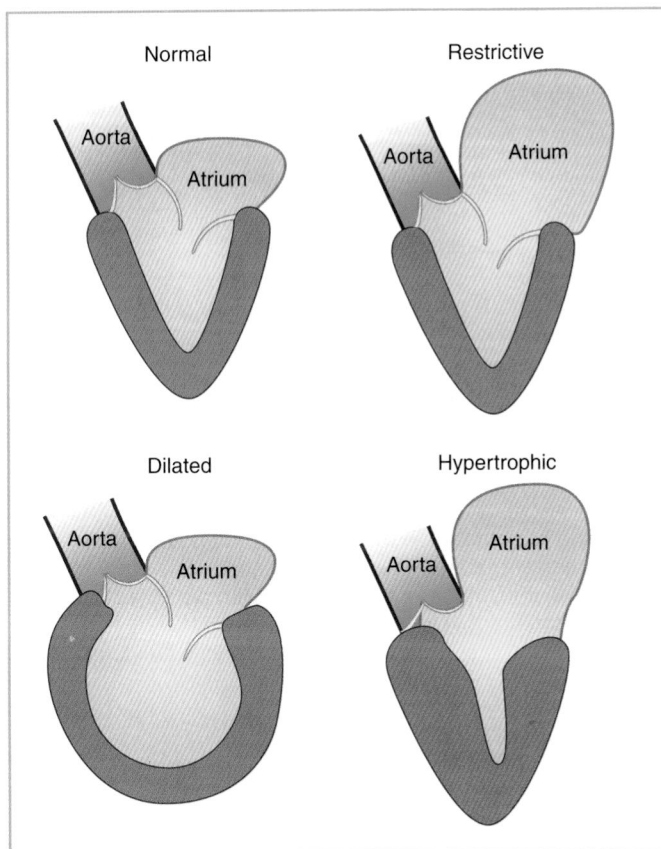

Figure 7-16. Cardiomyopathy.

Toxin exposure including heavy ethanol exposure and excess catecholamines also can produce dilated cardiomyopathy. Because of diagnostic limitations during life, a significant proportion of patients with a clinical diagnosis of dilated cardiomyopathy actually have chronic ischemic heart disease, which is much more prevalent than cardiomyopathy. Multiple small infarcts can produce a diffuse pattern of myocardial thinning that closely simulates dilated cardiomyopathy on two-dimensional echocardiography.

Restrictive Cardiomyopathy

Amyloidosis is the prototypical cause of restrictive cardiomyopathy in which there is deposition of abnormal protein with a β-pleated sheet conformation in the interstitium of the myocardium (see Figs. 7-17C and D). This interstitial material increases the stiffness (rigidity) of the wall and results in decreased compliance with impaired diastolic filling. Patients tend to have signs of right heart disease because of the backup of pressure into the pulmonary circulation. Systolic dysfunction increases as more and more amyloid is deposited in the interstitium. Other processes that result in the accumulation of interstitial or subendocardial connective tissue can also produce restrictive cardiomyopathy.

●●● RHEUMATIC HEART DISEASE

Rheumatic heart disease is caused by an abnormal host immune response (usually occurring in adolescents) to an infection with β-hemolytic group A streptococci.

The attack rate of myocarditis following such an infection (typically pharyngitis, i.e., "strep throat") is 1% to 3% and is dependent on HLA type, with strong HLA-DR2 and -DR4 linkage in the United States. Heart disease develops long after the infection has cleared (lesions are microbiologically sterile) (Fig. 7-18). Termination of the bacterial infection by antibiotic therapy prevents the development of myocarditis and has largely resulted in the eradication of this disease in the United States. Rheumatic heart disease remains an important cause of morbidity and mortality in the developing world, however.

The precise pathophysiology of rheumatic heart disease remains controversial. It is probably best understood as a transient autoimmune state. There is cross-reactivity between some myocardial and connective tissue proteins and bacterial antigenic determinants, but immunocomplexes do not appear to play a pivotal role in rheumatic heart disease (in contrast to poststreptococcal glomerulonephritis, which is caused by different bacterial serotypes with deposition of immuno-complexes in the glomeruli). The cellular infiltrate in rheumatic myocarditis is composed almost exclusively of helper T cells, and the identification of streptococcal M protein as a super-antigen (which results in the global activation of a subset of T lymphocytes expressing the Vβ-8 subclass of T-cell receptor) supports a cell-mediated autoimmune mechanism.

Rheumatic myocarditis develops 4 weeks after bacterial infection and begins with fibrinoid necrosis of collagen associated with a T-cell inflammatory infiltrate. This develops into the morphologically diagnostic lesion of rheumatic heart disease called an Aschoff body, which is composed of multinucleated histiocytes with unique nuclear features (dense striated chromatin bar surrounded by a zone of nuclear clearing). These myocardial lesions heal as small scars with minimal sequelae. In contrast, inflammation of the cardiac valves with verrucae composed of degenerating connective tissue and inflammatory cells has severe sequelae.

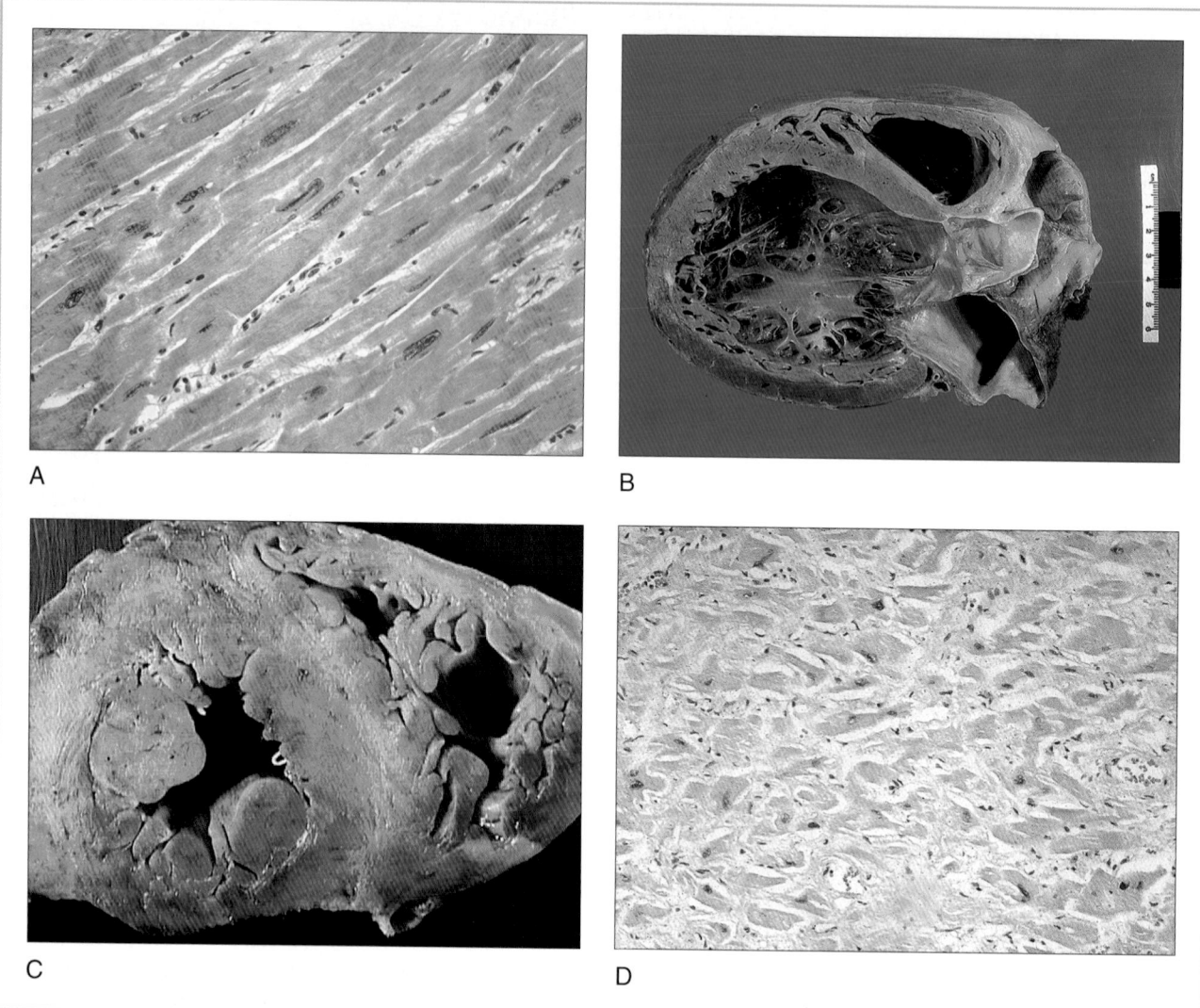

Figure 7-17. **A**, Hypertrophic cardiomyopathy. Microscopic section showing hypertrophied myocytes with marked nuclear enlargement (polyploid nuclei) and increased fiber diameter. **B**, Dilated cardiomyopathy. Gross coronal section showing marked dilatation of the left ventricle and aortic valve ring resulting in significant valvular insufficiency in a patient with alcoholic cardiomyopathy. **C**, Restrictive cardiomyopathy. Gross cross-section showing a massively thickened left ventricle that has a waxy appearance owing to amyloid deposition. **D**, Restrictive cardiomyopathy. Microscopic section showing interstitial amyloid deposition that has caused pressure atrophy of myocytes.

Verrucae form along the lines of valve closure (Fig. 7-19A) and result in neovascularization and scarring of the valve, often with fusion of the valve leaflets and severe stenosis. The mitral valve is most commonly affected, with only rare involvement of the right heart valves. Subsequent attacks of rheumatic fever (after recurrent streptococcal infection) tend to be more severe and cause progressive valvular disease (see Fig. 7-19B). Rheumatic heart disease can also result in self-limited involvement of other tissues, which produces signs and symptoms useful in establishing a diagnosis of rheumatic fever.

●●● VALVULAR HEART DISEASE

Because heart valves lack a vasculature and lymphatics their ability to respond to inflammation or infection is very limited.

Endothelial injury predisposes to the deposition of fibrin on the valve surface, which can serve as a nidus for bacterial infection. Congenital and acquired abnormalities of valves result in abnormal, turbulent flow that causes endothelial injury. Therefore, individuals with abnormal heart valves are at increased risk for developing bacterial endocarditis if they experience bacteremia. Prophylaxis with antibiotics for dental procedures in susceptible individuals can substantially reduce this risk.

Bacterial Endocarditis

Bacterial endocarditis acute or subacute depending on the organism involved. *Staphylococcus aureus* is the prototypical agent of acute endocarditis, resulting in rapid destruction of the valve substance and severe valvular insufficiency.

Regurgitation through damaged valves can produce diagnostic murmurs, and vegetations can be diagnosed by two-dimensional echocardiography. *Streptococcus viridans* is the prototypical organism of subacute bacterial endocarditis. Subacute endocarditis is associated with large vegetations on the valve surface (composed of fibrin, inflammatory cells, and bacteria) with slower destruction of the valve (Fig. 7-20). Septic emboli from these vegetations and autoimmune phenomena related to antigen-antibody complexes tend to dominate the clinical picture of subacute endocarditis, with valvular insufficiency occurring late.

Congenitally abnormal valves and valves previously scarred by rheumatic endocarditis are at markedly increased risk for the development of bacterial endocarditis. The left-sided heart valves are more commonly involved than the right except in intravenous drug abusers, in whom direct seeding of the right-sided heart valves may occur. In immunocompromised patients, fungal organisms may be a significant cause of endocarditis as well as unusual types of bacteria.

MICROBIOLOGY

Group A Streptococci

Group A streptococci are gram-positive bacteria that are usually seen in chains on gram staining. They can cause pharyngitis and skin or soft tissue infections (erysipelas or fasciitis) in immunocompetent individuals. Different serotypes are associated with rheumatic heart disease and poststreptococcal glomerulonephritis.

Streptococcal M protein can act as a superantigen to promiscuously activate a large number of T cells. M protein can also bind to and cause aggregation of fibrinogen. These macromolecular aggregates can then bind to receptors on platelets, inflammatory cells, and endothelial cells, causing vascular injury that can lead to septic shock.

Calcific Aortic Stenosis

Calcific aortic stenosis occurs in older individuals with dystrophic calcification in the valve substance beginning at the base of valves. Calcification results in the loss of valvular compliance and ultimately in high-grade stenosis of the aortic outflow tract. If a large pressure gradient across the valve is present, marked myocardial hypertrophy results as a compensatory mechanism. As this hypertrophy becomes severe, the risk of sudden death increases, and ultimately there is decompensation with overt heart failure. Calcific aortic stenosis is significantly more common in congenitally bicuspid aortic valves, which account for approximately half of aortic valve replacement surgeries.

Mitral Valve Prolapse

Mitral valve prolapse (MVP) is a relatively common condition (around 2.5% of the population) and is associated with degeneration of connective tissue (myxoid degeneration) within the valve substance. Mitral valve prolapse is almost universally present in Marfan syndrome owing to point mutations in the fibrillin gene that result in defective deposition of elastin within the valve substance. The valve and chordae become progressively elongated and balloon into the atrium during diastole. This abnormal valve motion is a risk factor for the development of bacterial endocarditis. Significant mitral regurgitation develops in a minority of patients with MVP that requires valve replacement.

Prosthetic Heart Valves

Two types of prosthetic heart valves are currently in use. Bioprosthetic valves are composed of animal valve tissue that is treated with glutaraldehyde and attached to a synthetic valve ring. These bioprosthetic valves cause less hemolysis and require less anticoagulation than metallic mechanical valves (mainly of the tilting disk type). Bioprosthetic valves

Figure 7-18. Chronology of events in rheumatic heart disease.

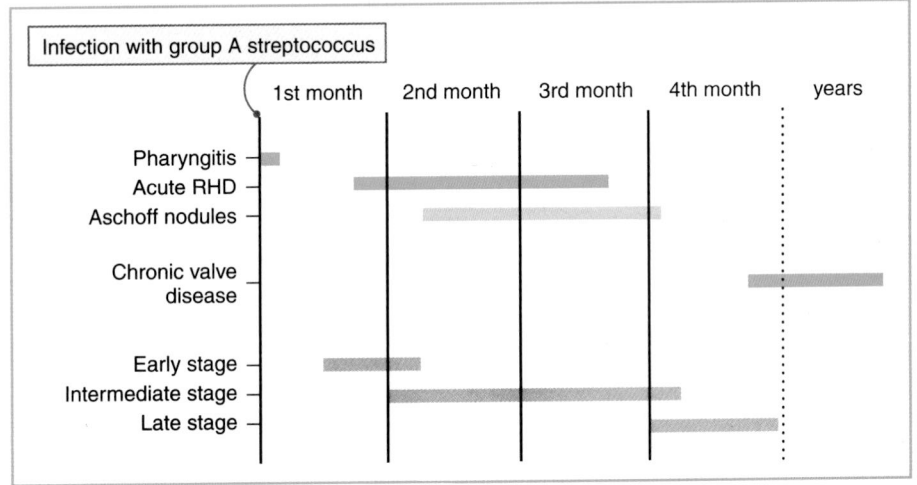

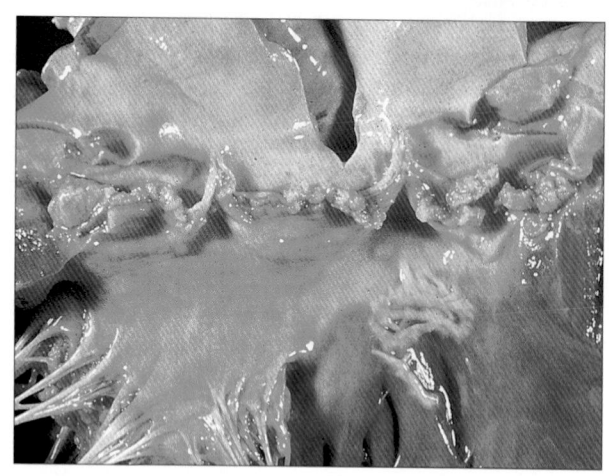

A

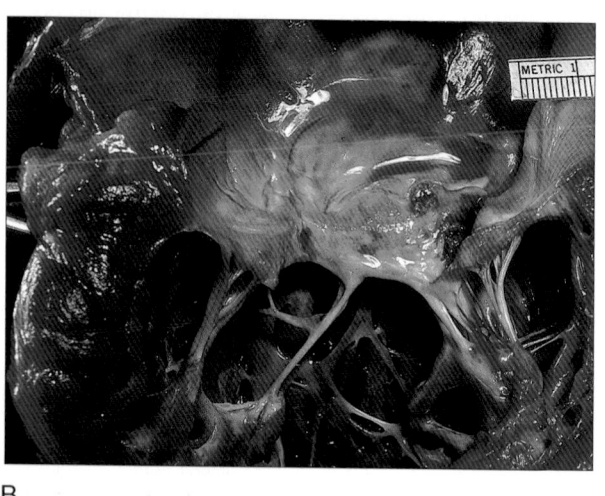

B

Figure 7-19. A, Acute rheumatic endocarditis. Gross photograph of an aortic valve with small vegetations (verrucae) along the lines of valve closure. **B**, Chronic rheumatic endocarditis. Gross photograph of a mitral valve with massive fibrosis and distortion of the leaflets and fusion of the chordae tendineae.

have a 10-year maximum life span, whereas synthetic valves many never require replacement. Both types of valve are associated with an increased risk of bacterial endocarditis.

Valvular Fibrosis

Significant valvular fibrosis has been observed in patients taking large amounts of fenfluramine-phentermine for weight loss. This is apparently a response to the high levels of serotonin induced by this treatment. A subset of these patients also developed severe pulmonary hypertension. The clinical magnitude of valvular disease resulting from this discontinued medication remains to be clarified.

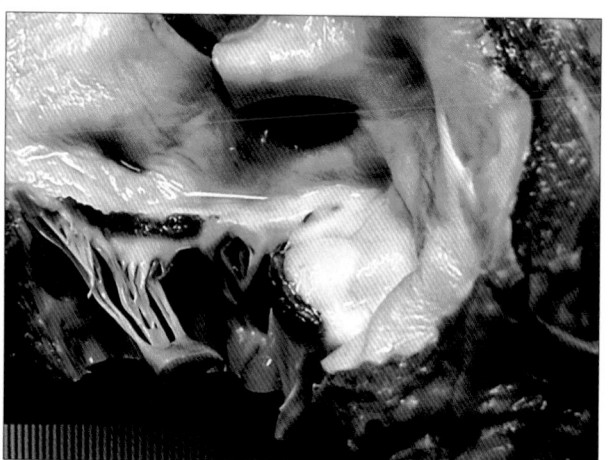

A

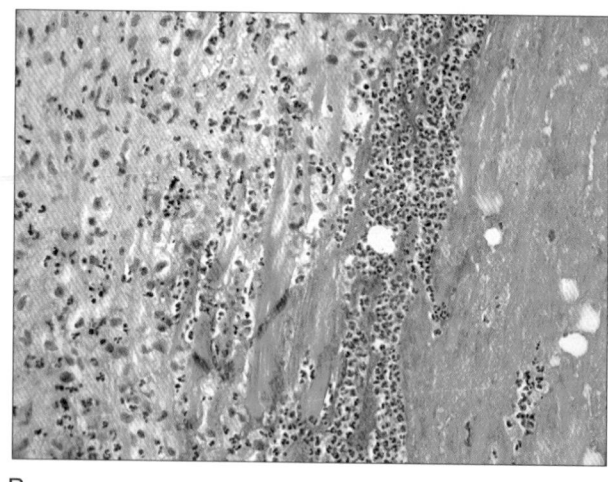

B

Figure 7-20. A, Infectious endocarditis. Gross photograph of a mitral valve with shaggy hyperemic vegetations resulting from bacterial growth, acute inflammation, and neovascularization of the valve substance. **B**, Bacterial endocarditis. Microscopic section showing vegetation with necrosis, acute inflammatory exudate, and numerous bacteria.

●●● PERICARDITIS

The pericardium is a simple structure composed of connective tissue lined by a single layer of mesothelial cells that encases the heart. The mesothelial cells secrete mucopolysaccharide, which lubricates the pericardium, allowing the heart to expand and contract with limited resistance. Fluid accumulations in the pericardium can result in impaired diastolic filling of the ventricles, but the rate at which fluid accumulates is critical. Slow accumulation (e.g., transudate in congestive heart failure) is accommodated by expansion of the pericardium, whereas rapid accumulation (e.g., ruptured myocardial infarct with hemopericardium) results in acute heart failure (tamponade), which usually is fatal.

Inflammation of the pericardium results in a disturbance of normal motion during the cardiac cycle. Deposition of fibrin on the pericardial surface causes severe pain and a characteristic pericardial friction rub that can be heard by auscultation. More severe inflammation and fibrosis due to metastatic cancer or bacterial infection usually results in contraction of the pericardium about the heart, causing impairment of diastolic filling (constrictive pericarditis), which can be life threatening.

●●● CONGENITAL HEART DISEASE

Congenital heart disease is relatively common abnormality occurring in just under 1% of live births. A minority of these cases are associated with specific genetic syndromes (around 10%) while most are isolated abnormalities of unknown cause. Most of these abnormalities are easily understood by reference to the normal embryogenesis of the heart and the transition from fetal to adult circulation at birth.

Prior to birth, oxygenated blood from the placenta flows through the inferior vena cava into the right atrium, and through the foramen ovale into the left atrium and subsequently into the left ventricle and into the systemic circulation (Fig. 7-21).

The ductus arteriosus provides a functional right-to-left shunt preventing excessive blood flow through the lungs prior to birth. The normal foramen ovale is a one-way valve that allows right-to-left blood flow but not left-to-right blood flow. At the time of birth, the foramen ovale is functionally blocked by increased left atrial pressure, and the ductus arteriosus constricts as a result of decreased levels of

prostaglandin E_2. Most types of congenital heart disease involve abnormal communications (shunts) between the right and left circulations. Almost all of these congenital abnormalities are surgically correctable.

Left-to-Right Shunt

Left-to-right shunts do not cause cyanosis at birth but can ultimately result in heart failure because of volume overload. The clinical significance of left-to-right shunts depends largely on their size and the volume of blood flow through them. Left-to-right shunts typically occur as a result of an atrial septal defect (ASD), a ventricular septal defect (VSD), or a patent ductus arteriosus (PDA) (see Fig. 7-21C). ASDs and VSDs result from incomplete septation during embryogenesis. PDA is a functional failure of constriction of the ductus arteriosus due to persistently high PGE_2 levels that can usually be corrected pharmacologically with indomethacin. PDA rarely requires surgical closure, whereas large ASDs and VSDs are surgical lesions.

Right-to-Left Shunt

Right-to-left shunts result in cyanosis at the time of birth and, if severe, will result in perinatal death unless corrected surgically. The most common type of right-to-left shunt is the tetralogy of Fallot, which accounts for up to 6% of congenital heart disease (see Fig. 7-21D). Tetralogy of Fallot corresponds to anatomic stenosis of the pulmonary outflow tract in the right ventricle in combination with a ventricular septal defect. This results in a blockage of flow to the lungs with shunting of poorly oxygenated blood into the left ventricle and the systemic circulation. The other components of tetralogy of Fallot include compensatory changes (e.g., right ventricular hypertrophy) resulting from the obstruction and shunt. Transposition of the great vessels (see Fig. 7-21E) occurs as a consequence of abnormal septation between the aorta and the pulmonary artery with the latter connected to the left ventricle and the former connected to the right ventricle. This abnormality must occur in combination with some type of ASD or VSD to be compatible with extrauterine life.

Coarctation of the Aorta

Coarctation of the aorta is a band-like constriction of the aorta that may occur either superior or inferior to the ductus arteriosus (see Fig. 7-21F). It has consequences similar to aortic valvular stenosis with resulting left ventricular hypertrophy but with diminished pressure in downstream vascular beds.

●●● CARDIOVASCULAR NEOPLASMS
Benign Vascular Neoplasms

Hemangiomas and lymphangiomas are benign tumors of endothelial cells that are often present at birth but rarely

---

EMBRYOLOGY

Cardiac Development

Cardiac development initiates at 12 weeks of gestation with the formation of the primitive truncus arteriosus. The truncus arteriosus loops on itself to create two parallel tubes in the thorax that ultimately form the right and left heart chambers. Septation of the ventricles, atria, and great vessels during embryogenesis transforms the primitive heart tube into a dual circulation with four chambers.

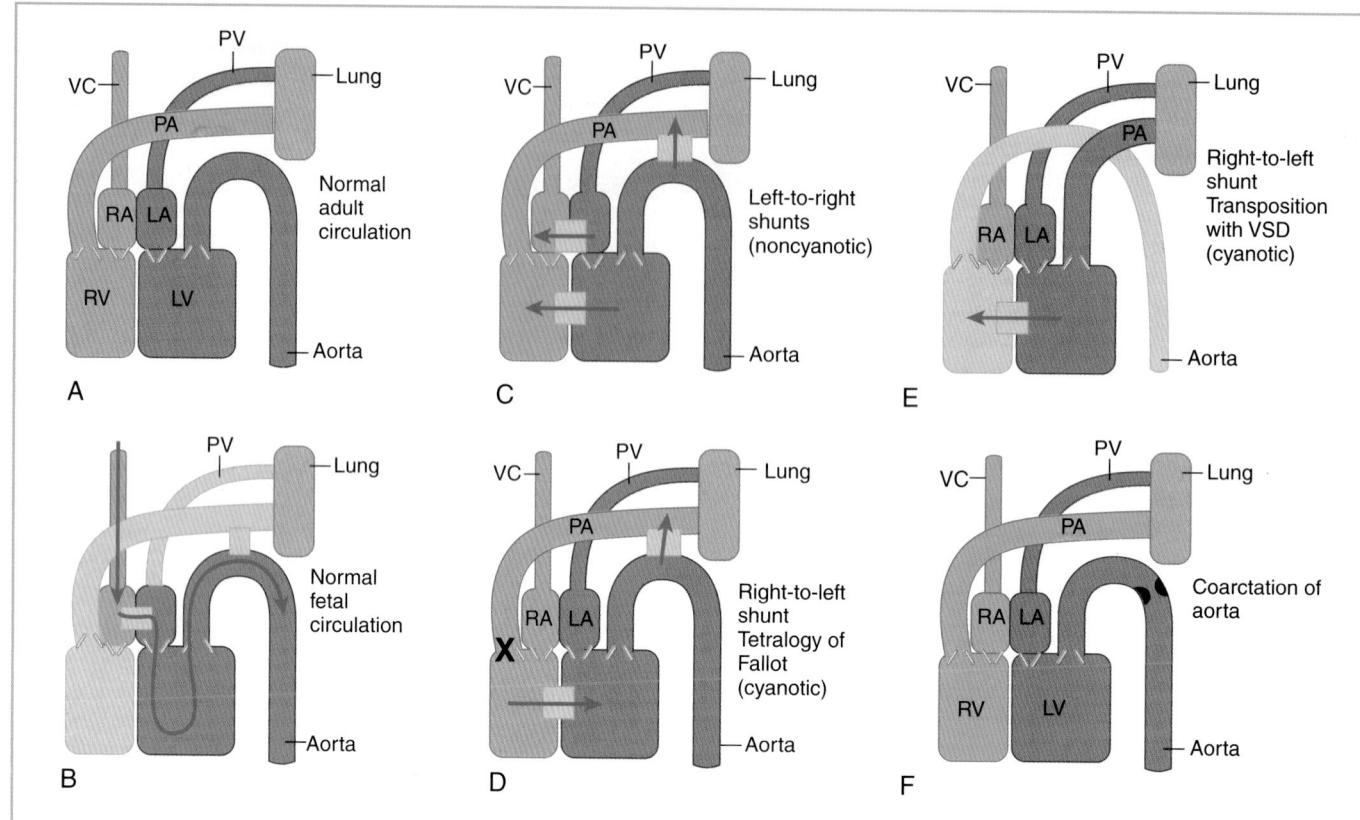

Figure 7-21. Congenital heart disease **A**, Normal adult circulation. **B**, Normal fetal circulation. **C**, Left-to-right shunts (noncyanotic heart disease). **D** and **E**, Right-to left-shunts (cyanotic heart disease). **F**, Coarctation of the aorta.

cause significant clinical problems. They may impinge on other structures, causing deformity or hemorrhage. Some are associated with genetic and chromosomal syndromes.

Angiosarcoma

Angiosarcoma is a highly malignant tumor of endothelial cells. Well-differentiated angiosarcoma retains obvious vascular morphology while poorly differentiated tumors may present as undifferentiated sarcomas (Fig. 7-22A). Angiosarcomas are often metastatic at presentation, and some are associated with prior chemical exposure. *Hemangioendotheliomas* are similar to angiosarcomas but are less malignant and tend to behave as locally aggressive neoplasms.

Kaposi Sarcoma

Kaposi sarcoma is an unusual vascular neoplasm that forms abnormal, slit-like vascular spaces containing compressed red cells (see Fig. 7-22B). Kaposi sarcoma was long recognized as an indolent tumor occurring on the lower extremities of elderly men of eastern Mediterranean origin. In contrast, AIDS-associated Kaposi sarcoma is an aggressive neoplasm that can metastasize and cause life-threatening hemorrhage. Both forms of Kaposi sarcoma are associated with infection by human herpesvirus 8 (HHV-8), which encodes cytokine-like proteins that apparently create autocrine feedback loops

that drive the abnormal proliferation of endothelial cells. Kaposi sarcoma can also develop in patients treated with immunosuppression for solid organ transplants. In this setting, lesions usually regress if immunosuppression is reversed.

Bacillary Angiomatosis

Bacillary angiomatosis can present with morphology similar to that of Kaposi sarcoma but is usually accompanied by a dense neutrophilic infiltrate. Bacillary angiomatosis is a direct result of bacterial infection with *Bartonella* species and is observed only in the setting of severe immunodeficiency. It responds to antibiotic therapy with eradication of vascular lesions.

Cardiac Neoplasms

Primary tumors of the heart are rare. Myxoma is the most common, typically involving the atrium as a ball-like mass tethered to the wall by a stalk. These tumors are composed of myxoid ground substance with scattered, stellate mesenchymal myxoma cells (see Fig. 7-22C). Although benign, they can result in mechanical damage to heart valves; transient blockage of ventricular filling, causing syncope; and systemic tumor emboli. Some cases are genetic. Rhabdomyomas are hamartomatous lesions of cardiac myocytes that form gray-white mass lesions in patients with tuberous sclerosis. Metastatic carcinoma to the heart is not uncommon in advanced cancer but is rarely clinically significant. In contrast, metastasis to the

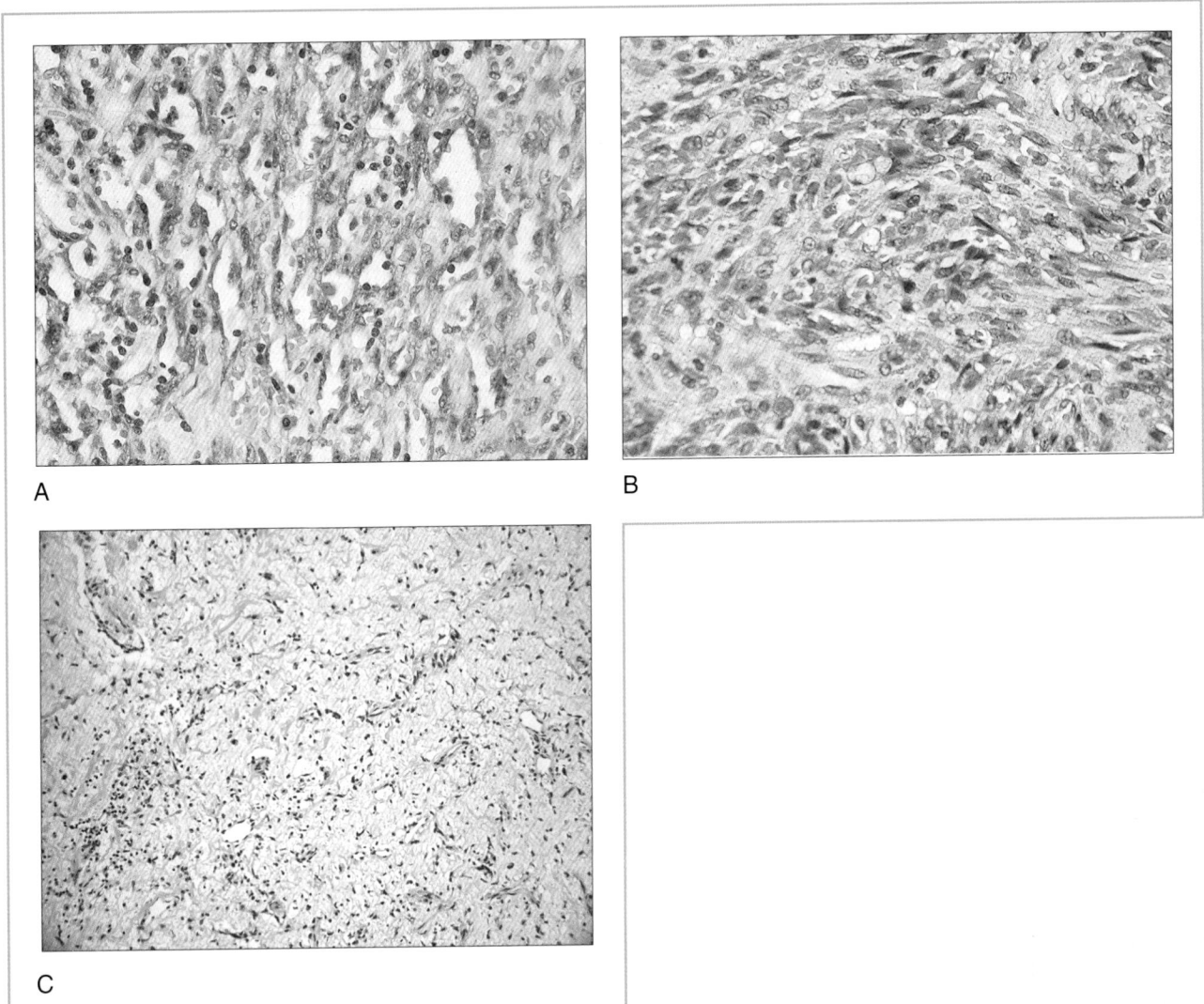

Figure 7-22. A, Angiosarcoma. Microscopic section showing pleomorphic tumor cells forming haphazard vascular spaces. **B**, Kaposi sarcoma. Microscopic section showing neoplastic spindle cells forming slit-like vascular spaces containing compressed (distorted) red blood cells. Tumor cells show moderate cytologic atypia in this aggressive lesion from a patient with advanced AIDS. **C**, Atrial myxoma. Microscopic section showing prominent myxoid stroma with scattered bland, stellate tumor

pericardium usually causes symptomatic constrictive pericarditis (see above).

●●● OTHER CONDITIONS

Lymphedema results from inadequate lymphatic drainage of an extremity. This can be secondary to congenital deficiency of lymphatic vessels, parasitic disease, or scarring, or it can be iatrogenic (e.g., secondary to axillary lymph node dissection for breast cancer). Varicosities of veins result from fibrosis of the vein wall associated with loss of normal valvular function and pooling of blood in lower extremities. Venous stasis predisposes to thrombosis, which is of particular clinical significance in the deep veins of the leg, where deep venous thrombosis is the main cause of life-threatening pulmonary emboli. Venous thrombi are excellent culture media for bacteria and can result in septic thrombophlebitis. Arteriovenous malformations (AVMs) are abnormal communications between the arterial and venous circulations that usually are dysmorphic and prone to bleeding or thrombosis. Mucosal or central nervous system AVMs can be life threatening. More rarely, AVMs may be large enough to cause significant left-to-right shunts. Some types of AVM are associated with genetic diseases and may suggest the diagnosis. Raynaud's disease is a symptom complex in which vasoconstriction occurs with subsequent pain and bluish discoloration of the fingers. In its most severe forms, it may be associated with digital infarction.

Respiratory Tract and Pleura 8

CONTENTS

Normal lung function depends on efficient gas exchange between the capillary network in alveolar septae and gases in the alveolar spaces. Gas exchange is compromised if fluid accumulates in alveolar spaces or if there is an increased amount of connective tissue in alveolar septae. In different pathologic conditions, impaired gas exchange may affect either oxygenation or removal of CO_2 more severely. Normal lung compliance (the stiffness of lung tissue) is important for normal pulmonary function. If lung tissue is abnormally stiff (as a result of fibrosis), the work of breathing increases markedly so that individuals may not be able to adequately oxygenate or remove carbon dioxide. Lung compliance can also be affected by intra-alveolar fluid accumulations or loss of surfactant (either can increase surface tension and increase the work of breathing). The same pathologic processes often affect both gas exchange and lung compliance. Loss of lung parenchyma (e.g., in emphysema) has a direct impact on the amount of surface area available for gas exchange but also reduces radial tension on airways that normally helps keep them patent during expiration. Premature collapse of these airways during expiration causes air trapping and can greatly reduce effective gas exchange (the dead space is larger). Because of these interactions, some relatively mild pathologic changes can result in significant pulmonary function abnormalities.

Since the lung communicates directly with the external environment, host defense mechanisms are essential to maintain normal pulmonary function and resist infection. Bronchi and bronchioles are lined by a ciliated columnar epithelium with interspersed goblet cells that secrete mucin. The cilia on the surface of these cells beat rhythmically, causing the directional movement of the mucin outward to the trachea, where it can be expectorated. Bacteria and particulates that make contact with the mucociliary blanket are effectively cleared from the lung. Individuals with genetic abnormalities of cilia and cigarette smokers have defective mucociliary blanket function and are at increased risk for infection. Particles that are small enough to reach the alveoli (beyond the mucociliary blanket) may not be effectively cleared from the lung. The size of particulate air pollutants and aerosolized infectious agents is a key factor in determining whether they reach alveoli to cause disease or infection. The normal gag reflex is also an important host defense mechanism that prevents aspiration of oral contents into the lower respiratory tract. Individuals with a deficient gag reflex (e.g., chronic alcoholics) are at risk for aspiration of oral secretions, which contain numerous microorganisms. Inherited and acquired immunodeficiency syndromes are significant risk factors for pulmonary infection.

●●● PULMONARY EDEMA

Pulmonary edema can result from abnormalities in the cardiovascular system that increase pulmonary arterial or venous pressure. High pressure in the pulmonary circulation favors the net movement of water into lung tissue. Since the volume of the lung interstitium is minimal, transudates rapidly move into alveolar spaces. Accumulation of a significant amount of fluid in alveolar spaces increases the work of breathing and blocks effective gas exchange. The amount of plasma proteins carried across with water in edema fluid is an index of the severity of the pulmonary edema. In severe cases, dense pink, frothy proteinaceous material is visible in alveolar spaces in tissue sections (Fig. 8-1A). Lungs with pulmonary edema are markedly increased in weight, and their cut surface appears frothy and exudes fluid. Long-standing pulmonary edema in patients with congestive heart failure results in microhemorrhages into alveoli. Red cells are ingested by macrophages and iron derived from hemoglobin

is converted to hemosiderin, which is only slowly cleared from alveoli. Inflammation associated with the small hemorrhages causes incremental fibrosis in alveolar septae, and chronic pulmonary edema can result in significant interstitial pulmonary fibrosis. Hemosiderin-containing alveolar macrophages are excellent markers of chronic congestive heart failure (so-called heart failure cells) but can also result from other types of pulmonary hemorrhage (see Fig. 8-1B). Edema fluid can also collect in the pleural spaces (i.e., pleural effusion), resulting in progressive collapse of the lungs and diminished gas exchange.

●●● DIFFUSE ALVEOLAR DAMAGE

Diffuse alveolar damage (DAD) is a stereotyped response to injury in lung tissue. DAD consists of an intra-alveolar exudate (often described as hyaline membrane) in association with marked hyperplasia of type II pneumocytes that may appear cytologically bizarre and pleomorphic (Fig. 8-2). Hyaline membranes consist of a mixture of proteinaceous exudate, surfactant from type II pneumocytes, and cellular debris. Diffuse alveolar damage can progress to organizing pneumonia (granulation tissue organizes the exudate), which may result in permanent pulmonary fibrosis or resolve with the restoration of normal lung architecture and function. The outcome depends on host factors, the severity of lung injury, and whether or not the inciting cause of DAD is corrected. Many different types of injury can produce diffuse alveolar damage including shock, some types of infection, chemotherapeutic agents, irradiation, and oxygen toxicity. Free radical damage from high levels of oxygen often required in an ICU setting is common cause of DAD in severely ill, hospitalized patients.

●●● PNEUMONIA

Pneumonia usually means an inflammatory process within the alveolar spaces and often implies an infectious etiology (e.g., bacteria, *Mycoplasma*, or viruses). The term pneumonitis is typically used for inflammatory diseases of lung tissue that result in significant interstitial inflammation and fibrosis and are immune mediated.

Viral Pneumonia

Many different types of viruses can produce pneumonia, but some viruses are more commonly associated with clinical pneumonia than others. Influenzavirus typically results in moderate to severe pulmonary involvement with a predominantly lymphoid infiltrate and exudation of proteinaceous fluid into alveolar spaces. Emerging agents of viral pneumonia include the so-called severe acute respiratory syndrome (SARS). SARS can rapidly produce a DAD-like pattern of injury that may result in death or permanent lung dysfunction.

Most forms of viral pneumonia do not cause death by themselves but can significantly predispose to the development of bacterial pneumonia, particularly in elderly patients

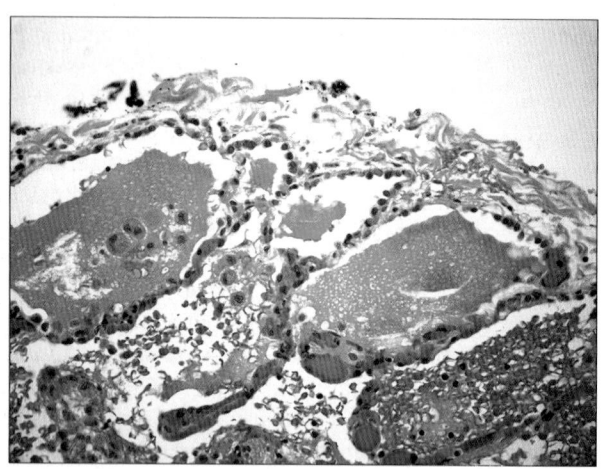

A

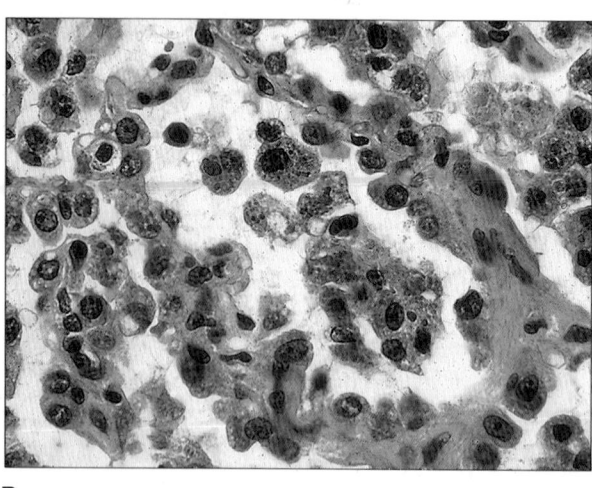

B

Figure 8-1. A, Pulmonary edema. Microscopic section of lung tissue showing dense eosinophilic proteinaceous material filling alveolar spaces. A few hemosiderin-containing macrophages are present. **B,** Pulmonary hemosiderosis. Microscopic section of lung tissue with numerous hemosiderin-containing macrophages from a patient with long-standing congestive heart failure.

or in patients with comorbid diseases such as congestive heart failure. Diminished lung function with protein-rich fluid in alveolar spaces strongly predisposes to colonization and infection by bacterial organisms present in the normal flora or in the environment. Some types of viruses tend to produce pneumonia only in immunocompromised hosts or neonates (e.g., cytomegalovirus [CMV]) but can produce a life-threatening pneumonia in these susceptible individuals.

Bacterial Pneumonia

Bacterial pneumonia can occur as a primary infection of the lungs or as a complication of sepsis. The former is more common in the outpatient setting. *Streptococcus pneumoniae* is the prototypic organism of community-acquired pneumonia. *S. pneumoniae* is spread by airborne droplets and has a well-formed capsule that resists phagocytosis by innate immune cells. *S. pneumoniae* tends to produce a bronchopneumonia in which intra-alveolar exudate is centered around bronchi and bronchioles that have been inoculated with bacteria. Individuals without functional spleens are at substantially higher risk for developing life-threatening sepsis during *S. pneumoniae* infection (the spleen can normally remove the small number of organisms circulating in the bloodstream in patients with pneumonia to prevent generalized infection).

Untreated bacterial pneumonia progresses through several morphologic stages of development, but these classical pathologic findings are now only rarely observed because of intercurrent antibiotic therapy. The inflammatory response to bacteria results in acute inflammatory exudate filling alveolar spaces. Inflammation progresses through a stage of "gray hepatization" with organization of the intra-alveolar exudate. The cut surface of involved lungs has nodular pattern of consolidation (solid areas in which alveoli are filled with acute inflammatory exudate) (Fig. 8-3A). If untreated, bronchopneumonia may progress to diffuse involvement of the entire lung lobe (lobar pneumonia; see Fig. 8-3B). The severity of acute respiratory compromise depends on the volume of lung tissue affected. If the patient survives, effective humoral and cellular immunity eventually clears the infection. Areas of consolidation progress to "red hepatization" because of hemorrhage that typically occurs during the organization of the intra-alveolar exudate. Usually, there is complete resolution with the restoration of normal lung architecture. Pneumonia in hospitalized patients treated with

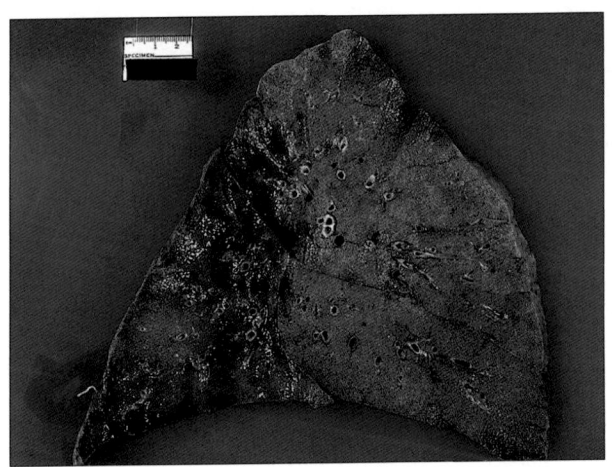

A

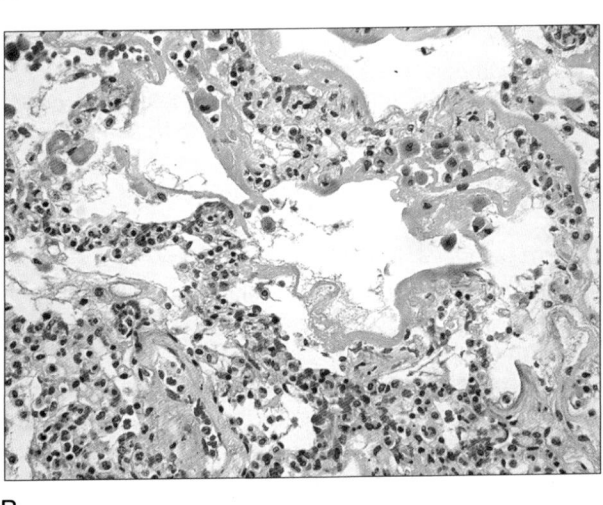

B

Figure 8-2. **A,** Adult respiratory distress syndrome. Gross cross-section of the lower lobe of the lung showing diffuse consolidation and hemorrhage. **B,** Adult respiratory distress syndrome. Microscopic section of lung tissue showing prominent hyaline membranes (eosinophilic exudate composed of fibrin and cellular debris) lining alveolar spaces. Scattered inflammatory cells are present.

MICROBIOLOGY

Severe Acute Respiratory Syndrome (SARS)

SARS was first recognized in late 2002 as a life-threatening respiratory disease in Guandong, China, with subsequent cases identified in Hong Kong and Canada, apparently as a result of transmission by airline passengers.

The SARS virus was initially cultured at the Centers for Disease Control and Prevention (CDC), and broad-spectrum RT-PCR primers homologous to the coronavirus polymerase gene were found to amplify viral RNA from patient samples. These PCR products showed a unique coding sequence that is most closely related to type II coronaviruses (approximately 60% sequence conservation). Serologic assays were subsequently developed for SARS.

Coronaviruses are enveloped RNA viruses with helical symmetry that are usually spread from person to person via aerosol and usually produce a common cold–like illness. The SARS coronavirus measures 80 to 140 nm in diameter by electron microscopy and has 20- to 40-nm complex surface projections at its periphery. Public health measures effectively contained the initial outbreak of this highly virulent new human pathogen.

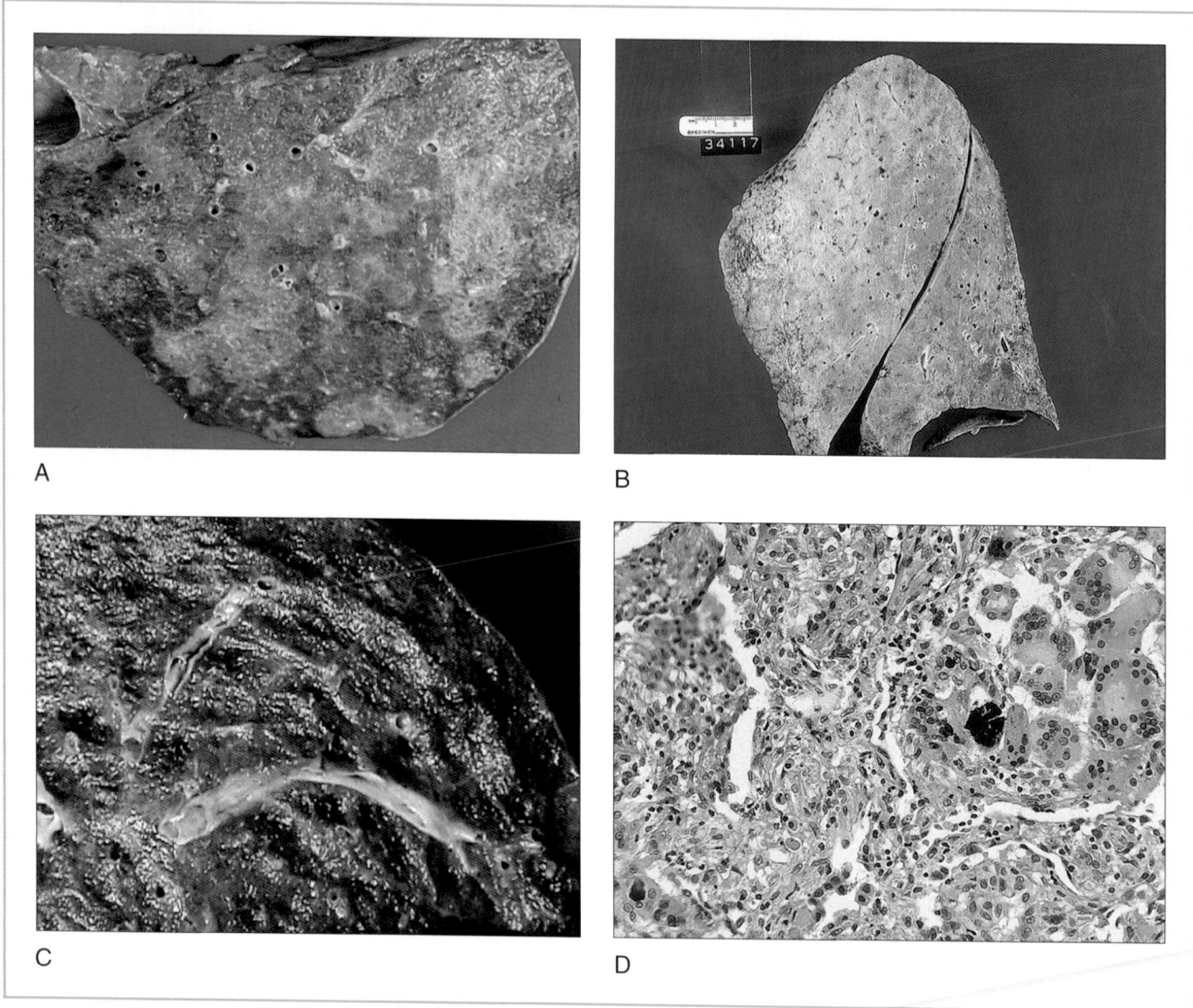

Figure 8-3. A, Bronchopneumonia. Gross cross-section of fixed lung tissue showing peribronchial consolidation. Consolidated areas appear slightly whiter and denser than aerated lung tissue. **B,** Lobar pneumonia. Gross cross-section of lung tissue showing diffuse consolidation of the entire lobe. **C,** Aspiration pneumonia. Gross cross-section of lung tissue showing focal early abscess formation in evolving aspiration pneumonia. **D,** Aspiration pneumonia. Microscopic section of lung tissue showing foreign body material with associated multinucleated giant cells and acute inflammatory exudate.

multiple antibiotics shows some of the pathologic changes described above but often has a DAD-like pattern resulting from combined infectious, immune, and oxygen free radical–mediated injury.

Pneumonia caused by more destructive bacteria, such as *Staphylococcus aureus,* tends to destroy the extracellular matrix supporting lung parenchyma, precluding the restoration of fully normal lung architecture and function. Lung abscess is a relatively common complication of Staphylococcal pneumonia.

Legionnaires' Disease

Legionella pneumophila is the causative agent of legionnaires' disease, which is an uncommon but potentially serious pneumonia, occurring predominantly in older individuals with comorbid disease. *Legionella* is named for a disease outbreak that occurred in association with an American Legion con-

vention. *Legionella* is a free-living organism that grows in water supplies of rooftop air-conditioning units. Large numbers of bacteria can be aerosolized from contaminated water, resulting in epidemic infections, usually in urban settings.

The incidence of legionnaires' disease has greatly diminished because of effective public health measures including environmental monitoring of cooling units. *Legionella* can cause pneumonia in normal individuals but is more likely to produce disease in persons with compromised lung function (e.g., chronic obstructive pulmonary disease or congestive heart failure).

Atypical Pneumonia

Mycoplasma pneumoniae is a prokaryote lacking a cell wall that causes so-called atypical pneumonia in immunocompetent hosts. *M. pneumoniae* is typically self-limited but may rarely be associated with complications, such as thrombotic thrombocytopenia purpura (see Chapter 11).

Aspiration Pneumonia

Aspiration pneumonia is usually caused by the aspiration of gastric contents that introduces bacteria and foreign material (including gastric acid) into alveolar spaces (see Figs. 8-3C and 8-3D). Acid causes direct injury to pneumocytes and disrupts normal host defenses, facilitating bacterial growth. The presence of foreign material also interferes with effective innate and acquired immunity so that most patients who aspirate will develop bacterial infection. Aspiration pneumonia is often polymicrobial, and gram-negative enteric organisms are common pathogens. These infections tend to be quite destructive (similarly to staphylococcal pneumonia) and frequently progress to lung abscess. Aspiration pneumonia is much more common in debilitated patients and in alcoholics with a diminished gag reflex. Aspiration of other materials such as barium in the setting of radiographic procedures or meconium during a complicated delivery can also cause a severe inflammatory reaction that irreversibly damages lung tissue.

Lung Abscess

Lung abscess is usually a complication of pneumonia with aggressive organisms such as *S. aureus* or gram-negative enteric organisms. Aspiration of foreign material also favors lung abscess formation. Hydrolytic enzymes released from bacteria and neutrophils digest the extracellular matrix in alveolar septae to form an abscess cavity within lung tissue (Fig. 8-4). Rupture of an abscess cavity into the pleural space can cause empyema (see below). Host immune responses are usually incapable of eradicating the infection unless the abscess cavity is drained (the abscess is an anaerobic environment in which inflammatory cells are minimally effective in killing bacteria).

Bronchiectasis

Bronchiectasis means the presence of abnormally large bronchi at the periphery of lung. Large bronchi are seen to extend to the pleural surface in cross-sections of lung tissue. Bronchiectasis usually results from repeated cycles of pulmonary infection during childhood. Repeated injury results in the loss of normal parenchyma and in the creation of abnormal, ectatic airspaces that then undergo bronchial metaplasia. The peripheral location and abnormal architecture of these air spaces results in impaired clearance of secretions, causing mucus plugging and new cycles of infection. Bronchiectasis is typical in patients with cystic fibrosis in which inspissated mucus causes bronchial obstruction and predisposes to infection and destruction of normal bronchial architecture. Bronchiectasis is a risk factor for pneumothorax and predisposes to empyema if pneumonia develops.

MICROBIOLOGY

Legionella pneumophila

Legionella is a free-living gram-negative bacillus (2–20 μm) that resides in surface and drinking water and can cause pulmonary infection if aerosolized. *L. pneumophila* is the usual agent of legionnaires' disease, but any of the 39 species of *Legionella* can cause human disease.

L. pneumophila is a facultative intracellular parasite that proliferates in alveolar macrophages and induces a marked acute inflammatory response to produce a destructive pneumonia that responds to erythromycin (legionnaires' disease). A less common clinical syndrome (Pontiac fever) caused by *L. pneumophila* produces a self-limited, influenza-like illness.

Effective host defense is largely cell mediated, and activated macrophages can kill or contain bacteria. Individuals with compromised adaptive or innate immunity are at increased risk for disease. Infection can be confirmed by culture on specialized agar plates. Decontamination of contaminated water that may be aerosolized (i.e., rooftop air-conditioning units) has reduced the frequency of human infection.

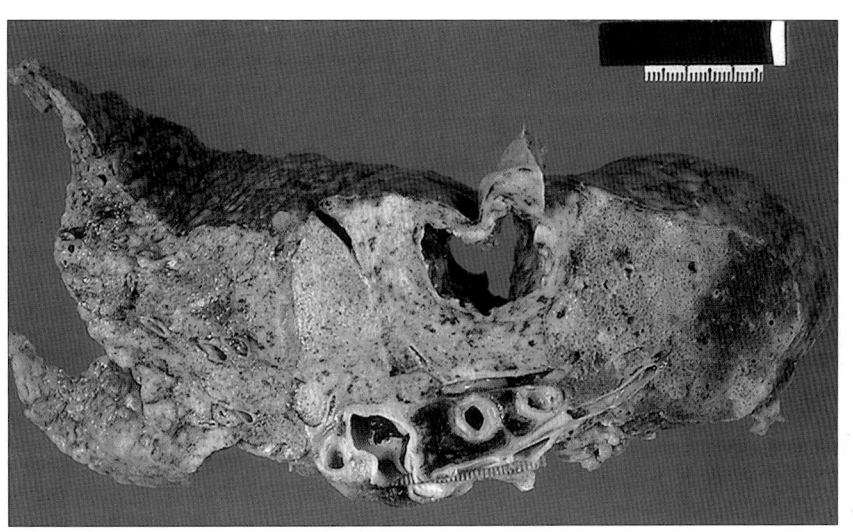

Figure 8-4. Lung abscess. Gross cross-section of lung tissue with a large abscess cavity. Surrounding lung tissue is fibrotic.

Mycobacterial Infections

Infection with *Mycobacterium tuberculosis* usually occurs through the respiratory tract. Patients with active tuberculosis can expectorate fomites (small particulates with viable bacteria), which can be inhaled by individuals in their close environment. If these fomites are small enough to reach beyond the mucociliary blanket, tuberculous infection may be initiated. Innate immune responses mediated by neutrophils are not effective in killing *M. tuberculosis*, which has a remarkably resistant cell wall. These organisms divide slowly but can grow effectively as intracellular pathogens after ingestion by macrophages. Effective killing of *M. tuberculosis* requires the initiation of a granulomatous inflammatory response in which stimulation of macrophages with IFN-γ (produced by T_H2 T cells) induces the formation of epithelioid histiocytes that have enhanced bactericidal

capacity. In many cases, activated histiocytes may successfully contain a mycobacterial infection but may not effectively kill all microorganisms. Viable mycobacteria may persist as intracellular parasites for many years. Compromise of the immune system (e.g., cancer, nutritional deficiency, and immunosuppressive therapy) can then permit reactivation of tuberculous infection.

Most individuals who develop primary pulmonary infection with *M. tuberculosis* have the so-called Ghon complex consisting of granulomatous lesions in lung tissue in conjunction with granulomas in draining hilar lymph nodes (Fig. 8-5A). If the organisms are contained at this stage, granulomas become fibrotic and undergo dystrophic calcification over the course of years. A Ghon complex is often visible on routine chest radiography because of these calcifications. If the host immune response in not sufficient to contain the mycobacteria, persistent active lung infection

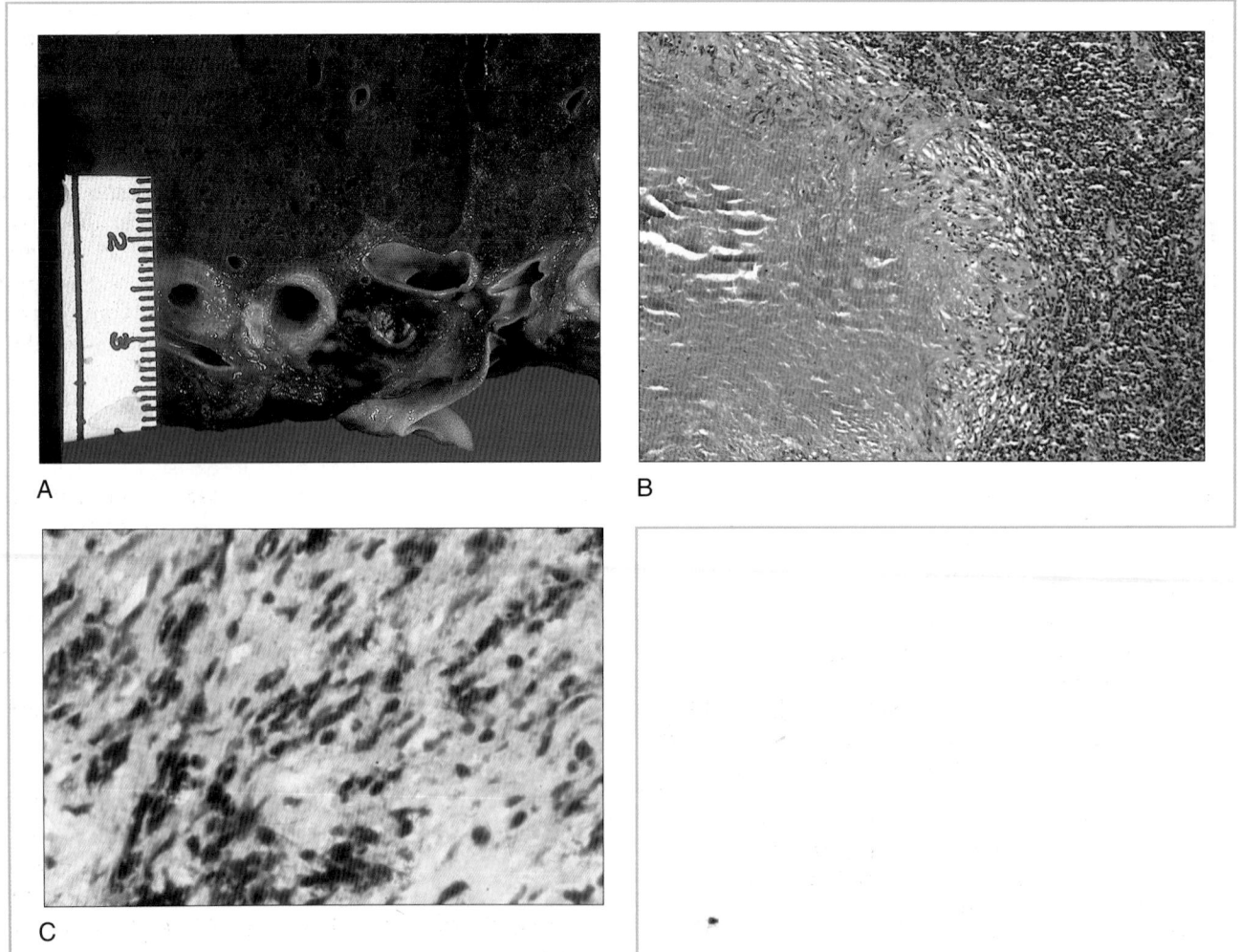

A

B

C

Figure 8-5. A, Calcified granuloma. Gross cross-section from lung hilum showing a calcified granuloma in an anthracotic (black) lymph node. Cross-sectioned bronchi are also visible. **B,** Necrotizing granuloma. Microscopic section of lung tissue showing a granuloma with central necrosis and palisading histiocytes about its periphery. **C,** Atypical mycobacterial infection. Microscopic section stained with Ziehl-Neelsen stain revealing large numbers of mycobacteria and histiocytes (red, rod-shaped organisms).

may produce cavitation (essentially an abscess with numerous mycobacteria present). Tuberculosis preferentially involves the apices of lungs, possibly because of the higher O_2 tension at this location.

In individuals with weakened immune systems, initial infection with *M. tuberculosis* can progress to a disseminated infection with involvement of many different organs (see Fig. 8-5B). Reactivation of latent infection in immunocompromised patients often results in a pattern of miliary tuberculosis in which innumerable small foci of infection develop within lung parenchyma and other organs. These miliary lesions consist of discrete masses of mycobacteria with associated histiocytes. The emergence of multiple drug–resistant *M. tuberculosis* poses a significant therapeutic challenge, and the spread of these organisms in patients with AIDS is an ongoing public health problem.

Atypical mycobacteria (all mycobacterial species aside from *M. tuberculosis*) produce a different pattern of lung disease.

Patients with chronic obstructive pulmonary disease are at increased risk for developing infection with these lower virulence organisms. Atypical mycobacteria often produce a pneumonic pattern of involvement with areas of cavitation. In the setting of AIDS, *M. avium-intracellulare* can cause infection of lung tissue as well as other organs in which numerous organisms distend the cytoplasm of histocytes, producing a characteristic granularity in routine histologic sections (see Fig. 8-5C).

Fungal Pneumonia

A small number of endemic fungal organisms commonly cause pulmonary infection in immunocompetent individuals.

MICROBIOLOGY

Atypical Mycobacteria

Atypical mycobacteria include approximately 10 species of mycobacteria that can produce disease in humans and animals that is less aggressive than *M. tuberculosis*. Some atypical mycobacteria are free living (in water) and may be confused with pathogenic mycobacteria if they contaminate tissue sections.

Mycobacterium avium complex (MAC) includes two species, *M. avium* and *M. intracellulare*, and can colonize normal individuals. In patients with immunodeficiency (usually AIDS), *M. intracellulare* can produce a disseminated infection in which it fills and distends macrophages in many organs without producing a marked inflammatory reaction.

M. scrofulaceum is a common cause of lymphadenitis in children (scrofula) that can progress to abscess formation.

M. kansasii is a photochromogenic organism that can produce chronic pulmonary disease similar to, but much less aggressive than, *M. tuberculosis*.

Skin infections can result from *M. ulcerans* and *M. marinum* acquired from aquariums or swimming pools. *M. fortuitum* complex is a species of free-living soil organisms that can cause wound infection.

Histoplasma capsulatum is a dimorphic fungus that is endemic to the Mississippi River valley and produces a flu-like illness in immunocompetent individuals, often resulting in the formation of calcified granulomas similarly to tuberculosis. Reactivation can occur during periods of immunosuppression with dissemination of disease. *Coccidioides immitis* is endemic in the southwestern United States and produces valley fever (Fig. 8-6C). *Blastomyces dermatitidis* is endemic in the southern United States and can produce skin and lung infection.

Immunocompromised Host

Immunocompromised patients are susceptible to infection with usual pathogens as well as organisms that do not typically produce disease in immunocompetent individuals. Infection may result from organisms that are ubiquitously present, such as *Pneumocystis carinii*, or from reactivation of prior viral or mycobacterial infection (e.g., CMV pneumonia) (see Figs. 8-6A, 8-6B, and 8-6D). Pneumocystis produces a characteristic foamy intra-alveolar exudate that can be seen on lung biopsy or in pulmonary cytology specimens.

Fungal pneumonia is a life-threatening complication in immunocompromised patients. *Aspergillus fumigatus* is a common organism in this setting. It forms septate hyphae and produces an aggressive pneumonia that leads to extensive tissue destruction and necrosis. Immunocompromised patients are also at risk for pneumonia caused by more typical human pathogens, such as *Histoplasma*, *Coccidioides*, and mycobacteria. Diabetic patients are predisposed to mucormycosis infection although the lung is not the usual portal of entry for the organism. Even with effective antimicrobial treatment, some of these infections are difficult or impossible to eradicate in the setting of severe immunosuppression.

●●● ASTHMA

Asthma is a form of chronic lung disease that is characterized predominantly by hyperreactivity of airways to various stimuli as well as increased mucus production by goblet cells in the bronchial mucosa. Peribronchial smooth muscle is usually hypertrophic. Asthma is often associated with eosinophilia, and Curschmann's spirals (casts of air spaces formed by the contents of eosinophil granules) may be observed in the sputum of some patients with asthma. Asthmatics frequently develop severe bronchoconstriction in response to various stimuli including heat, cold, exogenous allergens, and some chemicals including aspirin. Triggers for asthmatic attacks tend to remain relatively constant in individual patients throughout the course of their disease. The severity of symptoms in different patients with asthma varies greatly. Patients typically have wheezing and a decreased FEV_1 during attacks.

Abnormal lung function may predispose to infection that further exacerbates pulmonary dysfunction.

Several products of the 5′-lipoxygenase pathway (leukotrienes) are important mediators of vasoconstriction in patients with

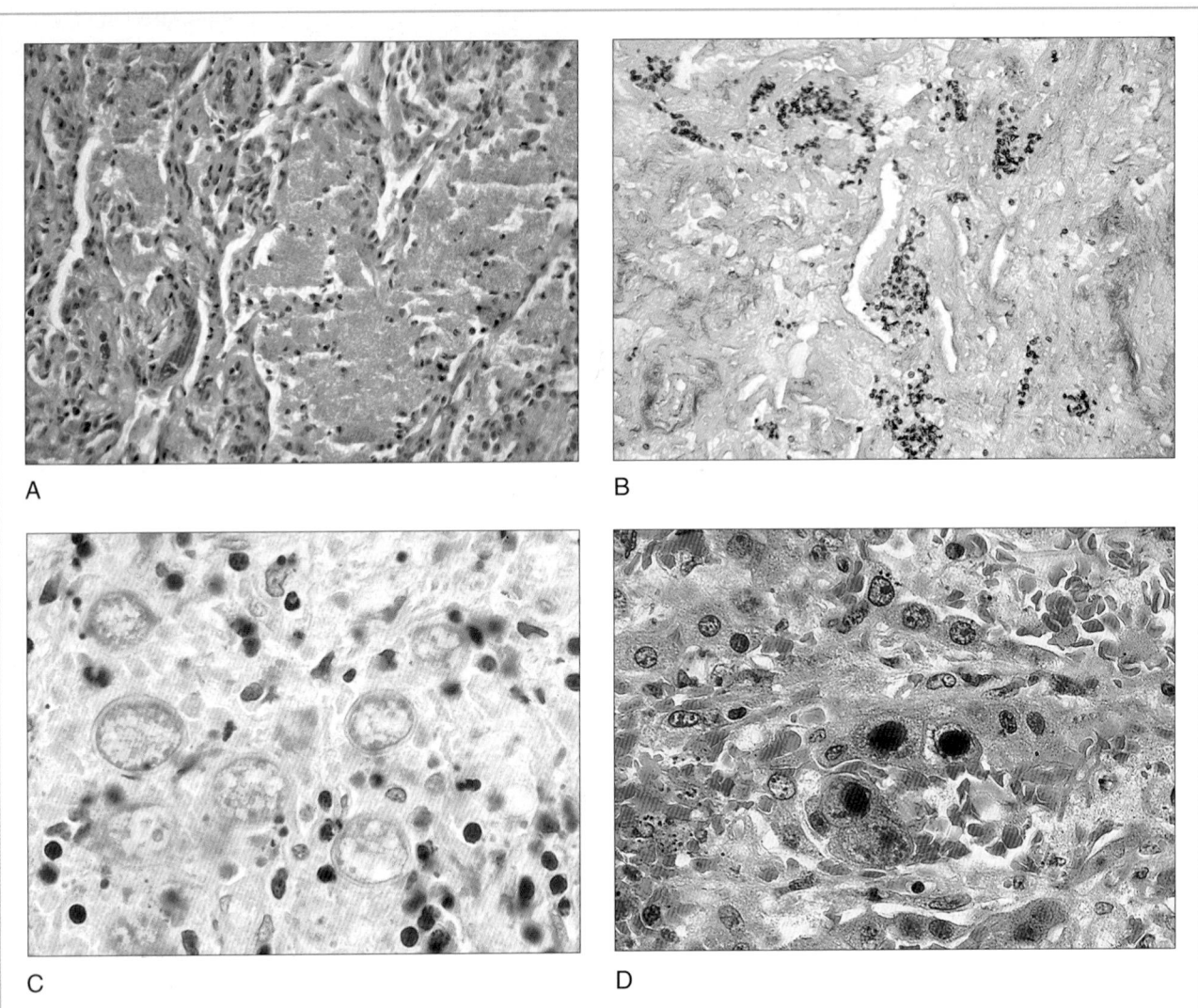

Figure 8-6. A, Pneumocystic pneumonia. Microscopic section showing lung tissue with granular eosinophilic exudate filling alveoli. **B,** Pneumocystic pneumonia. Microscopic section of lung tissue stained with Gomori methenamine silver stain showing numerous *Pneumocystis* organisms within the intra-alveolar exudate. Organisms have a characteristic cup shape. **C,** Coccidiomycosis. Microscopic section of lung tissue showing numerous cysts of *Coccidioides immitis* with refractile walls. Scattered inflammatory cells are present. **D,** Cytomegalovirus pneumonia. Microscopic section of lung tissue showing prominent eosinophilic intranuclear inclusions in infected pneumocytes. Smaller intracytoplasmic inclusions are also present as well as prominent hemorrhage.

asthma. Corticosteroid therapy (usually inhaled) has been a mainstay of therapy for severe asthma but can lead to significant metabolic and infectious complications. Theophylline is effective in diminishing bronchoconstriction in most patients with severe asthma and has been another mainstay of therapy. Recently, a specific inhibitor of 5′-lipoxygenase has become available as a treatment option, but its role in management is not yet clear.

The precise causes of asthma remain elusive and are almost certainly heterogeneous.

The prevalence of asthma is developed countries is clearly increasing at a substantial rate. Approximately half of asthmatics have atopic disease, and disease attacks are predominantly related to exposure to environmental allergens. The remaining half of asthmatic patients do not appear to have allergen-mediated disease. Population-based studies suggest that environmental allergen exposure in childhood is important (children with more limited allergen exposure have a greater likelihood of developing asthma). Polymorphisms in the IL-13 gene segregate with asthma risk, and this cytokine appears to be mechanistically involved in the persistent inflammatory reaction in many asthmatic patients.

●●● CHRONIC OBSTRUCTIVE PULMONARY DISEASE

Chronic obstructive pulmonary disease (COPD) usually results from the combination of several different architectural abnormalities of lung tissue. Many patients with COPD have significant emphysema resulting from destruction of the

MICROBIOLOGY

Pneumocystis carinii

P. carinii is ubiquitously present worldwide. *P. carinii* produces thick-walled cysts 6–8 μm in diameter that have a characteristic cup-like shape in silver stains. Up to eight sporozoites are present within cysts, but these are not visible in routine histologic stains. An extracystic trophozoite may also be present. *P. carinii* has features of both a protozoan and a fungus and has not been definitively classified.

Normal individuals are colonized with *P. carinii* through the respiratory route early in life, and organisms remain throughout life. *P. carinii* never produces disease in immunocompetent individuals, but if high-level immunosuppression occurs, pneumonia may develop over the course of weeks.

Humoral immunity is not protective against *P. carinii*, so vaccination is not helpful. Cell-mediated immunity is effective in preventing the development of disease. Prophylactic treatment of immunocompromised patients with trimethoprim-sulfamethoxazole usually prevents pneumonia.

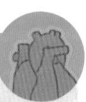

PHYSIOLOGY

Pulmonary Function Tests

Pulmonary function tests are conducted by means of spirometry, which measures how the lungs move air by recording the amount of air that is breathed in and out over a set time interval. Spirometric measurements can be performed with normal breathing or with forced inspiration and expiration.

Spirograms can be used to produce flow-volume loop graphs of inspiration and expiration that can be used to assess obstructive lung disease (e.g., asthma and COPD) and restrictive lung disease (e.g., pulmonary fibrosis and chest wall abnormalities). These results can be used to calculate FEV_1 (the amount of air exhaled in 1 second) and the FVC (total amount of air that can be inspired). If the ratio of FEV_1 to FVC is below 0.75, significant obstructive disease is present.

Lung volume can be measured with a plethysmograph. Total lung capacity (TLC) = residual volume (RV) + FVC. TLC is markedly increased in patients with emphysema and can impede effective gas exchange.

Diffusion capacity is usually measured by breathing a small amount of carbon monoxide, which avidly binds to hemoglobin. The difference in carbon monoxide concentration between inhaled and exhaled air provides an estimate of the efficiency of gas exchange.

IMMUNOLOGY

Asthma

Asthma incidence has increased markedly in developed countries, and its prevalence currently approaches 5% of the population. Approximately half of asthma cases develop before age 10 and more cases occur in disadvantaged persons living in urban environments.

IL-13 is necessary and sufficient to drive asthma in a mouse disease model. A complex interplay between multiple cell types and cytokine networks appears to underlie airway inflammation in most asthmatic patients.

IL-13 receptor variants have been shown to predispose to asthma, and IL-13 produced by T_H2 T cells plays a key role in stimulating macrophages and bronchial epithelial cells through these receptors. A common IL-13 polymorphism (present in up to 25% of individuals in some populations) produces an IL-13 that is more active than wild-type IL-13.

Prostanoid DP receptors (PTGDRs) mediate the chemotaxis of T cells in response to mast cell degranulation (prostaglandin D synthase products). PTGDRs have also been implicated in asthma via population-based studies linking SNP haplotypes in this gene with susceptibility to asthma. Mice deficient in PTGDR are unable to initiate airway inflammation in response to allergen challenge.

Most patients with COPD also have a degree of reactive airway disease similarly to asthmatics. In some patients it may be relatively minor, while in others, reactive airway disease is a major therapeutic target of bronchodilator therapy. Inflammation and fibrosis of small airways is an important in the pathophysiology of COPD in many patients. Minute decreases in the diameter of smaller airways result in significant decreases in air flow (cross-sectional area is proportionate to the square of the diameter). Recent studies suggest that the density of B cells in small airways is a strong predictor of progressive airway disease in patients with COPD, suggesting that acquired immune mechanisms are important in the pathophysiology of COPD.

Various types of chronic lung injury can cause or exacerbate COPD, most important of which is cigarette smoking. Cigarette smoke greatly decreases the effectiveness of the mucociliary blanket (squamous metaplasia of bronchial mucosa), increasing the likelihood of infection and decreasing effective clearance of pulmonary secretions. Over time, this can result in increased fibrosis in lung tissue, and repeated cycles of infection can worsen emphysema and interstitial fibrosis, eventually producing end-stage (honeycomb) lung disease (see Fig. 8-7C). Activation of inflammatory pathways by cigarette smoking can result in digestion of lung parenchyma by leukocyte metalloproteinases in the absence of intercurrent infection. Oxidants from cigarette smoke and inflammatory cells decrease the activity of histone deacetylase (HDAC2) in macrophages, resulting in increased histone acetylation and activation of some proinflammatory genes. IL-8 secretion recruits neutrophils that are primed by

lung's extracellular matrix by proteases (Figs. 8-7A and 8-7B). In emphysema, alveolar septae are lost, resulting in the consolidation of normal alveoli into larger dysfunctional airspaces. These enlarged airspaces result in increased total lung volume with a prominent increase in dead volume and decreased effective oxygen exchange. Destruction of lung parenchyma also results in a loss of external support for larger airways, causing premature airway collapse during expiration. Once developed, emphysematous changes are irreversible.

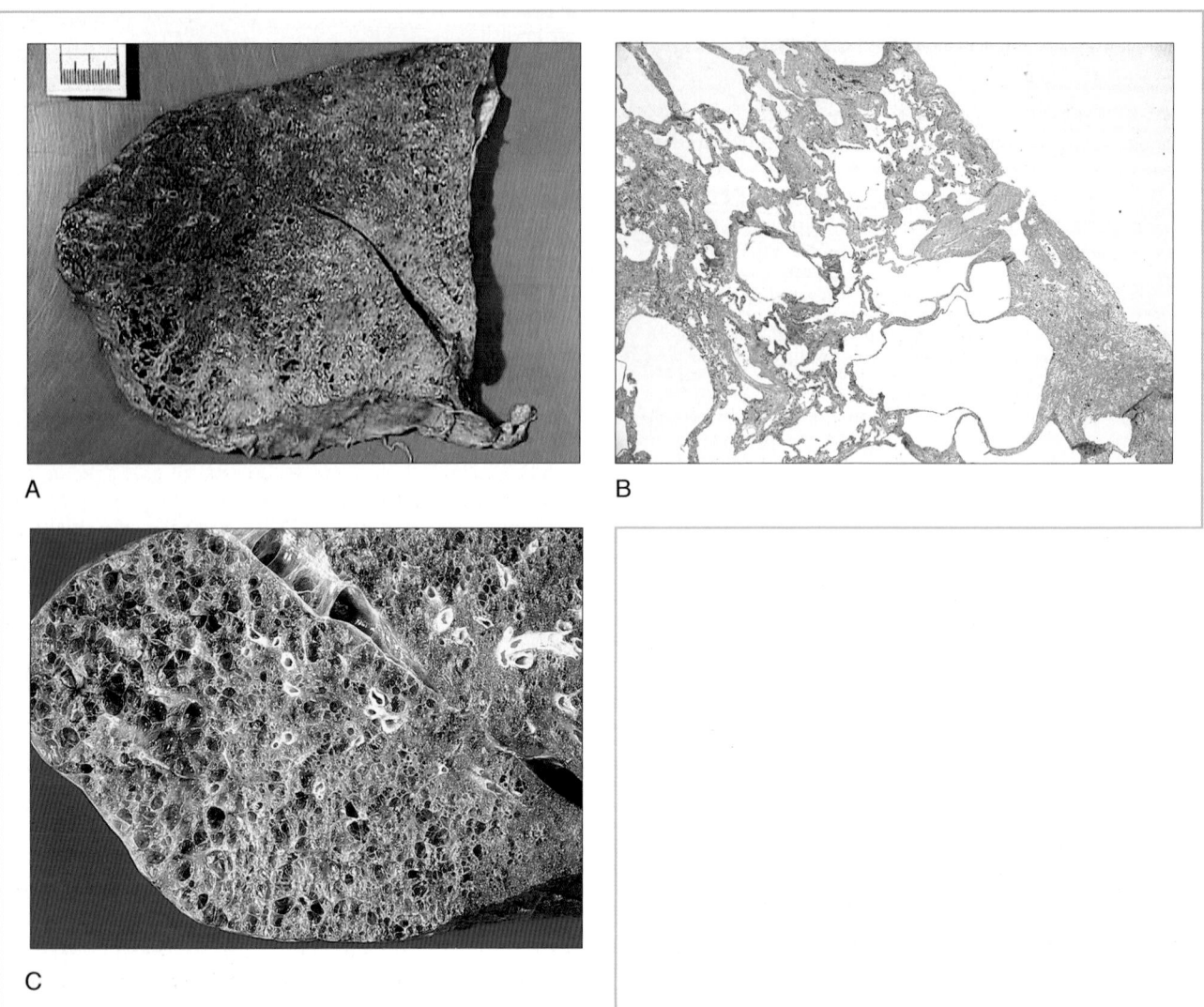

Figure 8-7. A, Pulmonary emphysema. Gross cross-section of lung tissue showing severe emphysema with massive enlargement of air spaces. **B**, Chronic obstructive pulmonary disease (COPD). Microscopic section of lung tissue showing abnormal air spaces (emphysema) that are more than 10 times the size of normal alveoli, with associated fibrosis in residual alveolar septae. **C**, End-stage lung disease. Gross cross-section of lung tissue showing honeycombing with large, abnormal air spaces.

TNFα and cause additional damage to the extracellular matrix. Derepression of matrix metalloproteinases 9 and 12 in macrophages results in increased elastase activity in lung tissue, which can destroy extracellular matrix and cause premature closure of airways during expiration (air trapping).

Individuals with α_1-antitrypsin deficiency have greatly accelerated development of emphysema because of genetic abnormality of this important protease inhibitor. Those with α_1-antitrypsin deficiency who smoke tend to develop emphysema early in life and usually succumb to respiratory insufficiency. Polymorphisms in protease and protease inhibitor genes may underlie less severe predisposition to COPD.

●●● PNEUMOCONIOSIS

Pneumoconiosis comprises a number of different types of occupational lung disease in which inhalation of particulates

or toxic chemicals results in pulmonary fibrosis or inflammation. Many different specific forms of pneumoconiosis are recognized. Some of the most important are related to exposure to asbestos fibers. Tiny asbestos fibers that are inspired beyond the mucociliary blanket are not effectively cleared by host defense mechanisms. These fibers remain permanently in lung tissue and may spread to the pleural spaces and peritoneal cavity via lymphatics. These particulates stimulate a chronic inflammatory/fibrotic process that results in the formation of pleural fibrous plaques and causes severe interstitial fibrosis in lung tissue (Figs. 8-8A and 8-8B). Asbestos was an important cause of pneumoconiosis in the past when heavy industrial exposure occurred, particularly in shipbuilders. Recognition of the important role of asbestos in the development of malignant mesothelioma has led to greatly reduced industrial exposure, and asbestos pneumoconiosis is now uncommon. Asbestos is also a significant

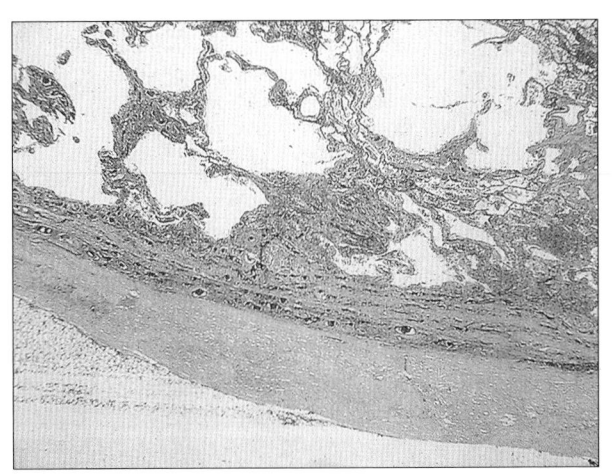

A

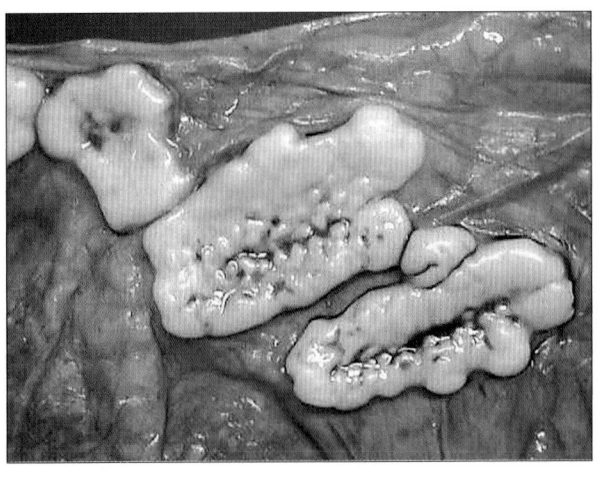

B

Figure 8-8. A, Asbestos pneumoconiosis. Section of lung tissue showing marked pleural fibrosis (*at bottom*) as well as mixed emphysema and interstitial fibrosis. **B**, Pleural plaques. Gross photograph of parietal pleura in a patient with asbestosis. The scalloped whitish-gray plaques are typical of heavy asbestos exposure.

risk factor for the development of bronchogenic carcinoma, particularly in individuals who smoke cigarettes.

Other forms of fibrogenic dust disease are associated with different kinds of occupations. Silicosis results from the inhalation of silica particles that are small enough to reach beyond mucociliary blanket, since these particles cannot be effectively cleared by host defenses. When these silica particles are ingested by inflammatory cells, they puncture their membranes to release hydrolytic enzymes and profibrotic cytokines that result in nodular fibrosis of lung tissue. Silicosis can occur in sand blasters without adequate respiratory protection and in miners of coal with high silica content.

Coal workers' pneumoconiosis is a fibrotic disease of lung tissue associated with the deposition of large amounts of carbon particles in lung (anthracosis). Anthracotic pigment is not as fibrogenic as silica or asbestos, and some anthracosis

is present in all city dwellers and prominently in cigarette smokers. Coal miners can be exposed to very high concentrations of coal dust and develop dust macules (nodular lesions composed of macrophages with ingested carbon pigment) over the course of years. Fibrosis associated with these deposits eventually causes sufficient interstitial lung disease to produce respiratory failure in susceptible individuals (black lung disease).

INTERSTITIAL LUNG DISEASE

Interstitial lung disease refers to a set of inflammatory conditions in which inflammation is localized predominantly within alveolar septae rather than in alveolar spaces. There is clinical and pathologic overlap between some of these entities and many are immune mediated. Some diseases produce sufficiently characteristic pathologic changes that lung biopsy is diagnostic, but most require careful correlation between radiographic findings on high-resolution computed tomography (CT) scan and clinical course to arrive at the specific diagnosis. Many of these diseases result in progressive interstitial fibrosis and can lead to respiratory failure.

Hypersensitivity Pneumonitis

Hypersensitivity pneumonitis is an inflammatory condition of lung tissue caused by an immune response to exogenous, inhaled allergens. Hypersensitivity pneumonitis may occur as an occupational disease or by exposure to substances in the home environment (e.g., "bird fanciers' lung," "hot tub lung"). Exposure to respiratory allergens in sensitized individuals can cause DAD with acute pulmonary failure or chronic progressive interstitial fibrosis. A careful exposure history is critical in establishing the diagnosis; removal of the allergen terminates the inflammatory response. Bronchoalveolar lavage usually shows prominent lymphocytosis with an inversion of the CD4:CD8 ratio. Lung biopsy usually shows non-necrotizing granulomatous inflammation.

Idiopathic Interstitial Lung Disease

Idiopathic interstitial lung disease encompasses a number of different clinicopathologic entities with somewhat characteristic clinical presentations. The cause of most of these diseases is unknown although recent evidence suggests that genetic abnormalities in surfactant protein may cause some familial forms of idiopathic pulmonary fibrosis. High-resolution CT is as important as or more important than lung biopsy in diagnosing many of these entities. These diseases have recently been reclassified as nonspecific interstitial pneumonitis (NIP), usually occurring in younger patients; idiopathic pulmonary fibrosis (IPF), formerly known as usual interstitial pneumonitis (UIP); and cryptogenic organizing pneumonia (COP), formerly known as bronchiolitis obliterans organizing pneumonia (BOOP) (Fig. 8-9). Respiratory bronchiolitis-associated interstitial lung disease (RB-ILD) is a disease of smokers with inflammation and

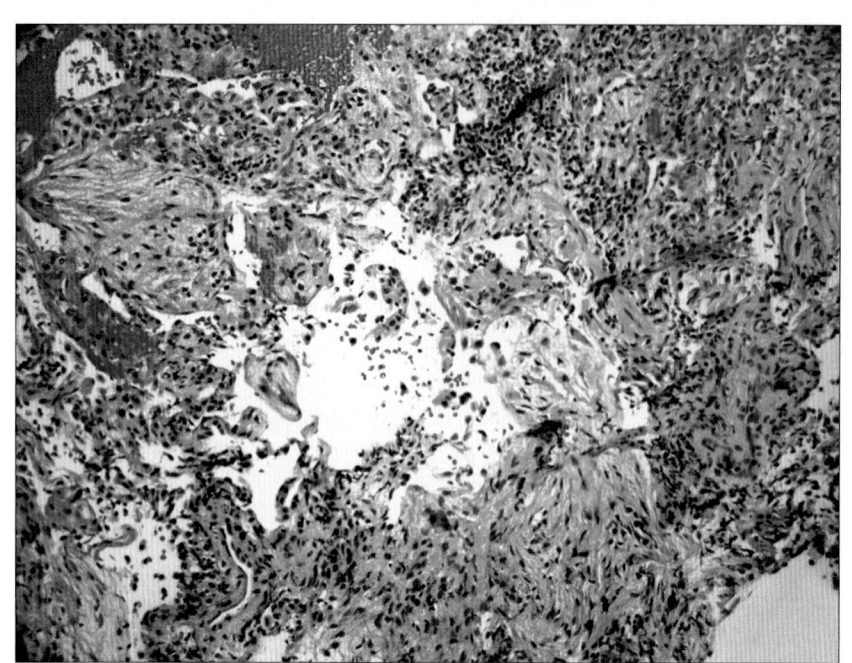

Figure 8-9. Organizing pneumonia. Microscopic section of lung tissue with focal Masson bodies (intra-alveolar granulation tissue). More mature interstitial fibrosis with collagen deposition is also present.

fibrosis of ter-minal bronchioles and prominent intra-alveolar histiocytes that share some features with desquamative interstitial pneumonia (DIP).

Sarcoid

Sarcoidosis is an idiopathic inflammatory disease characterized by the formation of discrete granulomas in multiple organ systems. The lung is usually involved in sarcoidosis, and lung biopsy or biopsy of mediastinal lymph nodes may be diagnostic (Fig. 8-10). The granulomas in sarcoid usually contain multinucleated giant cells that often contain asteroid bodies (crystalline cytoplasmic inclusions). These granulomas are typically compact and highly organized. Central necrosis is unusual, and no microorganisms are demonstrable by staining or culture. Individuals such as fire fighters who are exposed to particulates may be at increased risk for developing sarcoid, but the detailed pathophysiology of this disease is not well understood and may be heterogeneous. Sarcoid may be progressive and lead to significant pulmonary fibrosis with compromise of lung function as well as damage to other organ systems.

Immune-Mediated Lung Disease

Pulmonary interstitial fibrosis occurs in some patients as a manifestation of systemic autoimmune diseases (e.g., systemic sclerosis and systemic lupus erythematosus) (Fig. 8-11). Goodpasture's syndrome is caused by type II hypersensitivity in which anti–basement membrane antibodies react with the capillary basement membranes in lung tissue (as well as renal glomeruli) to produce pulmonary hemorrhage that may be life threatening.

●●● PULMONARY EMBOLI

Pulmonary emboli result from dislodgment of venous thrombi, which are then propelled into the pulmonary circulation. At least 90% of pulmonary emboli arise from deep venous thrombi in the thigh. Venous thrombosis in these larger deep veins is typically asymptomatic so that the diagnosis may not be suspected until pulmonary emboli develop. Small pulmonary emboli are frequently asymptomatic because of the dual pulmonary circulation but may cause hemoptysis. Involvement of more than 40% of lung parenchyma results in hypoxemia, even in normal individuals. Large pulmonary emboli that occlude the bifurcation of the pulmonary artery trunk are called "saddle emboli" (Fig. 8-12A) and are almost instantly fatal because they cause complete blockage of pulmonary blood flow with rapid and complete loss of cardiac output.

Over time pulmonary emboli are organized by tissue repair and thrombolysis, which recanalize affected blood vessels. These vessels often retain eccentric scars or a "spider web" of fibrous tissue, which are markers of chronic pulmonary emboli. Chronic pulmonary emboli can result in increased pulmonary artery pressure with strain on the right heart that may ultimately develop into cor pulmonale in the setting of pulmonary hypertension.

Pulmonary infarcts are rare except in patients with intrinsic pulmonary vascular disease or repeated episodes of pulmonary emboli. Pulmonary infarcts are typically hemorrhagic and wedge-shaped and produce symptoms related to pleural inflammation (see Fig. 8-12B). A pleural friction rub is produced owing to fibrin deposition on the pleural surfaces. Pulmonary emboli are usually not visible in routine chest radiography, but helical CT scan with contrast can identify

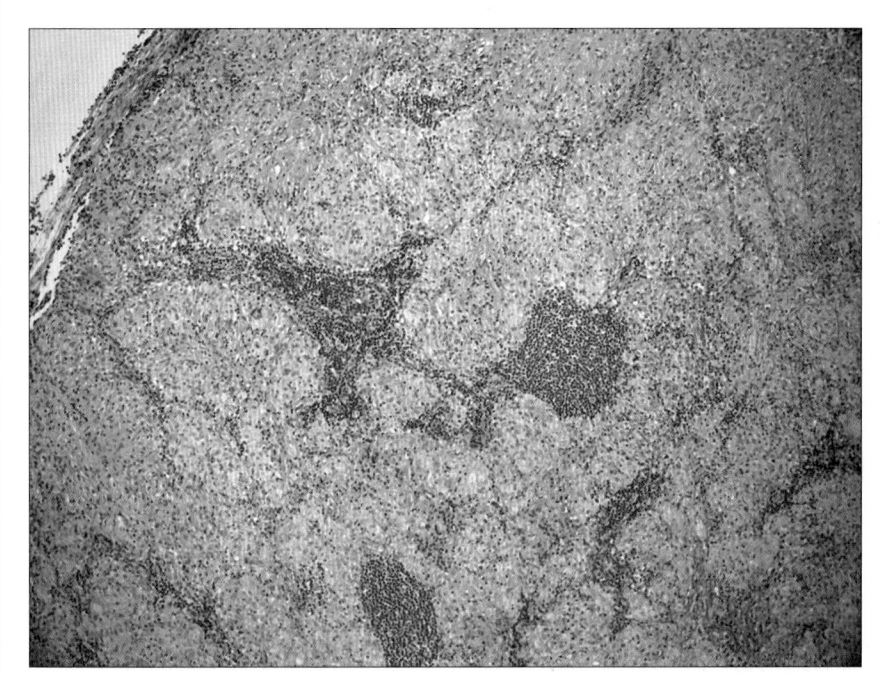

Figure 8-10. Sarcoid granulomas. Microscopic section showing numerous non-necrotizing granulomas. The tight concentric organization of granulomas is typical of sarcoidosis.

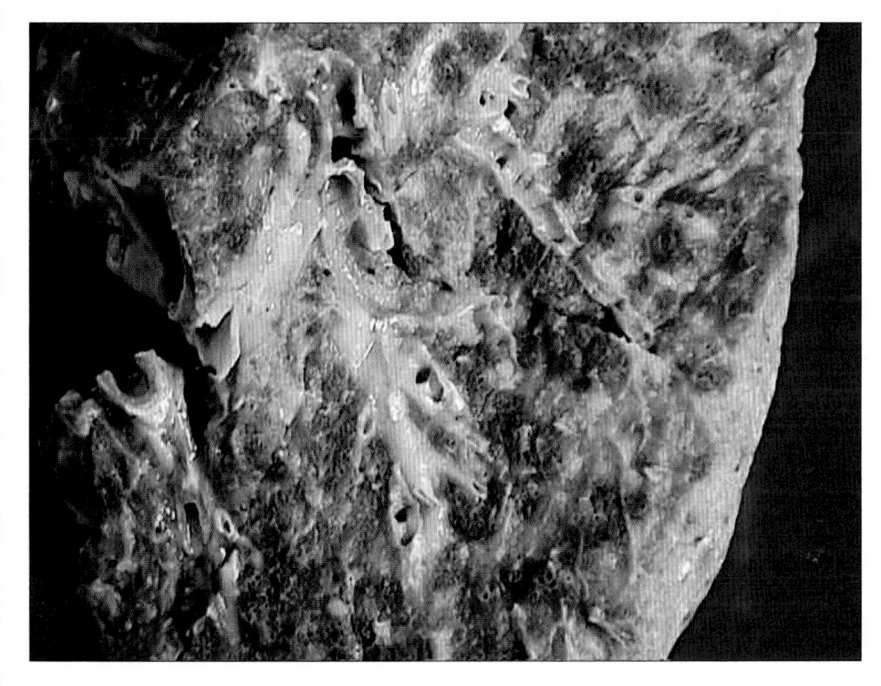

Figure 8-11. Pulmonary fibrosis in scleroderma. Gross cross-section of lung tissue showing severe septal fibrosis (strand-like whitish areas).

even small pulmonary emboli, in most cases permitting a specific diagnosis.

Pulmonary emboli are a major cause of morbidity and mortality in United States with over 200,000 deaths annually. Factors predisposing to pulmonary emboli are largely those favoring deep venous thrombosis. These include stasis, often associated with immobilization of elderly individuals for surgical procedures. Prophylactic treatment of

hospitalized patients at risk with low-molecular-weight heparin can significantly reduce the occurrence of pulmonary emboli.

●●● PULMONARY HYPERTENSION

Pulmonary hypertension is defined numerically as a mean pulmonary artery pressure greater than 40 mm Hg. Hypertension can result from recurrent pulmonary emboli,

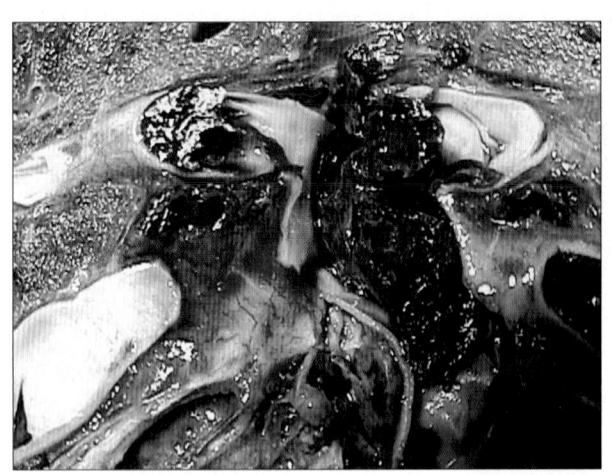

A

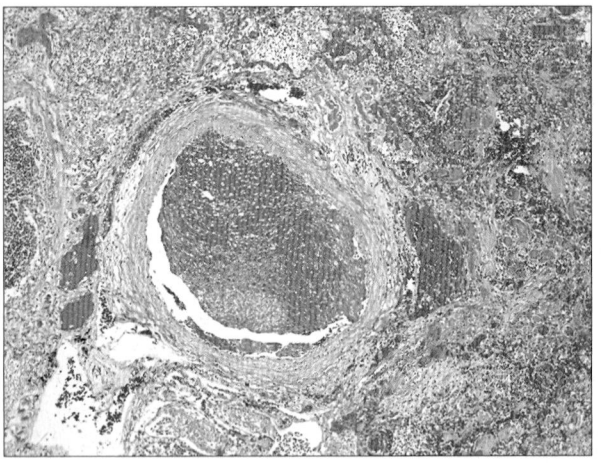

B

Figure 8-12. A, Pulmonary emboli. Gross cross-section from the lung hilum with an in situ acute pulmonary embolus blocking a large pulmonary artery trunk. **B,** Pulmonary infarct. Microscopic section of lung tissue showing in situ pulmonary embolus and associated hemorrhage and coagulative necrosis indicative of a pulmonary infarct.

from in situ thrombosis within the pulmonary vasculature, as a consequence of pulmonary fibrosis, secondary to increased left atrial pressure (in congestive heart failure or cardiomyopathy), or as an idiopathic condition (i.e., primary pulmonary hypertension). Over time, increased pulmonary artery pressures result in remodeling of the pulmonary vasculature with thickening of the walls of pulmonary arteries. In severe cases, necrosis of vascular walls may develop, and plexiform lesions may be observed. Once the pulmonary vasculature has been remodeled to accommodate high arterial pressures, adequate lung perfusion requires these high pressures. Increased pulmonary artery pressure produces strain on the right side of the heart and can cause cor pulmonale (Fig. 8-13).

●●● PULMONARY TUMORS AND TUMOR-LIKE CONDITIONS

Some bronchogenic tumors are highly associated with cigarette smoking while others show a weaker association.

Because of the large functional pulmonary reserve in normal lungs, tumors usually do not become symptomatic until they are large. Many lung cancers are not curable by surgery at the time they are discovered.

Bronchogenic Carcinoma

Bronchogenic carcinoma includes the most common lung cancers of adults and is classified into two major categories based on morphology and different clinical approaches to therapy. Non–small cell carcinoma includes squamous cell carcinoma and adenocarcinoma as well as large-cell carcinoma. These tumors often share morphologic features and, when feasible, are primarily treated by surgical excision. In contrast, small-cell undifferentiated carcinoma usually arises near the hilum of the lung and spreads to lymph nodes and other organs early in its course. For these reasons, small-cell carcinoma is not amenable to surgical therapy and is typically treated primarily with chemotherapy. Only a tiny fraction of tumors have features that overlap between small-cell and non–small cell carcinoma.

Non–Small Cell Carcinoma

Adenocarcinomas of the lung are less strongly associated with cigarette smoking than are other types of bronchogenic carcinoma. Adenocarcinomas tend to arise in the periphery of lung tissue and may have two different patterns of growth. Solid adenocarcinomas can arise in a preexisting scar (e.g., healed tuberculosis) or de novo (Fig. 8-14A). Well-differentiated tumors show obvious gland formation, but poorly differentiated tumors often show morphologic overlap with large-cell undifferentiated and squamous cell carcinoma.

Bronchioalveolar carcinoma is a distinct form of adenocarcinoma that does not form a solid mass. The malignant cells in bronchoalveolar carcinomas grow along existing alveolar septae, replacing normal pneumocytes (see Fig. 8-14B). This lepidic pattern of growth may begin as atypical alveolar hyperplasia (dysplasia of alveolar ring cells). Bronchioalveolar tumors may be small or large and are frequently multifocal. It is important to distinguish primary adenocarcinomas of lung from metastatic adenocarcinoma from other organs. Large-cell undifferentiated carcinoma does not show obvious glandular differentiation but shares many features with adenocarcinoma. Some pathologists view large-cell undifferentiated carcinoma as a form of poorly differentiated adenocarcinoma. The absence of neuroendocrine marker expression and the presence of vesicular nuclei with prominent nucleoli distinguish large-cell undifferentiated carcinoma from neuroendocrine carcinoma (see below).

Squamous cell carcinoma of lung tends to arise in the middle portion of the lung or near the carina, where carcinoma in situ develops in squamous metaplasia in larger

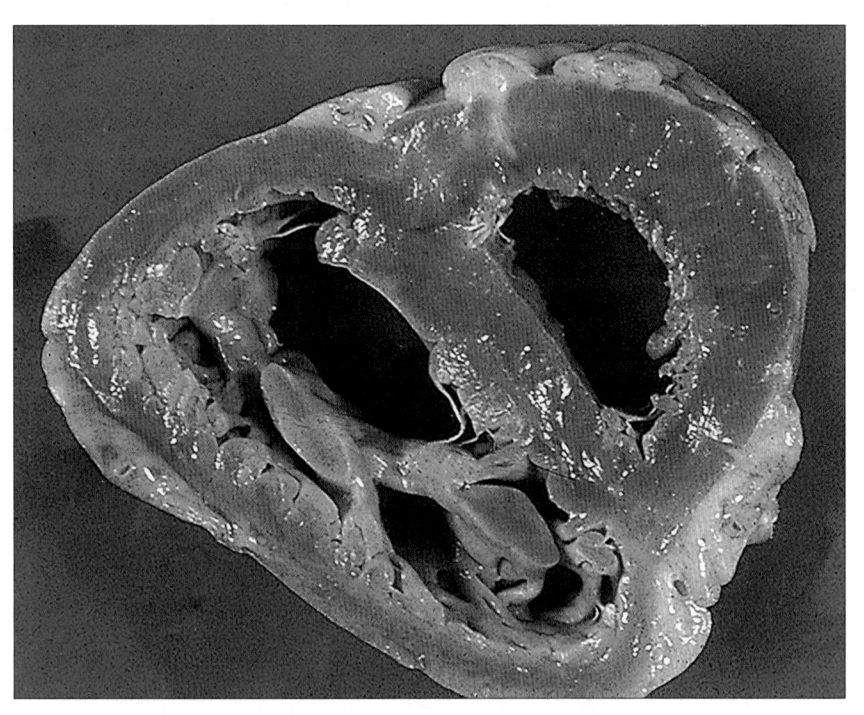

Figure 8-13. Cor pulmonale. Gross cross-section of a heart with massive right ventricular hypertrophy. The left ventricle (smaller chamber) is relatively normal.

BIOCHEMISTRY

Tobacco-associated Carcinogens

Tobacco smoke predisposes to a large number of different types of cancer, and at least 60 known carcinogens are present in cigarette smoke including nitrosamines, polycyclic aromatic hydrocarbons (PAH), and aromatic amines.

Metabolic processing of most tobacco-derived compounds is required before they become active carcinogens (e.g., benzo[a]pyrene (BaP), 4-(methylnitrosoamino)-1-(3-pyridyl)-1-butanone (NNK), N-nitrosodimethylamine (NDMA), N'-nitrosonornicotine (NNN), ethylene oxide, and 4-aminobipheynyl). In most cases, carcinogen activation is accomplished by cytochrome P-450 enzymes (see Chapter 3) that produce reactive electrophiles that can directly combine with DNA. Polymorphisms in cytochrome P-450 enzymes are associated with susceptibility or resistance to tobacco carcinogens and may underlie ethnic (racial) differences in susceptibility of smokers to lung cancer.

DNA adducts from tobacco carcinogens typically result in missense mutation, most commonly G→T and G→A. The presence of a large number of these base changes in a tumor is suggestive of tobacco-induced carcinogenesis.

bronchi. Squamous cell carcinoma is strongly associated with cigarette smoking. Tumors may be well differentiated with abundant keratin production or poorly differentiated (see Fig. 8-14C). Bronchogenic carcinomas with mixed squamous and glandular differentiation are common, and this mixed pattern is relatively characteristic of primary lung cancers.

The lung is a comparatively common site for metastasis, and it may be difficult to differentiate primary from metas-tatic adenocarcinomas. Immunohistochemical studies may be helpful in this regard, since most primary adenocarcinomas of the lung express thyroid transcription factor 1 (TTF-1), which is not expressed in most metastatic carcinomas from other organs. On gross examination, bronchogenic carcinomas tend to be stellate in configuration and typically contain anthra-cotic pigment (see Fig. 8-14D). In contrast, metastatic tumor deposits in the lung tend to be spherical in configuration and often do not contain grossly visible anthracotic pigment.

Non–small cell carcinoma usually spreads to hilar and mediastinal lymph nodes before metastasizing to other sites. Many tumors extend to the pleural surface, and they may extend through the visceral pleura to involve the parietal pleura. Tumors in the apex of the lung that extend into the chest wall can produce pain and paralysis by invading the brachial plexus (Pancoast's tumor). Non–small cell carci-nomas that have spread to contralateral mediastinal lymph nodes or to the parietal pleura are not curable by surgery. Combination chemotherapy and radiation therapy can effectively shrink some unresectable non–small cell carcino-mas and convert them to surgically resectable lesions. Even patients without demonstrable lymph node metastases at the time of lung resection are at risk for systemic metastasis. Non–small cell lung cancer is a fairly frequent cause of singular brain metastasis.

Small-Cell Undifferentiated Carcinoma and Neuroendocrine Tumors

Neuroendocrine tumors of the lung range from well-differentiated carcinoid tumors to small-cell undifferentiated carcinoma. Peripheral carcinoid tumors are relatively common in the lung and have features similar to carcinoid tumors arising

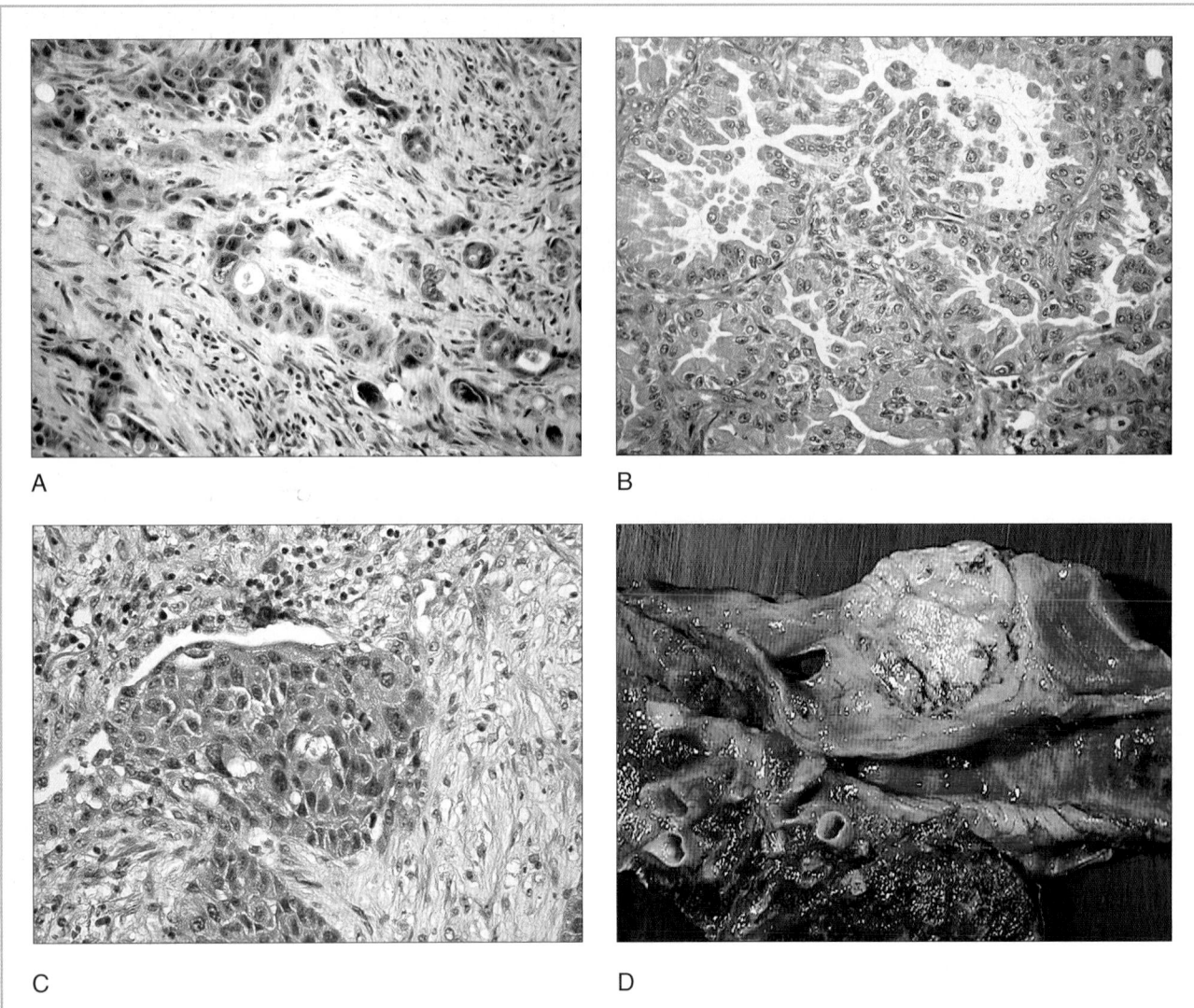

A

B

C

D

Figure 8-14. A, Bronchogenic adenocarcinoma. Microscopic section of lung tissue with a solid type adenocarcinoma with extensive associated fibrosis. Gland formation is evident. **B,** Bronchioalveolar carcinoma. Microscopic section of lung showing tumor growth along normal alveolar septae. This lepidic growth pattern is characteristic. **C,** Non–small cell carcinoma. Microscopic section of lung showing focal squamous differentiation in a typical non–small cell carcinoma. **D,** Non–small cell carcinoma. Gross cross-section of lung tissue showing a large non–small cell carcinoma (white lesion at the top) with scattered anthracotic pigment.

at other sites in the body. Carcinoid tumors typically show a nested pattern of growth with granular chromatin (so-called "salt and pepper" pattern) in the nuclei of tumor cells (Fig. 8-15A). Nucleoli are inapparent, mitotic figures are inconspicuous, and tumor necrosis is not observed. Some carcinoid tumors have a predominantly spindle cell pattern of growth. All carcinoid tumors strongly express neuroendocrine markers including chromogranin A, which is a component of dense core neurosecretory granules.

Although it is unusual for small carcinoid tumors to metastasize, all carcinoid tumors possess some metastatic potential. Larger tumors that show atypia are more likely to cause metastatic disease usually involving hilar or mediastinal lymph nodes.

Atypical carcinoid tumors are less well differentiated neuroendocrine tumors of the lung that are usually diagnosed as intermediate-grade neuroendocrine carcinoma. Morphologically, they show a less well developed nested architecture and tend to have a higher mitotic rate, often with foci of necrosis. The classification of neuroendocrine carcinoma reflects the lack of clear boundaries between well and poorly differentiated neuroendocrine tumors. Neuroendocrine carcinomas have a significantly higher potential for lymph node or hematogenous metastasis than do well-differentiated carcinoid tumors.

Small-cell undifferentiated carcinoma is a very poorly differentiated neuroendocrine carcinoma that usually arises in the central portion of the lung and involves hilar and mediastinal lymph nodes early in its course. The primary tumor itself may not be visible by radiography although enlarged lymph nodes suggest the diagnosis of metastatic disease. Small-cell undifferentiated carcinoma is almost

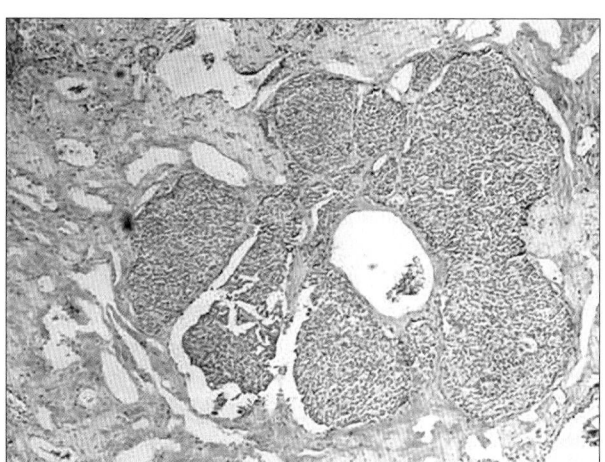

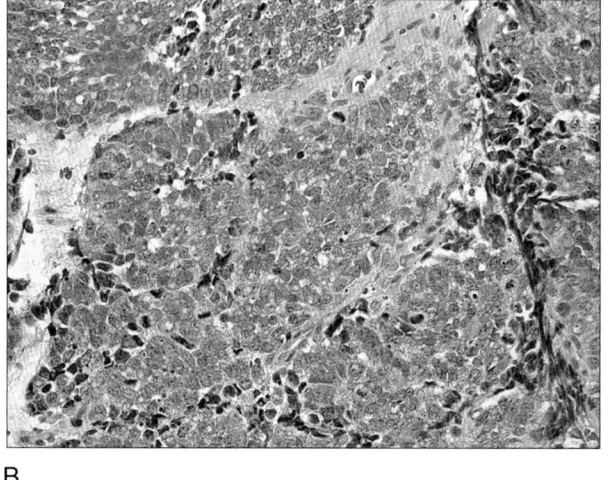

Figure 8-15. **A**, Pulmonary carcinoid tumor. Small peripheral carcinoid tumor composed of neuroendocrine cells with a nested growth pattern. **B**, Small-cell undifferentiated carcinoma. Microscopic section showing tumors cells with finely divided nuclear chromatin and prominent molding. Tumor cell cytoplasm is almost invisible in this section.

BIOCHEMISTRY

Neurosecretory Granules

Neurosecretory granules are membrane-bound vesicles that contain various hormones and chromogranin A. Neurosecretory granules have electron-dense cores bounded by membranes and are a characteristic and easily recognizable feature of neuroendocrine cells by electron microscopy. Synaptophysin was so-named because it was discovered in neuronal synapses, but it is a component of all neuroendocrine cells.

The membranes of neurosecretory granules have v-SNAREs (vesicle-associated soluble N-ethylmaleimide-sensitive factor attachment proteins) and regulatory proteins that control their docking and fusion with the cytoplasmic membrane in response to various stimuli (e.g., Ca^{++} influx or phosphorylation/dephosphorylation). v-SNARE proteins interact with t-SNAREs on the inner surface of the cytoplasmic membrane to mediate membrane fusion and exocytosis. Docking proteins are then recycled from the plasma membrane via clathrin-coated pits or other mechanisms.

Patients with small-cell undifferentiated carcinoma frequently have extensive liver metastases and usually are not treated surgically because of the likelihood of metastatic spread. Chemotherapy including cisplatin and etoposide often produce objective responses in patients with small-cell undifferentiated carcinoma, but none of these cases are ultimately curable. Effective chemotherapy may extend life significantly (months), but almost all patients succumb to their tumor over the course of several years.

Other Primary Lung Tumors

Other types of primary lung tumors are relatively uncommon. Tumors of endobronchial glands (similar to salivary gland tumors) and sarcomas can occur but are rare. Pulmonary hamartomas may simulate a lung tumor on radiographic analysis. Hamartomas are usually composed predominantly of mature cartilage but may include other cell types that normally occur in normal lung tissue. Pulmonary hamartomas are probably benign neoplasms rather than true hamartomas (i.e., developmental abnormalities), since they are not found in children. Primary lymphomas of the lung are unusual with low-grade non-Hodgkin's lymphomas (NHLs) of bronchial mucosa-associated lymphoid tissue (similar to the more frequent MALT lymphomas in the gastrointestinal tract) encountered most frequently. Pulmonary pseudotumor is a poorly defined entity composed of inflammatory cells and proliferating fibroblasts that may simulate a lung tumor.

Pulmonary Sequestration

Pulmonary sequestration is a developmental abnormality in which a portion of lung tissue is supplied by a systemic artery (rather than a pulmonary artery) and is not connected to the bronchial tree in a normal fashion. Sequestrations can develop

always a disease of heavy smokers and consists of small- to intermediate-sized tumor cells with scant cytoplasm and with finely divided nuclear chromatin. Tumor cells characteristically show nuclear molding in which one tumor cell may indent the nucleus of another tumor cell (see Fig. 8-15B). The fragility of nuclear membranes in small-cell carcinoma often leads to marked crush artifact in biopsy specimens of these neoplasms, which may be a useful diagnostic finding. Mitotic activity is brisk, and tumor necrosis is almost always present. Small-cell undifferentiated carcinoma typically has poorly formed cell junctions, making tumor cells poorly cohesive in cytologic preparations. Most small-cell undifferentiated carcinomas show some evidence of neuroendocrine differentiation by immunohistochemistry, but neurosecretory granules are usually scant in these poorly differentiated tumors.

infection and present as a lung mass lesion, mimicking a lung tumor. Angiography can usually demonstrate the abnormal vascular connections that are characteristic of sequestration, and surgical excision is curative.

LARYNGEAL PATHOLOGY

The larynx is surrounded by a cartilaginous wall that is an effective barrier to the spread of laryngeal tumors. The true vocal cords lack lymphatics as a consequence of their function in producing speech. As a result, the true cords are susceptible to lymphedema, which can result in so-called vocal nodules (singer's nodules caused by voice strain) that consist of accumulations of myxoid material in the stroma (Fig. 8-16).

Papillomatosis

Infection of the larynx with some strains of human papillomavirus (HPV) can result in the formation of numerous papillomas that can cause dysarthria (difficulty speaking) and may produce tracheal obstruction in extreme cases (Fig. 8-17A). Infection may be venereal in origin. A significant proportion of squamous cell carcinomas arising in the larynx contain HPV DNA, suggesting that this virus may be a predisposing factor for tumor development.

Carcinoma

The predominant malignant tumor of the larynx is squamous cell carcinoma, strongly associated with heavy alcohol consumption, cigarette smoking, or both. Tumors often develop in areas of epithelial dysplasia, and biopsy specimens of laryngeal mucosa before the development of an invasive tumor often show varying degrees of epithelial dysplasia (see Fig. 8-17B). Some carcinomas are associated with evidence of HPV infection. Invasive squamous cell carcinomas of the larynx tend to be confined by the laryngeal and thyroid cartilages (cartilage is hypoxic and is a poor substrate for tumor growth) so that spread into surrounding soft tissues occurs relatively late in their course. Since most tumors produce vocal symptoms early, patients often come to medical attention before there is extensive tumor spread. Primary radiation therapy is curative in some patients, and hemilaryngectomy is adequate for small tumors and allows preservation of relatively normal speech. Metastatic spread is typically to draining lymph nodes.

NASOPHARYNGEAL PATHOLOGY

Most nasopharyngeal pathology is related to tumors, and by far the most common is squamous cell carcinoma (either primary or by extension from the oral cavity or larynx). Mantle cell lymphoma can present around Waldeyer's ring (tonsillar and adenoid lymphoid tissue). A few tumors described below are unique to the nasopharynx.

Nasopharyngeal Carcinoma

Nasopharyngeal carcinoma has several different morphologic subtypes. The most characteristic is the so-called lymphoepithelial type in which tumor cells are intimately associated with infiltrating small lymphocytes. These tumors are usually associated with Epstein-Barr virus (EBV) infection and are

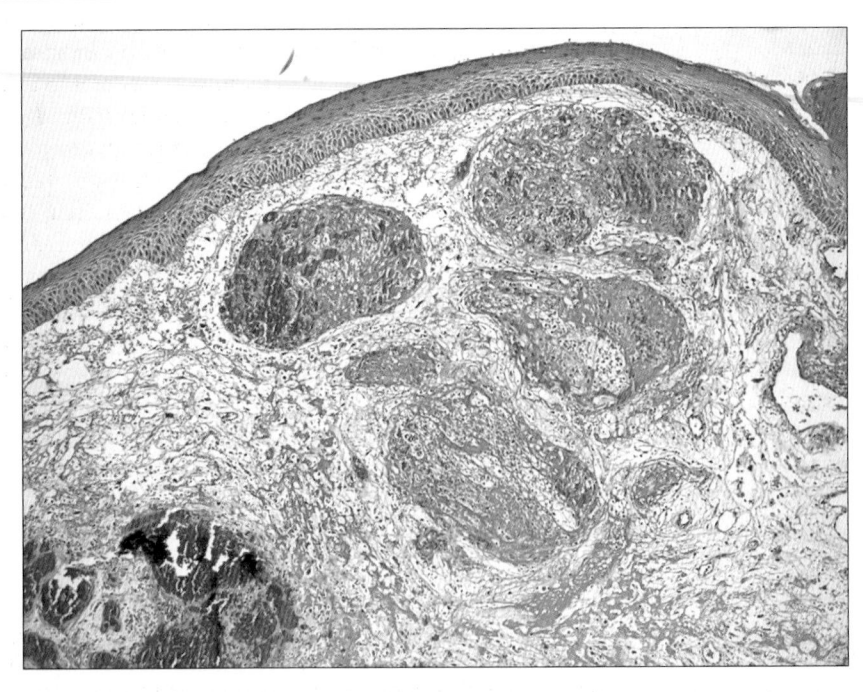

Figure 8-16. Vocal nodule. Microscopic section of true vocal cord showing the accumulation of myxoid material in the submucosa. The overlying squamous epithelium shows mild reactive changes.

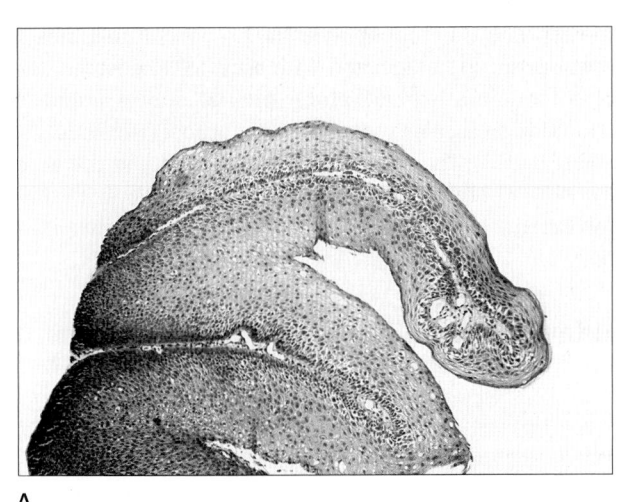

A

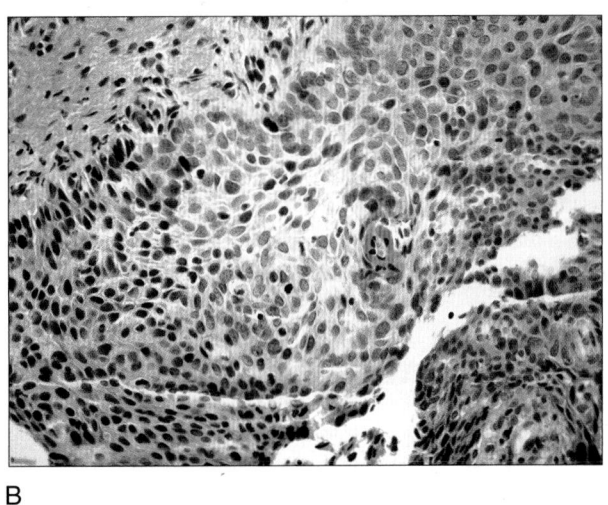

B

Figure 8-17. A, Laryngeal papilloma. Microscopic section of a papilloma showing features similar to condyloma of the uterine cervix. **B,** Squamous dysplasia in the larynx. Microscopic section of high-grade squamous dysplasia with loss of normal maturation pattern and pleomorphic preneoplastic cells. No invasion is evident in this section.

relatively common in individuals from Asia. Tumor cells express epithelial markers but do not show overt evidence of squamous differentiation. These tumors often present at an advanced stage but are highly responsive to radiation therapy, which often is curative. The precise role of EBV in the genesis of these neoplasms is not fully defined. Other subtypes of nasopharyngeal carcinoma that show overt keratinization are usually not curable with radiation therapy and behave similarly to squamous cell carcinoma.

Other Tumors

Angiofibroma is a vascular neoplasm of the nasopharynx that typically occurs in adolescent boys and can produce nasal obstruction or bleeding that may be severe. Angiofibromas are usually hormone (androgen) responsive, and excision is curative.

Aesthesioneuroblastoma is a malignant tumor of adults that arises from olfactory nerves in the nasopharynx, and its morphologic features and neuroendocrine differentiation are quite similar to neuroblastoma occurring in the adrenal gland.

●●● PLEURAL PATHOLOGY

Pleural Fluid Accumulations

Patients with pulmonary edema can accumulate fluid in the pleural spaces as well, resulting in progressive collapse of the lungs and diminished gas exchange. Prolonged lung collapse may be irreversible. Effusions resulting from congestive heart failure are usually bilateral and are characteristically transudates. Exudative pleural effusions can form in response to inflammation or neoplasia in the lung. Malignant pleural effusions are almost always exudates with increased protein concentration and specific gravity, and many are hemorrhagic. Cytologic examination may reveal clusters of tumor cells. Lung cancer frequently involves the pleura by direct extension and may lead to malignant effusion or chest wall involvement. Malignant effusions may be intractable, requiring therapeutic obliteration of the pleural space by sclerosing agents to maintain lung inflation. Patients with widely metastatic breast and ovarian carcinoma develop malignant pleural effusions with some frequency.

Tuberculosis can result in an exudative effusion with lymphocytes as the major cellular component. Bacterial pneumonia can produce an exudative pleural effusion with a neutrophilic infiltrate. Direct infection of pleural fluid can result in empyema that is essentially an abscess within the pleural space. Empyema most often develops in association with pneumonia caused by destructive organisms such as *Staphylococcus*. Empyema can also develop because of bacterial seeding of an existing pleural effusion of any cause. Empyema requires external drainage for the infection to heal. Healing usually results in extensive fibrosis with dense pleural adhesions or obliteration of the pleural space.

Pleurisy is an inflammation of the pleura that causes pleuritic chest paint (pain with breathing or coughing resulting from sliding of inflamed visceral and parietal pleura against each other). Inflammation often results in a fibrin exudate, which can produce a friction rub that can be heard on auscultation. The most common cause of primary pleural inflammation is viral infection. Patients with autoimmune disease and uremic patients may also develop clinically significant pleurisy. Pleurisy can occur secondary to pneumonia, pulmonary infarction, or malignancy.

Mesothelioma

Malignant mesothelioma is a highly aggressive neoplasm of mesothelial cells that usually arises in the pleural cavity but can arise in the peritoneum or pericardium. Tumors are often biphasic, with alternating papillary and spindle cell growth patterns (Fig. 8-18A). Biphasic tumors are morphologically characteristic, whereas pure papillary/glandular mesotheliomas can be difficult to differentiate from adenocarcinomas. Mesothelial cells express calretinin, which is only rarely expressed in epithelial tumor cells, and this immuno-histochemical marker provides a useful diagnostic test for mesothelioma in biopsy specimens. Mesotheliomas are almost universally associated with asbestos exposure.

Mesotheliomas spread along pleural surfaces and also extend along vascular and lymphatic spaces into lung tissue (see Fig. 8-18B). They are usually unresectable at the time of diagnosis and tend to progress relatively rapidly, with diffuse involvement of lung parenchyma producing respiratory failure.

Solitary Fibrous Tumor

The solitary fibrous tumor of pleura is a recently recognized entity composed of spindle cells that express CD34 and show random orientation (so-called patternless pattern) in histologic sections. Since the description of solitary fibrous tumor as a pleural neoplasm of intermediate biologic potential, this tumor has been recognized at many other sites throughout the body (many of these tumors were previously diagnosed as hemangiopericytomas). The majority of these tumors are cured by local excision, but a subset is associated with more aggressive biologic behavior and metastasis.

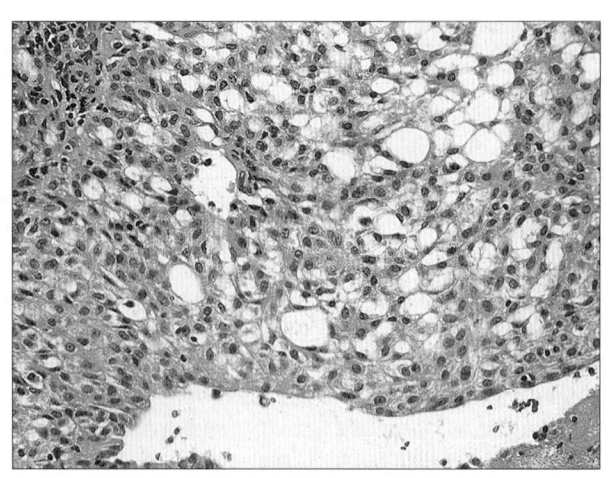

A

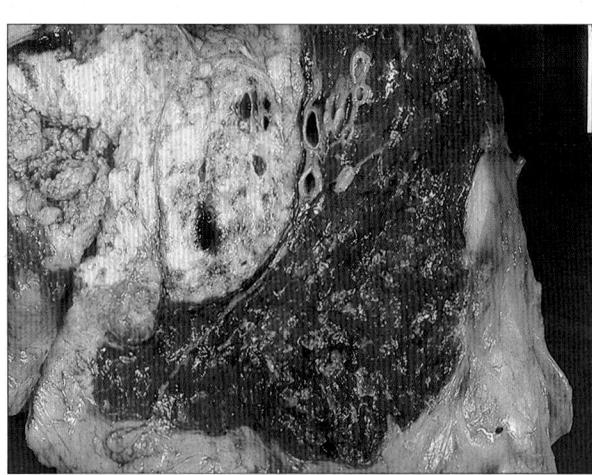

B

Figure 8-18. **A**, Malignant mesothelioma. Microscopic section of a predominantly papillary mesothelioma. It would be difficult to distinguish this tumor from a bronchogenic adenocarcinoma on histologic grounds. **B**, Malignant mesothelioma. Gross cross-section of lung with malignant mesothelioma. Whitish tumor extends along pleural surfaces and permeates lung parenchyma.

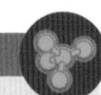

BIOCHEMISTRY

Asbestos

Asbestos is the name given to a collection of naturally occurring silicate minerals that can be separated to form long, flexible fibers and woven to form many useful materials. Asbestos is mechanically strong and extremely resistant to heat. These properties resulted in heavy industrial usage of asbestos until the mid twentieth century, when its biological hazards were recognized. Chrysotile asbestos is the most common form in industrial use and is still utilized in brake pads in automobiles.

Large asbestos fragments are not dangerous to humans, but small particles that are inhaled beyond the mucociliary blanket in the lung can produce pneumoconiosis and predispose to mesothelioma. Asbestos exposure need not be heavy to produce a mesothelioma, and individuals with even minor exposures are at some risk for developing this rare tumor. The exact mechanism by which asbestos produces mesotheliomas remains unclear. Asbestos exposure also greatly enhances the risk of lung cancer in cigarette smokers.

Gastrointestinal Pathology 9

CONTENTS

The gastrointestinal (GI) tract includes the tubular GI tract (which extends from the mouth to the anus) as well as the salivary glands, the liver and biliary tract, and the exocrine pancreas. The tubular GI tract has a common organizational structure that is important for understanding its normal function and pathologic changes.

The interactions of the GI mucosa with commensal bacteria in the gut lumen are essential for the maintenance of normal mucosal homeostasis, the production of some nutrients, and the enterohepatic circulation of bile. This relationship is complex, and the interaction of microorganisms with innate immune receptors on mucosal cells (including Toll-like receptors) appears to be essential for the development and maintenance of normal large and small intestinal mucosa.

● ● ● ORAL CAVITY

The oral cavity is lined by nonkeratinizing squamous mucosa and is bathed in secretions from both major and minor salivary glands. The oral mucosa is susceptible to most of the same types of inflammatory and neoplastic processes as the skin.

ANATOMY

Functional Anatomy of the Tubular GI Tract

The GI tract is lined by specialized squamous and glandular epithelia. The mucosal layer is composed of specialized squamous or glandular epithelium that overlies the lamina propria (loose connective tissue and resident chronic inflammatory cells). Underlying the mucosa is a thin muscularis mucosa that separates it from the submucosa composed of adipose tissue, vessels, and nerves. All these structures are surrounded by a muscularis propria composed of two layers of smooth muscle.

The GI tract has an intrinsic nervous system that controls peristalsis (rhythmic contractions that move food and fecal material through the GI tract) with both a submucosal and intermyenteric plexus of nerves and ganglia.

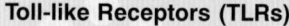

BIOCHEMISTRY

Toll-like Receptors (TLRs)

TLRs are a family (10 members) of innate immune receptors that recognize a variety of exogenous products (mainly bacterial products although the ligands for some TLRs have not been identified). Most TLRs signal by recruiting intracellular proteins MyD88 and IRAK to activate the NFκB signaling pathway and promote the expression of proinflammatory genes. TLRs appear to play a role in many disease processes (e.g., atherosclerosis) by increasing baseline inflammatory activity.

- TLR2 binds peptidoglycans, lipoproteins, glycopeptides, and lipopolysaccharide (LPS).
- TLR3 binds double-stranded RNA produced by viruses.
- TLR4 binds lipopolysaccharide LPS.
- TLR5 binds flagellin.
- TLR9 binds DNA (CpG), which is present in all bacteria.
- TLR1 and 6 act as cofactors for TLR2.

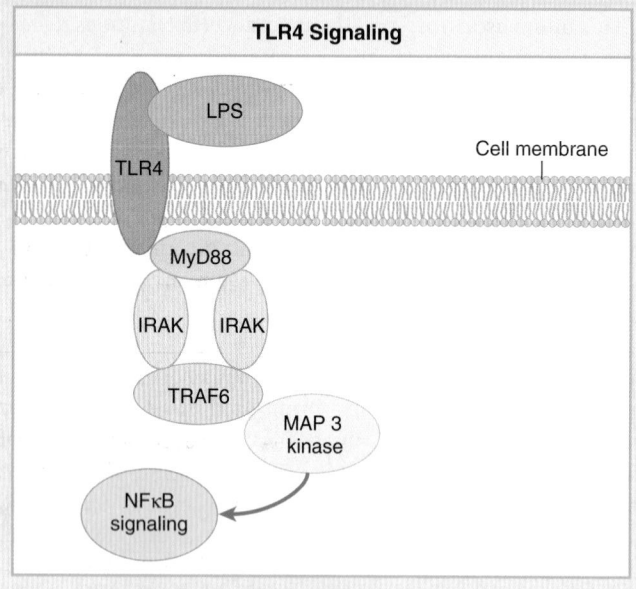

TLR4 Signaling

Inflammatory Conditions

Aphthous ulcers are small, discrete ulcerations of oral squamous mucosa that can be caused by multiple insults including different types of food as well as viral infection. They are typically self-limited but may be an indication of underlying systemic disease. More severe and painful ulcers can be caused by reactivation of herpes simplex virus type 1 or 2. *Lichen planus* is a chronic inflammatory process that can involve the skin or squamous mucosa of the oral cavity with a characteristic linear (band-like) chronic inflammatory cell infiltrate (see Chapter 6).

Tumors

The predominant tumor of the oral cavity is *squamous cell carcinoma*, which is strongly associated with tobacco use (smoking and smokeless tobacco) and high alcohol consumption. Epithelial dysplasia usually precedes the development of invasive squamous cell carcinoma. *Leukoplakia* is a clinical term referring to white patches in the oral squamous mucosa that correspond to acanthosis (thickening of the squamous mucosa) and hyperkeratosis or parakeratosis. Leukoplakia can result from inflammatory or reactive conditions but can also be a sign of epithelial dysplasia and squamous cell carcinoma. Invasive squamous cell carcinomas are characterized as keratinizing or nonkeratinizing, and different lymph nodes are at risk for metastasis depending on the location of the primary tumor. Squamous cell carcinoma of the oropharynx can present with metastatic disease in cervical lymph nodes before the primary tumor is identified.

●●● SALIVARY GLANDS

In addition to the major salivary glands (the seromucous parotid gland and the serous submandibular gland), innumerable minor salivary glands are present in the oral cavity and oropharynx. These small glands are composed of a few acini that drain via small ducts into the oral cavity and oropharynx.

Lithiasis

Stones can develop in the ducts of major and minor salivary glands, resulting in obstruction and inflammation. Prolonged obstruction results in atrophy, fibrosis, and destruction of glandular parenchyma (i.e., loss of acinar tissue). Mechanical trauma to minor salivary glands can disrupt individual glands, resulting in the formation of so-called mucoceles, which consist of inflammatory reactions to extravasated mucin from the ruptured minor salivary glands.

Sjögren's Syndrome

Patients with Sjögren's syndrome have an autoimmune disease that results in a chronic inflammatory reaction in their salivary and lacrimal glands that can ultimately result in the atrophy and loss of function of these glands, causing xerostomia (dry mouth) and xerophthalmia (dry eyes). The inflammatory cell infiltrate is composed predominantly of CD4+ T cells, but B cells are also present and may be prominent. Most patients have antinuclear antibodies that react with ribonucleoproteins (RNPs) SS-A(Ro) and SS-B(La). B cells frequently infiltrate the salivary gland epithelium to form lymphoepithelial lesions (small clusters of two to four B cells within the epithelium). The B-cell infiltrate is frequently monoclonal and shows features similar to MALT lymphomas in other organs (see below). This lymphoproliferative process usually remains localized to the salivary gland, but these patients are at risk for transformation to a high-grade B-cell lymphoma.

Tumors

Multiple benign and malignant tumors can arise in the major and minor salivary glands. *Pleomorphic adenoma* is the most common tumor of the major salivary glands. Pleomorphic adenoma is a tumor of myoepithelial cells that has a markedly varied microscopic appearance (Fig. 9-1A). The vast majority of pleomorphic adenomas are benign, although they can recur as multiple foci if they are ruptured during surgical excision. Rarely, recurrent tumors may undergo malignant transformation (so called carcinoma ex pleomorphic adenoma). *Warthin's tumor* is a benign neoplasm of the major salivary glands that is composed of oncocytic epithelium associated with dense lymphoid stroma (see Fig. 9-1B). Warthin's tumor results from the proliferation of oncocytic salivary gland epithelium within lymph nodes in the salivary gland.

Malignant tumors of the major and minor salivary glands include adenoid cystic carcinoma, mucoepidermoid carcinoma, and polymorphous low-grade carcinoma. All these neoplasms have characteristic morphologic features with glandular differentiation or a mixture of glandular and squamous differentiation. Acinic cell carcinoma arises from acinar cells and usually retains their characteristic cytoplasmic granularity. These tumors usually behave as low-grade malignancies that tend to invade locally and metastasize late. Malignant salivary gland tumors often present as painless masses although parotid tumors may cause facial nerve paralysis or pain. Perineural invasion is common in adenoid cystic carcinomas, and this mode of spread may allow tumor to extend directly into the central nervous system along cranial nerves. The primary treatment for all these tumors is surgical excision.

⬤⬤⬤ ESOPHAGUS

The esophagus is lined by nonkeratinizing squamous mucosa similarly to the oral cavity. Its wall contains well-developed muscle layers that propel swallowed food from the mouth into the stomach. The lower esophageal sphincter normally prevents reflux of gastric contents into the esophagus. Disorders of esophageal motility or strictures within the esophagus can result in difficulty in swallowing (*dysphagia*). *Achalasia* is a condition in which there is incomplete relaxation of the lower esophageal sphincter that results in functional esophageal obstruction.

Varices

Patients with portal hypertension (usually secondary to hepatic cirrhosis) develop abnormal dilated veins to bypass the obstruction to portal venous return. The esophagus is often prominently affected by this vascular ectasia (varices). Esophageal varices are usually located close to the mucosal surface and can be traumatized by swallowed food, resulting in massive bleeding into the GI tract. Rupture of esophageal varices can be a late and fatal complication of chronic alcoholism (Fig. 9-2A).

Infections

The squamous mucosa of the esophagus can be infected by fungal organisms such as *Candida albicans* (see Fig. 9-2B) and by viruses such as herpes simplex or cytomegalovirus (CMV). These infections are much more common in immunocompromised patients and can cause severe pain and dysphagia.

Gastroesophageal Reflux Disease and Barrett's Esophagus

Gastroesophageal reflux disease (GERD) results from the reflux of gastric contents into the tubular esophagus. This can occur as a result of abnormal function of the lower esophageal sphincter or in association with a hiatal hernia when a portion of the stomach is herniated through the dia-

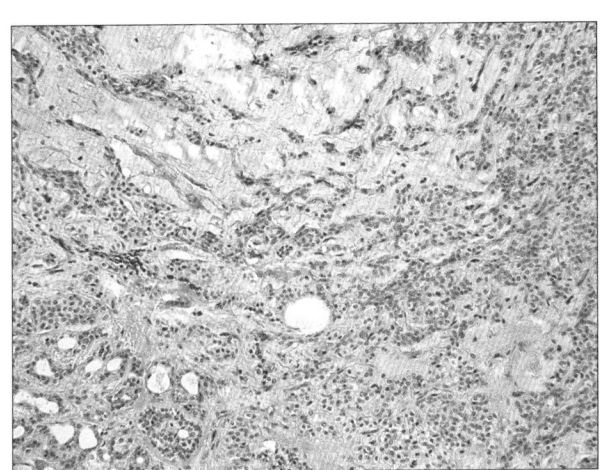

A

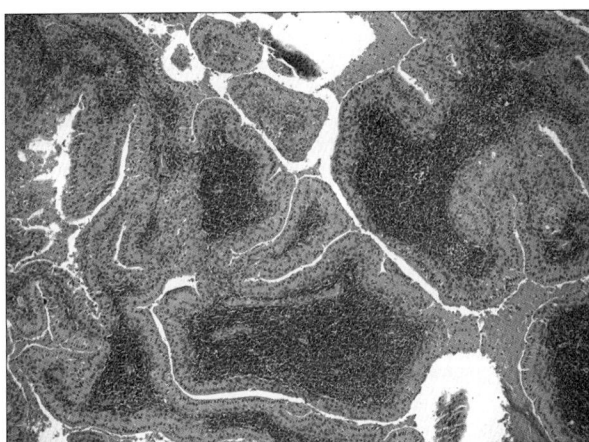

B

Figure 9-1. A, Pleomorphic adenoma. Microscopic section showing typical chondroid matrix with clusters of myoepithelial cells. The morphologic pattern of pleomorphic adenoma is as variable as its name implies. Some lesions closely resemble hyaline cartilage while others are much more densely cellular with little or no chondroid matrix. **B**, Warthin's tumor. Microscopic section showing dense lymphoid stroma with germinal centers lined by a layer of well-organized columnar cells with granular eosinophilic cytoplasm.

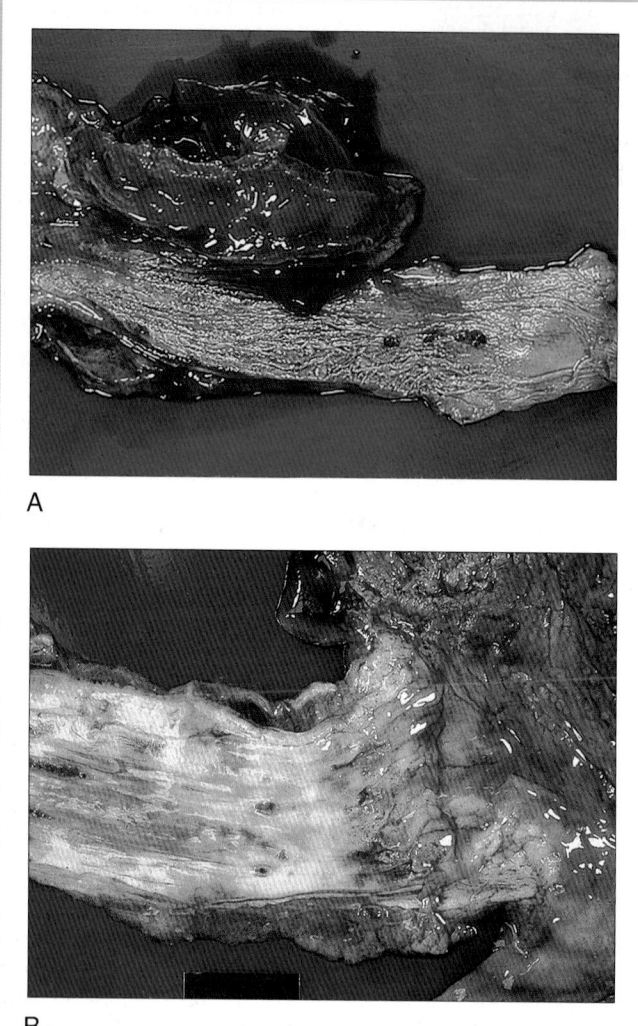

A

B

Figure 9-2. A, Ruptured esophageal varices. Gross photograph of an esophagus with ruptured and thrombosed variceal blood vessels resulting from portal hypertension in hepatic cirrhosis. **B**, Candidal esophagitis. Gross photograph of an esophagus from an immunosuppressed patient with severe candidal esophagitis. Exudate is adherent to the surface, and there is focal ulceration of the squamous mucosa. The gastroesophageal junction is visible near the bottom.

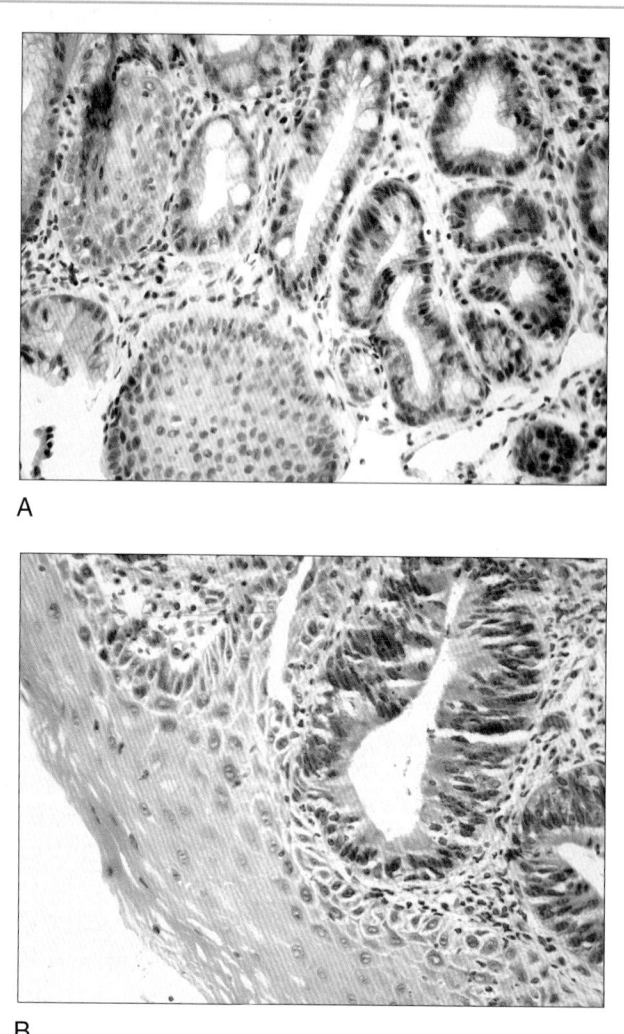

A

B

Figure 9-3. A, Barrett's esophagus. Microscopic section showing squamous mucosa abutting glandular mucosa with conspicuous goblet cells (diagnostic of intestinal metaplasia). Acute and chronic inflammation is present with reactive epithelial changes, but no dysplasia is evident. **B**, High-grade dysplasia in Barrett's esophagus. Microscopic section showing dysplastic glands beneath squamous mucosa. There is a marked increase in the nuclear:cytoplasmic ratio and no evidence of surface maturation. Goblet cells are no longer present in these dysplastic metaplastic cells (owing to mucin depletion).

phragm. The presence of acidic gastric contents in the esophagus results in a marked inflammatory reaction. This is initially manifested by intramucosal eosinophils and may progress to ulceration.

Prolonged reflux can result in metaplasia of the gastric mucosa from squamous to glandular similar to that in the small intestine. This type of metaplasia is referred to as Barrett's esophagus and is characterized by the presence of intestinal type goblet cells (Fig. 9-3A). Once specialized columnar epithelium is present in the tubular esophagus, it usually persists throughout life and may extend to involve the proximal esophagus. This metaplastic epithelium is at increased risk for transformation into adenocarcinoma, usually preceded by dysplasia.

Tumors

Squamous cell carcinoma of the esophagus is strongly associated with the same risk factors as oral cancer (smoking and heavy alcohol consumption). These tumors usually present with dysphagia, and lymph node metastases are frequently present at diagnosis. A significant proportion of these tumors show amplification of the cyclin D proto-oncogene that drives cellular proliferation through activation of cyclin-dependent kinase 4 (CDK-4). Squamous cell carcinoma is relatively common in some geographic areas outside the United States and may be associated with human papillomavirus (HPV) and/or environmental/nutritional factors in endemic areas.

Adenocarcinomas of the esophagus tend to develop in the lower portion of the esophagus in areas involved by intestinal metaplasia (Barrett's esophagus). Epithelial dysplasia usually precedes the development of invasive adenocarcinoma by months or years so that monitoring of Barrett's epithelium by serial endoscopic biopsy is usually employed to identify patients at highest risk for invasive adenocarcinoma (see Fig. 9-3B). Endoscopic ablation of high-grade dysplasia may delay or prevent the development of an invasive adeno-carcinoma. Once invasive adenocarcinoma develops, lymph node metastases can develop rapidly, rendering the tumor incurable by surgery.

●●●● STOMACH

The stomach is a receptacle for food that initiates digestion with pepsin and mechanically mixes food prior to emptying it into the duodenum. The stomach also helps kill ingested microorganisms by exposing them to gastric acid. Gastric dysmotility can result from nerve dysfunction in the setting of diabetic neuropathy (gastroparesis), and patients with long-standing diabetes may have markedly delayed gastric empty-ing with symptoms referable to retention of food in the stomach.

HISTOLOGY

Functional Gastric Anatomy

The stomach is composed of three major regions histologically: the gastric cardia (proximal), fundus (body), and antrum (pyloric, distal) all of which of have prominent depressions in their mucosa, which are known as foveolae (gastric pits). The base of each gastric pit receives several gastric glands, named for the region of the stomach housing them. These glands possess mucus-secreting cells that provide a protective layer to shield the gastric mucosa from luminal acid.

- The gastric body (fundus) contains chief cells (zymogenenic) and parietal (acid-producing) cells that are responsible for the acid and pepsin secretion. Chief cells have basophilic cytoplasm while parietal cells have granular eosinophilic cytoplasm because of their numerous mitochondria.
- The gastric cardia is a narrow zone of oxyntic mucosa that adjoins the tubular esophagus.
- The antrum contains mucus and neuroendocrine cells, which produce gastrin, but it does not contain chief cells.

Scattered neuroendocrine cells are present in the mucosa in all portions of the stomach and act to transduce hormonal signals (e.g., gastrin-secreting cells in the antrum stimulate enterochromaffin-like [ECL] cells in the body to produce histamine, which triggers acid secretion by parietal cells). The muscular wall at the gastric outlet in the pylorus is thickened and forms a functional sphincter that controls gastric emptying into the duodenum.

Acute Gastritis

Acute gastritis is an acute inflammatory reaction in the gastric mucosa that is often transient and self-limited (Fig. 9-4A). Acute gastritis can by caused by nonsteroidal anti-inflammatory drugs, heavy alcohol consumption, and other systemic diseases that predispose to a breakdown of the protective mucous layer (e.g., increased corticosteroid secretion by the adrenal gland can cause stress ulcers). Conditions that result in excessive acid secretion can also result in acute gastritis. If gastric acid breaks through the protective mucous layer, gastric epithelial cells are directly injured, initiating a superficial acute inflammatory reaction. Superficial mucosal erosions are usually self-limited pro-cesses that heal without sequelae. If the inciting cause of the erosion persists, however, deeper extension of the inflam-mation or necrosis can lead to the formation of a chronic peptic ulcer.

Chronic Gastritis

Chronic gastritis is a persistent inflammatory reaction in the gastric mucosa that is characterized by the accumulation of lymphocytes and plasma cells in the lamina propria. Chronic active gastritis implies that ongoing active inflammation is causing damage to epithelial cells. On gastric biopsy, chronic active gastritis shows acute inflammatory cells infiltrating gastric epithelium in addition to a chronic inflammatory cell infiltrate in the lamina propria (see Fig. 9-4B). By far the most common cause of chronic gastritis in the United States is chronic bacterial infection of the stomach by *Helicobacter pylori* (see Fig. 9-4C). *H. pylori* is adapted to live in the low pH environment of the gastric lumen, and infection is com-mon and often persists throughout life unless it is eradicated by treatment with antibiotics (often a combination of three antibiotics is employed).

H. pylori initiates a chronic immunoreaction that usually results in the formation of germinal centers in the gastric mucosa (antrum and fundus). While the bulk of organisms remain extracellular in the mucous layer adherent to gastric mucosa, the ongoing immunoreaction results in persistent acute and chronic inflammation with ongoing injury to the gastric epithelium. Over time, infection can result in meta-plasia of the gastric mucosa to small intestinal type mucosa or loss of specialized gastric epithelium (atrophy). Some strains of *Helicobacter* are associated with a more intense immune response, but host factors are probably also important. Eradication of the bacterium usually terminates the chronic gastritis but does not result in the regeneration of normal mucosa if atrophy has developed. Chronic *Helicobacter* gastritis and the resulting oxygen free radicals and inflammatory mediators predispose to the development of adenocarcinoma that can arise in metaplastic gastric mucosa.

Chronic gastritis can also result from autoimmune gastritis (e.g., pernicious anemia) that specifically destroys parietal cells and can ultimately result in gastric atrophy with the loss of all acid-producing parietal cells. Since the stomach is no

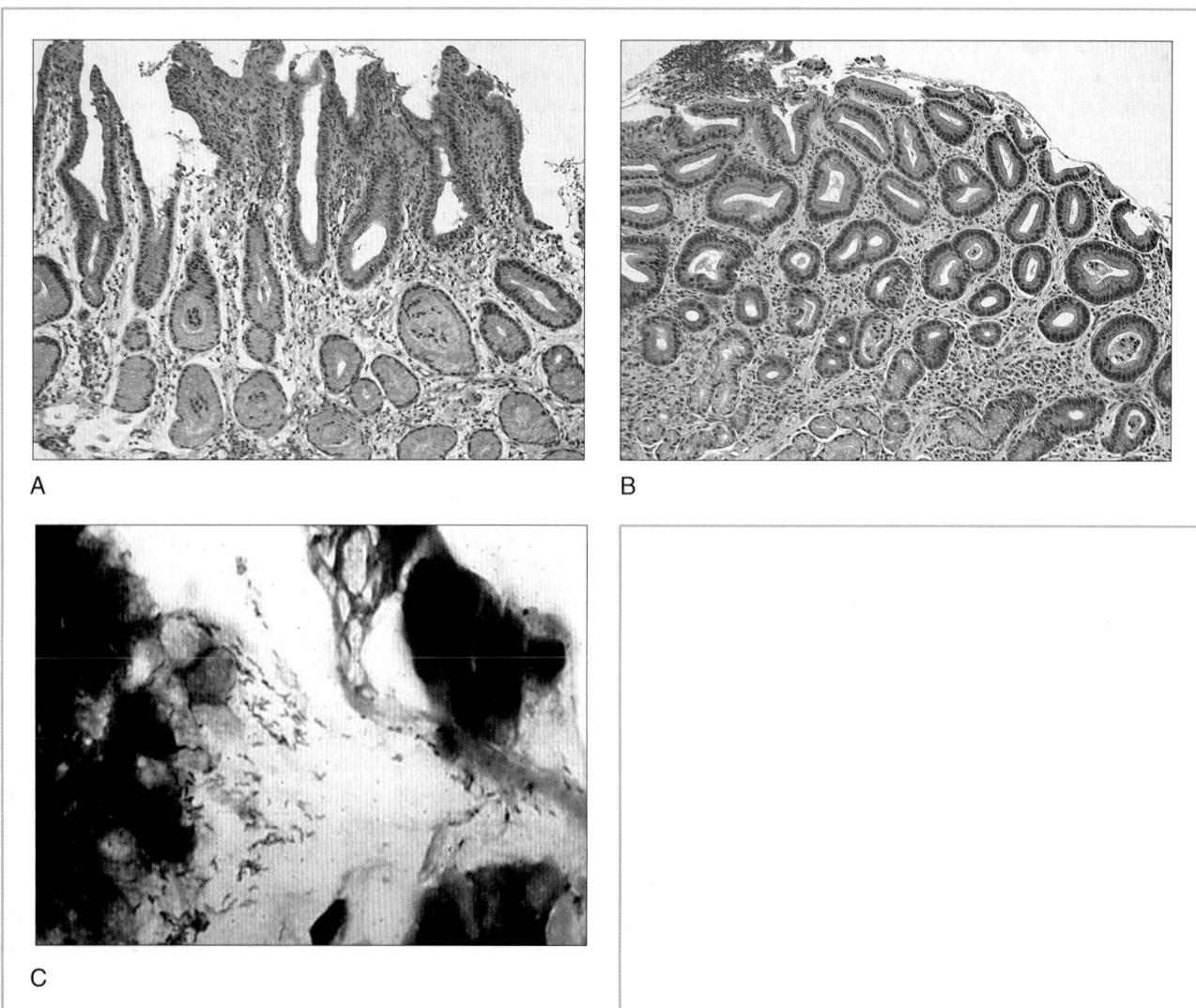

Figure 9-4. A, Acute gastritis. Microscopic section showing antral gastric mucosa with superficial acute inflammation. Significant chronic inflammation is not present. **B**, Chronic active gastritis. Microscopic section of gastric mucosa showing a dense chronic inflammatory cell infiltrate in the lamina propria and focal infiltration of gastric glands by neutrophils. **C**, *H. pylori* gastritis. Microscopic section of superficial gastric mucosa stained with a modified Giemsa stain. *Helicobacter* organisms (bacterial rods with a "gull wing" shape) are evident in the mucus adherent to gastric epithelial cells.

longer acidified, gastrin levels increase markedly in an attempt to stimulate acid secretion. High gastrin levels drive the hyperplasia of neuroendocrine cells in the gastric mucosa. Neuroendocrine hyperplasia is very prominent in pernicious anemia and may form microscopic neuroendocrine tumors (microcarcinoids). Neuroendocrine hyperplasia can also result from other forms of chronic gastritis but is usually much less severe.

Peptic Ulcer

Peptic ulcer disease consists of deep ulcers of the stomach or first portion of the duodenum that are caused by the action of gastric acid and proteolytic enzymes. There is a strong association between the formation of peptic ulcers and

H. pylori infection and chronic gastritis. Extensive damage to the gastric mucosa allows access of acid and pepsin to the deeper layers of the stomach that can lead to the incremental enlargement of an ulcer (Fig. 9-5). Chronic ulcers can erode through the entire wall of the stomach, resulting in perforation and release of gastric contents into the peritoneal cavity to cause peritonitis. Conversely, erosion of an ulcer into blood vessels in the gastric wall can result in chronic or massive GI hemorrhage.

Peptic ulcers are typically managed by reducing acid secretion with H_2 antagonists or in the case of intractable ulcers by surgical excision of the antrum and transection of the vagus nerves (to diminish the stimulus for acid production in the residual stomach). Gastric ulcers can also be produced by carcinomas, and careful endoscopic evaluation of gastric ulcers with biopsy is essential to detect ulcerating adenocarcinomas.

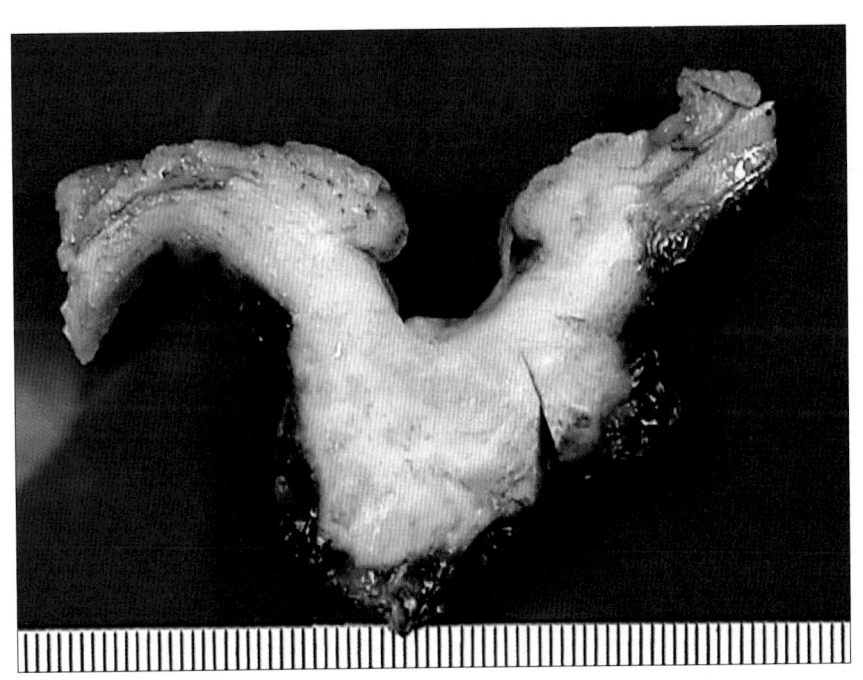

Figure 9-5. Chronic gastric ulcer. Gross cross-section of stomach showing a deeply excavated ulcer with associated fibrosis replacing muscularis propria and extending to the serosal surface.

Zollinger-Ellison Syndrome

Some patients with intractable peptic ulcers have Zollinger-Ellison syndrome, which results from the abnormal secretion of the hormone gastrin either from a neuroendocrine tumor of the pancreas or from hyperplastic gastrin-producing cells in the stomach. Gastrin stimulation of parietal cells results in very high levels of acid secretion, which can overwhelm normal mucosal defenses, leading to ulceration.

Tumors

Mucosal polyps can develop in the stomach as reactive conditions or as neoplastic processes similar to adenomatous polyps of the colon. Hyperplastic polyps are reactive in nature and correspond to thickening and hyperplasia of the mucosa. Fundic gland polyps correspond to dilatation of fundic glands. The vast majority of fundic polyps are benign but they can be dysplastic. Fundic polyps are common in patients with familial polyposis but also occur sporadically. Adenomatous polyps can be precursors of adenocarcinoma, but most gastric cancers in the United States are not associated with these precursor lesions.

MALT Lymphoma

Lymphomas also can develop as a result of chronic antigenic stimulation in the setting of chronic *Helicobacter* gastritis. These neoplasms are usually low-grade lymphomas called MALT lymphomas (i.e., lymphomas of mucosa-associated lymphoid tissue). Chronic antigenic stimulation of B lymphocytes by *H. pylori* is thought to favor expansion of B-cell clones that recognize bacterial antigens and that may eventually become independent of antigenic stimulation (by autocrine growth or resistance to apoptosis). In some cases of early gastric MALT lymphoma, eradication of *H. pylori* results in regression of the "lymphoma," suggesting that these are transitional lymphoproliferative lesions that have not acquired the ability to proliferate with complete autonomy. Some MALT lymphomas transform to diffuse large-cell lymphomas of the stomach.

Carcinoma

Two distinct types of gastric adenocarcinoma are recognized. The intestinal type usually develops in the setting of chronic *H. pylori* gastritis in mucosa that has undergone intestinal metaplasia (Figs. 9-6A and 9-6B). These tumors typically form a localized mass composed of glandular elements that secrete intestinal type mucin. Smaller, localized tumors are often cured by surgery, but most gastric adenocarcinomas present at relatively high stage. As with most adult solid tumors, the stage at diagnosis is the dominant prognostic factor. The incidence of gastric adenocarcinoma is much higher in Japan than in United States, and screening of asymptomatic individuals by endoscopy has been employed in Japan to detect tumors at an early stage, when most are curable by local surgical excision.

The diffuse form of gastric adenocarcinoma usually thickens the gastric wall without forming a discrete mass lesion. Diffuse infiltration by tumor cells produces the so-called "leather bottle" appearance of the stomach. Diffuse tumors are composed predominantly or exclusively of signet ring cells, which contain large mucin droplets that characteristically displace and indent their nucleus (see Fig. 9-6C). Signet ring cells are often cytologically bland and tend to invade the gastric wall as single cells without an associated

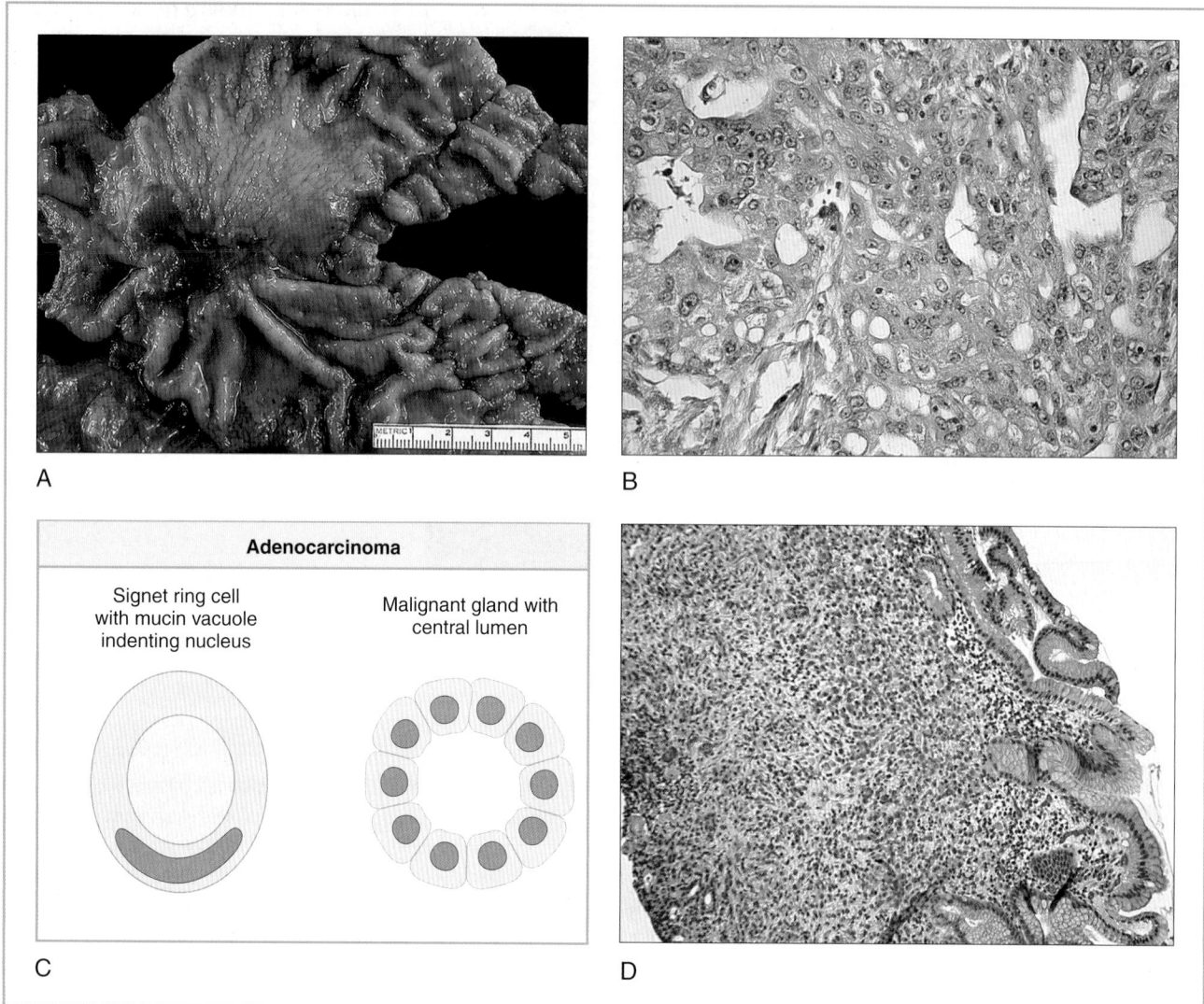

Figure 9-6. **A**, Gastric adenocarcinoma. Gross photograph of stomach with a central tumor that obliterates normal rugal folds. **B**, Intestinal type gastric adenocarcinoma. Microscopic section showing a poorly differentiated adenocarcinoma composed of irregular glands with an associated desmoplastic stromal reaction. **C**, Glandular and signet ring cell patterns in adenocarcinoma. **D**, Diffuse type gastric adenocarcinoma. Microscopic section showing diffuse replacement of gastric mucosa by a poorly differentiated carcinoma that infiltrates as single cells with signet ring morphology.

desmoplastic stromal response, making them difficult to recognize in endoscopic biopsy specimens (see Fig. 9-6D). Signet ring cells do not express E-cadherin protein and so are not capable of forming normal cell-cell junctions, rendering them poorly cohesive. The loss of E-cadherin protein expression also results in constitutive activation of Wnt signaling, which helps drive tumor cell proliferation. Signet ring cell tumors often permeate vascular and perineural spaces and are usually high stage at presentation with lymph node or distant metastases. Signet ring cell tumors frequently present with metastatic foci at distant sites including the ovary (Krukenberg's tumor) and other organs.

GIST

Gastrointestinal stromal tumors (GISTs) are rare, distinctive stromal (spindle cell) tumors that occur in the muscularis propria of the intestines and stomach. GISTs may result in

ulceration of overlying gastric mucosa. Gastric GISTs are usually low-grade tumors that remain localized and rarely metastasize, whereas GISTs of the small intestine are more aggressive (see below).

●●● SMALL AND LARGE INTESTINE

The primary function of the small intestine is food absorption, and its specialized villous architecture creates a large, absorptive surface area. Some portions of the small intestine have specialized receptors (e.g., a portion of the terminal ileum binds intrinsic factor secreted by parietal cells in the stomach to absorb vitamin B_{12}). Dysfunction of the small intestine can lead to malabsorption of nutrients but can also cause diarrhea, since passage of undigested food materials (particularly fats) into the large intestine results in abnormal bacterial proliferation. The large intestine functions predominantly to resorb water to create formed stool. Dysfunction of the large intestine results predominantly in diarrhea with associated fluid loss.

Celiac Disease

Celiac disease (also called sprue and protein-losing enteropathy) is an inflammatory process that results in atrophy of small intestinal villi to cause malabsorption. Patients with celiac disease have an abnormal immunoreaction to components of gluten, a protein that is present in wheat and wheat by-products. T-cell infiltration of the small intestinal epithelium (CD8$^+$ T cells) results in damage to the epithelium with flattening of normal villous architecture that markedly decreases absorptive surface area. Patients tend to have diarrhea and varying levels of malabsorption. Celiac disease is strongly associated with specific HLA class II alleles (particularly HLA-DQA1*0501 and DQB1*0201), which can effectively bind and present gluten breakdown products to CD4$^+$ cells present in the lamina propria. These CD4$^+$ T cells produce cytokines that drive crypt hyperplasia and activate the CD8$^+$ effector T cells in the epithelium.

Removal of gluten from their diet results in remission of disease in most patients, but even small amounts of gluten can cause disease recurrence. Some patients with mild forms of celiac disease may remain undiagnosed. The presence of antigliadin and antiendomysial antibodies in patient sera is helpful in establishing a diagnosis of sprue in concert with biopsy of the small intestine. Patients with chronic celiac disease are at increased risk for the rare complication of T-cell lymphoma of the small intestine.

Obstruction

Intestinal obstruction can result from blockage by luminal contents (such as occurs in cystic fibrosis of the pancreas), from tumor masses in the wall or mucosa of the intestine, and from extrinsic mechanical compression related to serosal adhesions, hernias, volvulus, and intussusception (Fig. 9-7). Serosal fibrosis and adhesions (from prior surgery or intra-abdominal trauma) can result in transient or fixed small intestinal obstruction. Herniation of small intestine into an inguinal or umbilical hernia can also result in obstructive or ischemic complications. Volvulus is a condition in which the intestine twists upon its own mesentery, causing luminal obstruction and frequently vascular compromise that can result in ischemia or infarction. In cases of intussusception, the intestinal wall herniates within its own lumen, causing obstructive and ischemic complications. Intestinal tumors can predispose to intussusception.

Ischemic Colitis

The arteries penetrating the muscular wall of the small and large intestine are functional end arteries that arise from the arcuate circulation in the mesentery. Obstruction of these perforating arteries usually results in segmental intestinal

IMMUNOLOGY

Antigliadin and Antiendomysial Antibodies

Gluten is a family of proteins present in the endosperm of cereal grains including wheat, rye, and barley. Minute amounts of gluten are present in oats.

Gliadin is a protein subfraction of gluten that is 16 to 40 kDa in size. Up to 50 different protein components may be present in gliadin. Gliadin can induce an immune response in susceptible individuals, causing celiac disease. Gliadins are divided into four fractions by molecular weight: α, β, γ, and ω.

Detection of serum antibodies against gliadin is suggestive of celiac disease but is not very sensitive or specific. IgA antibodies usually appear early and disappear rapidly if gluten is removed from the diet. IgG antibodies appear later and tend to persist even if gluten is withdrawn.

Serum IgA antiendomysial antibodies are a more sensitive and specific biomarker for celiac disease than antigliadin antibodies. Antiendomysial antibodies can be detected with an immuno-fluorescence assay using the muscular wall of the esophagus (endomysium) as a substrate for testing patient sera. Antiendomysial antibodies react with the enzyme transglutaminase, which is also expressed in intestinal epithelial cells and normally catalyzes the deamidation of gliadin proteins. Deamidated gliadin may be more effectively presented by the MHC class II alleles and strongly predispose to celiac disease.

IgA antibodies against tissue transglutaminase (tTG) are now the gold standard for the serologic diagnosis of celiac disease and dermatitis herpetiformis.

ischemia or infarction. The intestinal mucosa is much more metabolically active than the other layers so that ischemia affects the mucosa first and most severely. Mucosal ischemia can result in GI hemorrhage with mucosal ulceration. Endoscopic biopsies tend to show relatively characteristic features with "withering" of crypts and superficial necrosis (Fig. 9-8A) or formation of a pseudomembrane (see below). More prolonged or severe ischemia results in transmural necrosis, which usually is fatal unless the involved segment is surgically removed. Release of atheroemboli into the systemic circulation from atherosclerotic plaques or aneurysms can cause multifocal intestinal infarction. Atherosclerosis of the inferior and superior mesenteric arteries can result in chronic ischemia or acute infarction of the small and large intestine. Systemic hypotension can result in ischemia of watershed areas.

Infection

Many different types of viral and bacterial infection can result in colitis and diarrhea. Various viruses including rotavirus and adenovirus can cause viral gastroenteritis. Most viral infections produce transient diarrhea that heals without sequelae. Cytomegalovirus can produce chronic diarrhea, usually in immunodeficient patients (e.g., patients with HIV or undergoing cancer treatment).

Bacteria produce intestinal disease depending on their ability to (1) adhere to intestinal mucosal cells (to prevent

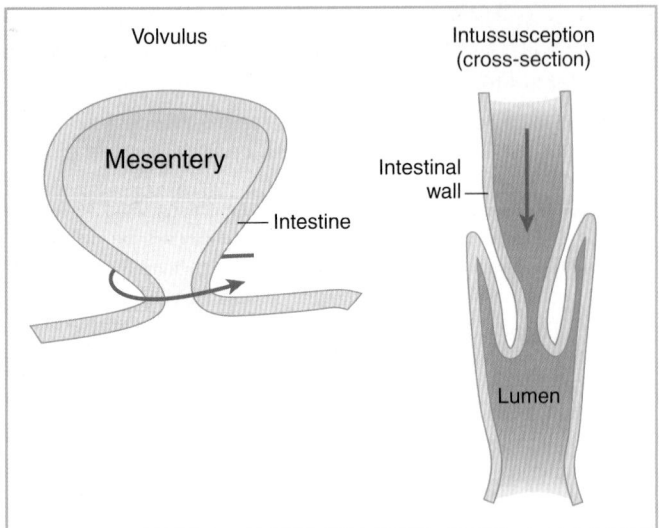

Figure 9-7. Intestinal obstruction. Schematic illustrations of volvulus and intussusception.

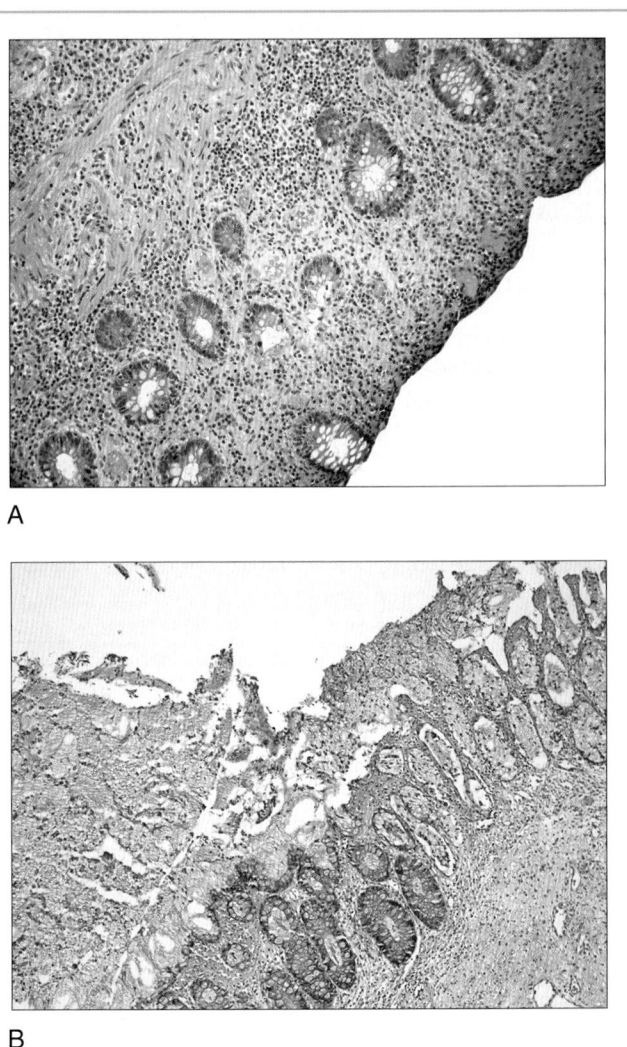

Figure 9-8. A, Ischemic colitis. Microscopic section of colon showing surface ulceration and "withering" crypts with associated mixed inflammatory infiltrate. **B,** Pseudomembranous colitis. Microscopic section of colon showing focal mucosal necrosis with an adherent pseudomembrane composed of mucin and necrotic cellular debris. A mixed inflammatory cell infiltrate is present in intact mucosa.

their removal by the fecal stream), (2) produce toxins, and (3) invade through the mucosal barrier to produce systemic infection. Most forms of bacterial gastroenteritis are spread via the oral-fecal route. Some bacterial food poisoning can result from the ingestion of preformed bacterial toxins (i.e., viable bacteria need not be present to cause disease). *Vibrio cholerae* is a noninvasive pathogen that results in a purely secretory diarrhea from toxin-mediated stimulation of adenylate cyclase in intestinal epithelium. Cholera typically results in massive fluid loss leading to shock unless fluids are effectively replaced.

Gram-negative bacterial pathogens including subtypes of enteropathogenic *Escherichia coli* can result in diarrhea that is largely secretory (secondary to the elaboration of toxins) but also have the potential to produce invasive infection with septicemia.

Shigella is a minimally invasive pathogen that usually produces bloody diarrhea by invading intestinal mucosa but in general does not cause systemic infection or involvement of mesenteric lymph nodes. *Salmonella typhi* and *Yersinia enterocolitica* are more invasive pathogens that frequently involve the full thickness of the intestinal wall as well as mesenteric lymph nodes and may produce septicemia.

Parasites (tapeworm and round worm) can cause diarrhea, malabsorption, and GI hemorrhage. *Giardia lamblia* is a protozoan microorganism that can reside in the small intestinal lumen and cause chronic watery diarrhea without producing invasive infection. *Cryptosporidium* and *Microsporidium* are protozoa that can produce diarrhea only in immunocompromised patients.

Pseudomembranous Colitis

Alterations in the normal intestinal flora induced by antibiotic therapy can cause diarrhea. Killing of commensal bacteria by antibiotics allows the expansion of resistant microorganisms that can cause disease. *Clostridium difficile*

colonizes many hospital patients and nursing home residents, and antibiotic treatment can allow it to proliferate in the intestinal tract. Toxin produced by *C. difficile* causes pseudomembranous colitis with mucosal necrosis and severe bloody diarrhea. A shaggy gray-green exudate is adherent to the mucosal surface and is composed of mucin and necrotic cellular debris (see Fig. 9-8B). While pseudomembranous colitis is typical in *C. difficile* infection, this pattern can be produced by ischemia and other infectious or inflammatory insults.

Inflammatory Bowel Disease

Inflammatory bowel disease (IBD) is a chronic inflammatory condition that primarily affects the large or small intestine

MICROBIOLOGY

Vibrio cholerae

V. cholerae is a gram-negative curved rod that is a γ-proteobacterium. It colonizes the gut by adhering to villous absorptive cells via filaments.

Cholera toxin is a peptide toxin secreted by *V. cholerae* that activates adenylate cyclase in enterocytes, resulting in increased cytoplasmic cAMP levels that trigger secretion of sodium, potassium, bicarbonate, and chloride, resulting in passive loss of water. Cholera causes severe dehydration and salt loss from diarrhea that rapidly can be fatal unless fluids are replaced. Fluid replacement can be accomplished intravenously; however, consumption of a mixture of salts and glucose that takes advantage of a glucose/sodium cotransport protein in enterocytes is also highly effective. This simple treatment can be effectively employed in developing countries, where it is lifesaving.

MICROBIOLOGY

Enteropathogenic *Escherichia coli*

Enteropathogenic *E. coli* (EPEC) is a major cause of severe and persistent diarrhea in infants in the developing world. EPEC infection typically produces so-called attaching and effacing lesions (A/E lesions) in the intestine that destroy the normal epithelial brush border, resulting in diminished absorptive surface. Enterohemorrhagic *E. coli*, which is the causative agent of hemolytic uremic syndrome (HUS), also produces A/E lesions. All four genes needed to produce A/E lesions are encoded in a single 35-kb DNA segment.

Initial EPEC adhesion to enterocytes is mediated by pili and is followed by secretion of bacterial proteins. Some of these proteins are delivered directly into the cytoplasm of host enterocytes (type III secretion) and induce signal transduction in these host cells. Intimin, which is present on the surface of EPEC, then forms a tight junction with the enterocyte membrane. Bacterial proteins disassemble the enterocyte cytoskeleton and redistribute its cytoplasmic actin to the bacterial attachment site, resulting in the loss of microvilli. The ensuing loss of functional absorptive surface can result in osmotic diarrhea.

(or both). Two forms are distinguished: Crohn's disease and ulcerative colitis (UC). Most patients have clinical and pathologic findings that are typical of either one, but a minority have intermediate clinical features (so-called indeterminate colitis). Intestinal inflammation tends to spontaneously wax and wane over the course of weeks to months in most patients with chronic IBD. The advent of highly effective anti-inflammatory therapies over the last 15 years has significantly modified the severity of disease symptoms and the nature of disease progression in many but not all patients. Some patients have intractable disease that requires surgical intervention.

Ulcerative Colitis

UC typically involves the large intestine and causes homogeneous and contiguous involvement of the large intestine from the anus proximally. The inflammatory process may terminate at any point in the large intestine (Fig. 9-9A). Involvement of the small intestine is exceptional in UC except for "backwash ileitis," which may affect the most distal portion of the ileum (see Fig. 9-9B). Backwash ileitis is observed only in patients who have cecal involvement and is thought to represent a bystander effect in which luminal inflammatory exudate in the cecum injures adjacent ileal mucosa. UC is not associated with skip areas (areas of normal mucosa between areas affected by IBD), and the presence of skip areas in a colon constitutes strong evidence against a diagnosis of UC.

The inflammatory process in UC tends to involve the mucosa predominantly and is usually associated with extensive cryptitis (neutrophils invading crypt epithelium) with the formation of crypt abscesses (collections of neutrophils within the lumina of crypts) (see Fig. 9-9C). Mucosal ulceration is common, but severe inflammation of the submucosa or muscularis propria is less common than in Crohn's disease. Ulcerative colitis tends to result in diffuse contiguous alterations of the large intestinal mucosa with the formation of pseudopolyps (residual mucosa between areas of mucosal ulceration) (see Figs. 9-9A and 9-9B). Because mucosal inflammation predominates, prominent thickening of the intestinal wall is usually not observed, and strictures or fistulas are exceptional.

Mucosal inflammation results in intestinal dysfunction with bloody diarrhea. Chronic injury to the mucosa eventually results in abnormal mucosal regeneration with the dropout (loss) of crypts and the formation of branched crypts (architectural distortion) (Fig. 9-10A). These architectural abnormalities are important morphologic clues that allow distinction between chronic IBD (either Crohn's or UC) and self-limited colitis (e.g., colitis resulting from bacterial infection). Fulminant cases of UC may present with toxic megacolon (massive dilation of the entire colon with diffuse ulceration and transmural inflammation), which requires immediate colectomy.

UC frequently is associated with disease manifestations in other organs including the skin and liver. These extracolonic manifestations are present in more than 50% of patents and may be helpful in establishing the diagnosis of UC. Some of these manifestations (e.g., primary sclerosing cholangitis) can result in significant morbidity themselves.

Mucosal T cells in UC initiate a cytokine cascade (predominantly T_H2 type with secretion of IL-4 and IL-13) that initiates a chronic inflammatory reaction resulting in tissue damage. This abnormal immune response may be related to defects in the mucosal barrier allowing penetration of commensal bacteria, or abnormalities of innate immunity resulting in an enhanced mucosal inflammatory response to commensal bacteria. Infection with pathogenic bacteria may trigger an abnormal inflammatory response in susceptible individuals that may persist after eradication of the pathogen.

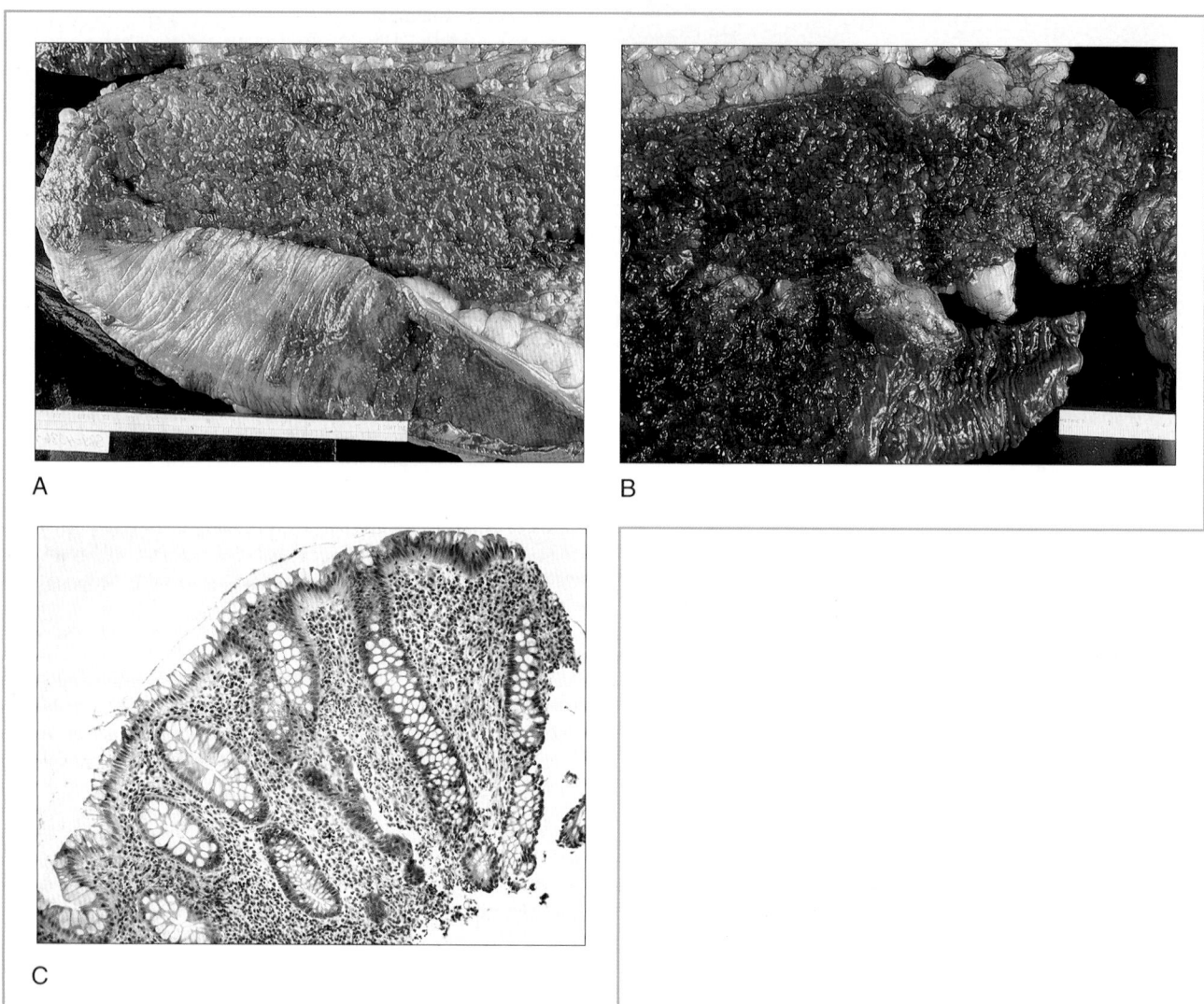

Figure 9-9. A, Ulcerative colitis. Gross photograph of large intestinal mucosa showing an abrupt cutoff between normal and diseased mucosa (*bottom*). Early pseudopolyp formation is evident in the extensively ulcerated mucosa. **B,** Gross image of right colon showing contiguous involvement by ulcerative colitis extending to the ileocecal valve (*bottom center*). Ileal mucosa (*bottom left*) is unremarkable. **C,** Microscopic section of colon showing chronic active ulcerative colitis. Note the extensive infiltration of crypt epithelium by acute inflammatory cells (cryptitis) with a dense chronic inflammatory cell infiltrate in the lamina propria.

The oxidative stress of chronic inflammation and the presence of cytokines and growth factors associated with this inflammatory process predispose to the development of epithelial dysplasia and adenocarcinoma. Dysplasia occurs in flat epithelium and does not usually form polyps (see Fig. 9-10B). This is in marked distinction to sporadic adenocarcinomas of the colon, which almost invariably develop from adenomatous polyps. Because areas of dysplasia in UC are flat and background inflammation distorts non-neoplastic mucosa, reliable endoscopic identification of preneoplastic dysplasia and small adenocarcinomas is often difficult or impossible. Prophylactic colectomy has often been performed in patients with long-standing UC with evidence of dysplasia.

Crohn's Disease

Crohn's disease (regional enteritis) can involve both the large and the small intestine, usually in a segmental manner. In contrast to UC, skip areas (segments of normal mucosa between diseased areas) are the rule in Crohn's disease. Crohn's disease involves the mucosa and also deeper layers of the intestinal wall, frequently resulting in transmural inflammation. The inflammatory process in Crohn's disease tends to be patchy and irregular compared with the diffuse homogeneous involvement in UC (Fig. 9-11A). Crohn's disease frequently produces linear, longitudinal ulcers in small and large intestinal mucosa that alternate with areas of grossly and microscopically normal mucosa. The most typical site of involvement is the terminal ileum although all regions of the small and large intestine may be involved. Unlike in UC, sparing of distal rectal mucosa is common. Perirectal fistula tracts may be present and help suggest the diagnosis of Crohn's disease.

Most patients with Crohn's disease have an inflammatory reaction that is predominantly of the T_H1 type involving

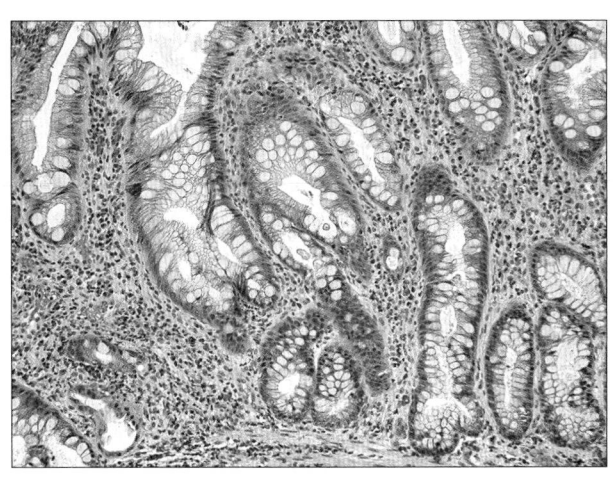

A

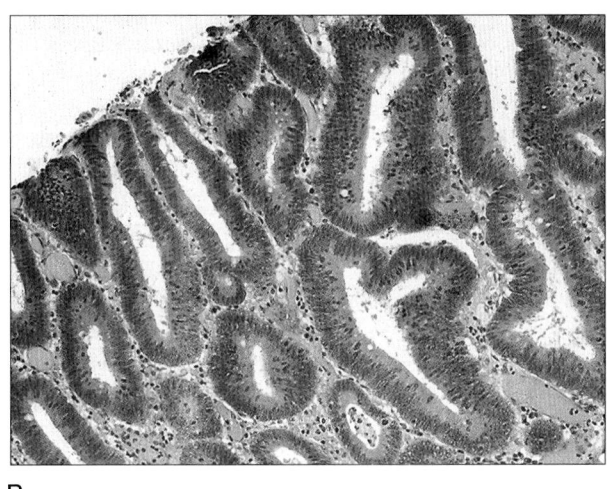

B

Figure 9-10. A, Architectural distortion in chronic inflammatory bowel disease. Microscopic section of colonic mucosa showing prominent crypt branching that is indicative of the chronicity of the inflammatory process. A moderately dense chronic inflammatory cell infiltrate is present as well as prominent active inflammation (cryptitis). **B**, High-grade dysplasia in chronic inflammatory bowel disease. Microscopic section of colon showing architectural distortion as well as a marked increase in nuclear:cytoplasmic ratio in dysplastic epithelial cells. There is no evidence of maturation as epithelial cells migrate to the surface of crypts and goblet cells are diminished in number (mucin depletion). This image could derive from either ulcerative colitis or Crohn's disease.

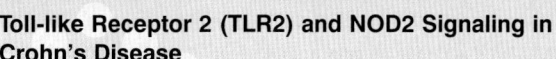

Toll-like Receptor 2 (TLR2) and NOD2 Signaling in Crohn's Disease

TLR2 normally binds to peptidoglycans present in the cell wall of commensal and pathogenic GI bacteria. TLR2 binding initiates signaling through the NFκB pathway to activate expression of proinflammatory genes. If peptidoglycan is ingested and degraded by enterocytes, a breakdown product (muramyl dipeptide, MDP) can bind to NOD2 protein in the enterocyte cytoplasm and down-regulate TLR2-mediated NFκB signaling. This negative feedback loop is thought to limit the amount of proinflammatory cytokines induced by commensal bacteria while preserving the ability to respond to pathogenic bacteria.

A small percentage of cases of Crohn's disease result from mutations in the NOD2 gene that prevent normal down-regulation of NFκB signaling. Increased production of proinflammatory cytokines then perpetuates and enhances the inflammatory reaction. Other components of this pathway may be targeted in subsets of patients with Crohn's disease.

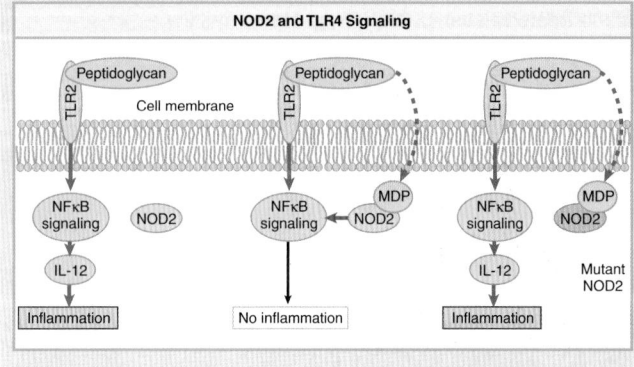

cytokines TNF α, IL-12, and IFN-γ. These cytokines are critical in perpetuating the inflammatory reaction in Crohn's disease, and therapies directed against TNF α and IL-12 (produced by activated macrophages) are effective in some patients. Some patients with Crohn's disease (up to 20%) have genetic alterations in molecules involved in modulating signaling by innate immune receptors (NOD2/CARD15), and abnormalities of innate mucosal immunity may be the inciting cause of inflammation in these patients.

Focal granulomatous inflammation is typical of Crohn's disease but is not observed in all cases (IFN-γ is part of the T$_H$1 cytokine cascade activated in Crohn's disease). Blockage of T-cell migration to the GI tract is effective in terminating this inflammatory pathway in some patients.

Transmural inflammation with fibrosis of the muscularis propria and mesenteric adipose tissue are the morphologic hallmarks of Crohn's disease. Mesenteric adipose tissue tends to expand around the full circumference of the intestine (fat wrapping). Because of the transmural nature of this inflammatory process, Crohn's disease predisposes to the formation of fistula tracts between the intestine and other organs (see Fig. 9-11B). This may result in fistulas between different segments of the intestines, between the intestine and the bladder (enterovesical fistula), or between the intestine and skin (enterocutaneous fistula). The marked serosal and muscular inflammation also promotes stricture formation, which can result in intestinal obstruction requiring surgical removal of the involved intestinal segment (see Fig. 9-11C).

Small intestinal involvement in Crohn's disease can cause malabsorption of nutrients, resulting in significant malnutrition. Surgical removal of large segments of the small intestine can exacerbate malabsorption, and some patients may become dependent on parenteral nutrition for survival (short-bowel syndrome). Crohn's disease can affect all regions of the GI tract, including the stomach and esophagus, often with foci of granulomatous inflammation. Manifestations of Crohn's disease outside the GI tract can also occur but are less common than in UC. Chronic oxidative stress in Crohn's disease results in a risk of flat dysplasia as in UC.

Diverticula

Diverticula are luminal outpouchings of the intestinal tract that are either congenital or acquired. The most common congenital diverticulum is Meckel's diverticulum, which usually is located in the distal ileum. Meckel's diverticulum may contain ectopic pancreatic or gastric tissue, which can give rise to inflammation and cause perforation.

Acquired diverticulosis tends to occur in patients with chronic constipation in whom increased intraluminal pressure from straining to defecate causes focal luminal herniation through the intestinal wall. This process typically is most marked in the distal large intestine (Fig. 9-12). Overgrowth of bacteria in these diverticula and luminal blockage by fecal material (fecaliths) can result in acute diverticulitis, which can progress to abscess formation and perforation with peritonitis. Chronic diverticulitis results in fibrosis and narrowing (stenosis) of the large intestinal lumen.

Dysmotility

Hirschsprung's disease results from congenital abnormalities of the intrinsic nervous system in the distal colon. The congenital absence of ganglion cells (aganglionosis) in the intermyenteric and submucosal nerve plexuses results in failure of peristalsis. Aganglionosis usually involves a contiguous segment extending from the anus proximally. Normal colon immediately proximal to the aganglionic segment is markedly dilated. Young children usually have intestinal obstruction and retention of stool. Removal of the aganglionic segment of intestine is curative. Acquired dysmotility of the GI tract is sometimes referred to as irritable bowel syndrome, and it remains controversial whether this is an organic or psychogenic illness.

Tumors

Adenocarcinomas are by far the most common tumors of the large intestine. Most carcinomas arise from precursor adenomatous polyps. Small intestinal adenocarcinomas are much less common but share many morphologic and biologic features with their large intestinal counterparts.

Polyps

Several different types of neoplastic colonic polyps are recognized. The two most common types are adenomatous and hyperplastic polyps. These polyps can develop either sporadically or in the setting of heritable genetic syndromes. Hyperplastic polyps arise because of point mutations in either the B-RAF proto-oncogene or less commonly in the K-RAS proto-oncogene. These alterations in the RAS signaling pathway result in abnormal proliferation in crypts, producing the characteristic "sawtooth" architectural pattern of hyperplastic polyps (Fig. 9-13A). Hyperplastic polyps usually remain small and rarely cause significant bleeding or develop into adenocarcinomas.

Tubular adenomas show typical adenomatous (dysplastic) features with increased nuclear size and nuclear hyperchromasia in tissue sections. They also show loss of nuclear polarity (mitotic figures are no longer confined to the base of crypts) and pseudostratification of nuclei at the luminal surface. There is usually also a decrease in the number of goblet cells (mucin depletion) in adenomatous epithelium (see Fig. 9-13B). Most tubular adenomas develop because of somatic point mutations in the APC tumor suppressor gene. These point mutations result in loss of functional APC protein with up-regulation of β-catenin. Abnormal β-catenin signaling causes increased cell proliferation with the formation of aberrant crypt foci that may eventually develop into adenomatous polyps. Adenomatous polyps are much more likely than hyperplastic polyps to acquire additional genetic mutations than can result in the formation of adenocarcinomas (see below).

Adenomatous polyps contain stromal cores that provide mechanical and vascular support for the neoplastic epithelium. Polyps may be relatively flat and broad-based compared

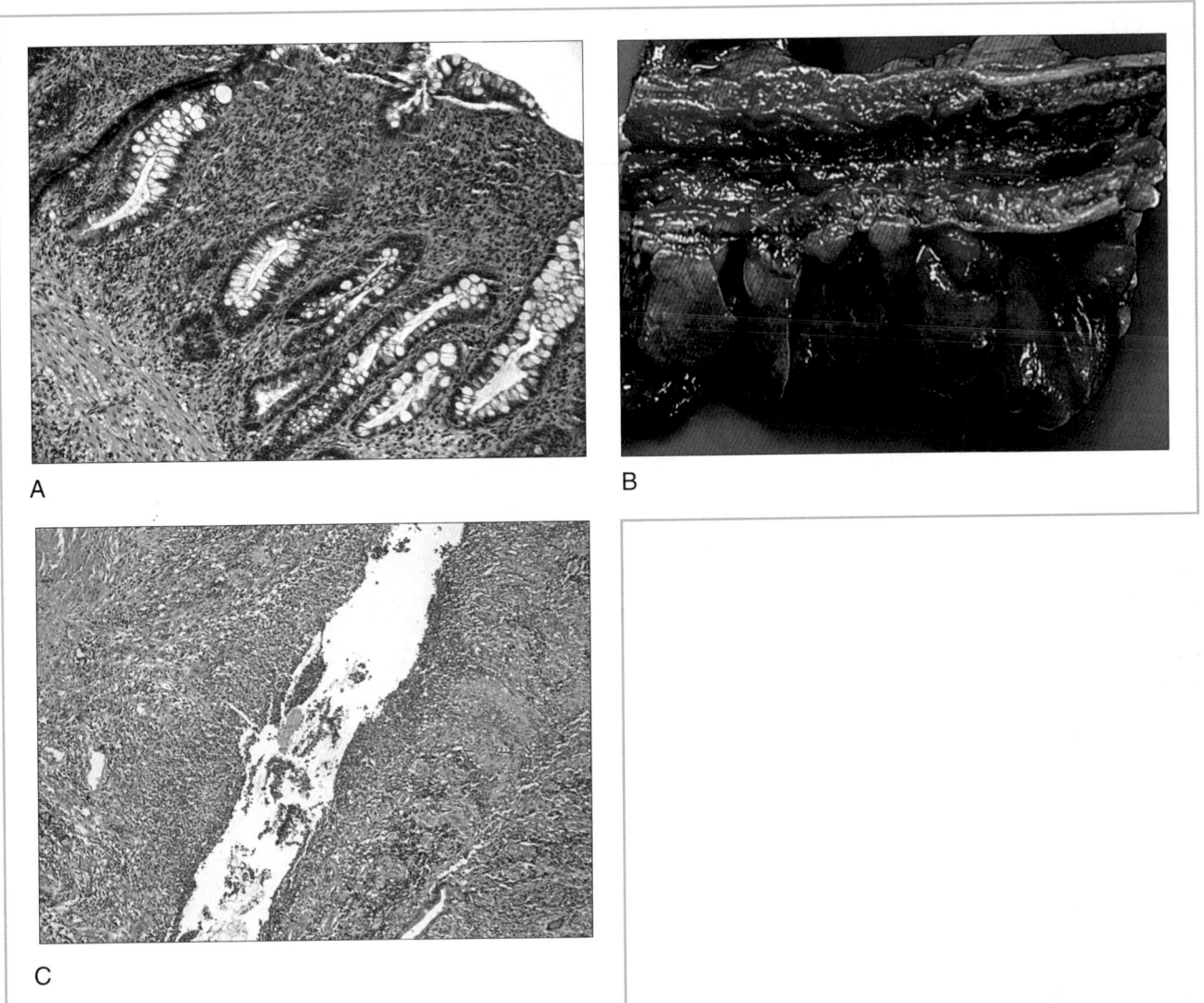

Figure 9-11. Crohn's disease. **A,** Microscopic section of colon showing severe chronic active inflammation extending into the submucosa. Architectural distortion is evident (crypt branching). **B,** Gross photograph of a segment of small intestine with marked wall thickening, luminal narrowing, and "creeping" of mesenteric fat around the entire serosal surface. This stricture was removed because of intestinal obstruction. **C,** Microscopic section of a fistula tract (*center*) lined by granulation tissue with a mixed inflammatory cell infiltrate.

with adjacent mucosa (sessile polyps) or may grow on a stalk (pedunculated polyps). Adenomatous polyps also vary in architectural pattern, with some forming predominantly tubules resembling normal colonic crypts (tubular adenomas) and others growing in a predominantly villous or papillary configuration (villous adenomas) (see Fig. 9-13C). Villous adenomas tend to have a greater potential for progression to adenocarcinoma than do tubular adenomas.

Patients with familial adenomatous polyposis (FAP) have an inherited abnormality of one copy of the APC gene and develop thousands of polyps in the large intestine (see Fig. 9-13D). By the time a patient with FAP reaches 35 years of age, some of these polyps usually have developed into invasive adenocarcinomas unless prophylactic total colectomy is performed. Patients with FAP can also develop less numerous adenomatous polyps of the small intestine and stomach, sometimes in association with tumors in other organs (Gardner's syndrome).

Other types of GI polyps can occur as a result of inflammation, in the setting of IBD, or in association with other genetic syndromes.

Adenocarcinoma

Adenocarcinomas of the large and small intestine are usually morphologically similar. The bulk of these tumors arise from adenomatous polyps. These precursor lesions may be obliterated by the tumor at the time of clinical presentation. Larger adenomatous polyps may sequentially acquire K-ras, SMAD4, and p53 gene mutations (Fig. 9-14). The precise order and identity of the genetic alterations that develop during tumorigenesis varies in different polyps, but the concept that there is a pathway to tumor formation has strong

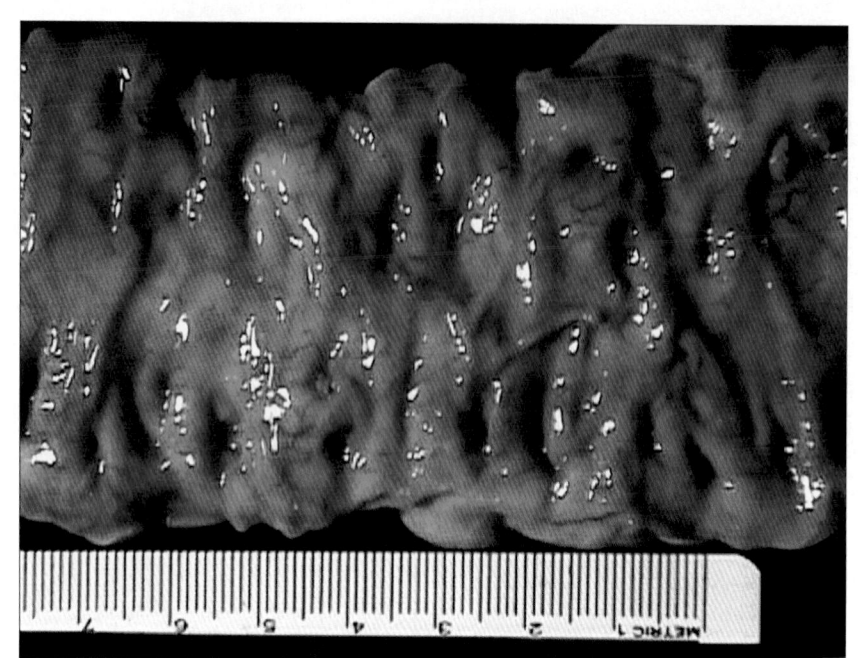

Figure 9-12. Colonic diverticulosis. Gross image of colon showing the openings to numerous diverticula in the mucosal surface.

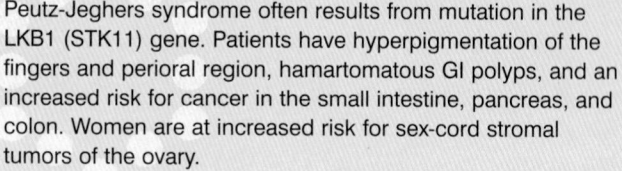

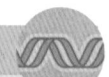

GENETICS

Familial Adenomatous Polyposis (FAP) Genetics

FAP results from mutations in the adenomatous polyposis coli gene (APC), which normally controls cell proliferation by down-regulating β-catenin and RAS signaling. Mutations in APC result in FAP (prevalence: 2 to 3/100,000), which is defined clinically as the development of more than 100 adenomatous polyps in the colon.

Many APC mutations produce stop codons that prematurely truncate the protein, and most truncating mutations are nearly 100% penetrant. The most commonly observed mutation is in codon 1349, and patients with this mutation tend to have hundreds of polyps with disease onset at approximately 16 years of age. Mutations in codons 1250 to 1463 tend to cause thousands of polyps. Other mutations, such as the 11307K polymorphism, which is prevalent in Ashkenazi Jews, have low penetrance and produce the clinical syndrome of FAP in only 10% to 20% of affected patients.

Attenuated familial polyposis results from mutations in three regions of the APC gene (5′ to codon 158, exon 9, or the distal 3′ portion). Patients with attenuated polyposis have between 30 and 100 polyps and tend to develop adenocarcinomas at a somewhat older age than usual FAP patients.

Mutations in codons 1395 to 1493 lead to a high frequency of fibromatoses (desmoid soft tissue tumors) in addition to polyposis, and this disorder is subclassified as Gardner's syndrome.

GENETICS

Other Familial Polyp Syndromes

Peutz-Jeghers syndrome often results from mutation in the LKB1 (STK11) gene. Patients have hyperpigmentation of the fingers and perioral region, hamartomatous GI polyps, and an increased risk for cancer in the small intestine, pancreas, and colon. Women are at increased risk for sex-cord stromal tumors of the ovary.

Familial juvenile polyposis causes hamartomatous GI polyps, and patients are at increased risk for GI carcinoma. Mutations in Smad4, PTEN, or BMPRIA can produce this syndrome.

Cowden's syndrome results from mutations in the PTEN gene that cause hamartomatous GI polyps and tumors of the thyroid, breast, uterus, and cutaneous trichilemmomas.

Bannayan-Ruvalcaba-Riley syndrome also results from alterations in the PTEN gene that cause microcephaly, fibromatosis, hamartomatous polyps, and hemangiomas.

Gardner's syndrome is a type of FAP in which patients also develop fibromatoses.

resulting in a cribriform pattern (i.e., high-grade dysplasia). High-grade dysplasia in the intestine is equivalent to carcinoma in situ in other organs. Cribriforming results from the solid growth of multiple layers of epithelial cells that are not supported by stroma (Fig. 9-15A). Apoptosis of individual tumor cells results in the formation of sharply "punched out" spaces in the epithelium that may contain apoptotic debris. Foci of high-grade dysplasia are at increased risk for invasion through the basement membrane to become full-fledged adenocarcinomas.

empiric support. The cytologic features of adenomatous polyps typically change as they acquire additional mutations with an increase in their nuclear to cytoplasmic ratio, loss of differentiated features, and more extensive apoptosis,

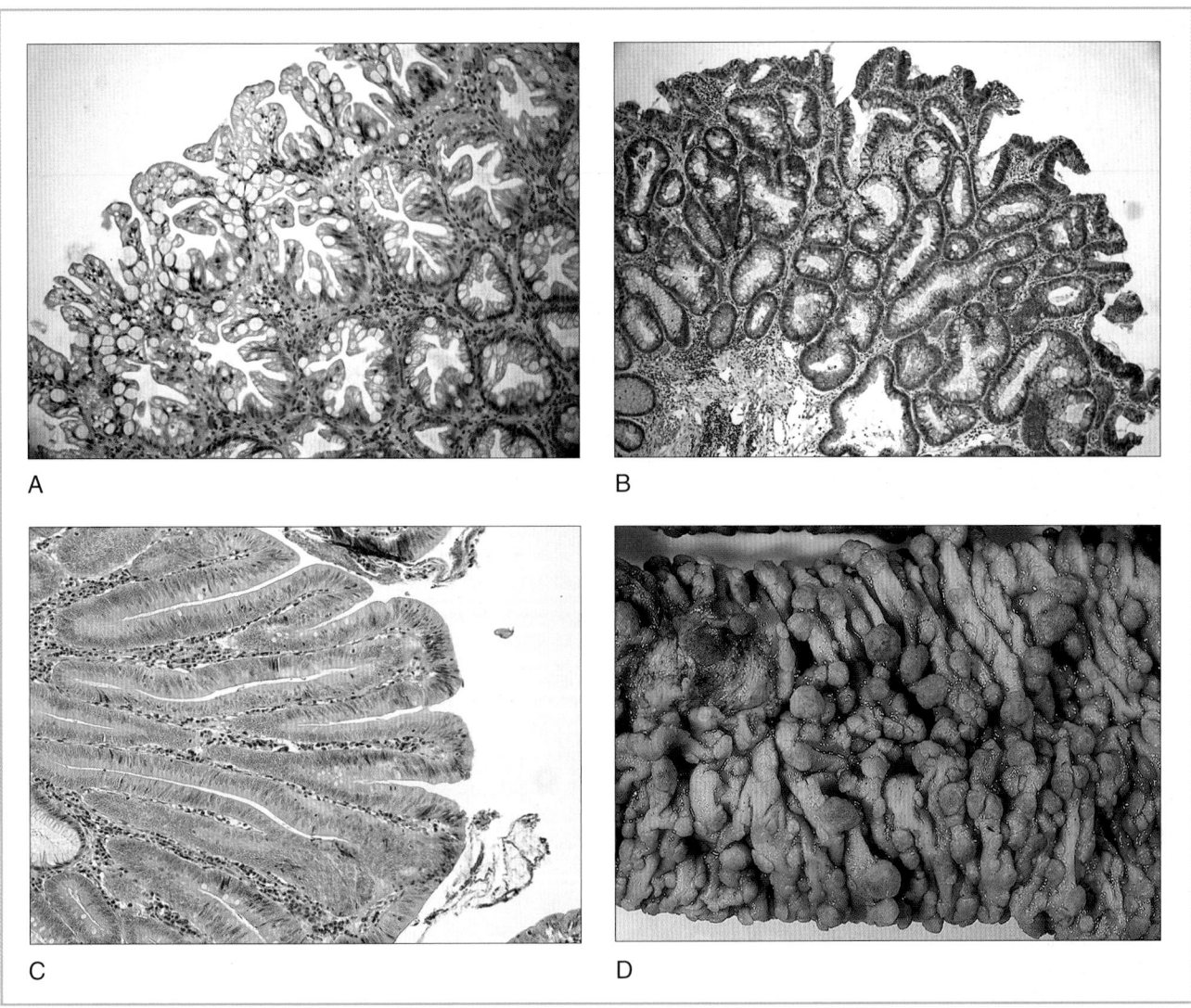

Figure 9-13. **A**, Hyperplastic polyp. Microscopic section showing typical "sawtooth" pattern in crypts. Nuclei are small and predominantly basal in orientation, and goblet cells are abundant. **B**, Tubular adenoma. Microscopic section showing marked nuclear enlargement, hyperchromasia, and pseudostratification extending to the surface of the polyp (i.e., no surface maturation is observed). Extensive mucin depletion (loss of goblet cells) is present. **C**, Villous adenoma. Microscopic section showing adenomatous colonic epithelium lining papillary fibrovascular cores. **D**, Familial polyposis. Gross photograph of colonic mucosa showing hundreds of small adenomatous polyps. Normal mucosal folds are almost completely obscured by polyps.

Most colonic adenocarcinomas form recognizable glands to some degree, and the extent of gland formation in intestinal adenocarcinomas determines their level of differentiation or tumor grade (poorly differentiated tumors show predominantly solid growth with <5% gland formation; see Fig. 9-15B). Colon cancer frequently has an exophytic growth pattern protruding into the intestinal lumen, and precursor polyp is often present at the periphery of invasive tumors (see Fig. 9-15C). Some adenocarcinomas have a predominantly ulcerating pattern of growth with deep invasion into the muscularis propria and mesenteric adipose tissue. The amount of mucin produced by these tumors is highly variable. Highly mucinous tumors containing signet ring cells tend to be more extensively invasive and are usually associated with a worse prognosis (see Figs. 9-15D and 9-15E).

Right-sided mucinous tumors arising in younger individuals that are associated with a prominent lymphoid infiltrate are often found to have a "high microsatellite instability" phenotype (MSI). These tumors appear to arise by a different pathway from the usual colonic adenocarcinomas that are associated with defects in DNA mismatch repair enzymes. These tumors accumulate numerous mutations in many genes and paradoxically have a better prognosis than the usual adenocarcinomas. This type of tumor is also observed in individuals with heritable abnormalities in mismatch repair genes (hereditary nonpolyposis colon cancer, HNPCC). Patients with HNPCC are at significantly increased risk for colon cancer but do not develop innumerable mucosal polyps.

The clinical behavior of intestinal adenocarcinomas depends predominantly on their stage. AJCC stage I tumors (tumors

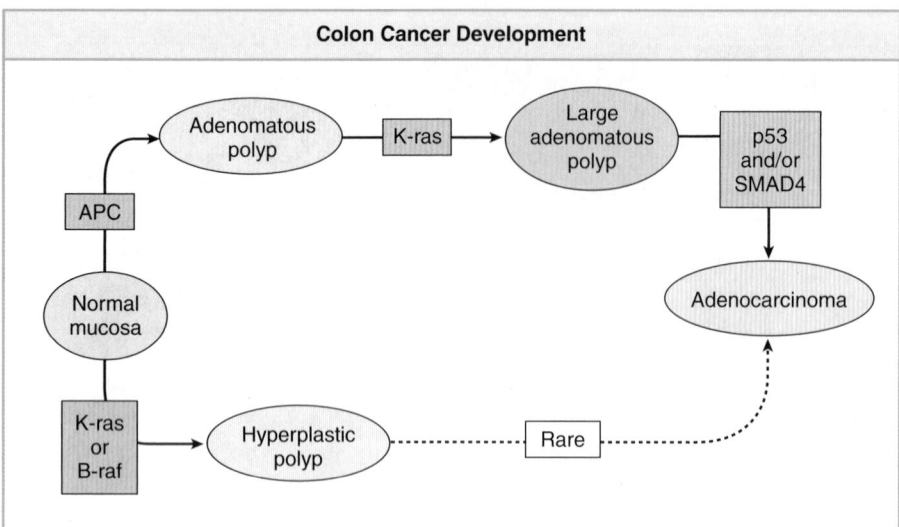

Figure 9-14. Colon cancer development.

that do not invade deeper than the submucosa) are almost always cured by surgical excision. Patients with lymph node metastases at the time of surgery (AJCC stage III) have a much more guarded prognosis and may benefit from adjuvant chemotherapy. Colonic adenocarcinoma typically spreads to regional lymph nodes prior to systemic metastasis, and a subset of patients have liver metastases. Metastatic colon cancer foci usually have a relatively characteristic morphology with gland-like spaces lined by columnar tumor cells that are filled with necrotic debris and neutrophils (so-called dirty necrosis).

Neuroendocrine Tumors

Neuroendocrine tumors arise from neuroendocrine cells, which are a normal but minor component of the intestinal mucosa. Most of these tumors take the form of carcinoid tumors, composed of well-formed nests of bland-appearing cells (Fig. 9-16A). Tumor cell nuclei have granular chromatin and other features of neuroendocrine differentiation including expression of chromogranin A (a component of dense core neurosecretory granules) as well as other neuroendocrine markers (see Fig. 9-16B). Most of these tumors are relatively indolent although a minority metastasize. Small carcinoid tumors of the large and small intestine are usually cured by local excision. A common site for the development of carcinoid tumors is the tip of the appendix. Large appendiceal carcinoids occasionally produce sufficient neuroendocrine mediators (predominantly serotonin) to cause the systemic carcinoid syndrome (flushing, hypotension, and watery diarrhea). Carcinoid syndrome is more often observed in association with carcinoid tumors outside the GI tract (most mediators released by GI carcinoids are immediately inactivated during passage through the portal circulation).

Gastrointestinal Stromal Tumor

Gastrointestinal stromal tumors (GISTs) are distinctive neoplasms that can arise from interstitial cells of Cajal. These tumors are composed of spindle or epithelioid cells and may show features of neural differentiation. GISTs may present with gastrointestinal hemorrhage or intestinal

obstruction if they cause mucosal ulceration or grow into the mesentery (Figs. 9-17A and 9-17B). Most of these tumors are of intermediate biologic potential and tend be locally aggressive but only rarely result in metastasis. Features associated with increased likelihood of metastasis are location in the small intestine, increased mitotic activity, and tumor cell necrosis. GISTs of the distal large intestine and stomach are much less frequently malignant.

Almost all GISTs overexpress the c-kit receptor (CD117), and many have point mutations in the CD117 gene that result in the constitutive activation of its tyrosine kinase activity. Many of these mutations result in a receptor tyrosine kinase that can bind the same small molecule drug (imatinib [Gleevec]) designed to block the bcr-abl fusion protein in patients with chronic myelogenous leukemia. This novel treatment has resulted in marked tumor regression in some patients with metastatic GISTs that are poorly responsive to other forms of therapy.

Lymphoma

The small and large intestine can be involved secondarily by most types of non-Hodgkin's lymphoma although Hodgkin's disease rarely involves the GI tract. Rare IgA-producing MALT lymphomas (similar to MALT lymphomas in the stomach) can arise in the small intestine in association with chronic *Campylobacter jejuni* infection. Mantle cell lymphoma can also arise primarily in the GI tract and present as mucosal polyps (because of the focal accumulation tumor cells in the lamina propria). Sporadic Burkitt's lymphoma in children frequently presents with involvement of the intestinal wall and mesenteric lymph nodes, which may cause intestinal obstruction. Large-cell non-Hodgkin's lymphoma can arise primarily in the intestine but more often involves it secondarily.

●●● APPENDIX

The narrow lumen of the appendix predisposes it to obstruction by fecaliths or foreign objects in the fecal stream. Obstruction results in bacterial overgrowth, which causes

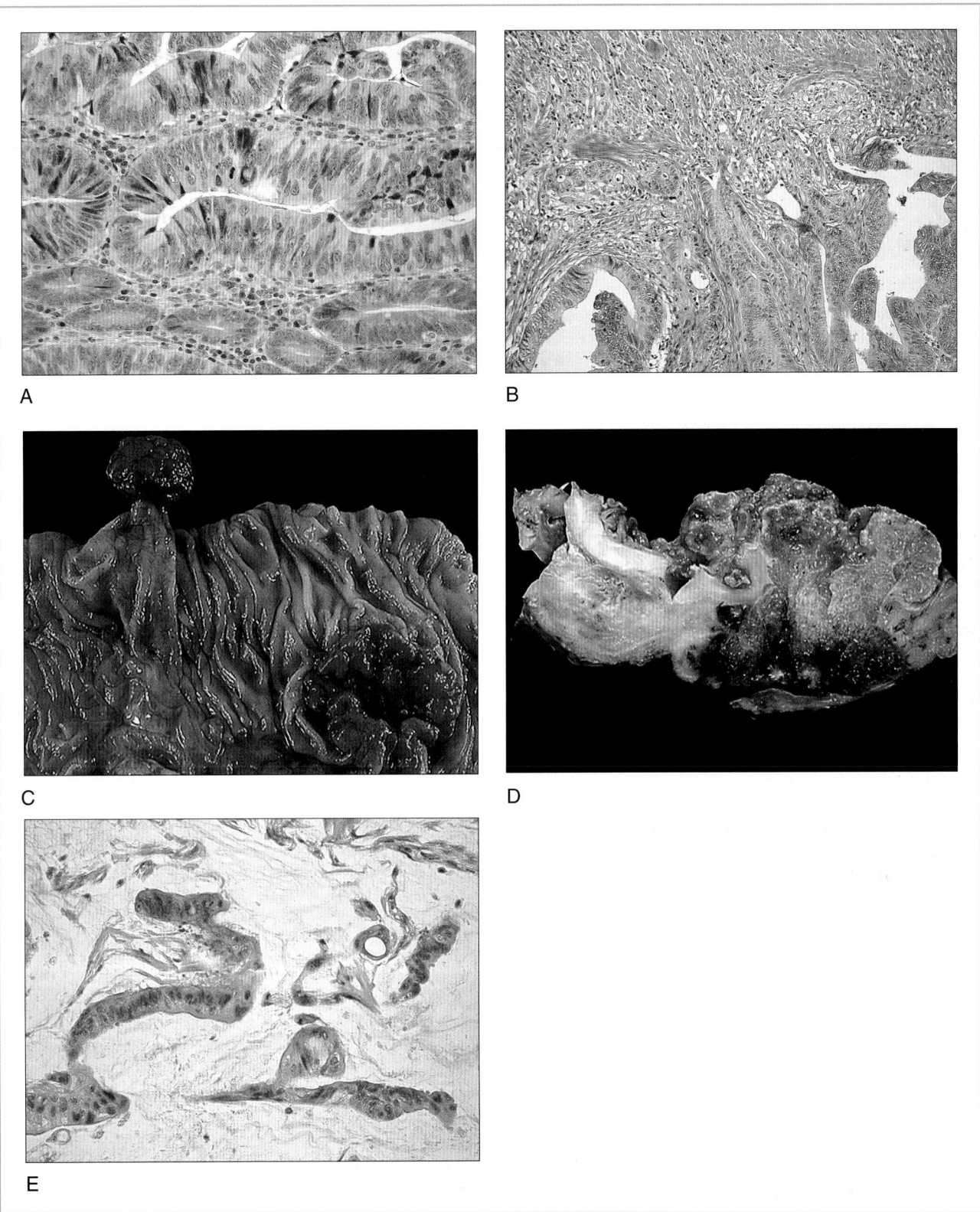

A

B

C

D

E

Figure 9-15. A, High-grade dysplasia in colonic mucosa. Microscopic section showing marked nuclear pleomorphism, nuclear pseudostratification, mucin depletion, and focal cribriform architecture. **B**, Colonic adenocarcinoma. Microscopic section showing irregular neoplastic glands invading muscularis propria. **C**, Colonic adenocarcinoma. Gross photograph of a colon showing a partially ulcerated adenocarcinoma with an exophytic growth pattern (*near bottom*). A pedunculated tubular adenoma is also visible (*upper left*). **D**, Mucinous colonic adenocarcinoma. Gross cross-section of intestinal wall infiltrated by a highly mucinous tumor. The tumor (*right*) appears gelatinous and shiny because of extensive extracellular mucin. Tumor extends entirely through the muscularis propria to the serosal surface. **E**, Microscopic section of a mucinous adenocarcinoma showing lakes of extracellular mucin containing strips and nests of tumor cells.

GENETICS

Hereditary Nonpolyposis Coli (HNPCC)

HNPCC (also known as Lynch syndrome) is an uncommon genetic disease that usually results from point mutations in one of the mismatch repair enzymes (MLH1, MSH2, MSH6, or PMS2). Lynch syndrome was defined clinically before the genetic lesions were identified. Patients typically developed colon cancer at a younger age than those with sporadic cancers, did not have the numerous polyps typical of familial polyposis (APC gene mutation), had polyps predominantly in the proximal (right) colon, and had a family history consistent with autosomal dominant inheritance.

Inherited loss of function of one allele of a mismatch repair gene results in an increased cancer risk because the remaining normal allele can be inactivated by somatic mutation or silenced by hypermethylation. Disruption of the mismatch repair pathway leads to an increased frequency of mutations in other genes, including oncogenes and tumor suppressor genes. Most colon cancers that develop in HNPCC patients have a high MSI (microsatellite instability) phenotype and a better prognosis than do non-MSI colon cancers.

Genetic screening for HNPCC is technically difficult and expensive so that clinical criteria remain important for identifying individuals at risk who should be more aggressively screened for colon cancer. The Amsterdam and Bethesda criteria for HNPCC are both used clinically but it is now clear that up to half of patients with documented germline mutations do not meet the criteria for the clinical diagnosis of HNPCC. Functional testing of colon cancers and polyps in suspected patients using immunohistochemistry to detect loss of expression of individual MSI genes is the currently favored approach although this does not allow discrimination of sporadic MSI tumors from those arising in patients with Lynch syndrome.

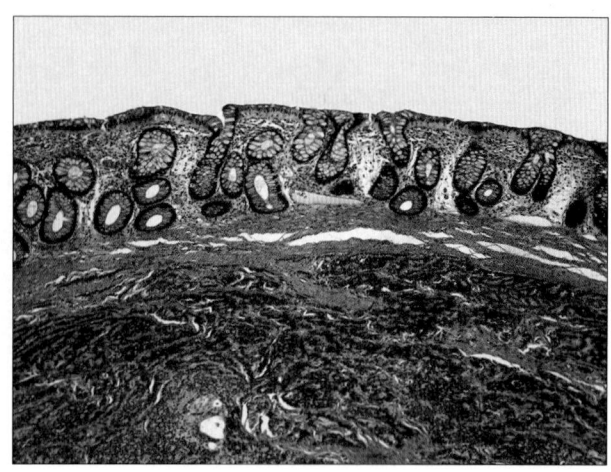

A

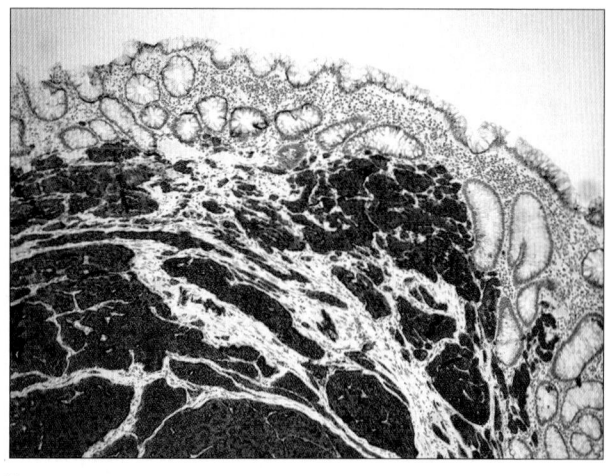

B

Figure 9-16. A, Carcinoid tumor. Microscopic section of colon showing a submucosal carcinoid tumor composed of nests of neuroendocrine cells with a trabecular growth pattern forming a polyploid mass beneath normal overlying mucosa. **B,** Microscopic section of the same tumor stained for chromogranin A (a protein component of dense core neurosecretory granules).

acute inflammation of the mucosa and may progress to acute appendicitis with transmural inflammation and perforation. Other inflammatory processes may also involve the appendix including IBD, diverticulitis, and endometriosis. Carcinoid tumors are relatively common in the tip of the appendix and may grow to a large size. Microscopic carcinoid tumors are an incidental finding in a minority of appendices removed for other reasons.

●●● LIVER AND BILIARY TRACT

The liver is responsible for the synthesis of many essential plasma proteins as well as for the detoxification of many natural and synthetic products. The liver also plays a critical role in processing lipid nutrients derived from the GI tract from chylomicrons into plasma lipoprotein particles. The production of bile and its enterohepatic circulation are essential for the normal absorption of lipids and for the detoxification of hemoglobin breakdown products.

Cholestasis and Biliary Obstruction

Cholestasis results from an interruption of normal hepatic secretion of bile and can occur by two major mechanisms: dysfunction of hepatocytes, resulting in their inability to secrete bile, and obstruction of the biliary tract. Either mechanism can result in jaundice (the deposition of bilirubin pigment in multiple organs and tissues secondary to high plasma concentrations). Jaundice can also result from the excessive production of bilirubin through the hemolysis of large amounts of red blood cells.

PHYSIOLOGY

Carcinoid Syndrome

Carcinoid syndrome tends to develop in patients with foregut or midgut carcinoid tumors that have extensively metastasized to the liver. It consists of a number of different manifestations resulting from the release of vasoactive substances (predominantly serotonin) by tumor cells.

Episodic flushing is the most common manifestation of carcinoid syndrome (flushing occurs at some point in up to 75% of patients) and may be spontaneous or induced by various stimuli (e.g., stress, alcohol). Diarrhea is also common and may be accompanied by flushing and abdominal pain.

Carcinoid heart disease results from the prolonged exposure of cardiac myocytes to toxic vasoactive peptides.

HISTOLOGY

Interstitial Cells of Cajal (ICCs)

ICCs are specialized cells that are sometimes called pacemaker cells and share features of muscle and nerve cells. ICCs contain numerous mitochondria, intermediate and thin filaments, caveolae, and smooth endoplasmic reticulum but are difficult to recognize based on ultrastructural features alone. They do not contain dense core neurosecretory granules and do not form typical synapses like neurons. ICCs express c-kit receptor and respond to its ligand, stem cell factor (SCF).

All tubular intestinal organs contain ICCs, which are important in controlling peristalsis in the GI tract although they may subserve other functions as well. ICCs are present in association with both the intermyenteric plexus and other ganglia and neural cells in the tubular GI tract. ICCs have come to be of great interest pathologically because they are now recognized as the parent cell of gastrointestinal stromal tumors (GISTs). Many GISTs have mutations in the c-kit receptor that result in abnormal cell proliferation and tumor formation. Many of these tumors respond to the RTK inhibitor imatinib (Gleevec), which was designed to treat leukemia with a novel fusion protein (bcr-abl) produced by chromosomal translocation.

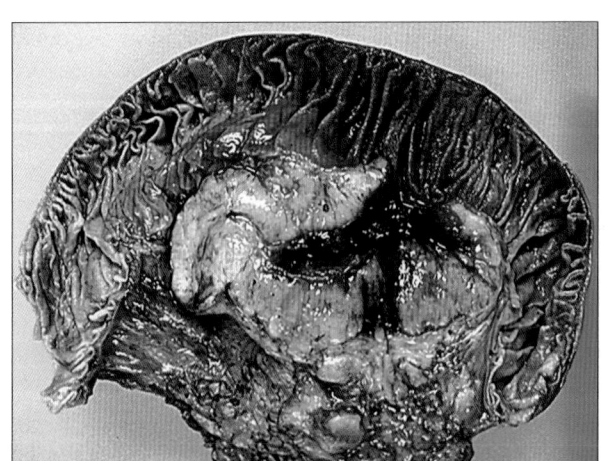

A

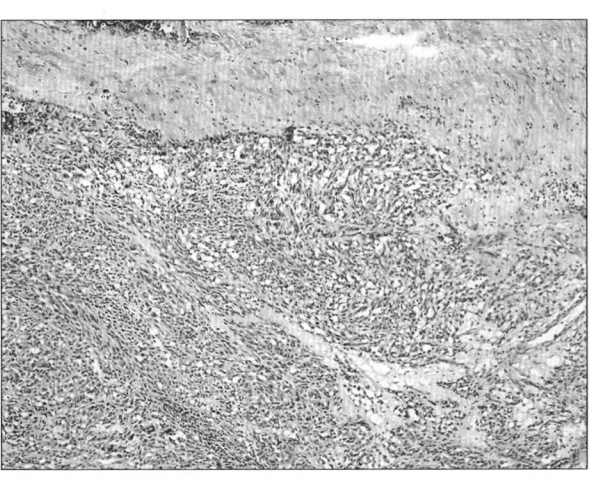

B

Figure 9-17. A, Gastrointestinal stromal tumor (GIST). Gross cross-section of small intestine showing a large, deeply ulcerated GIST focally replacing the intestinal wall and extending into the mesentery. The tumor has a whitish, slightly gelatinous cut surface. **B**, Microscopic section of a GIST showing plump spindle cells with a somewhat epithelioid appearance. Residual normal muscularis propria appears adjacent to the tumor (*upper right*).

Biliary obstruction and hepatocyte disfunction can usually be distinguished by clinical laboratory testing, and they show different features on liver biopsy. Cholestasis resulting from primary dysfunction of hepatocytes, so-called intracellular cholestasis, results in the accumulation of bile in the cytoplasm of hepatocytes without the formation of bile plugs in canaliculi or larger bile ducts (Fig. 9-18A). This may be associated with elevations of transaminases but is usually not associated with marked elevation of alkaline phosphatase. Intracellular cholestasis typically results from acute viral hepatitis, toxin exposure, and drug reactions.

Blockage of intrahepatic or extrahepatic bile ducts results in elevation of alkaline phosphatase in the serum and plugging of bile canaliculi with bile in liver biopsies. If this blockage becomes severe, intracellular accumulation of bile will be observed as well. Biliary tract obstruction can result from tumors that impinge on larger bile ducts (primary or metastatic tumors of the liver or the head of the pancreas), inflammatory processes that result in stenosis of the bile ducts, and luminal obstruction by stones (common bile duct stones from the gall bladder or less commonly intrahepatic lithiasis; see Fig. 9-18B). Inflammation of the bile ducts can result from autoimmune mechanisms as in primary sclerosing cholangitis or from bacterial infection of the biliary tract (ascending cholangitis). Mechanical obstruction of the biliary tract by stones or extrinsic compression predisposes to bacterial cholangitis. Some parasitic diseases can also result in obstruction to bile flow. Abnormal liver architecture in hepatic cirrhosis can produce significant functional obstruction to bile flow in the liver.

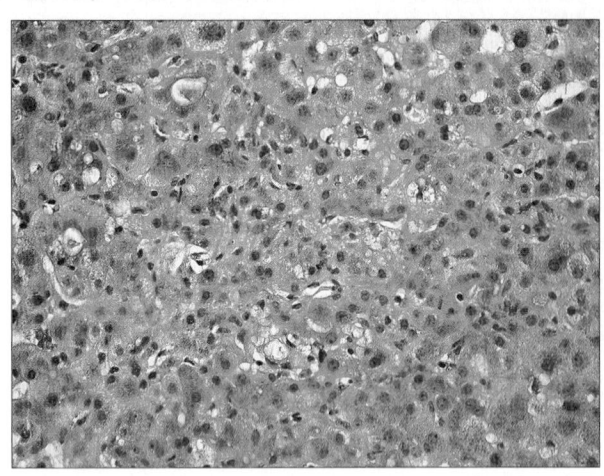

A

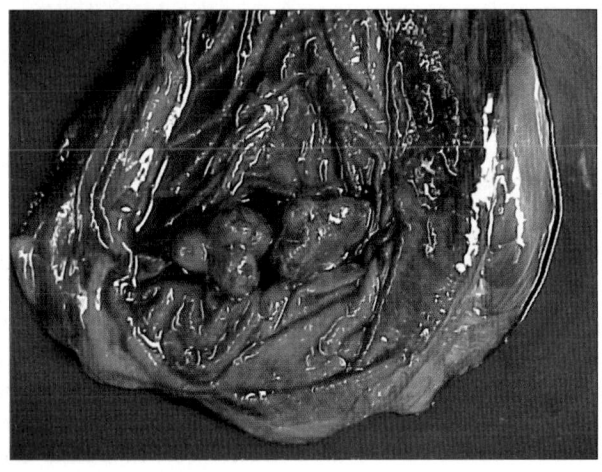

B

Figure 9-18. A, Hepatic cholestasis. Microscopic section of liver showing extensive intracellular bile accumulation (brown-green pigment) and focal bile plugs distending bile canaliculi. **B**, Cholelithiasis. Gross photograph of a gallbladder containing small cholesterol gallstones.

Acute and Chronic Cholecystitis

Some individuals are predisposed to form different types of stones within the gallbladder. Gallstones can be formed from bilirubin, cholesterol, and less commonly from other substances. Stones can result in chronic or intermittent obstruction of the cystic duct. This blockage results in hypertrophy and inflammation of the gallbladder wall (chronic cholecystitis). Complete obstruction of the cystic duct can result in acute cholecystitis, which may progress to transmural necrosis of the gallbladder. Acalculous cholecystitis is gallbladder inflammation in the absence of stones and usually is associated with significant comorbid disease and has a very poor prognosis. Small stones can reflux from the gallbladder and lodge in the common bile duct, resulting in acute biliary obstruction, acute pancreatitis, and jaundice. Less commonly large gallstones can be extruded into the small intestine, resulting in intestinal obstruction (gallstone ileus).

Cholangitis

Cholangitis is inflammation of the biliary tract, which can occur as an infectious process (acute ascending cholangitis) and is often seen in the setting of biliary tract obstruction. Primary sclerosing cholangitis is an autoimmune-mediated inflammation of the bile ducts that can occur in association with IBD, most often Crohn's disease. The clinical course is variable but may progress to cirrhosis.

Primary Biliary Cirrhosis

Primary biliary cirrhosis (PBC) is an autoimmune disease in which granulomatous inflammation within portal tracts destroys interlobular bile ducts. This inflammatory and destructive process progresses slowly (over months to years). It begins as compensatory proliferation of abnormal small bile ducts within portal tracts, followed by progression to cirrhosis with evidence of biliary tract obstruction. Most patients are female and have antimitochondrial antibodies in their serum, which is helpful in establishing the diagnosis.

Hepatitis

Hepatitis is an inflammatory process primarily involving hepatocytes and may result from viral infection, autoimmune disease, or chemicals or toxins.

Viral Hepatitis

Three types of hepatitis virus are responsible for most cases of human viral hepatitis—A, B, and C. Other hepatitis viruses are less common causes of human disease, and some (e.g., Epstein-Barr virus) can result in an acute, self-limited hepatitis although the dominant symptoms (acute mononucleosis) relate to involvement of other organs. Many forms of viral hepatitis result in significant dysfunction or apoptosis of hepatocytes, and the release of hepatocellular proteins from hepatocytes undergoing apoptosis results in marked elevations of serum transaminases, providing useful diagnostic markers. Acute viral hepatitis is a self-limited illness usually associated with transient jaundice. In uncomplicated acute viral hepatitis, the virus is cleared by the immune system with restoration of normal hepatic function within 6 months. In most cases, hepatocyte dysfunction or destruction does not exceed the regenerative capacity of the liver, and patients make a full recovery. A small minority of hepatitis A and B cases are severe enough to cause acute hepatic failure. Conversely, aggressive hepatitis viruses (e.g., yellow fever virus) frequently result in acute hepatic failure leading to death.

Chronic viral hepatitis is an inflammatory process that persists for more than 6 months after initial infection with a hepatitis virus and is associated with persistence of virus in the liver. Chronic hepatitis may be preceded by an episode of overt acute hepatitis or may develop after a subclinical acute infection. Chronic hepatitis can be associated with varying amounts of ongoing injury to the liver that may result in cirrhosis and increased risk for development of hepatocellular carcinoma (Fig. 9-19). In most forms of chronic viral hepatitis, T cells that recognize viral epitopes on the surface of hepatocytes mediate most of the damage to hepatocytes rather than direct viral cytopathic effects.

Hepatitis A

Hepatitis A virus is a single-stranded RNA virus that typically results in a self-limited illness. Infection is usually associated with transient, moderate-to-marked hepatic dysfunction. Hepatitis A never develops into chronic viral hepatitis and immunity is lifelong after infection. The incubation period is 2 to 6 weeks, and almost all individuals make a full recovery. The oral-fecal route usually spreads this virus, and individuals shed virus in their stool for several weeks prior to the onset of clinical hepatitis. The disease is usually manifested by the acute appearance of jaundice, and subclinical infection is uncommon.

Hepatitis B

Hepatitis B is a DNA virus that can cause acute hepatitis as well as chronic hepatitis. Some individuals mount an immune response during acute infection that completely clears the virus, whereas others develop chronic stable or chronic progressive hepatitis that can ultimately result in cirrhosis or hepatocellular carcinoma. Infection is typically spread via blood or secretions and can be spread venereally. Prior vaccination with recombinant vaccine results in significant immunity that usually is protective.

Approximately one fourth of patients infected with hepatitis B develop a stereotyped acute hepatitis with jaundice. Most of these individuals clear their infection and normalize hepatic function within 6 months (i.e., they do not develop chronic viral hepatitis). More than half of individuals infected with hepatitis B have subclinical disease and do not develop overt jaundice. Some of these may remain healthy carriers and can transmit the virus to others without developing liver disease. Approximately 20% of individuals who fail to clear hepatitis virus from their liver develop chronic liver disease (Fig. 9-20). In some cases, this results in a low-grade inflammatory reaction that is largely confined to portal tracts and does not progress to cirrhosis. Up to half of these individuals have a more significant chronic inflammatory reaction with ongoing hepatocyte injury that ultimately progresses to cirrhosis. The likelihood of developing cirrhosis may depend on immunologic factors in the host as well as environmental factors such as alcohol

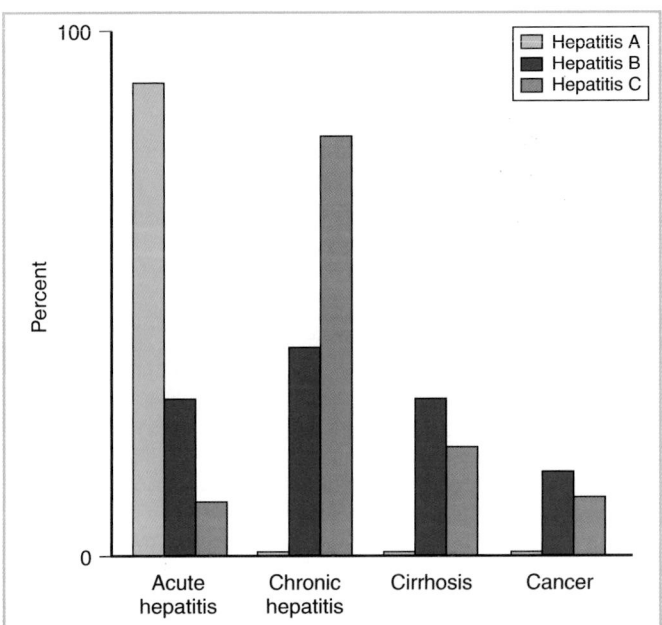

Figure 9-19. Sequelae of viral hepatitis.

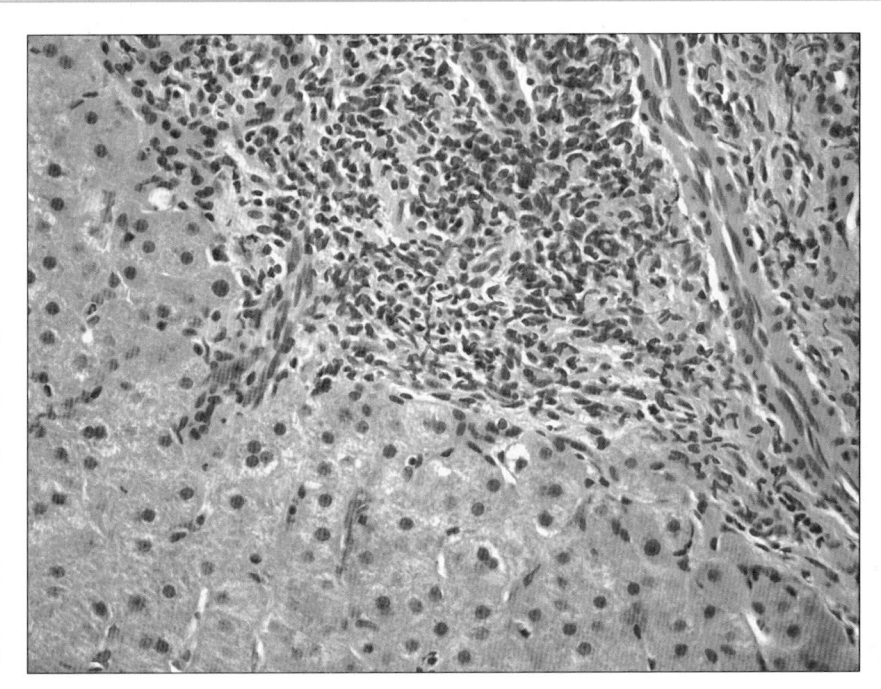

Figure 9-20. Chronic active viral hepatitis. Microscopic section of liver showing a dense chronic inflammatory cell infiltrate (almost exclusively T cells) in a portal tract (*upper right*). There is extension of the inflammatory infiltrate into the lobule, where T cells envelop and destroy individual hepatocytes (piecemeal necrosis).

consumption. Serologic assays that demonstrate antibodies to different viral components predict whether an individual is at risk for chronic liver disease.

Hepatitis C

Hepatitis C virus is an RNA virus that is significantly less contagious than hepatitis B virus and is usually spread through blood or blood products. The availability of a serologic assay for hepatitis C virus in the 1980s allowed the removal of contaminated blood products from the blood supply. Prior to this time, a significant number of individuals receiving blood transfusions developed either overt hepatitis C or, more commonly, subclinical disease that developed into chronic viral hepatitis. Most individuals (about 75%) infected with hepatitis C virus develop progressive liver disease (chronic viral hepatitis), and up to 20% of these ultimately develop cirrhosis and are at significantly increased risk for the development of hepatocellular carcinoma. Essentially all liver cell injury associated with hepatitis C infection is immune mediated in response to viral antigens expressed on the surface of hepatocytes.

Other Hepatitis Viruses

Delta virus or hepatitis D virus is a defective RNA virus that can only infect individuals with chronic hepatitis B virus infection. In these individuals, delta virus can result in fulminant hepatitis and liver failure. Hepatitis E virus causes a self-limited hepatitis that is relatively common in Asia and sub-Saharan Africa but is currently uncommon in the United States.

Autoimmune Hepatitis

Autoimmune hepatitis may be morphologically indistinguishable from some forms of chronic viral hepatitis. Plasma cells are typically prominent in the inflammatory infiltrate and can be a useful clue to the diagnosis. As with chronic viral hepatitis, immune-mediated injury to hepatocytes constitutes the main pathologic lesion. There is a significant female predominance and an association with other autoimmune diseases including rheumatoid arthritis and ulcerative colitis. Evaluation of serologic markers for immune disease (e.g., ANA) can be helpful in establishing the diagnosis. The course is variable but may progress to cirrhosis.

IMMUNOLOGY

Serology of Viral Hepatitis

The detection of IgM and IgG antibodies to various components of the hepatitis B virus (HBV) and hepatitis C virus (HCV) provides significant information about the chronicity and activity of an infection.

In HBV infection, IgM antibodies to hepatitis B core antigen (HBcAg) appear in the serum at the same time as viral DNA and surface antigen (HBsAg). In self-limited HBV infections, viral DNA and surface antigen disappear after clinical hepatitis ceases. IgM antibodies decline, and IgG antibodies appear at about 6 months. In chronic HBV infections, viral DNA and HBsAg do not disappear and IgG antibodies may not develop.

In HCV infection, IgM and IgG antibodies appear at about the same time as viral RNA and all diminish over time. Most patients have some degree of chronic infection with spikes of viral RNA in serum without accompanying changes in antibody titer.

Measurement of plasma viral load by PCR is an important determinant of disease activity and is used as a surrogate marker to evaluate the effectiveness of therapeutic interventions. Detection of antibodies directed against cellular components (e.g., antimitochondrial antibodies or anti–double stranded DNA antibodies) may be an indication of coexisting primary biliary cirrhosis or autoimmune hepatitis.

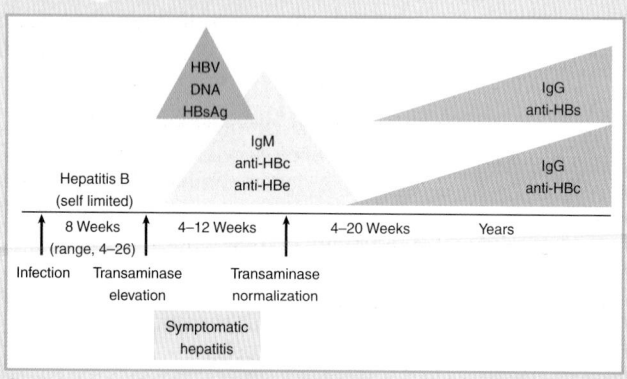

A

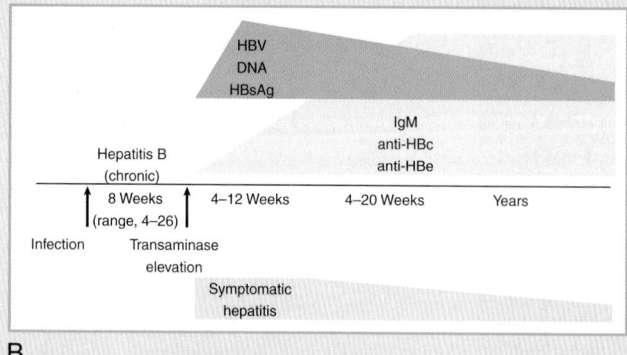

B

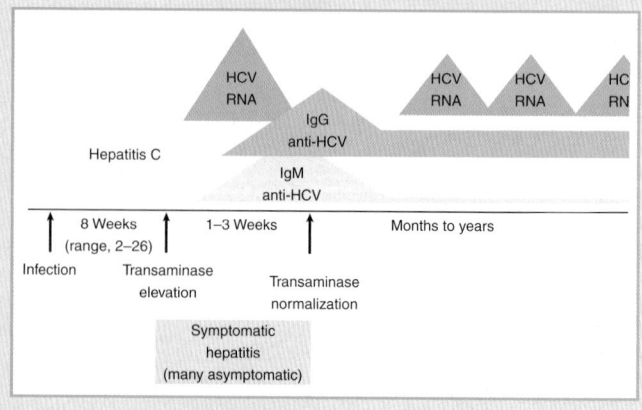

C

Chemical Hepatitis

Many different types of chemicals and drugs can cause hepatotoxicity. The liver metabolizes a wide variety of chemicals, and some of the reactive intermediates produced are responsible for hepatocellular damage and death. Genetic polymorphisms in cytochrome P-450 genes result in the formation of different types of chemical intermediates and different rates of drug metabolism, which may protect or predispose to hepatocellular injury. Carbon tetrachloride is a prototypical hepatotoxin that can result in massive hepatic necrosis and liver failure.

Alcoholic Hepatitis

Alcoholic liver disease is a major cause of morbidity and mortality throughout the world. Acute ingestion of large amounts of alcohol results in the accumulation of toxic intermediates (e.g., acetaldehyde) in hepatocytes that cause hepatocellular injury and result in alcoholic hepatitis. The resulting hepatocellular dysfunction results in the accumulation of dietary lipid in hepatocytes, producing steatosis. Alcoholic hepatitis is associated with a neutrophilic inflammatory infiltrate in hepatic lobules that results in further hepatocellular injury and dysfunction. There is increased regeneration of hepatocytes from oval cell precursors (to replace necrotic hepatocytes) as well as ongoing injury to surviving hepatocytes. Hepatocytes frequently accumulate intermediate filaments in their cytoplasm, forming gray-blue rope-like inclusions that are known as Mallory's bodies. These filaments are typical of alcoholic liver disease but may be seen in other conditions. Repeated episodes of alcoholic hepatitis result in chronic injury to the liver with the accumulation of collagenous fibrosis first in portal tracts. Over time, fibrosis progresses to form abnormal bands between portal tracts or between portal tracts and central veins (so-called bridging fibrosis). This fibrosis results in obstruction to bile flow and ultimately produces the micronodular pattern characteristic of alcoholic cirrhosis. In this setting, abnormal regenerative nodules of hepatocytes develop, completing the morphologic transformation to cirrhosis. The coexistence of viral hepatitis and exposure to other hepatotoxins in the setting of chronic alcoholism may greatly accelerate the development of alcoholic cirrhosis.

Iron- and Copper-induced Liver Disease

Heritable abnormalities in iron and copper metabolism can result in hepatic dysfunction and cirrhosis. Hemochromatosis is an autosomal recessive disease that results in the abnormal accumulation of iron in many organs including the liver (see Chapter 4). The accumulation of large amounts of iron in hepatocytes results in dysfunction and can ultimately cause the death of hepatocytes.

Wilson's disease results from the abnormal accumulation of copper in multiple organs. This can result in severe hepatocellular injury that causes cirrhosis or massive hepatic necrosis. Copper accumulation also results in neurologic injury and may be identified by the presence of greenish brown rings around the cornea of the eye (Kayser-Fleischer rings).

Drug-induced Hepatitis

Many drugs can produce varying degrees of hepatocyte dysfunction depending on their dose and individual variations in drug-metabolizing enzymes (e.g., cytochrome P-450 polymorphisms). Some drugs may result in idiosyncratic hepatotoxicity, which is immune-mediated in some cases. Drug-induced hepatotoxicity often results in the formation of small granulomas within the liver that may be helpful in establishing the diagnosis.

Nonalcoholic Steatohepatitis

Nonalcoholic steatohepatitis (NASH) usually occurs in obese individuals and individuals with diabetes and corresponds to varying degrees of steatosis (accumulation of lipid in hepatocytes) associated with a chronic inflammatory cell infiltrate (Fig. 9-21). These morphologic findings on liver biopsy may be indistinguishable from alcohol-induced liver disease. NASH progresses to cirrhosis in some patients, although its clinical course is variable. The incidence of NASH is rapidly increasing with epidemic obesity and type 2 diabetes mellitus in the United States. Over the next 10 to 20 years, NASH may become a numerically important cause of hepatic dysfunction and cirrhosis.

Other Causes of Hepatocellular Dysfunction

Reye's syndrome is a rare disease of uncertain pathogenesis that occurs in young children and is epidemiologically related to the ingestion of aspirin. It results in marked dysfunction of multiple organs including the liver (marked microvesicular steatosis) and central nervous system and frequently is fatal.

Hepatorenal syndrome is a symptom complex in which there is synchronous dysfunction of the liver and kidneys. Hepatorenal syndrome usually occurs in the setting of long-standing alcoholic cirrhosis and may be related to derangements of portal or systemic blood flow.

α_1-*Antitrypsin deficiency* is an autosomal recessive disease that results in emphysema because of the unopposed activity of proteolytic enzymes in the absence of this important protease inhibitor. These patients are also at markedly increased risk for the development of hepatic cirrhosis. Hepatocytes frequently contain PAS-positive cytoplasmic protein aggregates that correspond to abnormal α_1-antitrypsin protein.

Severe congestive heart failure results in increased central venous pressure that causes dysfunction of centrilobular hepatocytes (dilatation of central veins compresses adjacent hepatocytes). Severe congestion can result in necrosis of centrilobular hepatocytes, and chronic injury can eventually result in permanent centrilobular fibrosis and scarring, which interfere with normal hepatic function (so-called "cardiac cirrhosis").

Liver Abscess

Abscess formation within hepatic parenchyma is rare in the United States but is relatively common in developing countries, where it may be caused by pyogenic bacteria or

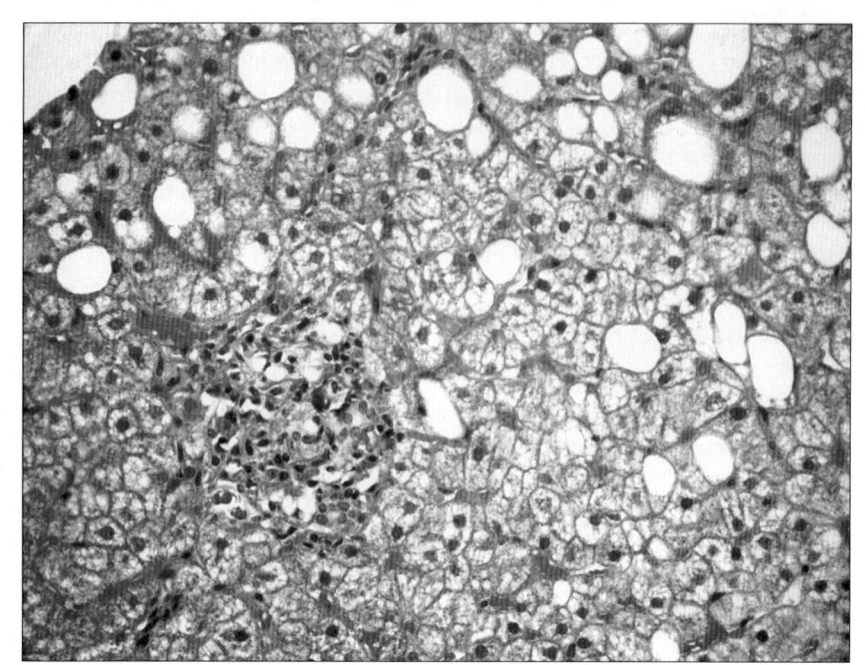

Figure 9-21. Nonalcoholic steatohepatitis (NASH). Microscopic section of liver showing extensive lipid accumulation in hepatocytes (lipid appears as optically clear micro- and macrovesicles). There is evidence of associated hepatocellular injury, and a mild chronic inflammatory cell infiltrate is present.

parasites. Liver abscess is usually associated with significant morbidity and mortality.

Cirrhosis

Cirrhosis is defined pathologically as the presence of marked hepatic fibrosis with the formation of architecturally abnormal regenerative nodules (Fig. 9-22A). These regenerative nodules lack associated portal tracts and are not connected to the biliary tree in a normal fashion (see Fig. 9-22B). Micronodular cirrhosis is typically observed in chronic alcoholic liver disease but may be seen as an end stage of chronic viral hepatitis or autoimmune hepatitis. Cirrhosis results in obstruction to portal venous blood flow as well as diminished or inadequate hepatocyte function, which may terminate in hepatic failure (see below). Patients with cirrhosis can develop jaundice owing to inadequate processing bilirubin into bile and intrahepatic abnormalities in biliary architecture. Mechanical obstruction to portal venous blood flow may be alleviated by the creation of a portal-caval shunt that bypasses portal venous circulation through the liver. This may diminish some of the vascular complications of cirrhosis but does not restore function. Over time, portal hypertension results in the compensatory dilatation and proliferation of veins with the development of varices (dilated veins) to bypass portal venous blood flow. GI bleeding from submucosal varices can further stress a cirrhotic liver (detoxification of hemoglobin breakdown products) and may lead to decompensation and hepatic failure. Cirrhosis is the most common cause of portal hypertension that can result from congenital abnormalities of the hepatic circulation or from portal vein thrombosis.

Hepatic Failure

Hepatic failure is the inability of the liver to adequately process endogenous toxins or produce adequate plasma proteins for the maintenance of oncotic pressure and normal blood coagulation. Drug metabolism is greatly impaired in patients with hepatic failure, and anasarca may develop as a consequence of decreased hepatic protein synthesis. Ammonia metabolism by the liver may be inadequate and contribute to the development of hepatic encephalopathy. Hepatic failure most often results from cirrhosis but can be caused by fulminant hepatitis or toxin exposure.

Vascular Obstruction

Hepatic vein thrombosis can occur acutely or develop progressively. This is referred to as Budd-Chiari syndrome and usually occurs in individuals in a hypercoagulable state. When severe, it can result in hepatic infarction and marked hepatocellular dysfunction.

Tumors and Tumor-like Conditions

Hepatic Adenoma and Focal Nodular Hyperplasia

Liver cell adenoma is an uncommon benign neoplasm that usually develops in young women and may be associated with use of oral contraceptive agents. Adenomas are composed of morphologically bland hepatocytes that form a mass lesion within the liver (Fig. 9-23). Adenomas may be complicated by hemorrhage. Focal nodular hyperplasia is a characteristic nodular proliferation of hepatocytes within the liver that is almost always associated with a central fibrous scar. Focal nodular hyperplasia is thought to represent an

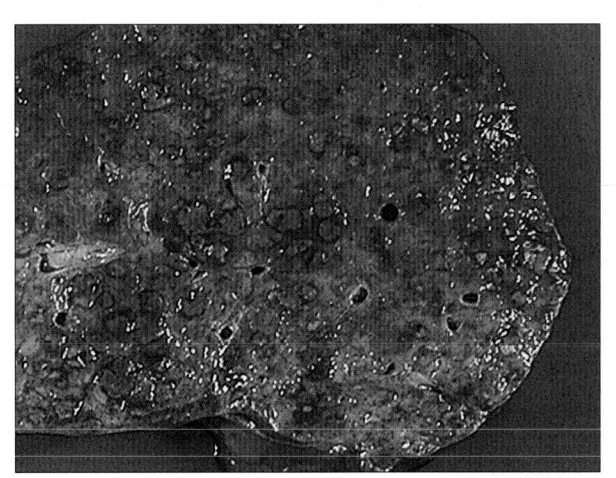

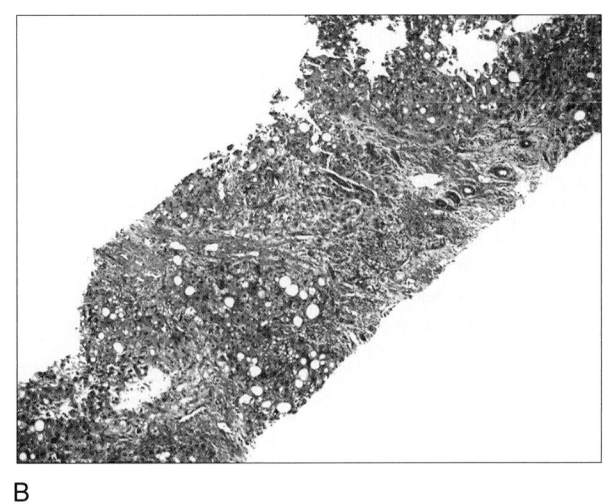

Figure 9-22. A, Hepatic cirrhosis. Gross cross-section of liver with small nodules replacing hepatic parenchyma. **B,** Microscopic section of liver tissue stained with a trichrome stain (hepatocytes appear red and fibrous tissue is stained blue). Fibrous septae are present between small, abnormal regenerative nodules of hepatocytes (micronodular cirrhosis).

exuberant response to injury and has no potential for malignant transformation.

Hepatocellular Carcinoma

Hepatocellular carcinoma is relatively uncommon in the United States but is one of the most common malignant tumors worldwide. There is a strong association between hepatocellular carcinoma and chronic viral hepatitis (both hepatitis B and C viruses). All types of chronic liver disease that result in cirrhosis increase a patient's risk for the development of hepatocellular carcinoma. Chronic exposure to oxidative stress, inflammatory cytokines, and growth factors probably underlie much of this predisposition to cancer. Transactivating proteins encoded by hepatitis B virus may directly contribute to tumorigenesis, and integration of hepatitis B viral DNA into the hepatocyte

genome may also be a factor in tumor development. Vertical transmission of hepatitis B virus (transmission from mother to fetus) results in a strong predilection for the development of hepatocellular carcinoma later in life. Vertical transmission is an important factor contributing to the high incidence of hepatocellular carcinoma in Asia. Certain environmental factors are directly associated with the development of hepatocellular carcinoma. In particular, aflatoxin (a product of peanut fungus that is present in some areas) causes a specific mutation in the p53 gene that predisposes to the development of hepatocellular carcinoma.

Well-differentiated hepatocellular carcinoma can closely resemble non-neoplastic liver tissue, and distinction from a regenerative nodule in the setting of cirrhosis may be difficult (Fig. 9-24A). Poorly differentiated tumors may be difficult to distinguish from metastatic tumors to the liver. Hepatocellular carcinoma is usually solitary, but extensive intraparenchymal dissemination may occur (see Fig. 9-24B). The primary treatment for hepatocellular carcinoma is surgical; however, this often is not technically possible if the tumor involves a significant percentage of the liver. Some patients with more advanced tumors may be cured by liver transplantation. Hepatocellular carcinoma frequently metastasizes to bone and lung. Tumors are usually discovered at late stage, and most are rapidly fatal.

Fibrolamellar carcinoma is a distinct tumor of hepatocytes that occurs in younger individuals and is linked with neither hepatitis virus infection nor alcohol consumption. As its name implies, this tumor is associated with marked fibrosis and tends to have pushing rather than infiltrative borders. For this reason, surgical resection is more often possible and can be curative.

Cholangiocarcinoma and Ampullary Carcinoma

Cholangiocarcinoma may arise within the liver or in extrahepatic bile ducts and is usually associated with marked fibrosis (desmoplasia). Morphologically, some cholangiocarcinomas may be indistinguishable from pancreatic ductal adenocarcinomas while others share many morphologic features with hepatocellular carcinoma. Oval cells are the precursors of both hepatocytes and bile duct epithelium, and their capacity for dual differentiation may underlie the genesis of such mixed tumors. Cholangiocarcinoma typically produces biliary obstruction that may be segmental or complete, and patients often have jaundice. The central location of most cholangiocarcinomas usually precludes curative surgery.

Carcinomas of the ampulla of Vater have a somewhat different clinical presentation and prognosis. They often arise from adenomatous polyps in the ampulla and tend to cause biliary tract obstruction early in their course. Because of this, they are more frequently amenable to surgical excision, and many may be cured by radical surgery.

Liver Transplantation

Liver transplantation has emerged as the definitive therapy for some heritable and congenital abnormalities of the liver

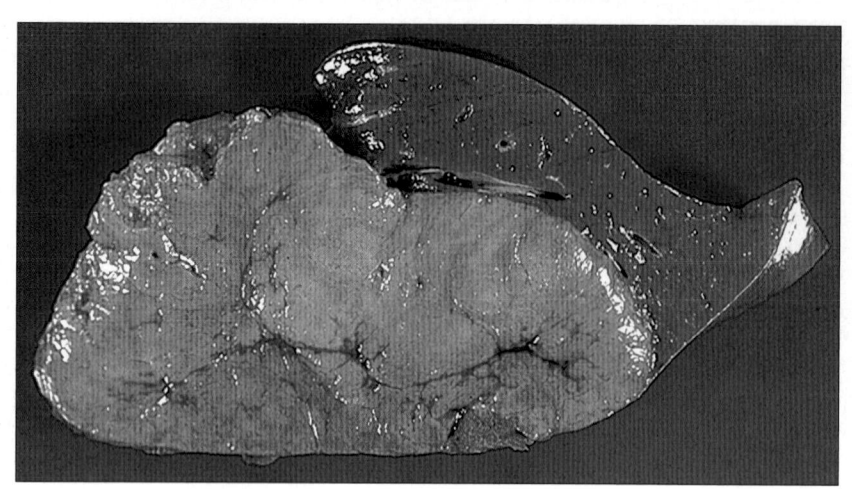

Figure 9-23. Hepatic adenoma. Gross cross-section of liver showing a large adenoma (pink tissue) that is sharply circumscribed from normal hepatic parenchyma (brown-red tissue at upper right).

as well as some localized tumors such as fibrolamellar carcinoma. Patients with hepatic cirrhosis are usually not candidates for liver transplantation owing to long-standing portal hypertension. Patients with liver failure as a result of viral hepatitis will often have recurrence of the hepatitis with the transplant.

●●● EXOCRINE PANCREAS

Acute and Chronic Pancreatitis

The exocrine pancreas is responsible for the synthesis and secretion of digestive enzymes that are stored as inactive zymogen granules in the cytoplasm of acinar cells. Premature activation of these zymogen granules in the setting of pancreatic ductal obstruction or trauma can result in acute pancreatitis. The release of activated hydrolytic enzymes results in tissue destruction and is often associated with fat necrosis in peripancreatic soft tissue (lipases cause saponification of adipose tissue, forming calcium salts) (Fig. 9-25A). Acute pancreatitis is associated with significant mortality and can be caused by gallstones obstructing the cystic duct, high concentrations of alcohol, or trauma (surgical or external). Chronic pancreatitis usually results from repeated episodes of acute pancreatitis that ultimately obliterate much of the pancreatic acinar tissue. A minority of patients with chronic pancreatitis do not have a history of acute attacks (see Fig. 9-25B). Some families have a heritable predisposition to pancreatitis, and these syndromes are associated with an increased risk for the development of adenocarcinoma. Chronic pancreatitis typically results in loss of normal exocrine function of the pancreas, which causes fat malabsorption and possible deficiency of fat-soluble vitamins. The pancreas is heavily innervated, and chronic pancreatitis is often associated with marked pain that may be intractable and require pancreatectomy. Islets are remarkably resistant to pancreatitis, and diabetes is an uncommon complication of chronic pancreatitis.

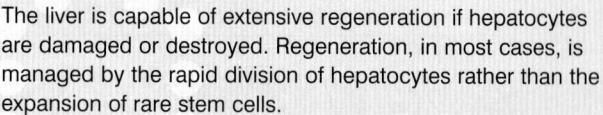

HISTOLOGY

Hepatic Oval Cells

The liver is capable of extensive regeneration if hepatocytes are damaged or destroyed. Regeneration, in most cases, is managed by the rapid division of hepatocytes rather than the expansion of rare stem cells.

Oval cells are defined as liver stem cells that are capable of differentiating into both hepatocytes and bile duct epithelial cells. The definition of oval cells largely derives from experimental paradigms in animals, and it seems clear that some hematopoietic stem cells are also capable of differentiating into hepatocytes. Stem cells play a role in regeneration after more severe forms of liver injury. Reconstitution of normal architecture depends on the integrity of the extracellular matrix (ECM). Damage or destruction of the ECM typically leads to cirrhosis.

Tumors

Adenocarcinoma

Most tumors of the pancreas are ductal adenocarcinomas. These are usually associated with marked fibrosis (desmoplasia) and are more common in the head than in the tail of the pancreas (Fig. 9-26). Because of this location, they frequently result in compression or obstruction of the common bile duct, and most patients have painless jaundice as their initial symptom. Most ductal adenocarcinomas are high-grade tumors that metastasize to regional lymph nodes or the liver relatively early in their course. Pancreatic ductal adenocarcinoma is often associated with perineural invasion, which may facilitate its dissemination to surrounding structures. Because of these features, radical surgical resection is rarely curative. Common duct obstruction can often be temporarily corrected by stent placement, but patients typically succumb to progressive tumor within 1 year of diagnosis.

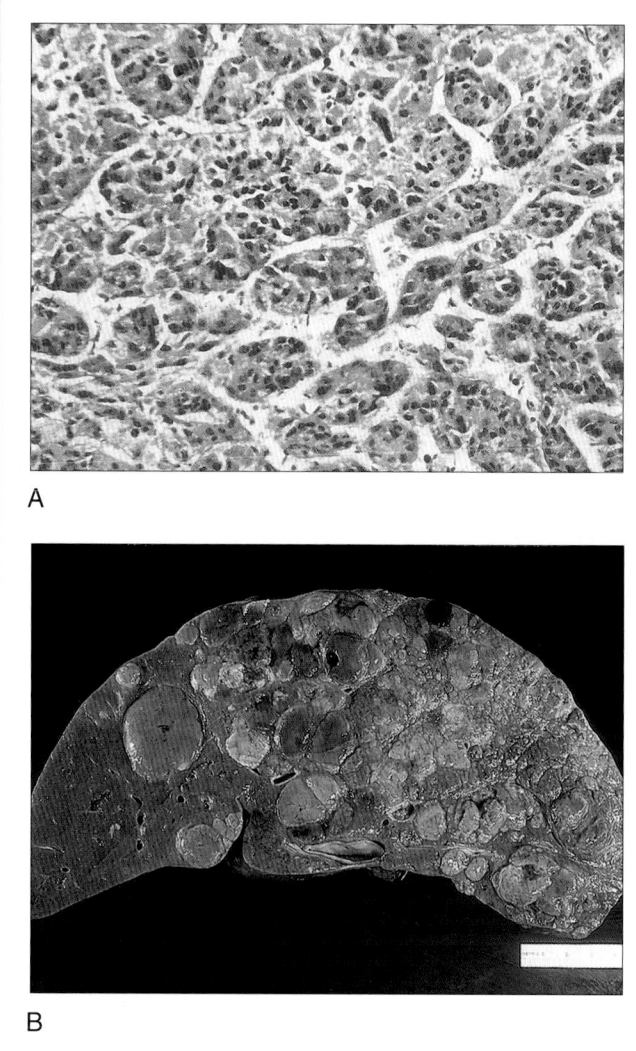

A

B

Figure 9-24. A, Hepatocellular carcinoma. Microscopic section showing moderately differentiated hepatocellular carcinoma with predominantly papillary architecture. Tumor cells resemble normal hepatocytes but have malignant cytologic features. **B**, Hepatocellular carcinoma arising in cirrhosis. Gross cross-section of liver showing a large, irregular, poorly circumscribed hepatocellular carcinoma (*upper center*). Multiple intraparenchymal metastases radiate outward from the main tumor. Uninvolved liver parenchyma is cirrhotic.

Intraductal papillary mucinous tumors (IPMTs) are low-grade mucinous tumors that grow within the pancreatic ducts from mucin-filled cysts within the pancreas. IPMTs may develop into full-blown adenocarcinomas, but most are slow growing and excision of early lesions is usually curative. Mucinous cystadenoma and cystadenocarcinomas of the pancreas are distinctive neoplasms that share many morphologic and biologic features with borderline mucinous tumors of the ovary.

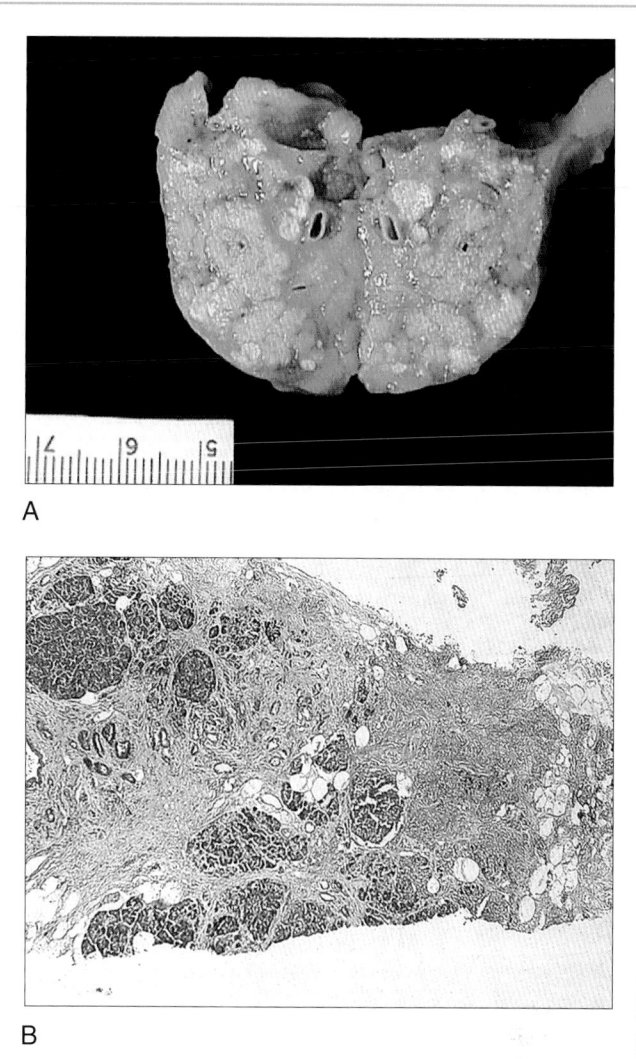

A

B

Figure 9-25. A, Chronic pancreatitis. Gross cross-section of pancreas showing punctate areas of whitish yellow fat necrosis in a background of fibrosis. **B**, Microscopic section showing extensive fibrous replacement of pancreatic acinar tissue and focal fat necrosis with dystrophic calcification.

Other Pancreatic Tumors

Unusual tumors of the pancreas include the so-called solid and cystic neoplasms of the pancreas that tend to occur in younger patients and follow a more indolent course than pancreatic ductal adenocarcinomas. Tumors of pancreatic acinar cells are quite rare. Serous cystadenomas of the pancreas are unusual benign neoplasms that are composed of cells with clear cytoplasm containing abundant glycogen. Neuroendocrine tumors of the pancreas arise from the islets of Langerhans (see Chapter 10).

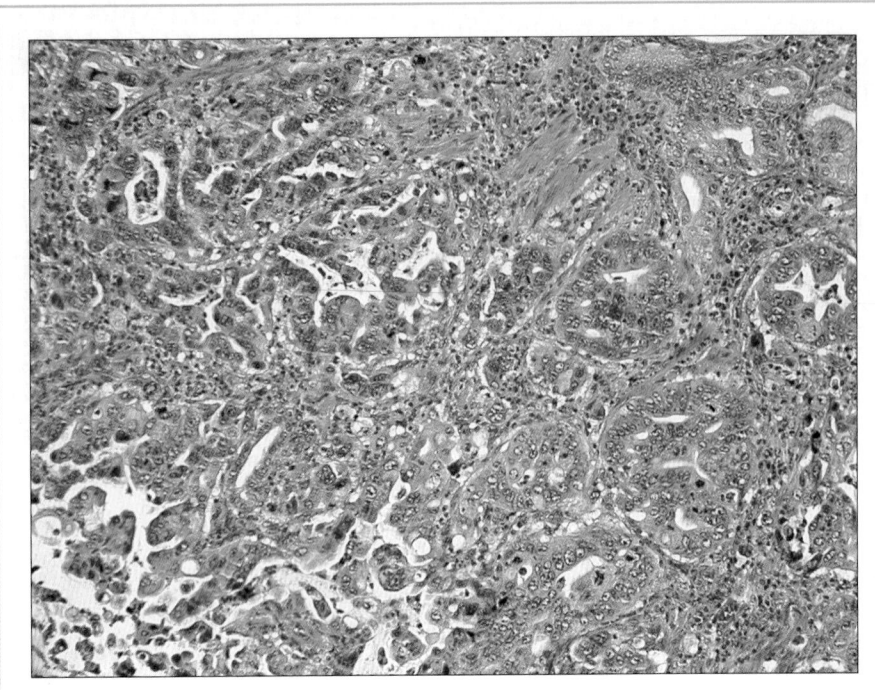

Figure 9-26. Pancreatic adenocarcinoma. Microscopic section of high-grade ductal pancreatic adenocarcinoma composed of pleomorphic tumor cells forming abortive glands with associated desmoplastic stromal response.

Endocrine Pathology 10

CONTENTS

Most pathologic conditions of the endocrine system are related to either deficiency or inappropriate secretion of specific hormones. Tumors, hyperplasia, or inflammatory lesions of the endocrine organs can cause endocrine hypofunction and hyperfunction. Since the hypothalamus and pituitary gland control hormone secretion by many endocrine organs, there is the potential for lesions at this level to result in abnormal hormone secretion by downstream endocrine organs. Identifying the root cause of abnormal hormone production is critical for establishing the correct diagnosis and managing treatment. Simultaneous measurement of the concentration of pituitary hormones (e.g., TSH or ACTH) and downstream hormones (e.g., thyroid hormone or cortisol) often allows localization of the endocrine abnormality. Assessing stimulation or inhibition of hormone release using various pharmacologic agents can also be helpful. Selective hormone measurement in different vascular beds or radiologic imaging using sestamibi scans can help localize endocrine adenomas.

Endocrine gland hyperplasia can result from excessive stimulation by trophic hormones (e.g., pituitary hormones in Cushing's disease) or abnormal concentrations of regulated metabolites (e.g., secondary hyperplasia of parathyroid glands as a consequence of abnormally high phosphate concentrations) in renal failure. Autoantibodies may also stimulate receptors on endocrine cells to cause hypersecretion.

Distinction of benign tumors of endocrine organs (adenomas) from focal or multifocal hyperplasia is often problematic clinically, and in some cases there may not be a clear biologic distinction between these processes. Adenomas tend to have a fibrous capsule and may result in feedback suppression of the normal gland if they are hyperfunctional. None of the pathologic criteria are fully reliable, however, and nodular hyperplasia may closely simulate adenomas. All endocrine organs are richly vascular to subserve their normal function of secreting hormones into the bloodstream. One consequence of this anatomic arrangement is that it is difficult to reliably assess vascular space invasion in endocrine neoplasms. Indeed, in some endocrine tumors, demonstration of metastatic disease is the only reliable criterion for malignancy. The pathologic and clinical staging of many endocrine tumors are markedly different than for most other solid tumors, with patient age and tumor grade being more important than the extent of tumor spread in some cases.

In addition to hormonal symptoms, some endocrine tumors are biologically aggressive and can result in death secondary to local tumor growth or metastatic disease. Neuroendocrine carcinoma can arise in many different organs, presumably from neural crest cells in these locations.

● ● ● PITUITARY

Loss of normal pituitary function can result from tumors or infections of the central nervous system that compress or destroy the sella turcica. Granulomatous diseases such as tuberculosis and sarcoid can cause global pituitary dysfunction. Cysts can cause pituitary compression with loss of normal function. Less commonly, pituitary dysfunction can result from abnormalities of the hypothalamus. The pituitary gland is composed of an adenohypophysis and a neurohypophysis. Hypothalamic stimulation of the neurohypophysis results in the release of specific hormones from the adenohypophysis. Antidiuretic hormone (ADH) is directly secreted by the neurohypophysis and acts on distal collecting ducts in the kidney to cause reabsorption of water. Inappropriate secretion of ADH (SIADH) can result from similar pathologic processes. SIADH can result from abnormalities of the posterior pituitary but more often occurs as a paraneoplastic syndrome in which tumor cells produce ADH. Loss of ADH secretion by the pituitary can cause diabetes insipidus with compulsive water drinking and dilutional hyponatremia, but renal abnormalities are more frequently the cause of nephrogenic diabetes insipidus.

Tumors

Benign tumors can arise from all cellular components of the adenohypophysis and can result in hypersecretion of the hormone corresponding to the tumor cell type (e.g., growth hormone–producing adenomas cause acromegaly in adults or gigantism in children). Pituitary tumors were characterized as chromophobe and chromophil adenomas in the past but are now more precisely classified based on the expressed hormone type (Fig. 10-1). Many pituitary adenomas are nonfunctioning, and their growth causes erosion of the sella turcica with pressure atrophy of normal pituitary cells, resulting in hormone deficiency. Some clinically silent tumors produce prolactin, which may result in infertility and galactorrhea in women but often produces symptoms owing to the loss of expression of other hormones. Most adenomas are microscopic (<1 cm) and can usually be removed by a transsphenoidal approach. Large tumors (macroadenomas >1 cm) can compress the optic chiasm, resulting in visual loss (bitemporal hemianopsia) as well as endocrine symptoms. Other primary tumors of the pituitary gland are less common than adenomas and include craniopharyngiomas, which are primitive tumors composed of epithelial and stromal components. Occasionally glial brain tumors arising in the hypothalamus cause pituitary dysfunction.

●●● THYROID

The thyroid gland is composed of follicles formed by lakes of colloid that are surrounded by a monolayer of cuboidal follicular cells. Follicular cells produce thyroid hormone by digesting colloid in response to stimulation by thyroid-stimulating hormone (TSH). Scattered C cells that secrete calcitonin are distributed throughout the thyroid gland and normally contribute less than 1% of its cellularity. C cells are the precursors of medullary carcinoma. Calcitonin opposes the action of parathyroid hormone to lower blood calcium, but C-cell hyperfunction rarely results in symptomatic hypocalcemia.

Hyperfunctional States

Graves' disease results in symptoms of thyroid hormone excess including rapid pulse and increased body temperature. Graves' disease is usually caused by autoantibodies that bind to receptors on follicular cells and stimulate them to produce thyroid hormone. These autoantibodies are often called long-acting thyroid stimulators (LATS) and functionally mimic the effects of TSH. As with many autoimmune diseases, Graves' disease is more common in first-degree relatives of patients. Long-standing Graves' disease can produce serious cardiovascular and ophthalmic complications (exophthalmos due to hypertrophy of the extraocular muscles). The thyroid gland in Graves' disease is hypervascular, and there is evidence of extensive thyroid hormone production with prominent scalloping of colloid (owing to its ingestion by individual follicular cells) and collapsed follicles (all consumed by colloid) (Fig. 10-2). Thyroid function can be suppressed with

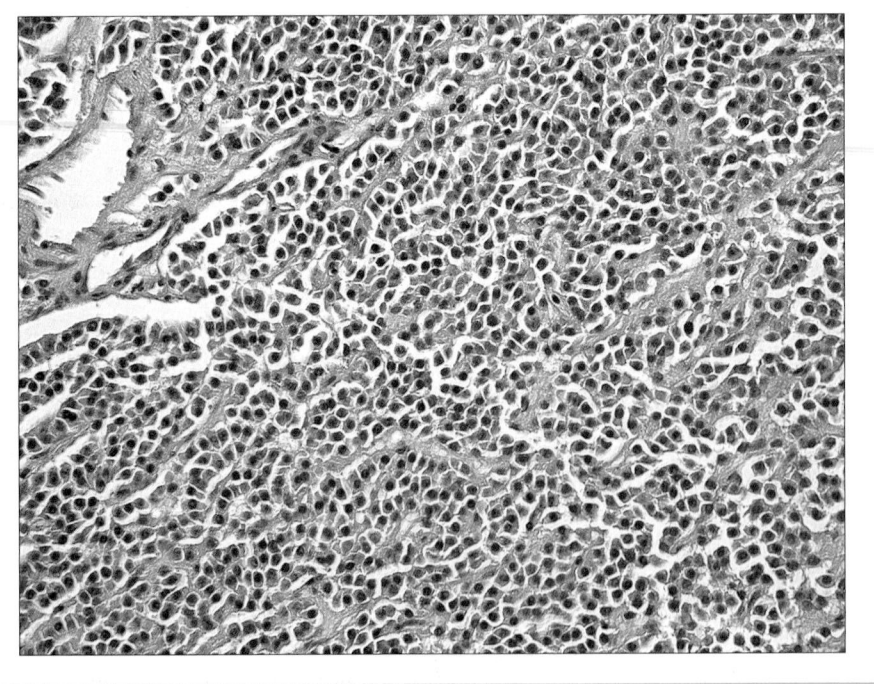

Figure 10-1. Pituitary adenoma. Microscopic section of pituitary showing bland monomorphous cells with neuroendocrine features replacing normal parenchyma.

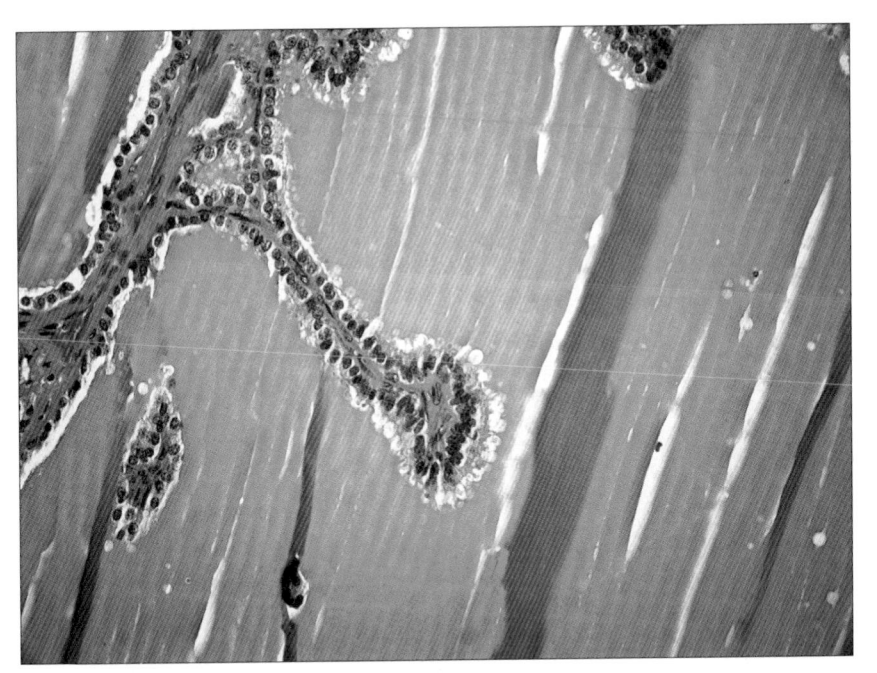

Figure 10-2. Graves' disease. Microscopic section of thyroid gland from a patient with Graves' disease showing scalloping of colloid by activated follicular cells.

propylthiouracil to prevent "thyroid storm" in severe cases of Graves' disease. Patients usually are treated with radioactive iodine, which partially or totally ablates thyroid function, or by thyroidectomy.

Thyroid hyperfunction can occasionally result from functional follicular adenomas (so-called "hot" adenomas), but the vast majority of adenomas do not secrete clinically significant amounts of thyroid hormone. Rarely, patients with multinodular goiter may show signs of thyroid hyperfunction ("toxic goiter"), but most patients are either euthyroid or hypothyroid. Patients with Hashimoto's thyroiditis may have transient thyroid hyperfunction in the early stages of their disease when active inflammation is ongoing (see below).

Hypofunctional States

The most common cause of thyroid hypofunction in the United States is Hashimoto's thyroiditis. *Hashimoto's thyroiditis* is an autoimmune disease caused by a cell-mediated immunoreaction that targets thyroid follicular cells. T-cell infiltration of thyroid gland with associated germinal centers and evidence of damage or reactive changes in follicular cells is typical in Hashimoto's thyroiditis. Many follicular cells show changes in Hürthle cells and develop more abundant, granular, eosinophilic cytoplasm in association with nuclear enlargement and prominent nucleoli. Hürthle cell change is not specific for Hashimoto's thyroiditis and occurs focally in other conditions as well as in some neoplasms. Diffuse Hürthle cell change with germinal centers is characteristic of Hashimoto's thyroiditis (Fig. 10-3).

Patients with Hashimoto's thyroiditis frequently develop autoantibodies to thyroid peroxidase or thyroglobulin.

These antibodies are helpful in establishing a diagnosis of Hashimoto's thyroiditis but may not be related to disease manifestations. The early stages of Hashimoto's thyroiditis are sometimes associated with thyroid hyperfunction (usually mild), but over time the thyroid gland is destroyed and replaced by fibrous tissue, resulting in thyroid insufficiency. Patients with Hashimoto's thyroiditis have an increased risk for developing thyroid tumors, particularly papillary carcinoma. Many cases of Hashimoto's disease have a demonstrable translocation between the RET and PTC genes in thyroid tissue, even in the absence of an identifiable papillary carcinoma (see below). For this reason, some clinicians advocate total thyroidectomy for all patients with Hashimoto's thyroiditis.

Other forms of chronic thyroiditis are less common. A lymphocytic infiltrate in the thyroid without associated Hürthle cell change or germinal centers is classified as nonspecific or lymphocytic thyroiditis; the clinical course is variable. Riedel's struma is a rare, primarily fibrosing thyroiditis that can result in tracheal compression.

Tumors and Tumor-like Conditions

Multinodular Goiter

Multinodular goiter (also called nodular hyperplasia) of the thyroid gland is one of the most common disease processes that bring a patient to medical attention. Multinodular goiter is characterized by the formation of multiple nodules in the thyroid gland that are irregular in shape and composed of small and large follicles (Fig. 10-4). Many of the follicles contain large lakes of colloid (so-called colloid nodules). Colloid nodules often undergo degeneration and hemorrhage

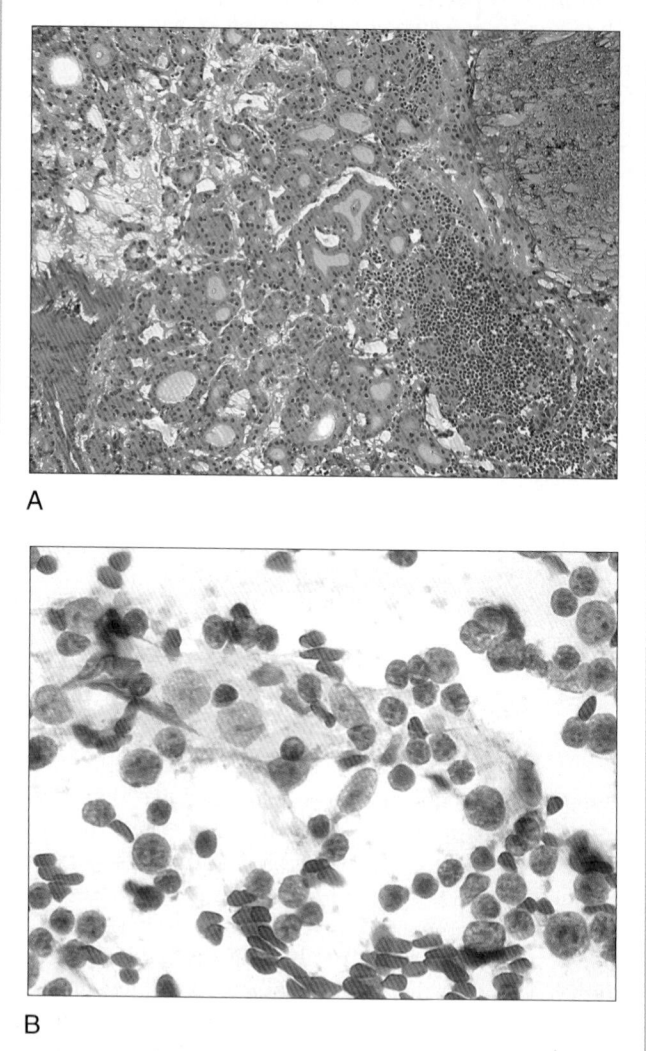

A

B

Figure 10-3. Hashimoto's thyroiditis. **A**, Microscopic section of thyroid gland showing diffuse Hürthle cell change in follicular cells with an associated dense lymphocytic infiltrate. **B**, Cytologic smear from a thyroid fine-needle aspiration (FNA) showing a mixture of Hürthle cells (large epithelial cells with granular cytoplasm and prominent nucleoli) and small lymphocytes typical of Hashimoto's thyroiditis.

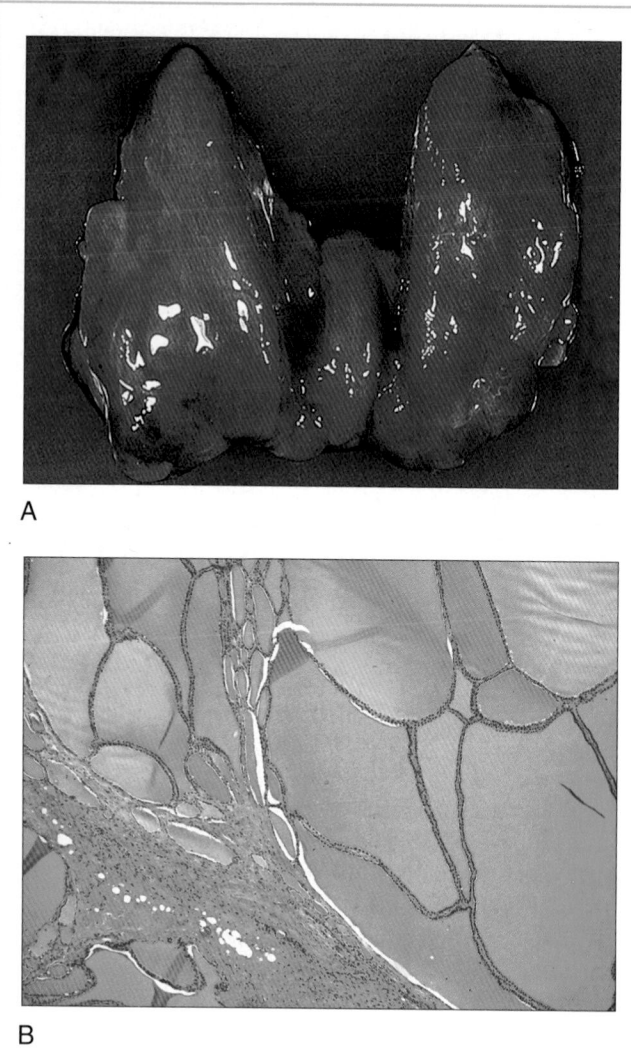

A

B

Figure 10-4. Nodular hyperplasia of the thyroid. **A**, Gross photograph of a thyroid gland showing irregular nodules bulging out the capsular surface. **B**, Microscopic section of thyroid tissue showing follicles of varying size and shape and focal hemosiderin-containing macrophages.

so that hemosiderin-containing macrophages are a common component of the thyroid gland in this disease. Hemorrhage and degeneration commonly lead to fibrosis and dystrophic calcification within this fibrous tissue. Focal (but not diffuse) Hürthle cell change is also frequently observed.

Patients with multinodular goiter often have a mixture of "hot" and "cold" nodules on radioactive thyroid scan. Since hot nodules almost never correspond to adenoma or tumors, cold nodules are frequently selected for evaluation by fine-needle aspiration (FNA).

The demonstration of typical features of nodular hyperplasia with abundant colloid, variable-sized follicles, and histiocytes containing hemosiderin can confirm the diagnosis

of nodular hyperplasia. Multinodular goiter can develop as a consequence of iodine deficiency, and this is a common cause of goiter in endemic areas in the developing world. The incidence of multinodular goiter increases with age in the United States, but its underlying cause is uncertain.

Papillary Carcinoma

Papillary carcinoma of the thyroid gland is usually a low-grade neoplasm that frequently is multifocal. Papillary carcinoma tends to grow as nodules composed of tumor cells that have characteristic nuclear features and show nuclear overlap in tissue sections (Fig. 10-5A). Tumor nuclei usually show prominent clearing, nuclear grooves, membrane-bound nucleoli, and pseudo-inclusions (see Figs. 10-5B and 10-5C). The presence of these nuclear changes in a focal lesion defines

Fine-Needle Aspiration (FNA)

FNA is a minimally invasive procedure that can provide diagnostic information about superficial or deep mass lesions. FNA is performed with a thin-bore needle (usually >22 gauge) and is usually done without local anesthesia. After the needle tip is placed in the lesion (either by palpation or radiographic guidance), back pressure is applied by syringe and the needle is moved in and out to cut small tissue fragments. The aspirated material (usually <50 µL) is smeared on a slide and stained to allow on-site evaluation of sample adequacy. Tissue fragments and cells make up the diagnostic material.

Thyroid FNA can be used to diagnose papillary carcinoma (based on nuclear features) and can provide clinically useful risk stratification for other thyroid lesions. Since thyroid nodules are present in up to 5% of the adult population and >95% are benign, FNA risk stratification is a useful approach that may avoid unnecessary surgery in many patients with benign disease.

papillary carcinoma, which generally is associated with abnormalities of the RET oncogene (germline or somatic). Most papillary carcinomas have a papillary growth pattern; however, it has become clear that follicular tumors with typical nuclear features of papillary carcinomas behave essentially identically to tumors with papillary architecture. For this reason, the "follicular variant of papillary carcinoma" is now recognized as a subtype of papillary carcinoma.

Most papillary carcinomas are associated with point mutations in the RET oncogenes, and patients with germline mutations in RET (MEN II [see Multiple Endocrine Neoplasia section]) often develop multiple tumors.

Papillary carcinomas frequently behave in an indolent manner and remain localized in the thyroid gland. Tumor metastasis is almost invariably to regional lymph nodes. Even in patients with lymph node metastases, tumors may remain localized in the neck region for many years. For this reason, the staging of papillary thyroid cancer is minimally affected by the presence of lymph node metastases. More important prognostic factors are patient age (with adverse tumor behavior seen in patients older than age 40). Some morphologic variants (e.g., tall cell) tend to behave more aggressively. Primary treatment is surgical (usually, complete thyroidectomy because of the frequency of multicentric tumors), with radioactive iodine reserved for metastatic disease. Even when disease is surgically incurable, it often remains relatively indolent with slow progression. A small number of patients have clinically aggressive tumors with systemic metastasis or tracheal obstruction.

Papillary microcarcinoma (encapsulated tumor <1 cm in diameter that is confined to the thyroid gland) has little or no clinical significance. Papillary microcarcinomas that are found incidentally (in thyroids removed for other reasons) are usually managed by watchful waiting.

Follicular Adenoma and Carcinoma

Follicular adenomas typically are encapsulated lesions of follicular thyroid tissue that are composed predominantly of microfollicles (see Fig. 5-1A). Distinction of adenomas from nodular hyperplasia is often operational in that adenomas are usually singular lesions while a thyroid with multiple nodules suggests a diagnosis of nodular hyperplasia. A small percentage of follicular adenomas show malignant features including destructive capsular invasion or evidence of vascular space invasion by tumor cells. Even in tumors that show some of these features, the clinical behavior is often indolent and metastatic disease is very rare. Minimally invasive lesions that are confined to the thyroid almost never behave aggressively. In contrast, true follicular carcinomas that invade beyond the thyroid capsule are clinically aggressive lesions that characteristically cause bony metastases. Hürthle cell carcinomas and adenomas can also occur, and there is some evidence that they are slightly more aggressive than other follicular lesions.

Anaplastic thyroid carcinoma is usually classified as a variant of follicular carcinoma that has transformed to a highly malignant neoplasm. Anaplastic carcinomas may be difficult to recognize as thyroid tumors because of their poor differentiation. Anaplastic carcinomas are classified as AJCC stage IV (usually reserved for patients with systemic metastasis) regardless of the extent of tumor spread. Tracheal invasion with respiratory insufficiency is a common presenting sign in anaplastic carcinoma.

Medullary Carcinoma

Medullary carcinoma is a tumor of C cells, which normally produce calcitonin. Medullary carcinoma is a typical neuroendocrine tumor with finely divided nuclear chromatin that may show nuclear molding (Fig. 10-6). A wide variety of morphologic variants of medullary carcinoma have been described, and some tumors are associated with an amyloid stroma. Many medullary carcinomas arise in the setting of multiple endocrine neoplasia (MEN) type I. These patients have germline mutations in the MEN gene, and tumors tend to arise in the setting of diffuse C-cell hyperplasia, which can be demonstrated immunohistochemically by staining for calcitonin. Medullary carcinomas can metastasize relatively early in their course. Calcitonin is a useful cellular and serum biomarker for these neoplasms and can be used to assess residual and recurrent disease.

●●● PARATHYROID

Four parathyroid glands are typically present in the neck, but some may be carried to intrathoracic locations by migration with the branchial arches. Normal parathyroid glands are composed of neuroendocrine cells that can appear as water clear cells, chief cells, and oxyphil cells depending on their functional state. Normal glands are quite small and usually contain lipid, whereas hyperfunctioning glands and adenomas are enlarged and tend to show lipid depletion.

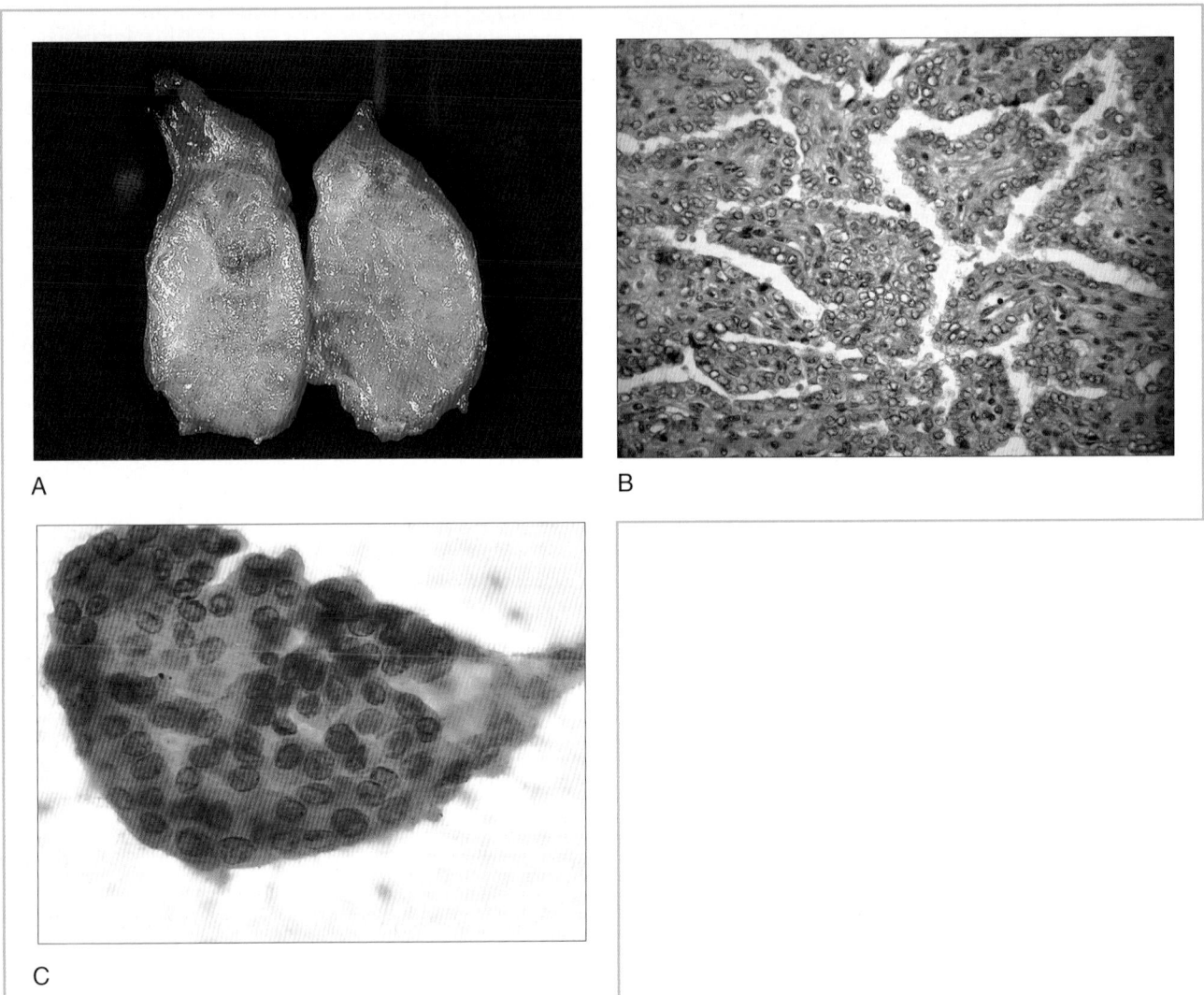

Figure 10-5. Papillary carcinoma of the thyroid. **A**, Gross cross-section of a thyroid gland that is largely replaced by a papillary carcinoma (pale ovoid mass at bottom). **B**, Microscopic section showing papillary structures lined by follicular cells with nuclear inclusions and occasional nuclear grooves. **C**, Cytologic smear from a thyroid FNA showing papillary tissue fragments with prominent nuclear grooves.

Primary Hyperparathyroidism

Primary hyperparathyroidism results either from an adenoma of one or more parathyroid glands or from hyperplasia of multiple parathyroid glands (Fig. 10-7). Pathologic distinction between hyperplasia and adenoma is not reliable. Intraoperative measurement of parathyroid hormone (PTH) levels allows a functional test of whether all hyperplastic or adenomatous parathyroid tissue has been removed (the serum half-life of PTH is measured in minutes). Hyperparathyroidism can develop in both MEN I and MEN II syndromes. Parathyroid adenomas are small (rarely more than 2 g) and so do not produce a significant mass effect. Carcinoma of the parathyroid gland is exceptionally rare.

Hypersecretion of PTH results in stimulation of osteoclastic bone resorption with elevated calcium levels. Patients typically have symptoms related to hypercalcemia, or hypercalcemia is incidentally discovered by clinical laboratory testing. Severe, long-standing hyperparathyroidism can result in substantial loss of bone mineral with osteopenia and pathologic fractures. In its most extreme form, tumor-like masses of osteoclasts (so-called brown tumors) can form within bones and present as osteolytic lesions. Therapy is aimed at removing the hyperfunctioning parathyroid gland or glands. PTH-like proteins are secreted by some tumors (particularly neuroendocrine tumors such as small-cell lung cancer). Paraneoplastic hypercalcemia is more often caused by different mediators such as osteoclast-activating factor (OAF), however.

Secondary Hyperparathyroidism

Secondary hyperparathyroidism results from hyperstimulation of normal parathyroid glands by abnormal concentrations of calcium and phosphorus in the blood. This most typically occurs in patients with end-stage renal disease in which hyperparathyroidism contributes to the metabolic bone disease (e.g., renal osteodystrophy).

●●● ADRENAL

The adrenal gland is a relatively common site for metastatic carcinoma from primary tumors of the lung and other organs. Mass lesions of the adrenal gland are found fairly frequently by computed tomography (CT) and MRI scans performed for staging of patients with various types of malignancies. For this reason, the evaluation of small adrenal lesions has become a relatively common clinical problem. Many of these mass lesions are found to be nonfunctioning (or minimally functioning) adenomas of the adrenal cortex.

Adrenal Cortex

Adrenocortical function is essential for the production of cortisol, aldosterone, and related hormones that manage stress, electrolyte balance, and blood pressure. Complete loss of adrenocortical function is rapidly fatal under conditions of severe stress (e.g., surgery, infection).

Hyperfunctional States

Hyperfunction of the adrenal cortex can result from Cushing's syndrome or Cushing's disease. *Cushing's disease* is caused by hypersecretion of adrenocorticotropic hormone (ACTH) by the pituitary (usually adenomas) with resulting adrenocortical hyperfunction. *Cushing's syndrome* usually results from a functioning cortical adenoma or from focal or diffuse cortical hyperplasia (Fig. 10-8A). Symptoms of Cushing's disease predominantly result from the effects of hypercortisolism. Redistribution of adipose tissue (predominantly to the upper back, where it forms a so-called buffalo hump) results from both excess cortisol stimulation of adipose tissue and cortisol-induced insulin resistance, which can cause overt diabetes mellitus. Individuals with high levels of cortisol are functionally immunosuppressed and are at increased risk for many types of infection. The mineralocorticoid effects of cortisol can result in sodium retention and hypertension that may exacerbate cardiovascular disease.

GENETICS

RET Proto-oncogene and Papillary Thyroid Cancer

RET is a receptor tyrosine kinase that is a member of the glial-derived neurotrophic factor family (GDNF). RET normally signals through the RAS pathway. The majority of papillary thyroid cancers have alterations that activate RAS signaling at some level.

The RET gene is rearranged (by chromosomal translocation) in up to 30% of spontaneous papillary thyroid cancers. RET can be involved in translocations with several different genes resulting in fusion proteins that tend to undergo autophosphorylation and activation in the absence of ligand. PTC3 is the most common RET translocation partner and is often found in irradiation-induced thyroid cancers.

A minority of papillary thyroid cancers have rearrangements of TRKA gene (a high-affinity receptor for nerve growth factor) or activating point mutations in RAS or BRAF.

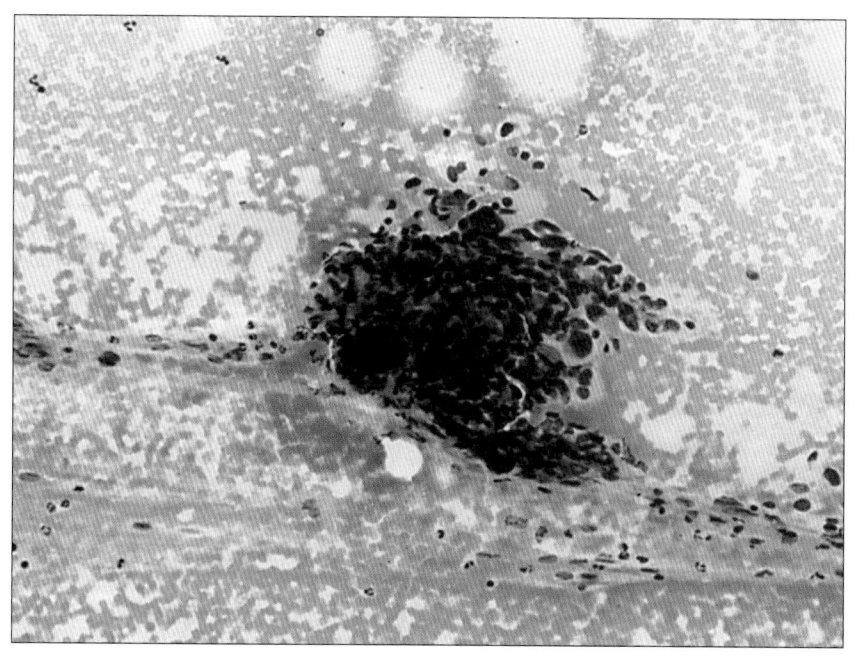

Figure 10-6. Medullary thyroid carcinoma. Air-dried cytologic smear from a thyroid FNA stained with Wright-Giemsa showing tumor cells with finely divided nuclear chromatin, inconspicuous cytoplasm, and nuclear molding (neuroendocrine features).

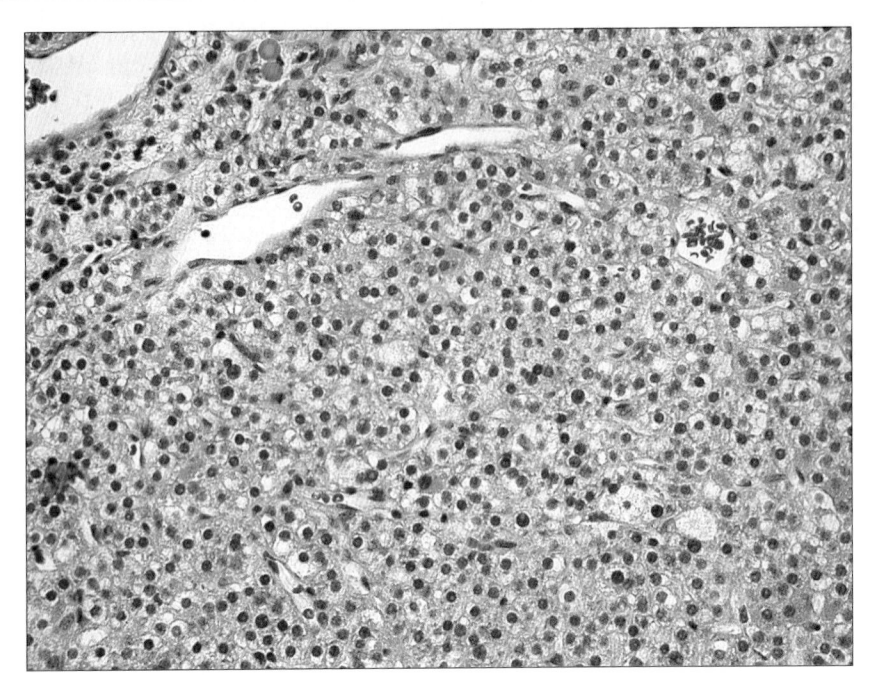

Figure 10-7. Parathyroid adenoma. Microscopic section showing solid sheets of monomorphous neuroendocrine cells with no residual adipose tissue.

Cortical adenomas and hyperplasia of the cortex each can result in hyperaldosteronism with marked potassium wasting (secondary to renal effects of aldosterone) and hypertension.

Congenital Adrenal Hyperplasia

Congenital adrenal hyperplasia can result from genetic abnormalities of 21-hydroxylase, which is essential for the synthesis of aldosterone and cortisol. Accumulated steroid hormone precursors are abnormally converted to androgens in the adrenal gland, and female infants may be pseudo-hermaphrodites.

Hypofunctional States

Hypofunction of the adrenal cortex can result from extensive tumor metastases to both glands although complete destruction of both glands is unusual and clinically significant hormone deficiency is rare. The most common cause of acute adrenal insufficiency is the so-called *Waterhouse-Friderichsen syndrome*, which can develop in patients with meningococcal infection. These acutely ill patients frequently develop bilateral adrenal gland hemorrhage that results in complete loss of gland function (see Fig. 10-8B). Loss of normal cortisol hastens circulatory collapse and death. Tuberculosis can occasionally cause chronic adrenal insufficiency.

Addison's disease is primary adrenocortical failure that is mediated by autoimmune mechanisms. Prolonged cortisol deficiency causes a compensatory rise in ACTH secretion by the pituitary, and high levels of ACTH and corticotropin-releasing factor cause hyperpigmentation of patients' skin (very high concentrations of this hormone with homology to melanocortin directly stimulates melanocytes).

Iatrogenic hypoadrenalism is more common than other forms of deficiency. Treatment of patients with intermediate or high doses of cortisol for a prolonged period of time results in suppression of the pituitary-adrenal axis, which may take days to weeks to recover after discontinuation of therapy. If patients have surgery or infection in this time window, life-threatening deficiency can result unless additional cortisol is supplied.

Carcinoma

Carcinoma of the adrenal cortex is rare. Distinction of large adenomas from carcinomas is operational and is based on the size of the neoplasm (almost always >5 cm) and the presence of necrosis or local invasion or metastasis. Most adrenocortical carcinomas do not produce a hormonal syndrome.

Adrenal Medulla

The adrenal medulla is a large paraganglion similar to paraganglia in the sympathetic chain. Catecholamines produced in the medulla are released directly into the bloodstream.

Paraganglioma

Pheochromocytomas are identical to paragangliomas arising in the sympathetic chain. Paragangliomas are tumors of neuroendocrine cells that produce catecholamines, and they may produce hormonal syndrome by releasing hormone chronically or episodically (see Figs. 10-8C and 10-8D). The episodic release of catecholamines results in a symptom complex with flushing and hypertension that is classically associated with pheochromocytomas. Extra-adrenal paragangliomas can also present with a hormonal syndrome or as mass lesions (e.g., carotid body tumor).

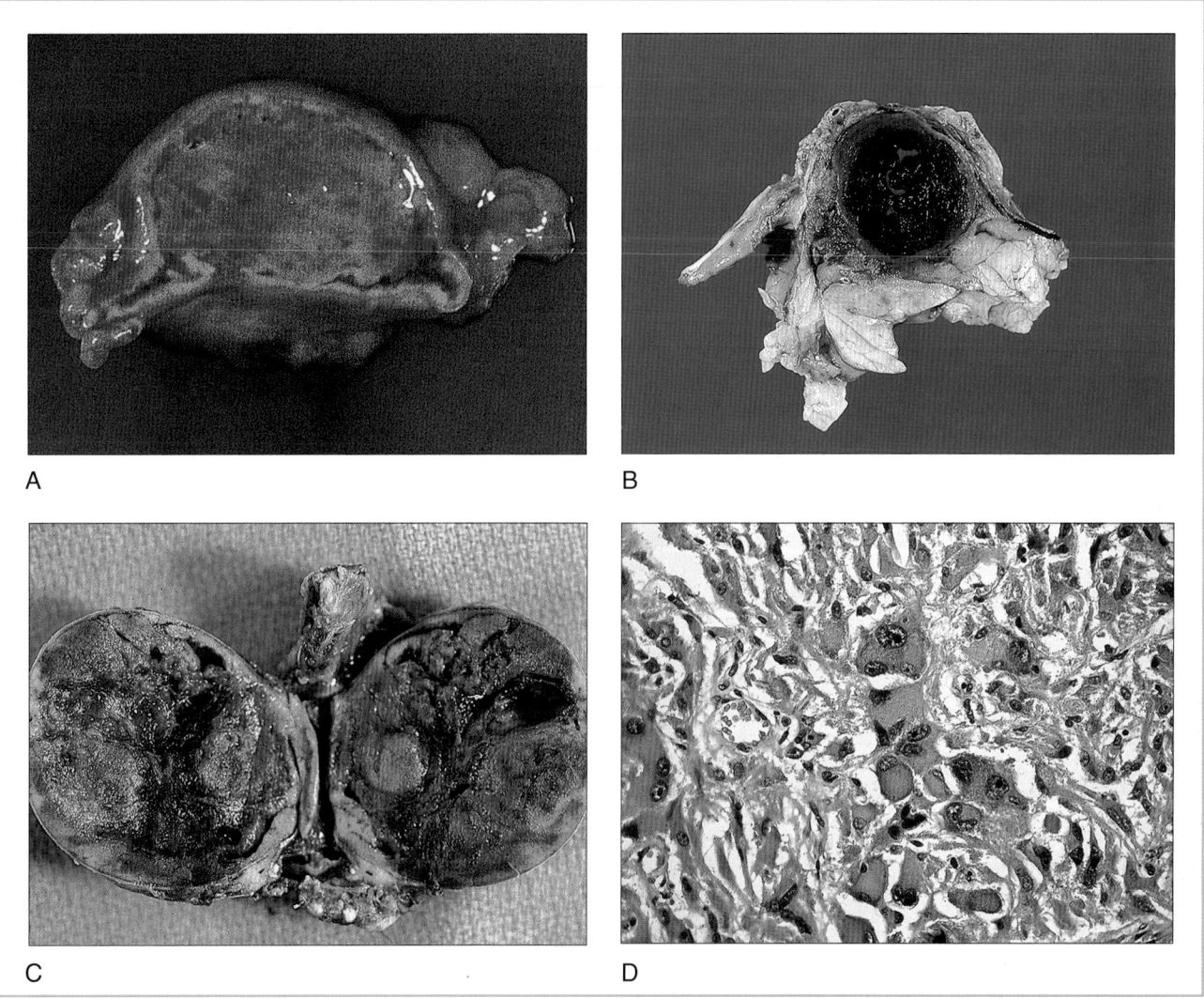

Figure 10-8. A, Adrenocortical adenoma. Gross cross-section of an adrenal gland showing a circumscribed yellow nodule arising from the cortex. **B,** Adrenal hemorrhage. Gross cross-section of adrenal gland showing extensive hemorrhage that has resulted in acute adrenal failure in a patient with meningococcemia. **C,** Pheochromocytoma. Gross cross-section of adrenal gland showing a large pheochromocytoma in the medulla with a variegated appearance and focal hemorrhage. **D,** Microscopic section of a pheochromocytoma showing pleomorphic tumor cells forming nests.

Neuroblastoma

Neuroblastoma is a tumor of childhood that frequently arises in the adrenal medulla but can also occur in the sympathetic chain or at other sites where paraganglia are present (Fig. 10-9A). Neuroblastoma is a primitive tumor composed predominantly of neuroblasts that may show rosette formation (arrangement of tumor cells in a circular fashion resembling an embryonic neural tube; see Fig. 10-9B). Neuroblastoma is one of the small blue-cell tumors of childhood, and a retroperitoneal mass in a young child suggests this diagnosis, which can often be confirmed by the finding of increased catecholamine metabolites in the urine.

Some neuroblastomas show gene amplification of the N-myc proto-oncogene. N-myc gene amplification is associated with a poor prognosis in neuroblastoma and is one of the first molecular prognostic markers identified.

Patient age is an important prognostic factor in neuroblastoma, and presentation in infancy or very early childhood is usually associated with the favorable prognosis, whereas diagnosis after 4 years of age carries a grim prognosis. Pathologic tumor staging is of limited importance in neuroblastoma compared with patient age and N-myc gene status. A special tumor stage (IVS) corresponds to infants with small primary neuroblastomas and evidence of microscopic bone marrow metastases. Despite extensive tumor spread, IVS patients have an excellent outcome and are usually cured by chemotherapy. The propensity of some neuroblastomas to undergo terminal differentiation is a dominant factor in determining prognosis in this disease. Effective chemotherapy may induce susceptible neuroblastomas to undergo terminal differentiation as well as kill tumor cells. The occasional finding of ganglioneuromas in adults is likely a marker of neuro-

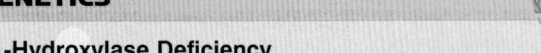

21-Hydroxylase Deficiency

Patients with severe genetic deficiency of 21-hydroxlyase (1/15,000 births) cannot complete the conversion of cholesterol to cortisol or aldosterone and accumulate steroid intermediates in the adrenal cortex. The increased concentration of steroid intermediates can produce several syndromes depending on the severity of the enzyme deficiency. Most cases of this autosomal recessive disorder are caused by rearrangement between the CYP21A2 gene and a pseudogene, leading to a nonfunctioning CYP21A2 gene.

There are three clinical types of 21-hydroxylase deficiency, two of which result in significant clinical symptoms. In the simple virilizing form, patients have some residual 21-hydroxylase activity but the accumulation of steroid intermediates results in increased androgen synthesis that virilizes female fetuses so that they are born with masculinized external genitalia (the internal genital organs form normally). The simple virilizing type accounts for 90% of congenital adrenal hyperplasia (CAH). Approximately 10% of patients with CAH have nearly complete 21-hydroxylase deficiency that results in profound hyponatremia because almost no aldosterone can be formed to stimulate renal sodium resorption.

The third form of 21-hydroxylase deficiency (so-called nonclassical form) is quite common (1/100 births) but produces only mild symptoms. These individuals have only moderately decreased levels of 21-hydroxylase activity, and some (both males and females) show evidence of androgen excess after birth.

blastomas that underwent spontaneous terminal differentiation to ganglioneuromas. Patients with partially differentiated neuroblastomas (ganglioneuroblastomas) have a substantially better outcome than do patients with undifferentiated neuroblastomas.

Other Tumors

Myelolipomas are tumors of the adrenal gland composed of adipose tissue and hematopoietic cells (often multiple lineages). Myelolipomas may become large and can produce life-threatening hemorrhage but have no metastatic potential.

●●● ENDOCRINE PANCREAS

The endocrine pancreas consists of the islets of Langerhans. Islets are more numerous in the tail of the pancreas than in the head. Islets are composed of a mixture of different types of neuroendocrine cells that secrete insulin, glucagon, somatastatin, gastrin, as well as other hormones. Inflammation of the exocrine pancreas in acute and chronic pancreatitis may result in islet dysfunction although islets are surprisingly resistant to pancreatitis. Surgical excision of the pancreas because of tumors or disease of the exocrine pancreas can result in secondary hypoinsulinemia and diabetes mellitus. Some infants have diffuse hyperplasia of

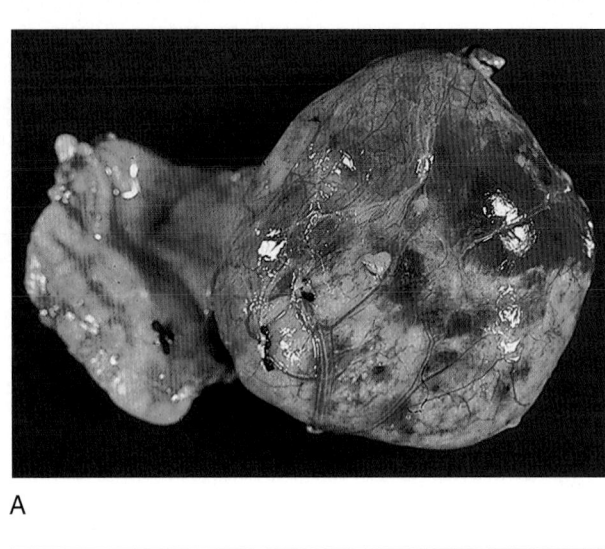

A

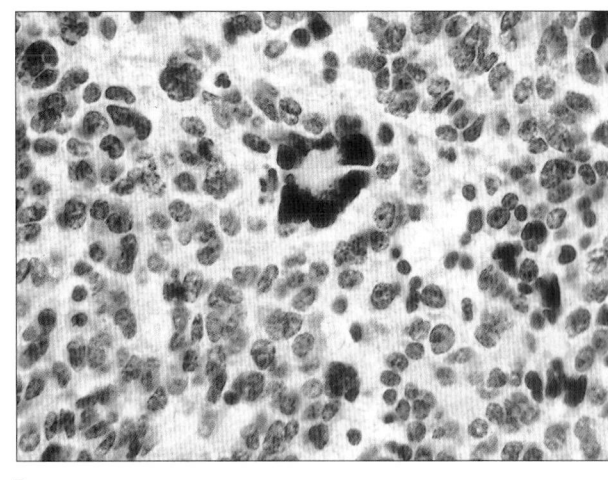

B

Figure 10-9. Neuroblastoma. **A,** Gross cross-section of an adrenal gland replaced by neuroblastoma. The tumor has a gross appearance similar to primitive brain tissue with foci of hemorrhage and necrosis. **B,** Microscopic section of a neuroblastoma showing primitive neuroendocrine cells forming a rosette.

β-cells throughout the pancreas (nesidioblastosis) and develop severe hypoglycemia.

Diabetes Mellitus

Diabetes mellitus comprises two distinct diseases that have overlapping features and complications. Hyperglycemia is the major abnormality in both type 1 and type 2 diabetes, and the degree and duration of hyperglycemia determine the severity of most long-term complications. The diagnosis of diabetes mellitus is usually based on a random blood glucose measurement in excess of 200 mg/dL or a fasting blood glucose greater than 150 mg/dL.

Type 1 diabetes (also called juvenile diabetes) results from hypoinsulinemia (Fig. 10-10). Most patients with type 1 diabetes develop a cell-mediated autoimmune reaction

GENETICS

N-myc Gene Amplification in Neuroblastoma

Gene amplification (the presence of more than two copies of a single-copy gene in a cell) usually leads to increased expression of the amplified gene. Amplification can occur as tandem duplication of the gene in situ (i.e., at its normal chromosomal location) to produce a homogeneously staining region (HSR) visible in cytogenetic spreads of metaphase chromosomes. Alternatively, amplification can occur as an extrachromosomal element called a double-minute chromosome (DM), which lacks centromeres and is randomly distributed during cell division.

HSR and DM terminology derives from classical cytogenetics but can also be detected by interphase fluorescence in situ hybridization (FISH), which is now the method of choice for assessing gene amplification in clinical samples.

For N-myc, both DM and HSR patterns of amplification have the same effect—increasing N-myc gene expression by increasing gene dosage. Overexpression of N-myc is a strong adverse prognostic indicator in neuroblastoma.

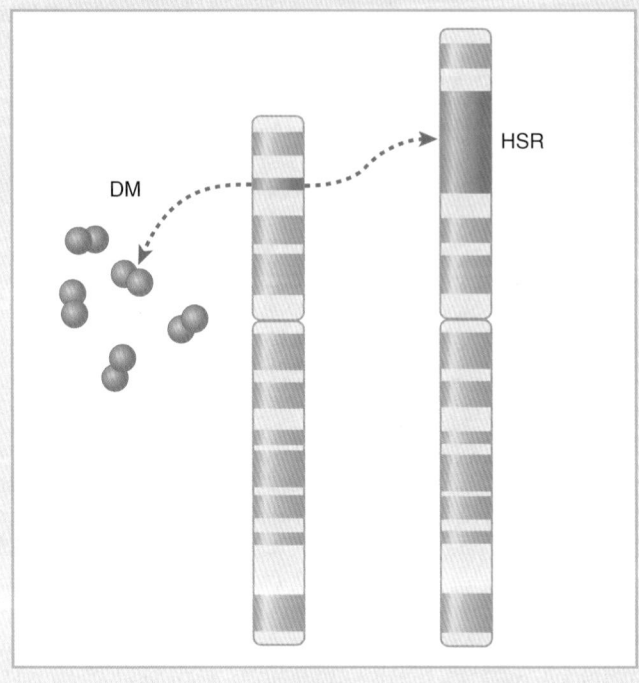

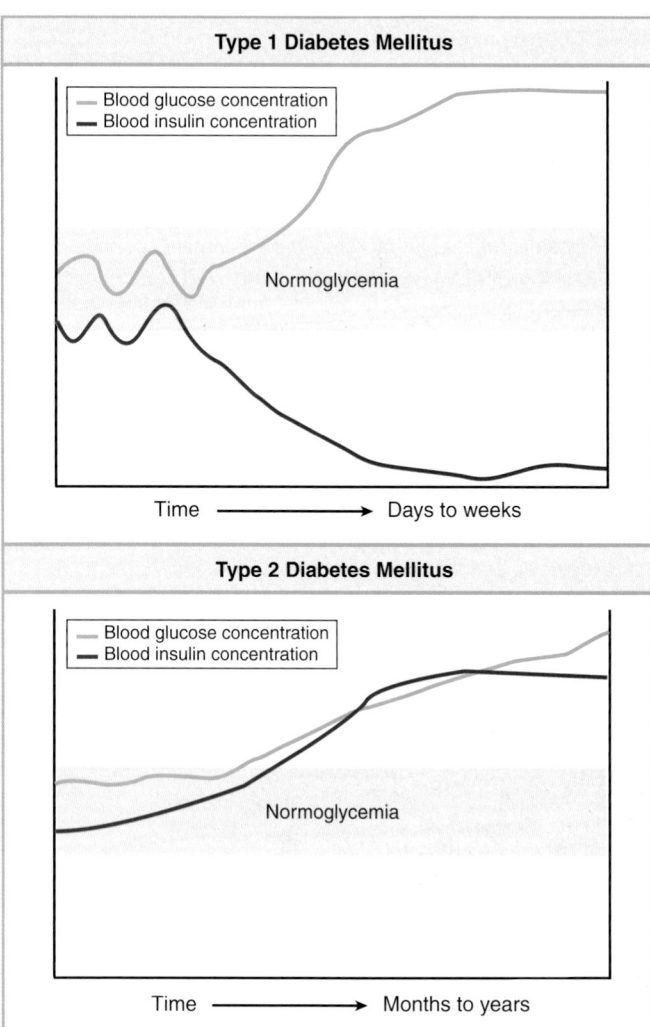

Figure 10-10. Serum concentration of glucose and insulin in type 1 and type 2 diabetes mellitus.

against β-cells in pancreatic islets. This is usually an acute or subacute process that results in the destruction of β-cells over the course of days or weeks. The risk of developing type 1 diabetes is strongly associated with MHC class II immune response genes, and disease almost always develops during childhood or adolescence. It is likely that transient viral infection activates this autoimmune process in susceptible individuals, and rapid initiation of immunosuppression may preserve some β-cell function in these patients. Patients with the most severe type 1 diabetes have essentially no β-cells and can produce almost no insulin. These patients are usually difficult to regulate with exogenous insulin (i.e., "brittle

diabetics") because they have no endogenous insulin secretion to help modulate peaks and valleys in insulin dosing.

Patients with type 1 diabetes may have severe hyperglycemia and often have associated ketoacidosis. The inability to normally import glucose into cells (because of insulin deficiency) causes a switch to ketosis in the liver.

Ketosis results in increased acid production and decreased blood pH, producing the manifestations of diabetic ketoacidosis, which can be rapidly fatal. Patients typically become dehydrated as a result of severe glycosuria and resulting osmotic diuresis. Dehydration exacerbates the metabolic abnormalities in these patients.

Type 2 diabetes results from insulin resistance rather than hyposecretion of insulin (see Fig. 10-10). Type 2 patients are typically obese, and their adipose tissue and skeletal muscle have an abnormally weak response to normal levels of insulin. As a result, these patients typically have higher than normal circulating levels of insulin with coexistent hyperglycemia (i.e., insulin resistance). The effects of increased adipose tissue in obesity are twofold. First, there is a simple

BIOCHEMISTRY

Insulin Synthesis and Secretion

Insulin gene transcripts code for a precursor protein called pre-proinsulin, and removal of its signal peptide in the endoplasmic reticulum of pancreatic β-cells converts it to proinsulin. Proinsulin is cleaved by endopeptidases in the endoplasmic reticulum that remove the internal C peptide linking the α- and β-chains. Mature insulin and C peptide are packaged in neurosecretory granules that accumulate in the cytoplasm as membrane-bound vesicles.

Glucose enters β-cells via facilitated diffusion (GLUT2 transporter). Elevated intracellular glucose increases the ATP/ADP ratio, resulting in blockage of the ATP-sensitive K^+ channel in the plasma membrane, which triggers depolarization to cause an influx of calcium. Increased intracellular calcium triggers docking and fusion of neurosecretory granules with the plasma membrane, resulting in exocytosis of insulin into the extracellular environment.

Insulin secretion is bimodal; the second phase is mediated by reserve vesicles that must first be activated by phosphorylation (protein kinases A and C) before they can undergo membrane fusion and exocytosis.

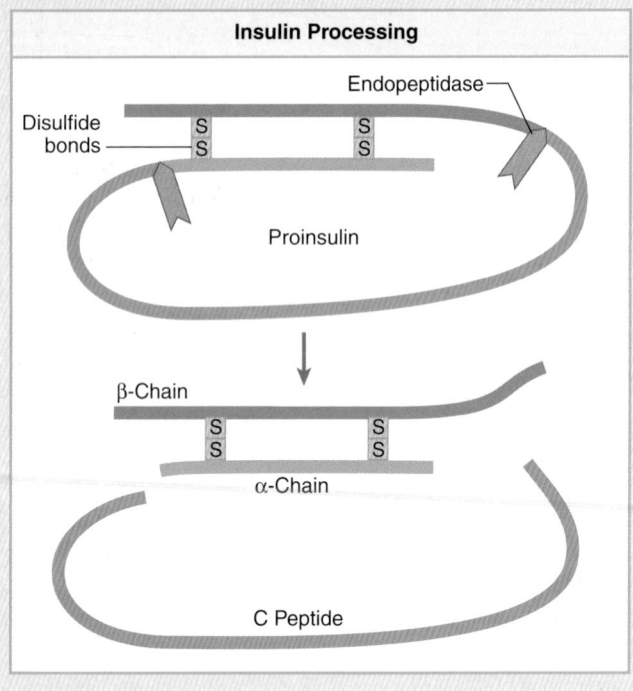

Insulin Processing

Endopeptidase

Disulfide bonds

S S

S S

Proinsulin

β-Chain

S S

S S

α-Chain

C Peptide

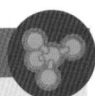

BIOCHEMISTRY

Ketone Bodies

Ketone bodies (acetoacetate, acetone, and β-hydroxybutyrate) are normally formed from acetyl coenzyme A in liver mitochondria during starvation by catabolism of fatty acids.

Ketogenesis is favored at low intracellular glucose concentrations, which block the entry of acetyl CoA into the citric acid cycle by depleting citric acid cycle intermediates. Profound insulin deficiency in type 1 diabetes prevents entry of glucose into hepatocytes and activates ketogenesis in the same manner as starvation (low intracellular glucose).

Ketone bodies are acids, and their accumulation in blood results in metabolic acidosis. Acetone forms spontaneously from the decarboxylation of acetoacetate and results in the characteristic fruity odor of the breath of patients in diabetic ketoacidosis.

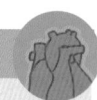

PHYSIOLOGY

Osmotic Diuresis

The ability of renal proximal tubular cells to resorb glucose from the glomerular ultrafiltrate is limited, and when serum glucose concentrations exceed this capacity, glycosuria results. This threshold concentration can be somewhat different in different individuals and is diminished in patients with chronic renal insufficiency. The presence of concentrated glucose in urine causes an osmotic diuresis by preventing normal reabsorption of water. Patients with marked hyperglycemia typically have polyuria and may become severely dehydrated if blood glucose levels remain high.

Patients with type 2 diabetes tend not to develop ketoacidosis (because they have sufficient insulin to allow glucose utilization by critical tissues) but may have silent, prolonged hyperglycemia that results in severe complications. Treatment in type 2 diabetes is directed at reducing insulin resistance (dieting and pharmacologic treatments) and increasing insulin secretion (by pharmacologically stimulating β-cells. Some treatments such as PPARγ antagonists may decrease resistance and increase secretion.

Over time, patients with type 2 diabetes frequently develop secondary dysfunction of β-cells because of secretory exhaustion. Patients with long-standing type 2 diabetes develop amyloid deposits in pancreatic islets composed of amylin, which is co-secreted with insulin by β-cells. The epidemic incidence of obesity and children in the United States is associated with a marked increase in the development of type 2 diabetes early in life.

The long-term complications both type 1 and type 2 diabetes are similar and are directly related to the severity and duration of abnormal serum glucose concentrations (Fig. 10-11). Measurement of hemoglobin A_{1C} concentration is a useful measure of diabetic glucose control in both type 1 and type 2 patients. Hemoglobin A_{1C} is formed

increase in the number of potential receptors available for insulin because of enlargement of adipose tissue so that more insulin may be required to saturate receptor binding. Second, important qualitative changes in adipose tissue occur in obesity. The number of macrophages present in adipose tissue deposits in obese individuals is markedly increased (i.e., the ratio of macrophages to adipocytes changes). Macrophages are the main producers of resistin and tumor necrosis factor α (TNF-α) in adipose tissue. Both of these substances modulate the sensitivity of adipocytes and skeletal muscle to effect insulin resistance.

BIOCHEMISTRY

Resistin

Resistin is a small protein composed of 108 amino acids that is produced predominantly in adipose tissue. Resistin was originally thought to be an adipocyte-specific hormone, but it is now clear that it is also produced by other cells, most importantly, macrophages. Resistin decreases the sensitivity of a number of different target tissues to insulin by poorly defined mechanisms.

Resistin is elevated in most patients with type 2 diabetes and is a potentially important therapeutic target in this disease. Resistin levels are also elevated in obese mice and can be reduced by treatment with PPARγ agonists.

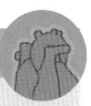

PHARMACOLOGY

Thiazolidinediones

Thiazolidinediones are a class of compounds that can sensitize cells to the effects of insulin stimulation. They bind to the nuclear transcription factor peroxisome proliferator gamma (PPARγ) to modify gene expression.

PPARs undergo conformational changes when they bind ligand that can result in their dimerization with RXR and binding to response elements in sensitive genes to activate transcription or to block the access of other transcription factors to inhibit transcription.

Three PPARs (α, β, and γ), which bind to endogenous ligands such as fatty acids and bile acids, are currently known. PPARα is the target of fibrates such as gemfibrozil, which is used to reduce triglyceride levels and increase HDL-cholesterol levels in hyperlipidemia.

PPARγ is prominently expressed in adipose tissue, endothelial cells, macrophages, and pancreatic β-cells and is required for adipocyte differentiation and uptake of fatty acids. PPARγ is the main target of thiazolidinediones, which can increase insulin sensitivity. While some effects of thiazolidinediones can be explained by their actions in adipose tissue that enhance insulin effects (e.g., decreased resistin and leptin expression), they also have direct effects on gene expression in other tissues, including the liver, that likely are mediated through changes in the expression of different target genes.

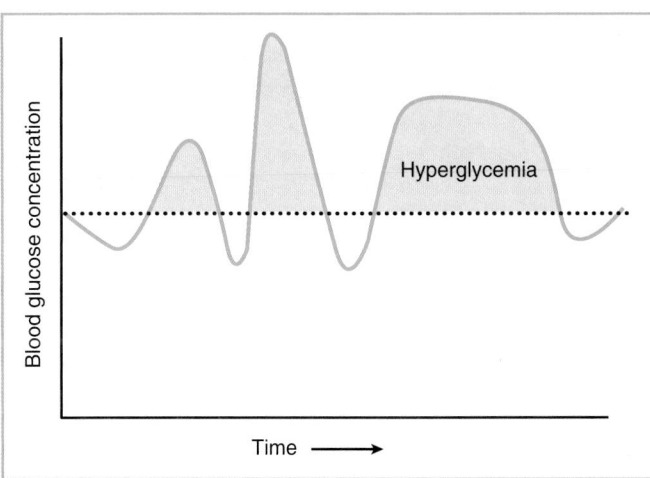

Figure 10-11. Level of serum glucose in a patient with diabetes mellitus treated with insulin injections.

by the nonenzymatic glycosylation of hemoglobin, which occurs at a rate proportionate to glucose concentration. Hemoglobin A_{1C} can provide a measure of long-term (days to weeks) control of serum glucose that is correlated with the development of significant complications. Elevated serum glucose also results in nonenzymatic glycosylation of many other proteins and macromolecules. Abnormally glycosylated proteins are often resistant to degradation and can result in dysfunction in multiple organs. The kidney is particularly affected by these glycosylation end products, which result in thickening of the glomerular basement membrane, causing abnormal glomerular filtration (Fig. 10-12). Hyperglycemia also accelerates atherosclerosis, and these macrovascular abnormalities can exacerbate renal microvascular disease as well as cause death due to cardiovascular disease. Diabetes mellitus is the most common cause of end-stage renal disease requiring dialysis or kidney transplantation in the United States. Accelerated atherosclerosis and microvascular disease caused by accumulation of glycosylated proteins in arterioles and capillaries are major causes of lower extremity ischemia. Diabetes mellitus is the most common indication for limb amputation in this country. Diabetic foot damage is often exacerbated by the coexistence of peripheral neuropathy (loss of sensation results in excess trauma). Unattended foot ulcers can progress to osteomyelitis, requiring amputation. Diabetic neuropathy results from direct toxicity of glycosylation end products in combination microvascular disease.

Hyperglycemia also results in abnormalities in the polyol pathway that predispose to the development of cataracts of the lens of the eye. Microvascular disease in the retina produces ischemia, which in turn stimulates neovascularization of the retina (so-called proliferative retinopathy). Newly formed small blood vessels are prone to hemorrhage, which can progress to retinal detachment with the rapid loss of vision.

Islet Cell Tumors

Islet cell tumors derive from neuroendocrine cells in the pancreatic islets, which tend to grow in a ribbon pattern (Fig. 10-13). Tumors with a hormonal syndrome may present with hyperglycemia due to glucagon-secreting tumors, hypoglycemia due to insulin-secreting tumors, or gastric ulcers due to gastrin-secreting tumors as well as less common syndromes. Removal of localized tumors is usually curative. Most islet cell tumors are nonfunctional and often reach a large size before being discovered. Most islet cell tumors develop in the tail of the pancreas and do not produce common duct obstruction and jaundice as is common in ductal pancreatic adenocarcinomas. Some islet cell tumors are malignant and

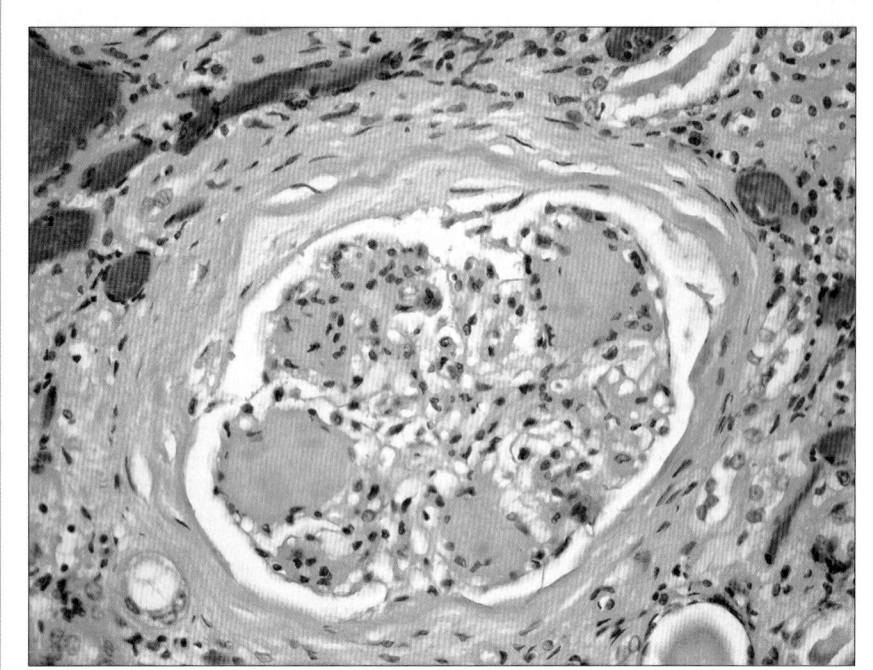

Figure 10-12. Diabetic glomerulosclerosis. Microscopic section of kidney showing severe thickening of the glomerular basement membrane with the formation of Kimmelstiel-Wilson nodules.

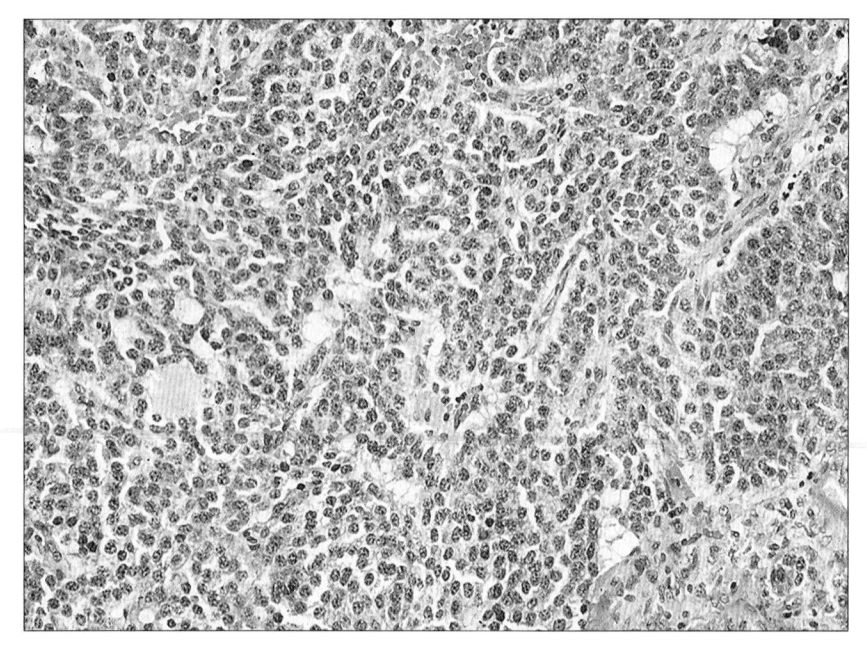

Figure 10-13. Islet cell tumor. Microscopic section showing neuroendocrine cells forming ribbon-like patterns.

often present with multiple metastatic tumor deposits in the liver. Treatment of metastatic tumors with octreotide may ameliorate hormonal symptoms but does not result in cure. Carcinoid tumors can also develop in the pancreas and behave similarly to other carcinoid tumors of the gastrointestinal tract (see Chapter 9).

●●● MULTIPLE ENDOCRINE NEOPLASIA

Multiple endocrine neoplasia (MEN) comprises two different genetic diseases in which point mutations of the MEN1 gene (in MEN I syndrome) or the RET gene (in MEN II syndrome) result in hyperplasia or tumor formation (or both) in several different endocrine organs. Both MEN I and MEN II syndromes are inherited in an autosomal dominant pattern. MEN I results from alterations in the MEN I tumor suppressor gene that controls SMAD signaling in the TGF-β and other pathways that can inhibit cell proliferation. These patients tend to develop hyperplasia or adenomas of parathyroid glands, islet cell tumors of the pancreas, as well as pituitary adenomas, which usually are not prolactinomas but may occasionally produce growth hormone.

MEN II is caused by mutations in the RET proto-oncogene, which is altered in the majority of sporadic papillary thyroid cancers (see Papillary Carcinoma section). MEN II patients have activating mutations in RET, and almost all develop medullary carcinomas of the thyroid gland as they age. Some patients have pheochromocytomas as well. MEN II patients are usually managed by prophylactic thyroidectomy because of the near certainty of their developing medullary thyroid carcinoma (a potentially deadly cancer). Two different forms of MEN II are recognized (Table 10-1), and differences may be related to the nature of the RET gene mutations in different kindreds. Some MEN IIA patients develop hyperparathyroidism, but MEN IIB patients do not. MEN IIB patients develop ganglioneuromas in the gastrointestinal tract.

TABLE 10-1. Multiple Endocrine Neoplasia (MEN) syndromes

Disease	Incidence		
	Type I	Type IIA	Type IIB
MEN I (MEN1 gene)			
Parathyroid hyperplasia	Almost all		
Pancreatic endocrine tumor	1/3		
Pituitary adenoma	1/3		
MEN II (RET gene)			
Medullary thyroid carcinoma		All	All
Pheochromocytoma		1/2	1/2
Parathyroid hyperplasia		1/3	None
Ganglioneuroma		None	Most

Hematopoietic Pathology   11

CONTENTS

The hematopoietic system is unique in that many of its cellular components routinely traffic between different organs and tissues throughout the body. Integrins and other specialized receptors on the surface of lymphoid and myeloid cells recognize receptors on activated endothelium (at sites of inflammation) or on specialized endothelium. Neoplasia of the hematopoietic system is usually widespread at the time of diagnosis, since many neoplastic hematopoietic cells retain the ability to travel throughout the body. For this reason, the concept of metastasis is less relevant for most types of hematopoietic neoplasms than for solid tumors. Intensive study of the immune system has identified many different antigens that are expressed at specific stages of lymphoid and myeloid differentiation. These markers allow precise characterization of both normal and abnormal populations of hematopoietic cells by flow cytometry or immuno-histochemical techniques. These specialized techniques play a critical role in the diagnosis of most hematopoietic neoplasms and permit a level of tumor subclassification that is not possible for carcinomas or sarcomas.

●●● BONE MARROW

The bone marrow is the primary organ producing hematopoietic cells in postnatal life. Extramedullary hematopoiesis (hematopoiesis occurring outside the bone marrow) normally ceases by the time of birth but can be reactivated in certain pathologic conditions. Normal hematopoiesis is dependent on the availability of an appropriate bone marrow microenvironment that allows proliferation and maturation of erythroid, myeloid, lymphoid, and platelet progenitors. This microenvironment consists of specific cellular interactions as well as an appropriate milieu of cytokines and growth factors that promote and direct normal hematopoietic differentiation. Hematopoietic bone marrow is located in trabecular bone and is normally between 20% and 70% cellular, decreasing with advancing age. The remainder of the marrow space is composed of adipose tissue with blood vessels and sinusoids, which permit the ingress and egress of hematopoietic cells. The relative proportion of myeloid and erythroid precursors usually is between 2:1 and 5:1 with a small number of megakaryocytes (usually one is present per high-power microscopic field) and scattered lymphocytes with a few perivascular plasma cells. The bone marrow

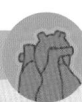

PHYSIOLOGY

Flow Cytometry

Flow cytometry can be used to count and characterize individual cells or particles suspended in solution on the basis of scattered or emitted light. A single cell suspension is forced through a narrow fluid stream so that single cells pass between a single wavelength light source (a laser beam) and photodetectors. The nature of the light scattered by the particle is a measure of its size.

If antibodies with fluorophores are attached to cell surface proteins, the intensity of emitted fluorescence is a measure of the number of proteins expressed on each cell. The use of multiple detectors and antibodies labeled with different fluorophores allows measurement of the coexpression of two or more different proteins on individual cells. Flow cytometry permits the rapid analysis of many thousands of cells to allow detailed analysis of even rare cell populations.

Flow cytometry can also be used to assess DNA content in individual cells (using propidium iodide to stain DNA). This type of assay can detect aneuploidy and estimate the percentage of cells in S phase. Specialized techniques can be used to make cells permeable to allow antibodies to bind to and detect intracellular proteins.

normally has a fine reticulin meshwork that makes up its extracellular matrix. Scattered macrophages containing hemosiderin provide an immediate reservoir of iron for erythropoiesis. In children, both the axial and appendicular bone marrow are active in hematopoiesis, but in adults hematopoiesis normally is limited to the axial skeleton.

All hematopoietic cells derive from pluripotent stem cells that undergo division and differentiation into committed progenitor cells (Fig. 11-1). These progenitor cells first commit to either lymphoid or nonlymphoid differentiation, and dividing progenitor cells then undergo further differentiation. As these progenitor cells mature, their capacity to replicate is progressively diminished. Myeloid cells complete their maturation in the bone marrow while lymphoid progenitors migrate to lymphoid organs (thymus or lymph nodes) to complete their maturation and undergo antigenic selection. The phenotype of most hematopoietic neoplasms closely resembles that of normal cells at some point in their differentiation. Since the hematopoietic system is a labile tissue, active replication of progenitor cells is essential to maintain homeostasis. Changes in the size of different progenitor pools can markedly increase or decrease the number of mature cells produced in each lineage. Examination of the bone marrow can show changes in the size and degree of maturation of these progenitors and combined with clinical data can permit considerable insight into the nature of different disease processes.

Anemia

Anemia is defined as diminished oxygen-carrying capacity in blood secondary to a decrease in the number of erythrocytes or in the amount of hemoglobin, or both. Anemia results from abnormal erythroid homeostasis and can be caused by increased red blood cell (RBC) destruction, inadequate RBC production, or a combination of these two factors. Understanding the dynamics and morphology of normal RBC production provides insight into the causes of many types of anemia. Normal erythrocytes have a life span of approximately 120 days, and processes that shorten this life span can cause anemia if RBC production does not keep pace. Erythroid precursors in the bone marrow tend to grow in clusters (erythrons), which are easily visible in tissue sections. As RBC precursors mature beyond the normoblast stage, they extrude their nucleus, converting themselves into reticulocytes with still active hemoglobin synthesis. Reticulocytes enter the circulation and complete maturation into mature erythrocytes and then cease hemoglobin synthesis. Increased peripheral destruction of blood cells stimulates the egress of immature erythroid cells into the circulation, and a reticulocyte count is a useful measure of the proliferative stress on the erythroid bone marrow. In extreme circumstances, nucleated RBCs may appear in the circulation as a reactive adaptive process although this may also result from pathologic processes in the marrow.

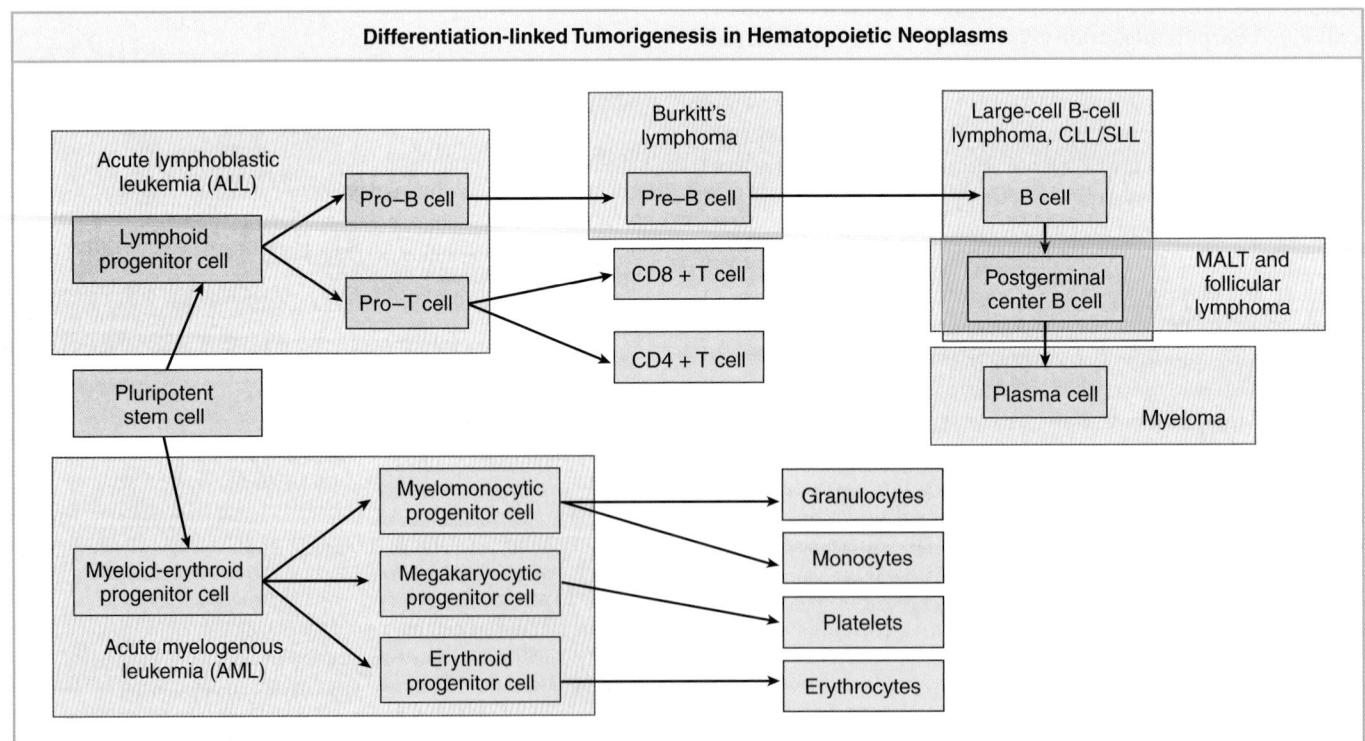

Figure 11-1. Schematic representation of hematopoiesis from hematopoietic pluripotent stem cells to fully differentiated cells. The correspondence of different tumors to particular levels of differentiated progenitor cells is highlighted.

Anemia can result from acute or chronic blood loss by hemorrhage or by intravascular destruction of RBCs. Lost or destroyed erythrocytes can potentially be replaced (within limits) by the expansion of erythroid progenitors in the bone marrow if the marrow is normal and if adequate nutrition (including iron) is present. Abnormalities in the synthesis of hemoglobin resulting from nutritional or genetic causes can interfere with erythroid maturation. Abnormalities in stem cells or progenitor cells may also result in abnormal RBC production. The resulting erythrocytes may be deficient in hemoglobin concentration or of abnormal size (macrocytic or microcytic).

Nutritional Anemia

Two major types of nutritional anemia occur. Iron deficiency anemia is a common disease that usually results from a combination of increased blood loss and inadequate iron stores. Iron deficiency anemia occurs in many types of chronic disease and often is present in menstruating women with suboptimal nutrition. One of the most common causes of iron deficiency anemia is chronic occult blood loss from the gastrointestinal (GI) tract. Mild-to-moderate degrees of iron deficiency result in hypochromic microcytic RBCs, which are smaller and contain less hemoglobin than normal RBCs. These changes can be appreciated on blood smears when they are marked but are more sensitively measured by laboratory instruments. Supplementation with iron corrects these abnormalities if the anemia is mild and ongoing blood loss is not severe. Body iron stores can be evaluated by measurement of serum total iron-binding capacity and ferritin levels as well as by staining for iron in bone marrow aspirates or biopsy specimens.

HISTOLOGY

Red Blood Cell Indices

Red blood cell number, volume, and hemoglobin content can be measured by passing a thin stream of blood treated with anticoagulants through a device with optical and electric impedance sensors (i.e., a Coulter counter). Coulter counters provide a readout of RBC parameters including the hematocrit and hemoglobin concentration.

The mean cell volume (MCV) is measured in femtoliters. Macrocytes are usually classified as RBCs with MCV >100 fL and microcytes <80 fL.

MCH (mean cell hemoglobin) is the average amount of hemoglobin in each RBC in picograms.

MCHC is the mean corpuscular hemoglobin concentration (normal, 31–36 g/dL).

RDW is a measure of the variation in size between different RBCs and is normally less than 15%. Increased RDW may indicate the presence of abnormal RBCs (e.g., sickled cells or RBC fragments).

Microscopic examination of blood smears permits identification of specific RBC abnormalities (e.g., schistocytes in microangiopathic hemolytic anemia).

The other main form of nutritional anemia is megaloblastic anemia, which results from either vitamin B_{12} or folate deficiency. Deficiency of these vitamins results in ineffective erythropoiesis, and the mature RBCs produced have abnormally large cellular volumes (macrocytes). Deficiency of these nutrients also results in abnormalities in neutrophil maturation that cause hypersegmentation (more than five lobes per nucleus of neutrophils), which may be a clue to the diagnosis of megaloblastic anemia. B_{12} deficiency most often results from autoimmune gastritis that destroys parietal cells in the stomach. The loss of intrinsic factor produced by parietal cells causes pernicious anemia with the inability to absorb B_{12} (see Chapter 3). Unlike B_{12}, folate stores are quite limited so that dietary deficiency of folate (found in fresh green vegetables) can result in depletion relatively quickly. In extreme forms, megaloblastic anemia may be morphologically confused with some forms of leukemia on bone marrow aspiration and biopsy (markedly hypercellular bone marrow with enlarged, abnormal erythroid precursors). Careful attention to RBC indices and clinical history is important to avoid an incorrect diagnosis. B_{12} (but not folate) deficiency can also result in irreversible neurologic complications, so prompt diagnosis is critical.

Anemia of Chronic Disease

Anemia of chronic disease is typically a normochromic normocytic anemia that frequently results from a combination of functional nutritional deficiency and abnormalities in growth factor production that contribute to diminished erythropoiesis (Fig. 11-2). Diminished erythropoietin secretion and direct inhibition of erythroid precursors by IL-1, TNF-α, and IFN-γ may all contribute to anemia in various clinical settings. In most patients, multiple factors including blood loss contribute to anemia as well.

Genetic Anemia

The most common genetic causes of anemia are abnormalities of hemoglobin (hemoglobinopathy and thalassemia; see Chapter 4). Heritable structural abnormalities of RBCs (e.g., spherocytosis) are less common genetic causes of anemia. Deficiency of enzymes that normally protect RBCs from oxidative stress (e.g., glucose-6-phosphate dehydrogenase [G6PD] deficiency) can also result in severe anemia under some circumstances.

Hereditary Spherocytosis

Hereditary spherocytosis results from mutations in spectrin-associated proteins. Spectrin is an intracellular protein that normally forms a matrix with other proteins to stabilize the biconcave shape of RBCs. Mutations (dominant or recessive) in several of these proteins can result in RBCs that are spherical rather than biconcave. Spherocytes are less deformable than normal RBCs and are prone to damage in the microcirculation. As a result, the life span of spherocytes is reduced and they are removed from the circulation by the spleen. Patients with hereditary spherocytosis usually

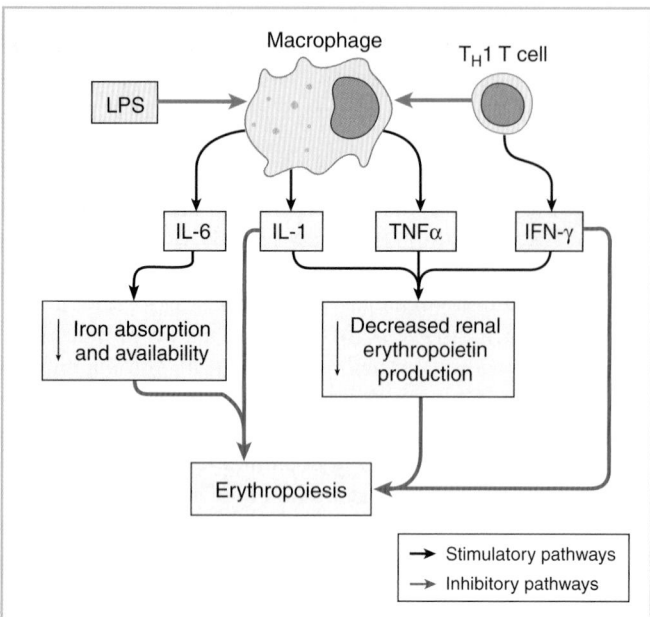

Figure 11-2. Anemia of chronic disease.

have splenomegaly, and splenectomy may lessen anemia in these patients by extending RBC life span.

Glucose-6-Phosphate Dehydrogenase Deficiency

G6PD deficiency can result in an acute hemolytic anemia if RBCs are exposed to oxidative stress. Since G6PD is located on the X chromosome, males are hemizygous for this gene, resulting in a sex-linked recessive pattern of inheritance. Many different mutations are known, but the A variant is common in blacks (prevalence approximately 10%). This mutation results in a decreased life span of G6PD so that older RBCs are at increased risk for oxidative damage and hemolysis. Female heterozygotes are usually asymptomatic. Some drugs and foods may trigger a hemolytic crisis (e.g., fava beans).

Paroxysmal Nocturnal Hemoglobinuria

Paroxysmal nocturnal hemoglobinuria (PNH) is an acquired disease that results from somatic mutations in the phosphatidylinositol glycan (PIGA) gene on the X chromosome. This gene encodes a protein that provides a membrane anchor for a number of cell membrane proteins that normally inhibit early complement components and protect RBCs from complement-mediated lysis. Loss of expression of phosphatidylinositol glycan prevents membrane localization of these proteins, and affected RBCs are susceptible to lysis by spontaneous complement activation. Patients typically have episodic attacks of hemolysis, which often occur at night and may be triggered by proinflammatory stimuli. Somatic mutations occur in hematopoietic stem cells, since all myeloid cells carry the mutation. Most normal individuals have a small number of hematopoietic stem cells with PIGA mutations, apparently as a consequence of immune-mediated selection for cells that lack surface expression of some

of these proteins. Patients with PNH have mutations in a significant fraction of their hematopoietic stem cells and so can develop severe episodes of hemolysis. Individuals with stem cell failure or aplastic anemia are at increased risk for developing PNH because of immune-mediated destruction of normal hematopoietic stem cells.

Immune-mediated Hemolytic Anemia

The most common types of immune-mediated hemolytic anemia are caused by type II hypersensitivity reactions in which antibodies bind directly to antigens expressed on RBC membranes. This results in the fixation of complement, which may cause intravascular lysis of RBCs via its membrane attack complex or opsonization of RBCs leading to their removal by histiocytes in the spleen.

Transfusion Reaction

Iatrogenic transfusion reactions are an important cause of immune-mediated hemolytic anemia. Transfusions with mismatch of major transfusion antigens such as ABO or Rh cause an acute febrile hemolytic reaction because of preformed antibodies present in the transfusion recipient. Donor RBCs are lysed over the course of hours, resulting in massive hemoglobin release in the bloodstream that can cause renal failure. The release of cytokines initiates a systemic inflammatory reaction that often is fatal. This type of transfusion reaction is extremely uncommon and usually results from a medical error (e.g., patient identification error).

Transfusion with mismatch of minor transfusion antigens tends to result in much slower hemolysis unless the recipient has been previously sensitized to those antigens (i.e., antibodies are not preformed and develop only after exposure to RBCs in the transfusion). The slow hemolysis in this situation does not usually produce the acute, systemic inflammatory reaction typical of a major acute transfusion reaction but ultimately results in destruction of all transfused RBCs.

Autoimmune Hemolytic Anemia

Autoimmune hemolytic anemia (AIHA) can develop in the setting of autoimmune disease or as a transient phenomenon that is initiated in susceptible individuals by exposure to drugs or other agents. Drug haptens can bind to RBC membrane proteins, rendering them immunogenic to initiate an antibody or cell-mediated immune response. In this situation, hemolysis abates when the modified RBCs are cleared from the circulation.

Microangiopathic Hemolytic Anemia

Abnormalities of the microvasculature can produce microangiographic changes on a peripheral blood smear that result from damage and fragmentation of RBCs. Characteristic schistocytes as well as other deformed RBCs and RBC fragments are usually seen on the peripheral blood smear. Thrombotic thrombocytopenic purpura generally produces microangiopathic changes, but these changes also can be observed in disseminated cancer and other pathologic conditions.

Aplastic Anemia

Aplastic anemia is a rare disease of unknown cause that results in a failure of production of one or, more frequently, multiple lineages of hematopoietic cells from the bone marrow. The most serious consequences of aplastic anemia are usually in the loss of granulocytes, since these cannot be readily replaced by transfusion, and marked neutropenia frequently leads to fatal infection. Most cases of aplastic anemia are thought to be mediated through immune or autoimmune mechanisms, since immunosuppression results in remission or partial remission in many cases. Bone marrow transplantation may be curative in some patients, but in others, abnormalities of the bone marrow microenvironment prevent effective engraftment. A minority of patients with aplastic anemia have germline mutations in the telomerase gene or in the DNA encoding the template RNA that is part of the telomerase holoenzyme. In these patients, progressive telomere shortening in hematopoietic stem cells apparently leads to replicative failure of stem cells with increasing age (see Chapter 3). Cases of aplastic anemia caused by telomerase mutations do not respond to immunosuppressive therapy.

Infectious Hemolytic Anemia

A number of different microorganisms can infect RBCs and result in their lysis. Malaria is the most common RBC parasite worldwide and is a major cause of morbidity and mortality in endemic areas in the developing world. Malaria is usually spread by a mosquito vector (the definitive host) although blood transfusion can also result in infection. Some forms of malaria such as *Plasmodium ovale* tend to produce a relatively mild, low-grade hemolytic anemia. Aggressive parasites such as *Plasmodium falciparum* can produce massive hemolysis causing renal failure and death secondary to anemia. Malarial parasites have a cyclic division cycle that results in the synchronous lysis of RBCs, producing recurrent hemolysis and fever. Malaria can usually be diagnosed by careful examination of blood smears, but the cyclic life cycle of the parasite results in low levels of RBC parasitemia after hemolysis. Host factors are important in resistance to malaria, and individuals with sickle cell trait have milder disease than those with hemoglobin A.

Babesia microti has a life cycle similar to that of malaria and is also spread via a mosquito vector. *Babesia* is endemic in some portions of the northeastern United States. Infection typically results in a low-grade hemolytic anemia, but high levels of parasitemia in patients without a functional spleen can result in fatal disease.

Thrombocytopenia

Thrombocytopenia indicates that an abnormally low number of platelets are present in circulating blood. Very low levels of platelets are associated with extensive petechial hemorrhage owing to wear and tear–induced defects in the microvasculature. Patients with fewer than 5000 platelets per cubic millimeter (normal, 200,000/mm^3 to 400,000/mm^3) are at high risk for spontaneous, life-threatening hemorrhage into the central nervous system. An important cause of thrombocytopenia is cancer chemotherapy. Severe thrombocytopenia can be treated with platelet transfusion, but the short life span of platelets (<2 days) makes chronic treatment difficult.

Idiopathic Thrombocytopenia Purpura

Idiopathic thrombocytopenia purpura (ITP) is an immune-mediated process that results in a marked decrease in the number of platelets in the circulation. Binding of antibodies to platelets causes them to be removed from the circulation by the spleen. Plasmapheresis can remove antiplatelet antibodies and may be effective in some patients. Corticosteroid therapy may also induce remission, but some patients may require splenectomy to decrease platelet destruction. Bone marrow biopsy in patients with ITP typically shows megakaryocytic hyperplasia as a compensatory response to peripheral platelet destruction (Fig. 11-3).

Thrombotic Thrombocytopenia Purpura and Hemolytic Uremic Syndrome

Thrombotic thrombocytopenia purpura (TTP) and hemolytic uremic syndrome (HUS) share many clinical and pathologic features but usually affect different patient populations. TTP is typically a disease of adults while HUS tends to occur in children. In both conditions there is an inappropriate activation of platelets (probably by antiplatelet IgG), often in association with activation of the coagulation system. This results in formation of microthrombi in the vasculature, most prominently in the kidney and lungs, that decrease effective perfusion, resulting in ischemia and hypoxia. Activation of platelets also releases inflammatory mediators that cause damage to target organs, producing adult respiratory distress syndrome (ARDS) or acute renal failure (or both) (Fig. 11-4). Consumption of platelets and coagulation factors can ultimately result in severe hemorrhagic complications. Patients typically show a microangiopathic pattern on a blood smear with schistocytes resulting from damage to RBCs in the microvasculature. Treatment includes plasmapheresis and supportive measures.

Myeloproliferative Syndromes

Most myeloproliferative disorders result from acquired genetic abnormalities in myeloid cell progenitors that lead to excessive proliferation and diminished function. Most of these syndromes affect myeloid cells, but many also involve erythroid and megakaryocytic lineages derived from the same committed progenitor cell. The monocytic lineage is less frequently affected. In many of these diseases, the abnormal function of the inflammatory cells predisposes to serious infection. Heritable genetic causes of myeloid cell dysfunction are discussed with immunodeficiency syndromes in Chapter 2.

Acute Myeloid Leukemia

Acute myeloid leukemia (AML) can develop in both adults and children but much more commonly in adults. AML occurs

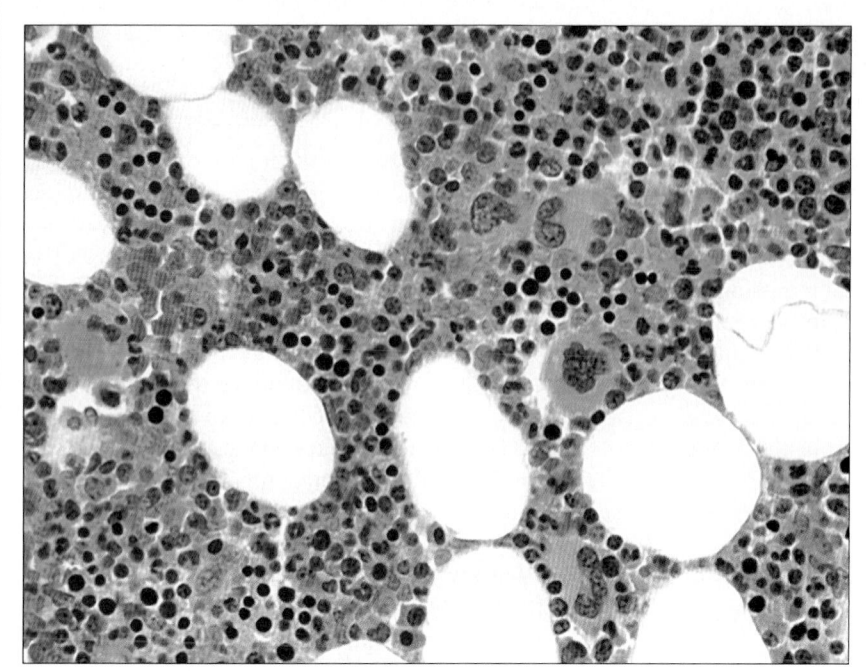

Figure 11-3. Idiopathic thrombocytopenia purpura (ITP). Microscopic section of bone marrow showing marked compensatory hyperplasia of megakaryocytes in response to increased peripheral platelet destruction.

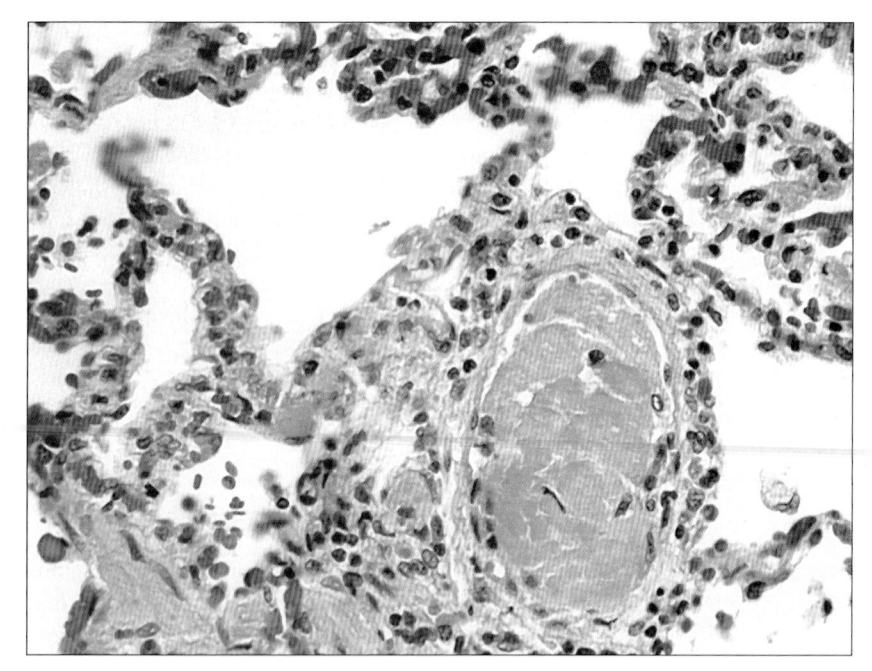

Figure 11-4. Thrombotic thrombocytopenia purpura (TTP). Section of lung tissue showing microthrombi in small blood vessels.

in two distinct settings. In younger patients, AML frequently results from specific chromosomal translocations that code for novel fusion proteins. Expression of these fusion proteins is often sufficient to transform progenitor cells to produce "de novo" leukemia. The other form of AML develops in the setting of myelodysplasia or chronic myeloproliferative syndrome. These tumors tend to occur in older patients, and many genetic changes are present in tumor cells at the time of diagnosis. These leukemias are usually much less respon-

sive to conventional chemotherapy than are "de novo" leukemias.

AML demonstrates primitive hematopoietic cells (blasts) with finely divided chromatin, prominent nucleoli, and scant cytoplasm. Myeloid leukemia usually presents with numerous leukemic cells (blasts) in the peripheral blood (sometimes >100,000/mm³), which may cause hemorrhage or tissue ischemia (by sludging and blocking blood flow in capillary beds). A peripheral blast percentage above 20% is diagnostic of acute leukemia (Fig. 11-5A). All patients with overt leukemia have bone marrow involvement, but a minority of patients have only bone marrow involvement (>20% blasts are required for a diagnosis of acute leukemia) without blasts in their peripheral blood (see Fig. 11-5B). All acute leukemia patients have cytopenia of normal hematopoietic cells because of disruption of the bone marrow. In advanced disease, leukemic infiltration of organs and tissue is common and results in dysfunction (see Fig. 11-5C). Involvement of the central nervous system occurs in acute myeloid leukemia but is less common than in acute lymphoblastic leukemia (see below). A minority of patients develop solid tumor deposits composed of leukemic cells (extramedullary myeloid cell tumor), and rare patients may have an extramedullary myeloid cell tumor before leukemia develops.

Acute myeloid leukemia has eight subtypes based on morphologic and phenotypic features (French-American-British [FAB] classification: M0 through M7) (Table 11-1). M0 and M1 correspond to an immature myeloid phenotype without differentiated features. M2 leukemia has differentiated myeloid cells with Auer rods, and many tumor cells express myeloperoxidase. M3 shows more evidence of myeloid differentiation with morphologic similarity to promyelocytes with numerous cytoplasmic granules and is often associated with prominent thrombotic complications. M3 is defined by a specific translocation (t[5;17] PML [promyelocytic leukemia] to RAR [retinoic acid receptor] α gene), which renders these tumors cells sensitive to treatment with retinoic acid. M4 is myelomonocytic leukemia in which tumor cells show features of monocytic and myeloid cells, and M5 shows

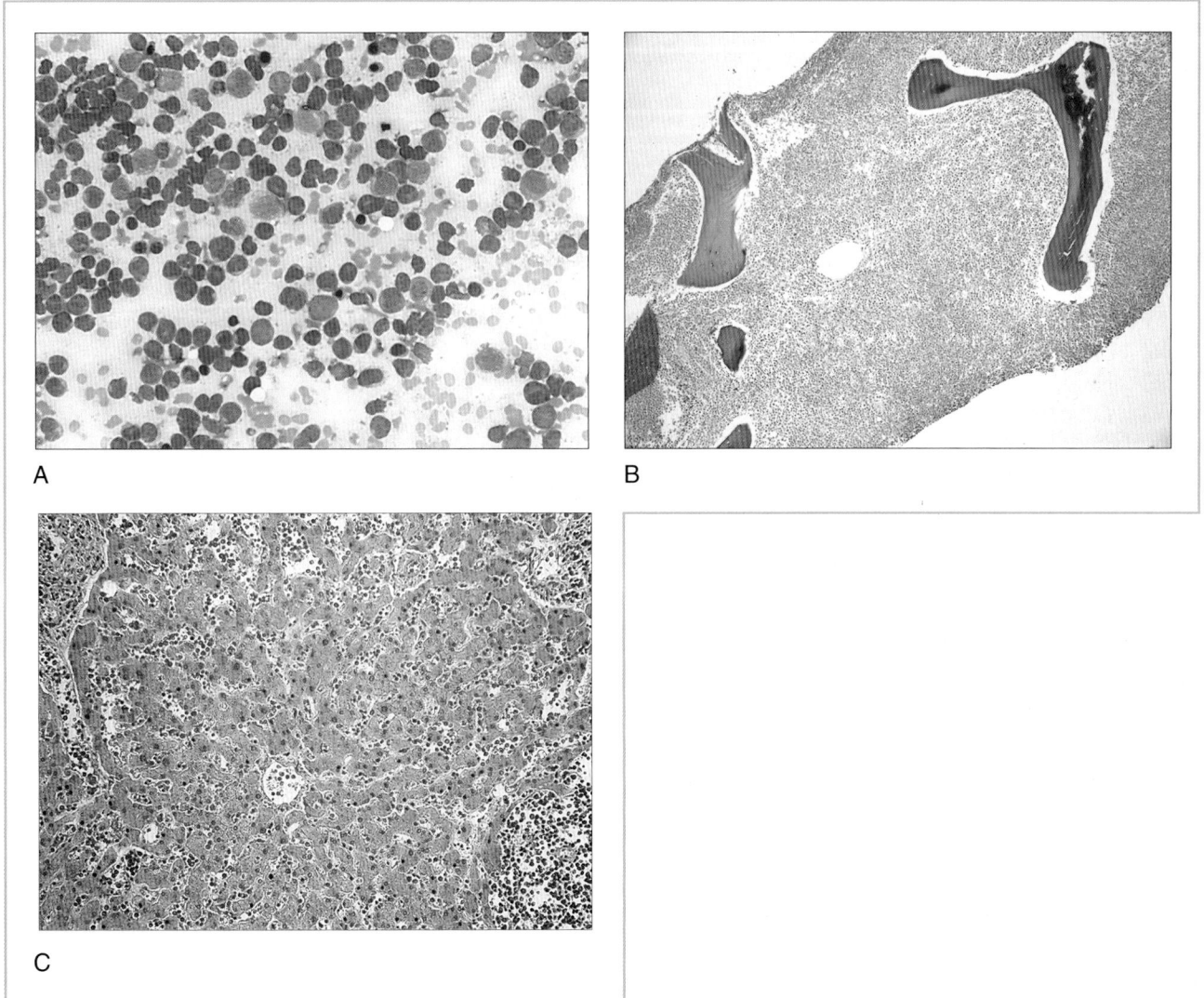

A

B

C

Figure 11-5. Acute myelogenous leukemia (AML). **A**, Peripheral blood smear showing numerous myeloblasts with primitive, finely divided chromatin and a high nuclear:cytoplasmic ratio. Granules and Auer rods are not visible in tumor cell cytoplasm at this magnification. **B**, Microscopic section of bone marrow replaced by AML. Normal hematopoietic elements are completely effaced. The leukemic blasts have a very high nuclear:cytoplasmic ratio and show essentially no differentiated features. **C**, AML involving the liver. Microscopic section of liver showing infiltration of sinusoids by leukemic cells.

TABLE 11-1. French-American-British (FAB) Classification of Myeloid Leukemia

FAB Class	Abbreviation	Features	Frequency
M0	AML	Minimal evidence of myeloid differentiation (no Auer rods)	Rare
M1	AML	No differentiated myelocytes present (few Auer rods)	20%
M2	AML	Differentiated myelocytes present in addition to blasts (Auer rods present)	Most common (30% to 40%)
M3	APL	Acute promyelocytic leukemia; t(5;17)	10%
M4	AMML	Acute myelomonocytic leukemia (mixture of myeloblasts and monoblasts)	15%
M5		Acute monocytic leukemia	10%
M6		Acute erythroleukemia	Rare
M7		Acute megakaryocytic leukemia	Rare

predominantly monocytic differentiation. M6 and M7 are rare forms of leukemia with predominantly erythroid or megakaryocytic differentiation.

Superimposed on the FAB subtypes of AML are newer classification schemes based on DNA microarray analysis of mRNA expression in acute leukemias. Supervised and unsupervised clustering analyses of these data have identified putative new subtypes of leukemia that may have different prognoses and responses to specific types of chemotherapy. Tumors with characteristic translocations (such as M3 AML with PML-RAR translocation) tend to emerge as distinct subtypes in this genetic analysis, but other nontraditional subtypes can also be identified, particularly in patients with a normal karyotype. The clinical and prognostic utility of these newer categories is currently undergoing validation and may alter the traditional diagnostic categorization of AML. The identification of specific biologic targets (such as FLT-3 gene alterations that are present in a small subset of de novo AML patients) also drives the precise molecular characterization of individual tumors to arrive at optimal treatment strategies (i.e., utilization of predictive tumor markers).

The prognosis of untreated AML is grim, with death usually resulting in days to weeks. Treatment results in remission in many patients, but recurrence is common. Some of these patients can be salvaged with high-dose therapy and bone marrow transplantation. The graft-versus-host disease associated with allogeneic transplants is almost certainly of therapeutic benefit in these patients.

Chronic Myeloid Leukemia

Chronic myeloid leukemia (CML) is a chronic myeloproliferative disorder in which large numbers of morphologically mature (but functionally abnormal) myeloid cells are produced without a marked increase in the number of myeloblasts. This is accomplished by expansion of myeloid precursor pools by progenitor cells with a characteristic chromosomal translocation. Patients with CML have markedly increased numbers of myeloid cells in their bone

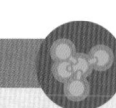

BIOCHEMISTRY

Retinoic Acid

9-*cis* Retinoic acid can bind to both the retinoic acid receptor (RAR) and the retinoid X receptor (RXR). All-*trans* retinoic acid (ATRA) binds only to RXR. Receptor binding triggers dimerization of RAR and RXR, which may form homodimers or heterodimers and bind to response elements in various genes to either enhance or repress transcription.

The RAR-PML fusion protein in M3 AML causes a differentiation block at the promyelocyte stage. ATRA binding to the fusion protein removes this block, allowing leukemic cells to complete differentiation into granulocytes. Many of the complications of M3 AML (see text) result from the physical properties of promyelocytes, including a marked prothrombotic tendency. Maturation of leukemic cells diminishes these effects and also provides at least partially effective granulocytes that help decrease the risk of infection.

marrow and peripheral blood. Neutrophils predominate, but less mature forms are also increased. These neutrophils have lower than normal alkaline phosphatase activity and are dysfunctional, making these patients susceptible to infection despite their high neutrophil count.

CML is one of the first diseases to be associated with a specific chromosomal translocation. The Philadelphia chromosome results from a translocation between the bcr gene on chromosome 21 and the abl proto-oncogene on chromosome 9, t(9;21) (Fig. 11-6A). This translocation produces a novel fusion protein (with exons derived form both the bcr and abl genes) that has novel functions in signal transduction and transcriptional control (see Fig. 11-6B). Some cases of ALL also have bcr-abl translocations, but the resulting fusion protein contains different exons from those of the fusion protein. These translocations in CML can be identified by interphase FISH (fluorescence in situ hybridization) or by molecular methods (e.g., RT-PCR) that can detect the fusion

GENETICS

FLT3 Gene

FLT3 (FMS-like tyrosine kinase 3) is a receptor tyrosine kinase with homology to platelet-derived growth factor (PDGF) that contains five immunoglobulin-like motifs in its extracellular domain. FLT3's ligand FL modulates the proliferation and differentiation of primitive hematopoietic cells. The FLT3 gene is quite large and contains 24 exons spanning approximately 96 kb of DNA. A large intron is present between exons 2 and 3 that is >50 kb in length.

FLT3 is normally expressed on bone marrow progenitor cells and fetal liver cells, but it is also expressed by most myeloid leukemias and B-cell ALLs. Alterations in FLT3 are the most frequent genetic changes identified in acute myeloid leukemia. A common FLT3 alteration is an internal tandem DNA duplication in exon 11 or in exons 11 and 12 adjacent to the coding sequences for the juxtamembrane domain. This duplication results in an FLT3 protein that is constitutively active in signaling owing to ligand-independent autophosphorylation. Tandem duplication is associated with adverse prognosis in leukemia but provides a potential tumor-specific drug target (similar to the bcr-abl kinase in CML that is inhibited by imatinib [Gleevec]).

Point mutations can also occur in the second tyrosine kinase domain of FLT3, but their clinical significance is less clear.

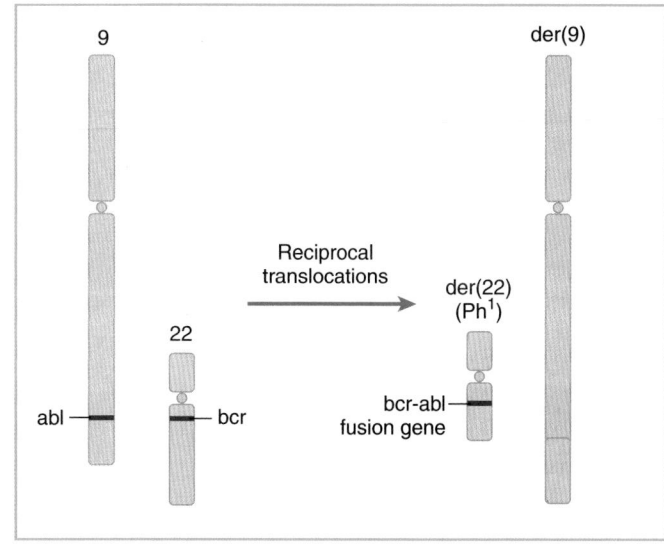

A

B

Figure 11-6. A, Philadelphia chromosome (chromosome 22). **B**, BCR-ABL fusion protein interactions and effects.

transcript. The presence of this specific translocation defines CML, and patients with clinical features suggestive of CML who lack this translocation tend to have a very different clinical course. The Philadelphia chromosome is present not only in mature myeloid cells but also in early progenitor cells. The bcr-abl fusion protein results in increased proliferation in these progenitor cells, expanding the size of these precursor pools in the bone marrow to permit the production of a large number of mature granulocytes.

Suppressive treatment with low-dose chemotherapeutic agents can lower the white blood cell (WBC) count in CML but is not curative. Indeed, the mutagenic effects of alkylating agents or irradiation may hasten the development of acute leukemia, which eventually occurs in many CML patients. With or without treatment, most patients show slowly increasing immaturity of the myeloid cells, which is associated with the accumulation of additional genetic changes. Some patients eventually reach a blast count that is diagnostic of acute leukemia. Acute leukemia may show either lymphoid or myeloid differentiation consistent with the idea that the underlying genetic abnormalities exist in early progenitor or stem cells. Recent evidence suggests that the Philadelphia chromosome is usually present in progenitor cells but not in pluripotent stem cells.

Polycythemia Vera, Essential Thrombocythemia, and Primary Myelofibrosis

These three myeloproliferative disorders each show varying elements of hyperplasia of one or more hematopoietic lineages combined with fibrosis and destruction of the bone marrow space. Recent reports suggest that most patients with polycythemia vera as well as some patients with essential thrombocythemia and primary myelofibrosis have missense mutations in the JAK-2 gene. JAK proteins are second messengers that participate in cytokine receptor signal transduction to activate STAT proteins, which ultimately effect changes in gene transcription. The precise pathophysiologic consequences of these recently described genetic changes are not fully elucidated at this time. All three disorders eventually lead to bone marrow failure, with death resulting from infection or transformation to acute leukemia.

Polycythemia vera is always associated with prominent hyperhplasia and dysplasia of the erythroid lineage, but many cases demonstrate concurrent hyperplasia and dysplasia of myeloid cells and megakaryocytes. The bone marrow is usually markedly hypercellular and usually shows evidence of increased reticulin fibrosis as the disease progresses. This abnormality of the microenvironment in the bone marrow may eventually progress to a disease with features identical to those of primary myelofibrosis (see below). Patients with polycythemia vera may require phlebotomy to decrease their RBC mass to prevent sludging in the microcirculation. Essential thrombocythemia shows features similar to those of polycythemia vera, but the megakaryocytic lineage is prominently hyperplastic, leading to a hypercoagulable state.

Primary myelofibrosis presents with extensive reticulin fibrosis of the bone marrow that destroys the microenvironment necessary for normal hematopoiesis. As a result, hematopoiesis shifts to extramedullary sites, usually first involving the spleen (so-called myeloid metaplasia). Splenomegaly may be one of the presenting symptoms in patients with primary myelofibrosis. Ultimately, hematopoiesis may also involve the liver, lymph nodes, and other nonlymphoid organs (Fig. 11-7). Some patients with myelofibrosis almost certainly have a late stage of undiagnosed polycythemia vera.

BIOCHEMISTRY

Janus-associated Kinases (JAKs)

The JAK gene family contains four members (JAKs 1–3 and TYK2), which function in signal transduction between membrane receptors and other signaling molecules, particularly STATs (signal transducers and activators of transcription). Activated JAKs phosphorylate the SRC homology domain on STATs, which causes them to dimerize and migrate to the nucleus to act as transcription factors. JAKs all have two tandem kinase domains, but the internal kinase domain is nonfunctional (pseudokinase domain). This tandem structure suggests the two-faced ancient Roman god of home and hearth for which JAKs are named. The JAK pseudokinase domain acts as an inhibitor of the functional kinase so that mutations in the pseudokinase domain can result in constitutive kinase activation.

Many hematopoietic growth factors signal through JAKs, and some JAKs are fusion partners in leukemias with chromosomal translocations.

Myelodysplastic Syndromes

Myelodysplastic syndromes result from genetic abnormalities in progenitor or committed hematopoietic stem cells that cause serious abnormalities in the differentiation and maturation of red and white blood cells and platelets. In some cases, abnormalities of myeloid cells predominate, whereas in others erythroid or megakaryocytic dysplasia is most prominent. Most patients have anemia and diminished WBC count owing to ineffective hematopoiesis. Examination of bone marrow smears typically shows cytologic abnormalities (dysplasia) of progenitor cells of several lineages with hyperplasia or hypoplasia of various lineages. Flow cytometry analysis of the DNA content in bone marrow cells usually shows evidence of aneuploidy, which corresponds to the presence of multiple chromosomal abnormalities. Some subtypes of myelodysplasia (e.g., refractory anemia with excess blasts) are transitional stages in evolving acute leukemia, and some patients with myelodysplasia will eventually have overt acute leukemia. Most patients with myelodysplasia die as a result of infection because of the abnormal function of their myeloid

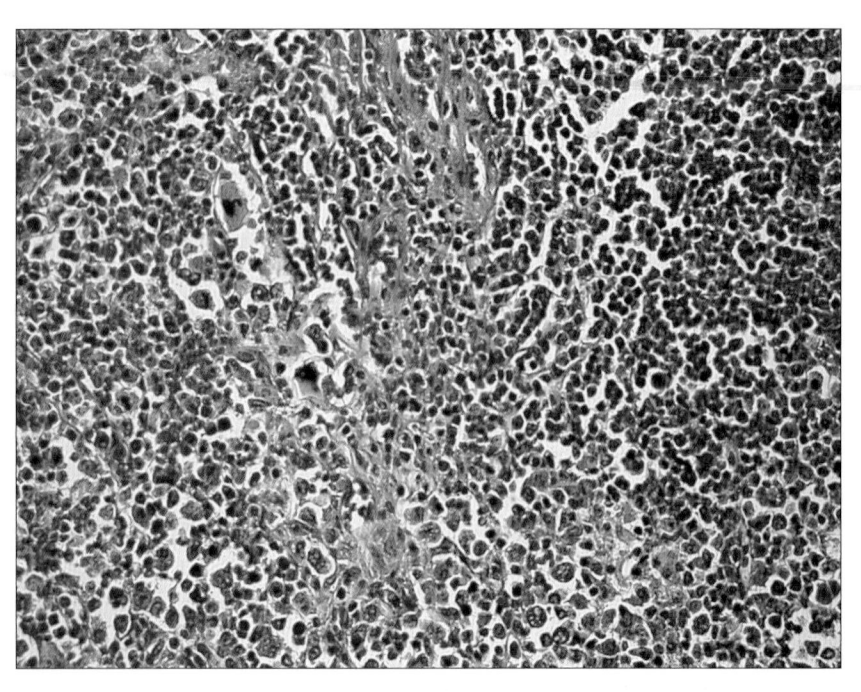

Figure 11-7. Extramedullary hematopoiesis. Microscopic section of spleen showing prominent megakaryocytes (multinucleated cells) as well as other hematopoietic progenitors filling-in the splenic red pulp.

cells. Myelodysplasia can arise in patients without known risk factors but can also occur as a late complication of chemotherapy, particularly with regimens that include alkylating agents.

Bone Marrow Transplantation

Bone marrow transplantation is an effective therapy for aplastic anemia and some nonhematopoietic genetic diseases in which defective proteins can be replaced through the bloodstream. Bone marrow transplantation is an important form of salvage therapy and sometimes of primary therapy for patients with aggressive solid tumors, leukemias, lymphomas, and myeloma. Autotransplantation of stem cells derived from the patient's bone marrow or peripheral blood (after expansion in vitro) can be employed after high-dose therapy (usually a combination of radiation therapy and chemotherapy designed to kill tumor cells) that destroys normal marrow function. This type of autologous transplantation is more common in patients with solid tumors, who tend to have few circulating tumor cells in the blood or bone marrow. The main therapeutic advantage of bone marrow transplantation in patients with nonhematopoietic neoplasms such as breast cancer is that very-high-dose chemotherapy can be utilized to eradicate the patient's tumor. This level of radiation therapy and chemotherapy would normally be fatal because of bone marrow failure. The ability to expand stem cells from the peripheral blood in vitro offers the possibility of purging residual neoplastic cells from this population to provide tumor-free stem cells for autologous transplantation.

Allogenic transplants (from an MHC-matched donor) are more commonly employed as therapy for leukemia and lymphoma. Donor-derived T cells cause a degree of graft-versus-host disease that has important therapeutic effects in eliminating residual tumor cells. Severe graft-versus-host disease can be fatal so that the degree of donor-patient mismatch and the extent of immunosuppression after transplant are critical in determining the success of this therapy. Other more complex therapies involving minitransplants alternating with chemotherapy may extend life in some patients with aggressive myeloma.

●●● LYMPH NODE AND MUCOSA-ASSOCIATED LYMPHOID TISSUE

Lymph nodes are the main organ in which antigen selection of B cells occurs in germinal centers. Lymph nodes usually have a well-defined architecture with germinal centers surrounded by mantle and marginal zones that are separated by intrafollicular zones composed largely of small T cells. Germinal centers contain small B cells and larger transformed B cells (centroblasts) as well as dendritic histocytes and a few T cells. Secondary germinal centers show active proliferation and apoptosis of B cells as a consequence of ongoing antigenic selection. The marginal sinus at the periphery of lymph nodes connects with sinusoids that extend to the lymph node hilum (Fig. 11-8). Afferent lymphatics connect to the marginal

sinus, and lymph percolates through the sinus and the substance of the lymph node before draining into efferent lymphatic vessels. Draining lymph flows through more proximal lymph nodes and ultimately into the thoracic duct. This architectural arrangement ensures that antigens are available for interaction with B cells.

Most lymphomas destroy (efface) lymph node architecture as they grow. Inflammatory and infectious conditions can modify and distort lymph node architecture, but they do not efface it, so that retention of normal architectural pattern is a critical finding in the histopathologic examination of lymph nodes. Metastatic solid-tumor deposits in lymph are usually first trapped in the marginal sinus and, if they survive, grow to form metastatic foci that may ultimately destroy the lymph node. Micrometastases are usually present within or adjacent to the marginal sinus because this is the first point of contact for tumor cells migrating through lymphatic vessels.

Mucosa-associated lymphoid tissue (MALT) typically contains germinal centers and interfollicular T cells, but no sinuses or other lymph node–like structures are usually present. Peyer's patches correspond to larger deposits of MALT typically found in the terminal ileum. MALT functions similarly to lymph nodes in the GI tract as well as the lung.

Reactive hyperplasia may mimic the morphologic appearance of some lymphoproliferative diseases. Clear pathologic distinction between reactive and neoplastic processes is essential for appropriate therapy. Flow cytometric analysis of single-cell suspensions from lymphoid tissues allows precise delineation of the phenotype of different cell populations. Coexpression of three or more antigens can be evaluated on individual cells using specific antibodies labeled with different fluorophores. The availability of molecular diagnostics has significantly improved the diagnostic accuracy and sensitivity of lymphoma diagnosis. This is particularly true for small-needle biopsy of lymphoproliferative disorders. Assessment of the clonality of antigen receptor gene rearrangement in both T cells and B cells can be helpful in discriminating a neoplastic (monoclonal) from a reactive (usually polyclonal) process. The identification of specific translocations by PCR or by FISH is also helpful in establishing a specific diagnosis for a number of different types of lymphomas and leukemias.

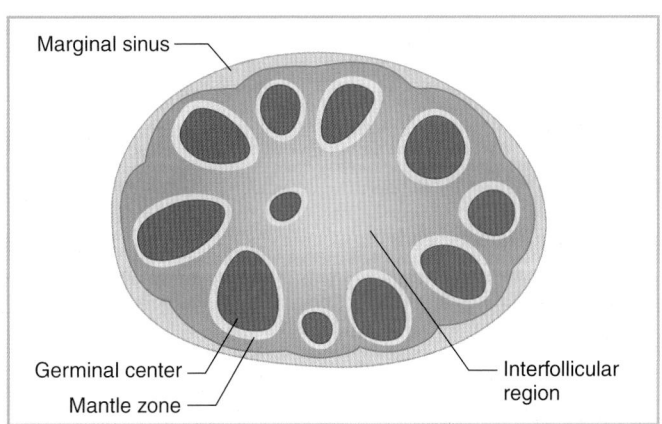

Figure 11-8. Lymph node architecture.

Lymphadenitis

Many types of infection result in prominent hyperplasia of lymph nodes. The presence of lymphadenopathy may raise the possibility of lymphoma or metastatic carcinoma, and biopsy specimens of unexplained, enlarged lymph nodes are often the means to establish a specific diagnosis.

Mononucleosis

Infectious mononucleosis is caused by acute infection with Epstein-Barr virus (EBV). The full-blown syndrome typically occurs in adolescents, who develop marked splenomegaly as well as lymphadenopathy. Demonstration of IgM specific for EBV is diagnostic in these patients (the Monospot test) and can prevent the morbidity associated with lymph node biopsy. This is also important because the morphologic changes in lymph nodes in mononucleosis can closely resemble a high-grade lymphoma with massive expansion of germinal centers and virtual disappearance of interfollicular T cells. Mononucleosis is a self-limited disease although EBV infection remains latent in some lymphoid cells for life. Some types of lymphoproliferative disorders as well as neoplasms of other tissues are associated with Epstein-Barr viral infection (e.g., nasopharyngeal carcinoma, endemic Burkitt's lymphoma, and probably some cases of Hodgkin's disease).

MICROBIOLOGY

Epstein-Barr Virus (EBV)

Ninety-five percent of adults between 35 and 45 years of age show serologic evidence of prior EBV infection. Infants become susceptible to EBV when maternal antibodies decline, and many children develop subclinical EBV infection in early childhood. Initial EBV infection during adolescence or early adulthood produces the full-blown clinical syndrome of infectious mononucleosis in one third to one half of those infected.

Primary EBV infection can be diagnosed if IgM antibodies to capsid proteins are present but antibodies to EBV nuclear antigen (EBNA) are absent. Detectable antibodies typically remain for many years, and reactivation of infection is characterized by the presence of IgG anti-EBNA antibodies with antibodies against EBV early antigens.

EBV predominantly infects lymphocytes and epithelial cells in the salivary gland, resulting in high virus titers in saliva, which is highly infectious. EBV's tropism for these cell types is related to its role in lymphoma and nasopharyngeal carcinoma. EBV produces approximately 100 antigenic proteins during active infection, but only 10 proteins are produced in latent infection including EBNAs 1–6 and latent membrane proteins (LMPs) 1–3.

The exact role of EBV in the genesis of tumors remains unclear although EBV encodes a number of different transactivating proteins (e.g., LMP) that can modify host cellular transcription. EBV can be used to "immortalize" peripheral blood B cells in vitro so that they continue to proliferate in tissue culture.

Toxoplasma Lymphadenitis

Toxoplasma gondii is a protozoan pathogen that can cause infection of lymph nodes draining the site of inoculation. A puncture wound (often associated with soil exposure during gardening chores) can inoculate organisms and result in enlargement of the draining lymph node (usually axillary). Lymph node biopsy typically shows loose clusters of histiocytes (poorly formed granulomas) and foci of so-called monocytoid B cells (i.e., B cells with kidney bean–shaped nuclei) (Fig. 11-9). This full-blown morphologic pattern is characteristic, and the diagnosis can be confirmed by serologic tests for antibodies against *Toxoplasma* antigens.

Cat-Scratch Lymphadenitis

Cat-scratch lymphadenitis is similar in clinical presentation to toxoplasmosis, often with enlargement of an axillary lymph node after a scratch from a domestic cat. Lymph node biopsy shows hyperplasia with microabscess formation within germinal centers. This morphologic pattern is characteristic, and the diagnosis can be confirmed by demonstrating the presence of the causative bacterium (*Bartonella* species) in lymph node tissue by DNA-based PCR.

Bacillary Angiomatosis

Bacillary angiomatosis occurs only in severely immunocompromised patients and is also caused by *Bartonella*. Infection of endothelial cells results in vascular proliferation in lymph nodes that may mimic metastatic Kaposi's sarcoma. Since most patients with bacillary angiomatosis have advanced HIV, this differential diagnosis is clinically important because bacillary angiomatosis can be cured by antibiotic therapy. Bacillary angiomatosis is typically associated with a prominent neutrophilic infiltrate that is not present in Kaposi's sarcoma, and the diagnosis can be confirmed by PCR of DNA isolated from lymph node tissue.

Mycobacterium avium-intracellulare

Mycobacterium avium-intracellulare (MAI) is an intracellular pathogen that can cause massive but usually indolent infection in immunocompromised patients, most often in patients with advanced HIV. MAI infection often produces lymphadenopathy but also may involve the GI tract and other sites. Lesions consist of expansile masses of histiocytes that are filled with mycobacteria, giving their cytoplasm a granular or beaded appearance. Stains for acid-fast bacteria are diagnostic.

Lymphoproliferative Disease

Lymphoproliferative diseases may take the form of leukemia (predominantly with blood and bone marrow involvement) or lymphomas (solid tumors growing in lymph nodes, lymphoid organs, or less frequently nonlymphoid organs). A mixed pattern of leukemia and lymphoma often occurs at some point during the clinical course in many patients (e.g., leukemia is common in advanced lymphomas, and tissue infiltration is often observed in advanced leukemias) but gen-

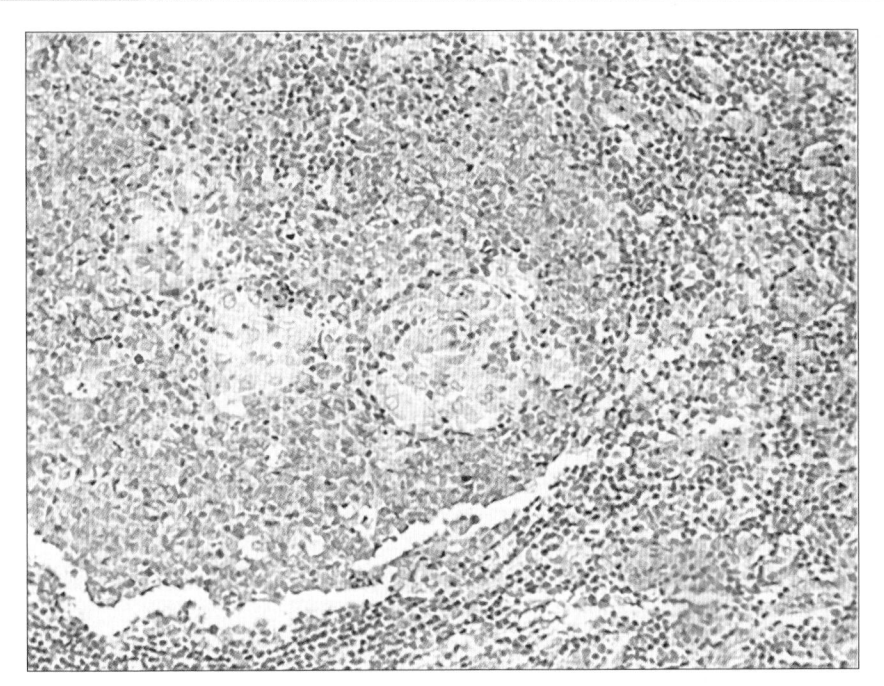

Figure 11-9. Toxoplasmosis. Microscopic section of lymph node showing loose aggregates of histiocytes typical of toxoplasmosis.

MICROBIOLOGY

Bartonella

Bartonella is a genus of small, weakly gram-negative bacteria that are difficult to culture in vitro. Detection of bacterial DNA in tissue by PCR is useful diagnostically.

Bartonella quintana is the agent of "trench fever," which was epidemic in World War I and was spread by body lice. *B. quintana* rarely has been reported as a cause of human disease since that time but is now recognized as a cause of bacterial endocarditis in debilitated individuals.

Bartonella henselae can cause cat-scratch fever, producing clinically worrisome lymphadenopathy. Domestic cats are a reservoir for *B. henselae,* and up to 40% are persistently infected. Humans become infected by a scratch or via a tick vector (*Ixodes pacificus*). *B. henselae* can also cause bacillary angiomatosis in immunocompromised patients (typically advanced HIV) that can mimic Kaposi's sarcoma morphologically.

Bartonella bacilliformis is endemic in some regions of South America, where it is spread via sand flies and produces Oroya fever.

erally presents as either leukemia or lymphoma. Hodgkin's disease is a unique form of lymphoma with distinctive clinical behavior and clinical presentation and is discussed separately from other forms of lymphoproliferative disease (i.e., non-Hodgkin's lymphomas).

The classification of non-Hodgkin's lymphoma (NHL) is work in progress with the integration of clinical, morphologic, immunophenotypical, and molecular data. The REAL (revised European American lymphoma) classification attempts to incorporate most of these data into specific diagnostic entities. NHLs have been classified as low-, intermediate-, or high-grade neoplasms (in the NCI working formulation), and this stratification provides useful information about their clinical behavior (Table 11-2). Low-grade tumors have a relatively low proliferative rate and do not show tumor necrosis. Most low-grade lymphomas are composed of relatively small cells (slightly larger than normal small lymphocytes) and clinically progress very slowly. They usually present at a high clinical stage with involvement of the bone marrow and multiple organs. Paradoxically, most low-grade lymphomas are not curable with conventional therapy although patients with low-grade tumors may live for many years, even without treatment. Persistent growth of low-grade lymphomas eventually results in effacement of the bone marrow and other organs, leading to death due to infection or hemorrhage.

High-grade lymphomas have a high proliferative rate, and tumor necrosis is usually present. Most high-grade lymphomas are composed of large cells. High-grade lymphomas are clinically aggressive and can kill a patient over the course of days or weeks if untreated. Patients usually have elevated serum LDH, which can be a marker of tumor burden. Radiation therapy with or without chemotherapy usually causes significant tumor regression (high-grade lymphomas are inherently sensitive because of their high mitotic rate), and some patients are cured by modern chemotherapy.

Intermediate-grade lymphomas share some features of low-grade and high-grade tumors. Some represent low-grade tumors in transition (transformation) to high-grade tumors. Most tend to involve multiple sites at presentation, and their

TABLE 11-2. Non-Hodgkin's Lymphoma (NHL)

Grade	Subtype	Typical Features
Low	MALT and marginal zone lymphoma	Small cells
	Chronic lymphocytic leukemia and small lymphocytic lymphoma	Low proliferation rate
	Follicular lymphoma, grade 1	No necrosis
Intermediate	Mantle cell lymphoma	
	Follicular lymphoma, grade 2	
High	Follicular lymphoma, grade 3	
	Large-cell B-cell lymphoma	Large cells
	T-cell lymphoma (most types)	High proliferative rate
	Acute lymphoblastic leukemia	Necrosis
	Burkitt's lymphoma	

proliferation rate makes them less uniformly responsive to chemotherapy than high-grade lymphomas. Intermediate-grade lymphomas are usually treated at diagnosis, but responses are often disappointing and patients frequently succumb to their disease over the course of a few years.

B-cell leukemias and lymphomas are much more common than their T-cell counterparts. Immunoglobulin gene rearrangement and hypermutation that take place during the development of B cells likely predisposes to neoplasia because of the potential for abnormal rearrangement events producing translocations (e.g., BCL-1 and BCL-2 gene translocations to immunoglobulin heavy chain gene locus in follicular and mantle cell lymphoma). Indeed, BCL-2 translocations can be observed in a small percentage of normal tonsillar cells by means of a very sensitive PCR assay (nested PCR). Since BCL-2 is a weak oncogene, this single translocation event is not sufficient to produce a tumor, but the antiapoptotic effects of BCL-2 protein overexpression permit cells to survive for long time intervals in which additional mutations may be acquired to complete tumorigenesis.

A few other specific forms of lymphoid hyperplasia are tumor-like in their behavior but are not usually classified as leukemias or lymphomas. These include Castleman disease, which may be associated with autoimmune disease (CREST syndrome) and frequently shows evidence of human herpesvirus 8 (HHV-8) infection. Posttransplant lymphoproliferative disorders are discussed with immunodeficiency in Chapter 2.

Chronic Lymphocytic Leukemia

Chronic lymphocytic leukemia (CLL) is a low-grade neoplasm of small B lymphocytes that coexpress CD5 (normally a T-cell differentiation antigen) and CD23. Peripheral blood and bone marrow involvement are readily diagnosed by flow cytometry (abnormal CD5 and CD23 coexpression on B cells), and peripheral counts are usually in the range of $20,000/mm^3$ to $50,000/mm^3$ at diagnosis but increase over time. The bone marrow shows either focal or diffuse infiltrates

of small lymphocytes. Involved lymph nodes usually show complete effacement of normal architecture by a diffuse infiltrate of small lymphoid cells (slightly larger than normal B cells with minimal nuclear membrane irregularities). Proliferation centers (areas with increased cell division composed of larger cells are usually evident on low power as pale areas containing slightly larger cells. Scattered paraimmunoblasts (large cells) are also present (Fig. 11-10).

CLL is not associated with specific chromosomal translocations, but all tumors have undergone immunoglobulin gene rearrangement. About half these tumors show evidence of antigenic selection in germinal centers (i.e., the presence of somatic mutations in the hypervariable regions of their immunoglobulin genes).

Tumors that have undergone antigenic selection have a better prognosis. Most cases of CLL without evidence of antigenic selection also express ZAP-70 protein, and this may be a more convenient biomarker for more aggressive tumors that may benefit from more intensive therapy. The clinical course of untreated CLL is usually prolonged, with a slow increase in tumor burden over the course of years that eventually displaces normal hematopoietic cells in the bone marrow and lymphoid organs to produce cytopenia and immunodeficiency. Many patients ultimately die as a result of opportunistic infection.

CLL frequently involves lymph nodes, and some patients have a mixed pattern of leukemia and lymphoma. Morphologically similar disease that is predominantly lymph node based is referred to as small lymphocytic lymphoma (SLL). Some patients may develop a more aggressive form of CLL in which neoplastic small lymphocytes contain nucleoli similar to lymphoid progenitors (also called prolymphocytic leukemia). A small percentage of CLL tumors undergoes transformation to a high-grade large-cell lymphoma that can be rapidly fatal ("Richter's transformation").

MALT Lymphoma

Most so-called MALT lymphomas and the closely related marginal zone lymphomas appear to develop in the setting

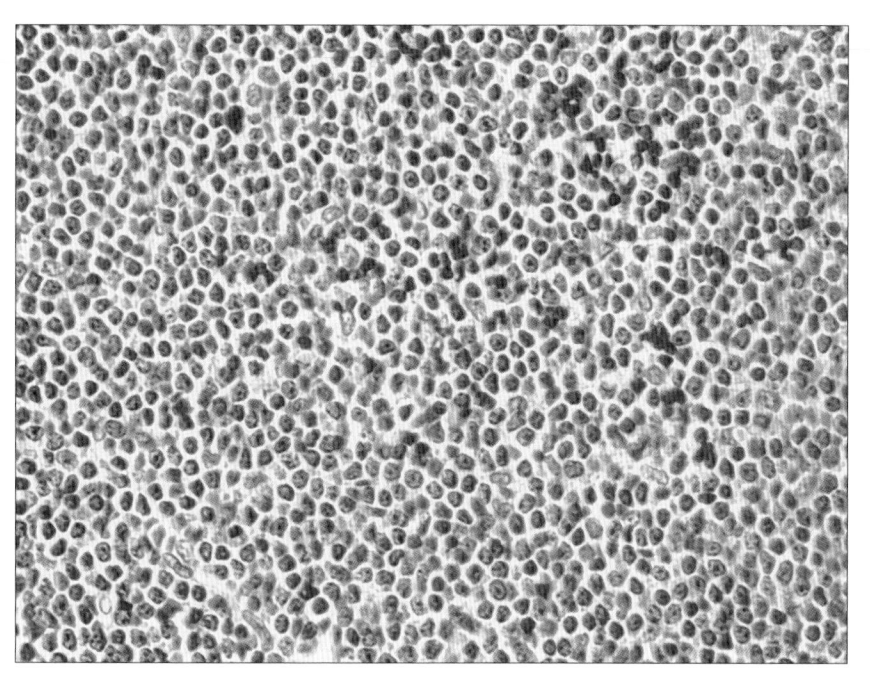

Figure 11-10. Chronic lymphocytic leukemia (CLL). Microscopic section of lymph node showing a diffuse infiltrate and small lymphocytes with occasional larger cells (paraimmunoblasts). Normal architecture is completely effaced.

IMMUNOLOGY

Antigen Selection

Antigen selection occurs in secondary follicles, where B cells expressing antibody compete for antigen binding. B cells that fail to bind antigen trigger apoptosis (BCL-2 protein is not normally expressed in germinal center B cells so that their apoptotic pathways are fully active).

Re-challenge with antigen results in the proliferation of memory cells that can bind antigen, and these cells localize to germinal centers. These B cells activate hypermutation, which is largely confined to the complementarity-determining regions (CDRs) in the variable regions of their immunoglobulin genes. Some mutations occur in framework regions as well.

B cells with mutations that result in stop codons or in nonfunctional immunoglobulin structure cannot bind antigen and are rapidly eliminated by apoptosis. This selection process results in the expansion of B-cell clones with higher affinity for antigen (i.e., "affinity maturation") to produce effective immunity.

Mutations in CDRs and framework regions serve as permanent markers (divergence from germline sequences) that these B cells have undergone antigen selection and identify them as post–germinal center B cells.

Mutations in nonimmunoglobulin genes during hypermutation may contribute to neoplasia in these B cells.

of chronic antigenic stimulation. The development of MALT lymphomas of the stomach in association with chronic *Helicobacter pylori* infection is discussed in Chapter 9. MALT lymphomas can develop in other organs (e.g., the salivary gland, often in association with Sjögren's syndrome). Lymph node–based tumors with morphologic features similar to MALT lymphomas also occur. All MALT lymphomas tend to be indolent and remain localized although a small percentage ultimately transform to high-grade lymphomas. A minority of MALT lymphomas show trisomy for chromosome 3 or a translocation between the immunoglobulin heavy chain locus and the MALT1 gene, t(11;14).

Follicular Lymphoma

Follicular lymphoma is one of the most common types of lymphoma in middle-aged and older individuals. Follicular lymphomas produce a nodular infiltrate in lymph nodes that eventually effaces normal germinal centers. Most patients with follicular lymphoma seek medical attention with relatively high stage disease (usually with bone marrow involvement that is characteristically paratrabecular). Tumor cells in low-grade follicular lymphoma (grade 1) are small with prominent nuclear angulations (also called *small cleaved cells*) and have phenotypic features of follicular center B cells (typically CD10$^+$) (Fig. 11-11A). Most follicular lymphomas have a specific translocation in which the coding region of the bcl-2 proto-oncogene is juxtaposed with the immunoglobulin heavy chain locus (14;18 translocation) (see Fig. 11-11B). This translocation results in overexpression of BCL-2 protein that allows cells to escape apoptosis. As low-grade follicular lymphomas persist and progress, they may loose their nodular architecture and appear as diffuse sheets of small, cleaved lymphocytes.

Low-grade follicular lymphomas are usually indolent tumors that may persist for many years producing bulky adenopathy. Bone marrow infiltration may eventually result in cytopenia. Follicular lymphoma is organized into three

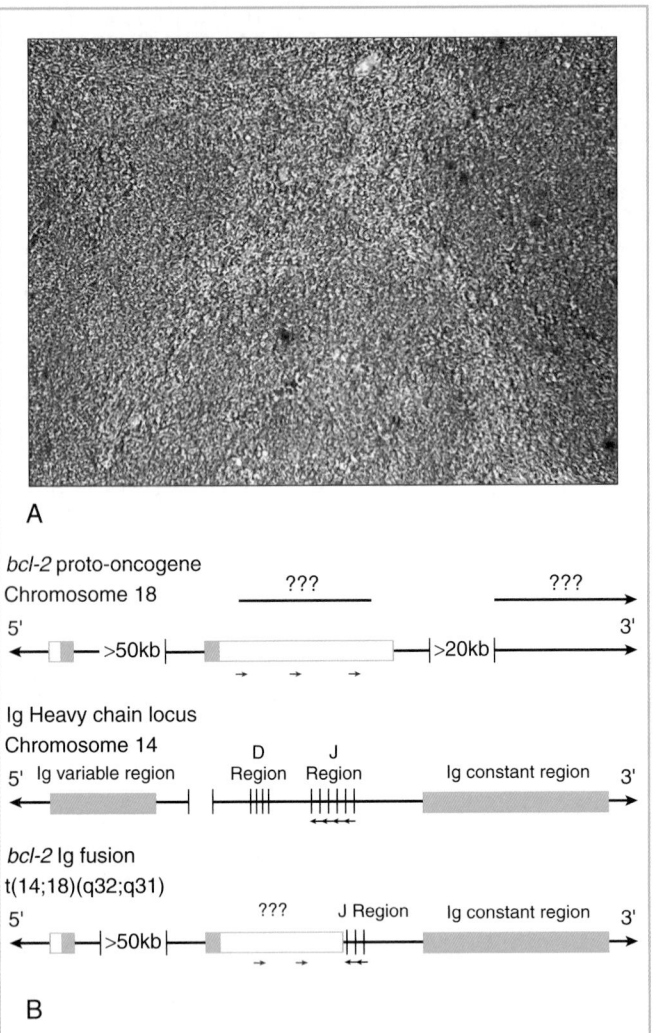

A

bcl-2 proto-oncogene
Chromosome 18

B

Figure 11-11. A, Follicular lymphoma, grade 1. Microscopic section of lymph node showing a nodular infiltrate of angulated, small B cells effacing normal architecture. **B,** bcl-2 Translocation in follicular lymphoma. The germline configurations of the bcl-2 and immunoglobulin heavy chain genes are shown at the top and middle of the figure, with a typical translocation shown below. The locations of PCR primers used to diagnose this translocation are indicated. No PCR product is produced from germline DNA while DNA from tumor cells with this translocation generate a discrete-length PCR product.

grades in the REAL classification with grade 1 corresponding to predominantly small cleaved cells and grade 3 corresponding to predominantly large cells that are mitotically active. Grade 1 tumors behave in a low-grade manner in terms of clinical aggressiveness while grade 3 tumors are all clinically aggressive. Grade 2 tumors are often aggressive and may represent transformation from grade 1 to grade 3. A significant percentage of grade 1 follicular lymphomas ultimately progress to large-cell lymphoma, and acquired alterations in p16 and p53 genes frequently are involved in this transformation. Most high-grade lymphomas that develop from low-grade lymphomas tend to be resistant to chemotherapy. Some large-cell lymphomas (see below) likely represent transformed follicular lymphomas.

Mantle Cell Lymphoma

Mantle cell lymphoma is a tumor of small lymphocytes that has an aggressive clinical course with low 5-year survival. Mantle cells resemble normal B cells in the mantle zone around germinal centers and have a cell surface phenotype similar to that of CLL with coexpression of normal B-cell markers and CD5. Unlike CLL, mantle cell lymphomas

usually do not express CD23, and they have a specific translocation between the bcl-1 proto-oncogene (i.e., the gene that encodes cyclin D) and the immunoglobulin heavy chain gene. This translocation results in overexpression of cyclin D, which drives cell proliferation through the G_1S cell cycle checkpoint. Mantle cell lymphoma is an intermediate-grade lymphoma and although it usually responds to chemotherapy, cure is rare. Mantle cell lymphoma can present around Waldeyer's ring (peritonsillar area of the oropharynx), in lymph nodes, or in the GI tract, where it may produce polyps composed of neoplastic small lymphocytes. Low-level involvement of the peripheral blood (i.e., subleukemic involvement) is fairly common, and involvement of extranodal sites such as skin is not unusual (Fig. 11-12). It is essential to distinguish mantle cell lymphoma from less aggressive neoplasms such as CLL and grade 1 follicular lymphoma.

Large-cell, B-cell Lymphoma

Some large-cell, B-cell lymphomas arise from low-grade lymphomas, but others probably develop de novo. Tumor cells are large, and tumor cell nuclei are typically vesicular with relatively prominent single or multiple nucleoli (Fig. 11-13).

Cyclin D

D type cyclins (cyclins D1–D3) are essential for cell cycle progression at G_1S, where they bind to and activate cyclin-dependent kinases (CDK4 and CDK6) to trigger phosphorylation of the retinoblastoma protein and initiation of DNA synthesis. Cyclin proteins are normally synthesized de novo at the appropriate time in the cell cycle and are then rapidly degraded after cell cycle progression is initiated.

Translocation of the cyclin D1 gene to the immunoglobulin heavy chain locus in neoplastic B cells results in constitutive overexpression of cyclin D1, which drives cell proliferation in the absence of growth factors or other normal growth stimuli. This translocation results from aberrant immunoglobulin gene rearrangement similarly to bcl-2 gene translocations in follicular lymphoma.

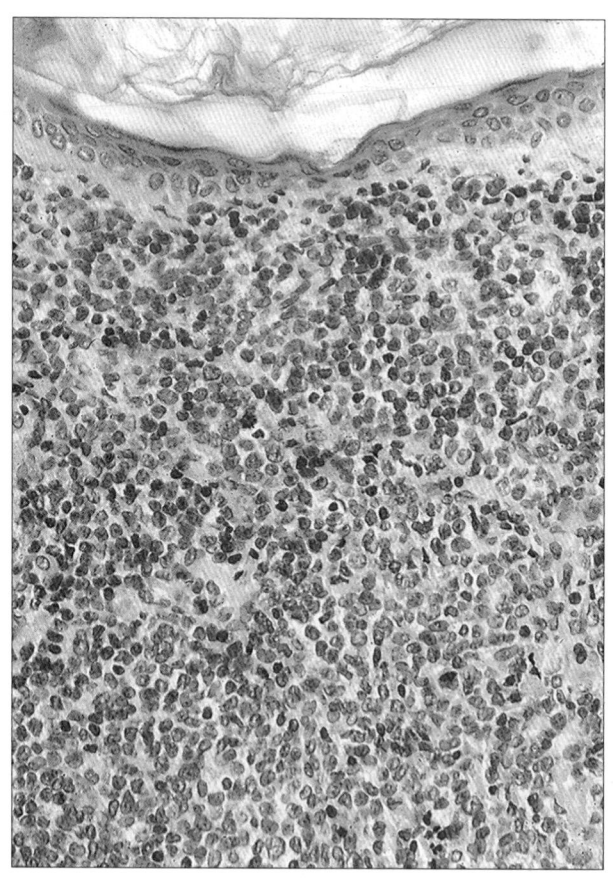

Figure 11-12. Mantle cell lymphoma. Microscopic section of skin (epidermis at top) with a diffuse infiltrate of small lymphocytes with rounded nuclei and somewhat primitive (blastic) nuclear chromatin.

These tumors tend to form masses within lymph nodes or other organs that may mimic metastatic carcinoma morphologically. Almost all large-cell, B-cell lymphomas express pan-B-cell antigens, and many show nuclear expression with BCL-6 (point mutations are frequently present in the bcl-6 gene as well). Distinction of lymphoma from carcinoma can be readily accomplished with immunohistochemical markers or by analysis of antigen receptor gene rearrangement by PCR.

Untreated large-cell lymphoma is rapidly fatal, but many tumors show a dramatic response to chemotherapy because of their high proliferative rate. Recently, different subtypes of large-cell, B-cell lymphoma have been defined by means of transcriptional profiling with supervised and unsupervised clustering analysis. Some of these subcategories appear to have relatively specific prognostic features (e.g., post–germinal center B-cell phenotype). Validation studies are in progress; while promising, the ultimate clinical utility of this form of classification is not proved as yet.

Burkitt's Lymphoma

Burkitt's lymphoma is a high-grade lymphoma composed of pre–B cells that occurs in both endemic and sporadic forms. Burkitt's lymphoma is endemic in Africa, where it develops predominantly in children and frequently presents as a tumor mass in the jaw. Endemic Burkitt's lymphoma is almost always associated with EBV infection. Sporadic Burkitt's lymphoma is more common in the United States, and most cases are not clearly associated with EBV. Most patients in the United States have lymph node disease or involvement of the GI tract.

Sporadic Burkitt's lymphoma is usually a disease of early childhood although it can occur in adults and is a relatively common morphologic presentation of lymphoma in patients with advanced AIDS. Most Burkitt's lymphomas show a translocation between the c-MYC proto-oncogene and the immunoglobulin heavy chain gene. This translocation deregulates c-MYC transcription, and overexpression of c-MYC protein drives rapid tumor cell proliferation. c-MYC is a powerful oncogene that contributes to the morphologic

appearance of Burkitt's lymphoma, which is referred to as a "starry sky" pattern (Fig. 11-14). The rapid proliferation of medium-sized lymphoid cells and extensive tumor cell apoptosis produce this pattern, which is typical but not pathognomonic of Burkitt's lymphoma. Burkitt's lymphoma is an extremely aggressive neoplasm that can kill a patient within days without chemotherapy. Most tumors are responsive to chemotherapy, although durable remissions are less common.

Acute Lymphoblastic Leukemia and Lymphoblastic Lymphoma

Acute lymphoblastic leukemia (ALL) is usually a disease of childhood. Tumors are of B- or T-cell lineage, mixed T- and B-cell phenotype, or null for T- and B-cell differentiation antigens, expressing only more primitive lymphoid markers and CD10 (common acute lymphoblastic leukemia antigen, or CALLA). ALL cells usually express terminal deoxynucleotidyl transferase, which normally is expressed only in primitive lymphoid cells (Fig. 11-15). Patients typically have extensive bone marrow involvement and numerous blasts in peripheral blood.

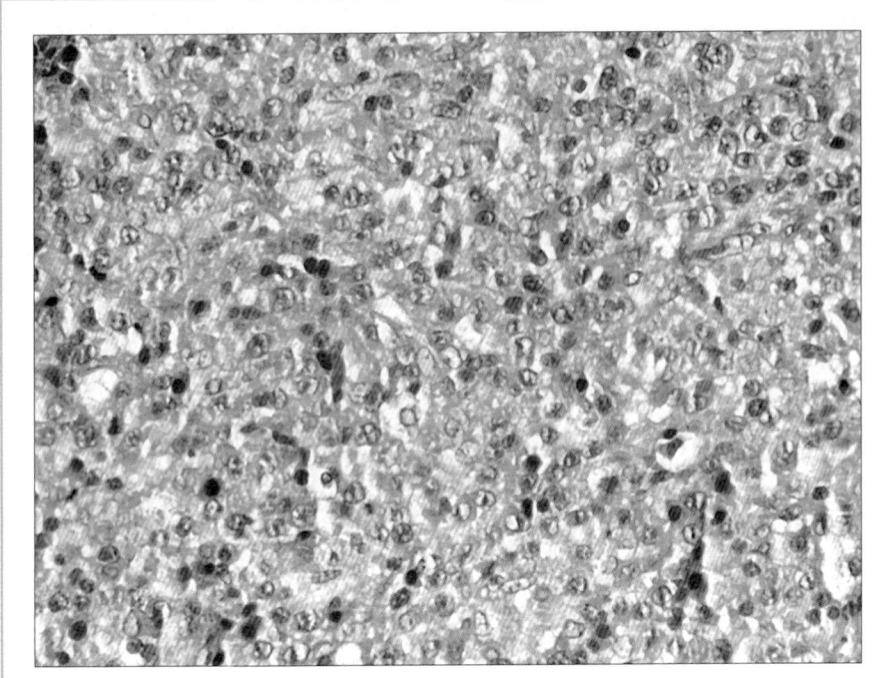

Figure 11-13. Large-cell, B-cell lymphoma. Microscopic section of lymph node showing a diffuse infiltrate of large lymphoid cells with vesicular nuclei and prominent nucleoli. No discernible architectural pattern is present. Mitotic activity is brisk.

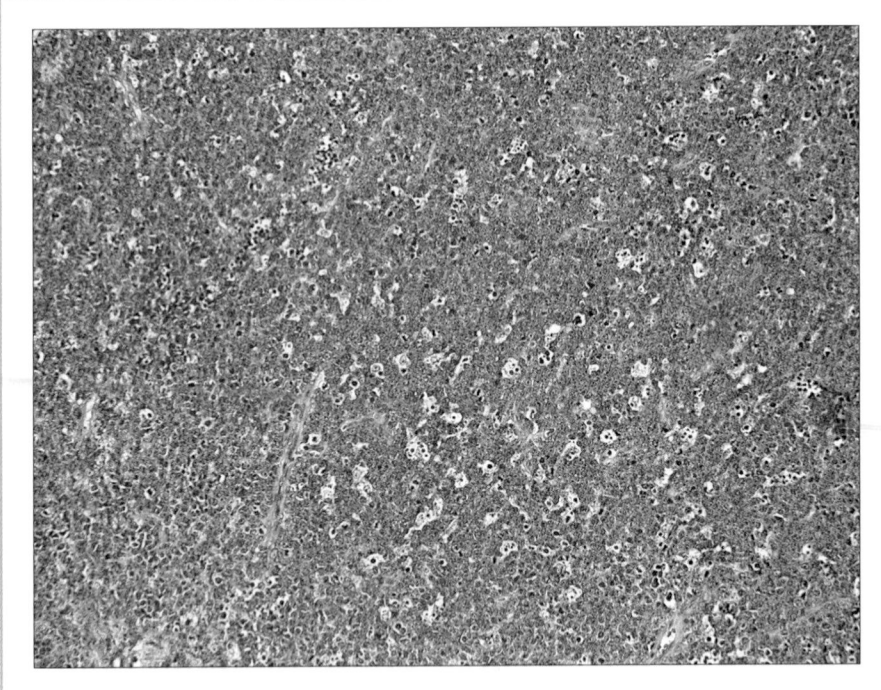

Figure 11-14. Burkitt's lymphoma. Diffuse infiltrate of intermediate-sized lymphoid cells with blastic chromatin. Mitotic activity is intense, and apoptosis of tumor cells is prominent, creating the "starry sky" pattern.

Treatment of ALL is one of the major successes of medical oncology over the last half-century, with the great majority of patients achieving durable remission and cure. ALL frequently involves the central nervous system, and direct treatment of the cerebrospinal fluid with chemotherapeutic agents (intrathecal chemotherapy) is usually necessary to eradicate all tumor cells. The central nervous system and testis can act as "sanctuary" sites where tumor cells can escape the effects of chemotherapy (e.g., the blood-brain barrier) and lead to recurrence.

ALL can be classified into different prognostic groups based on expression of specific differentiation antigens, DNA ploidy, and cytogenetic analysis. Many cases of ALL have specific chromosomal translocations, which often involve developmental control genes (such as HOX) that are normally expressed during embryogenesis. ALL is separated into three

GENETICS

c-myc Translocations in African and American Burkitt's Lymphoma

All c-myc translocations in Burkitt's lymphoma result in the activation of c-myc transcription by juxtaposing the c-myc oncogene and immunoglobulin gene enhancers (E) that are active in B lymphocytes.

In most cases of endemic (African) Burkitt's lymphoma, the c-myc gene (chromosome 8) is translocated to the 5' region of the immunoglobulin heavy chain locus (chromosome 14) in a head-to-head configuration.

In most cases of sporadic (American) Burkitt's lymphoma, c-myc exons 2 and 3 (including the complete protein coding sequence) are translocated to the switch region of the immunoglobulin heavy chain gene. A cryptic promoter adjacent to exon 2 is then utilized to overexpress c-myc protein.

Less common variant translocations also occur in which the c-myc gene is translocated to the kappa or lambda light chain loci (chromosome 22 or 2).

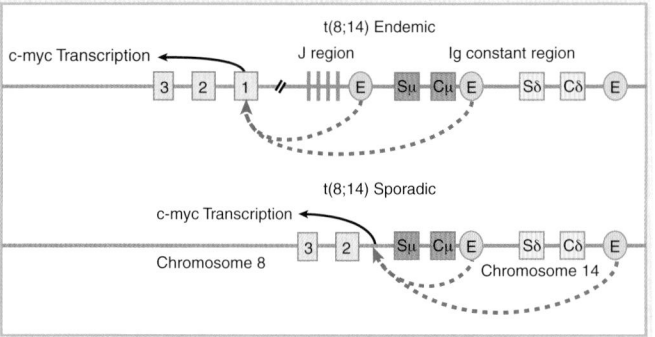

BIOCHEMISTRY

Terminal Deoxynucleotidyl Transferase (TdT)

Terminal deoxynucleotidyl transferase (TdT) is a template-independent DNA polymerase that is normally active only during antigen receptor gene rearrangement in primitive B and T cells. 3' Phosphate groups formed during recombination catalyzed by RAG (recombinase activating gene) proteins provide an appropriate substrate for TdT, which adds a variable number of random nucleotides before rejoining occurs. Insertion of these nucleotides in CDR III increases antigen receptor diversity.

TdT has the potential to act as a potent mutagen, and its expression is tightly controlled. Immunofluorescence or immunohistochemical stains for nuclear TdT can be useful in identifying lymphoblasts in ALL and lymphoblastic lymphoma.

GENETICS

Translocations in ALL

Different translocations occur in B- and T-cell ALL, and some specific translocations are associated with favorable or adverse prognoses and with specific clinical syndromes. Many of the genes involved in these translocations are developmental control genes, and the fusion proteins created are thought to interfere with cellular differentiation and trap these cells in a primitive or precursor state. Some of these translocations are capable of transforming naïve precursor lymphoid cells while others are not, suggesting that additional genetic alterations are required to complete tumorigenesis. Constitutive activation of recombinase and TdT in lymphoid precursor cells may allow rapid selection for additional genetic alterations in partially transformed cells.

Translocation t(1;19) is present in 25% of pre–B cell ALLs (tumor cells are positive for cytoplasmic Ig but not for cell surface Ig) and fuses a portion of the E2A gene (a basic helix-loop-helix transcription factor) to PBX1 (a homeobox gene involved in controlling developmental gene expression during embryogenesis). The resulting fusion protein prevents maturation of tumor cells beyond the pre–B cell stage.

The MLL gene on chromosome 11 is a zinc finger transcription factor that has more than 25 different known translocation partners in different types of leukemia. MLL translocations are common in ALL presenting in infants and are associated with a poor prognosis.

Translocation t(12;21) is present in 25% of childhood ALL and fuses the TEL helix-loop-helix domain with the DNA binding or transactivation domain of AML1, which is altered in some types of myeloid leukemia. The fusion protein interferes with normal homeobox gene function to block differentiation.

Many translocations in T-cell ALL involve transcription factor genes that are rearranged to the T-cell receptor loci (β, α, or δ), resulting in their overexpression and downstream alterations in the expression of their target genes.

FAB subtypes, L1 to L3. L1 corresponds to small monomorphic blasts while L2 blasts are larger and have more cytoplasm. L2 blasts show prominent nucleoli and are less monomorphic than L1 blasts. L3 corresponds to a Burkitt's lymphoma–like morphology, with large blasts with dispersed chromatin, multiple nucleoli, and vacuolated cytoplasm. ALL occurring in adults tends to have a substantially poorer prognosis than childhood ALL.

Lymphoblastic lymphoma shares many features with ALL. Lymphoblastic lymphoma is usually a tumor of T cells that has a convoluted nucleus and expresses TdT. Most patients have a thymic tumor often composed of double-positive T cells (CD4$^+$ and CD8$^+$).

T-cell Lymphomas

T-cell lymphomas are much less common than their B-cell counterparts (approximately 4:1 ratio). Most T-cell lymphomas are quite variable in morphologic appearance and clinical presentation. They often present at extranodal sites (much more frequently than B-cell lymphomas). The morphologic findings in many T-cell lymphomas suggest an inflammatory condition rather than a malignant lymphoma.

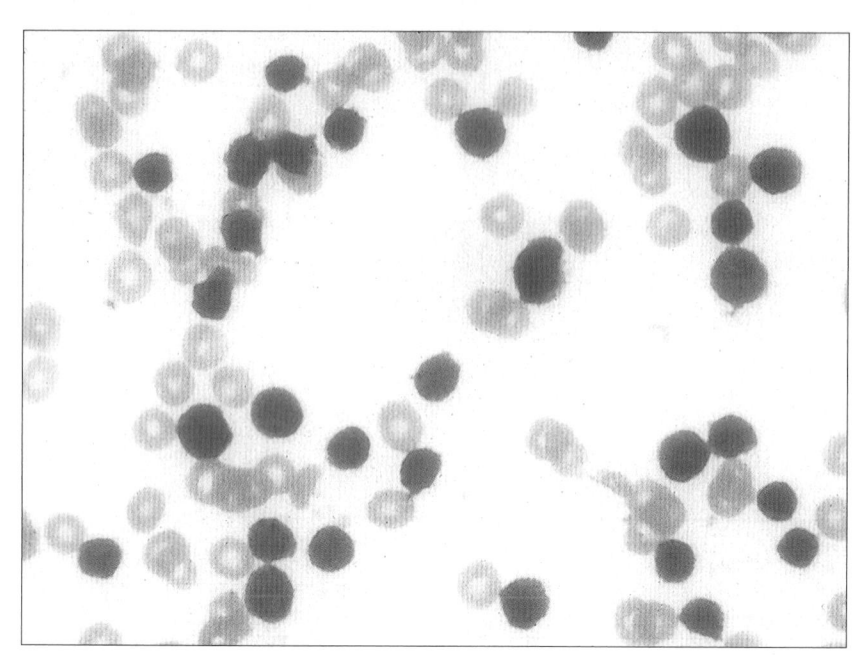

Figure 11-15. Acute lymphocytic leukemia (ALL). Peripheral blood smear showing numerous lymphoblasts. These blasts may be difficult to distinguish from AML blasts morphologically.

Neoplastic T cells often produce large quantities of cytokines and chemokines that attract other inflammatory cells. Since only a small number of neoplastic T cells may be present, morphologic identification may be problematic. Clonality of T cells cannot be demonstrated by flow cytometry as in many B-cell tumors (light chain restriction) although the ratio of CD4 to CD8 cells and the loss of expression of some normal T-cell differentiation antigens may be helpful in establishing a diagnosis of lymphoma. Evidence of T-cell antigen receptor gene rearrangement by PCR can also provide critical information about clonality in difficult cases.

Specific subtypes of T-cell lymphoma include mycosis fungoides (MF), which is a primary lymphoma of skin (Fig. 11-16), anaplastic large-cell lymphoma (ALCL), and peripheral T-cell lymphoma. Human T lymphotropic virus 1 (HTLV1) can produce T-cell tumors that present with diverse symptoms and often show mixed features of leukemia and lymphoma. HTLV1 is endemic in the Caribbean and Southeast Asia but is uncommon in the United States. Demonstration of antibodies to the virus or of viral nucleic acid in tumor cells can assist in making the diagnosis.

Hodgkin's Disease

Hodgkin's disease is a morphologically distinct form of lymphoma that can usually be cured with modern therapy. Prior to effective radiation therapy and chemotherapy, Hodgkin's disease was uniformly fatal. The number of neoplastic cells in most forms of Hodgkin's disease is small, and these cells (Hodgkin's cells) are greatly outnumbered by infiltrating inflammatory cells as well as a prominent fibroblastic reaction. In this way, Hodgkin's disease shares some features with T-cell lymphomas that recruit normal cells by secretion of cytokines, chemokines, and growth factors. Many cases

of Hodgkin's disease occur in young adults, who usually have localized disease (confined to one or several lymph node groups). Most forms of classical Hodgkin's disease present with adenopathy above the diaphragm, but occasional patients may have different patterns of disease. Involvement of nonlymphoid organs is less common than in NHLs but does occur in patients with larger tumor burdens. For all these reasons, Hodgkin's disease is distinguished from other "non-Hodgkin's" lymphomas. Hodgkin's disease is separated into two major categories: classical Hodgkin's disease and other forms of Hodgkin's disease. Cases of classical Hodgkin's disease usually demonstrate a moderate number of Hodgkin's cells with easily identifiable Reed-Sternberg cells (Box 11-1).

Reed-Sternberg cells are generally easy to identify in cases of classical Hodgkin's disease, having a characteristic morphologic appearance with a bilobed nucleus and prominent eosinophilic nucleoli and a moderate-to-abundant amount of cytoplasm (Fig. 11-17A). Identification of diagnostic Reed-Sternberg cells is required for a diagnosis of Hodgkin's disease. Hodgkin's cells do not express leukocyte common antigen or most pan-B-cell markers but typically express the activation marker CD30 as well as CD15 and fascin in many cases (see Fig. 11-17B). Some cases of Hodgkin's disease show evidence of clonal rearrangement of the immunoglobulin heavy chain gene, but this is not a diagnostically useful finding, since many cases do not show evidence of clonality. No specific chromosomal translocations have been associated with classical Hodgkin's disease.

Reed-Sternberg cells and Hodgkin's cells produce cytokines and growth factors that stimulate fibrosis and recruit a mixture of different types of inflammatory cells. In nodular sclerosis Hodgkin's disease (NSHD), broad bands

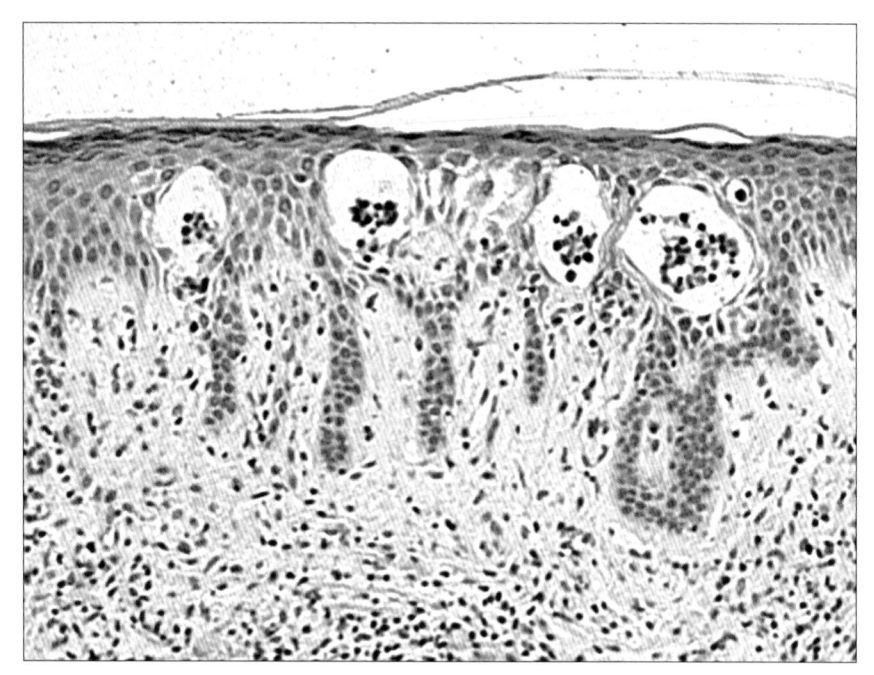

Figure 11-16. Mycosis fungoides. Microscopic section of skin showing multiple Pautrier microabscesses along the dermal-epidermal junction. These abscesses are filled with neoplastic T cells with vesicular nuclei and prominent nuclear folds.

MICROBIOLOGY

Human T Lymphotropic Virus 1 (HTLV1)

HTLV1 is a type C retrovirus with a single-stranded RNA genome that encodes three major classes of genes: reverse transcriptase; envelope glycoproteins; and gag structural proteins. HTLV1 is trophic for CD4$^+$ T cells but can infect other cell types. The glucose transport protein GLUT1 has recently been implicated as a cellular receptor for HTLV1 although the expression pattern of GLUT1 does not explain its tropism for T cells. Another as yet uncharacterized coreceptor may be involved, as in HIV (CD4 and chemokine receptor).

HTLV1 is prevalent in southern Japan (15% to 30% of the population) and in the Caribbean (3% to 6%). HTLV1 is transmitted by blood or sexual contact, and vertical transmission by nursing mothers is critical in endemic areas. HTLV1 replicates via chromosomal insertion through a DNA provirus and usually produces inapparent, latent infection. Approximately 1 in 500 infected individuals eventually develops acute T-cell leukemia/lymphoma (ATLL), usually after an incubation period of more than 10 years. Other cofactors or genetic alterations are likely involved in tumorigenesis. HTLV1 infection can also cause a progressive neuromuscular disorder called tropical spastic paraparesis (TSP) in the Caribbean and South America.

Box 11-1 HODGKIN'S DISEASE SUBTYPES

- Classical Hodgkin's disease
  - Nodular sclerosis Hodgkin's disease (NSHD)
  - Mixed cellularity Hodgkin's disease (MCHD)
  - Lymphocyte-rich classical Hodgkin's disease (LRCHD)
- Lymphocyte-depleted Hodgkin's disease (LDHD)
- Lymphocyte-predominant Hodgkin's disease (LPHD)

called "lacunar cells" (Hodgkin's cells surrounded by a halo of cytoplasmic retraction) are typical of NSHD (see Fig. 11-18B). NSHD typically presents as mediastinal disease in young women and has an excellent response to modern therapy, with cures in the vast majority of patients.

Mixed cellularity Hodgkin's disease (MCHD) has a less characteristic clinical presentation than NSHD does. Although fibrosis is present in MCHD, dense bands of collagen are usually absent and eosinophils and Hodgkin's cells are usually more numerous than in NSHD (Fig. 11-19). Hodgkin's cells in MCHD frequently express EBV antigens, and this can be diagnostically helpful in some cases. MCHD often has a slightly more aggressive clinical course than NSHD but still has an excellent chance for cure with modern therapy. Cases of classical Hodgkin's disease that do not meet the diagnostic criteria of either NSHD or MCHD are classified as lymphocyte-rich classical Hodgkin's disease. These tumors usually have a predominance of small lymphocytes and a clinical behavior similar to that of NSHD and MCHD.

Lymphocyte-predominant Hodgkin's disease (LPHD) shows morphologic and clinical features more in keeping

of collagenous fibrosis are formed that efface normal lymph node architecture (Fig. 11-18A). Background cells (normal inflammatory cells recruited by cytokines) consist predominantly of small lymphocytes with a scattering of plasma cells and eosinophils. Diagnostic Reed-Sternberg cells are usually easy to identify although they may constitute less than 1% of the cells present. Morphologic variants of Hodgkin's cells

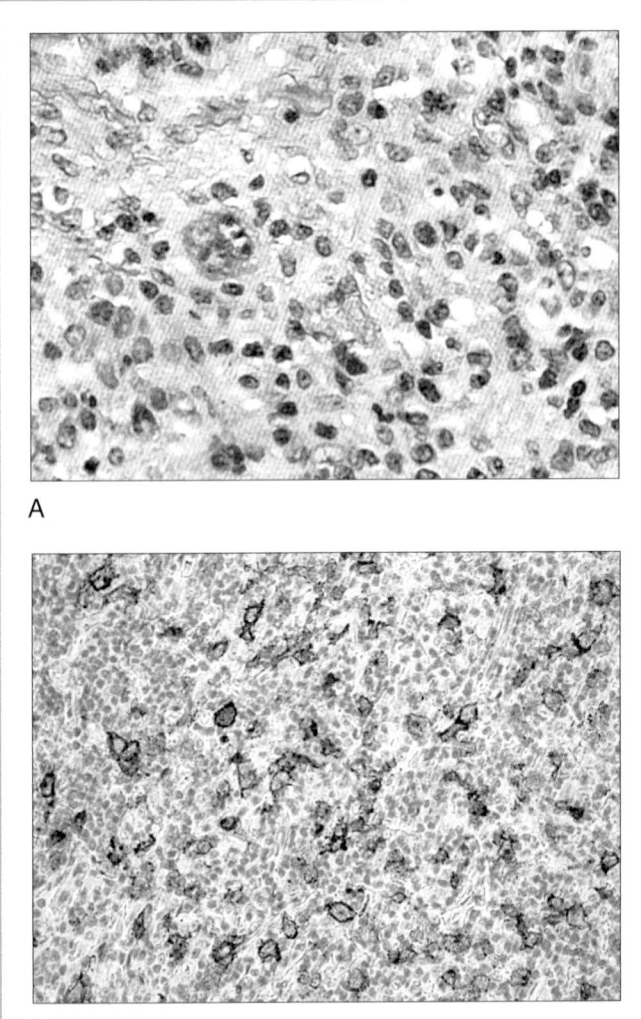

A

B

Figure 11-17. **A**, Reed-Sternberg cells. Microscopic section showing Reed-Sternberg cells with bilobed vesicular nuclei with prominent nucleoli. **B**, CD30$^+$ Reed-Sternberg cells. Immunoperoxidase-stained section highlighting CD30$^+$ Hodgkin's cells in a lymph node with classical Hodgkin's disease.

IMMUNOLOGY

Reed-Sternberg (RS) Cells

Reed-Sternberg cells have been convincingly shown to be of B-cell lineage although they have an unusual and characteristic phenotype (CD30$^+$, CD15$^+$, fascin+, LCA–).

CD30 expression is results in activation of NFκB signaling in RS cells. RS cells often express CD40 on their surface, and binding of CD40 ligand (soluble or expressed on T cells) can also activate NFκB signaling. IκB mutations are present in up to 20% of RS cells, further implicating enhanced NFκB signaling in the pathobiology of these tumor cells. In addition, IL-13 is produced by many RS cells and can bind to IL-13 receptor on their surface, resulting in an autocrine loop that promotes cell proliferation.

Most RS cells show evidence of extensive somatic mutation in their immunoglobulin genes, indicating that they are post–germinal center B cells. Some of these immunoglobulin genes contain stop codons, suggesting that RS cells have escaped apoptosis (since they are incapable of binding antigen).

RS cells produce a variety of cytokines and chemokines (IL-6, IL-10, IL-13, TGF-β, and TARC), which recruit the normal inflammatory cells that constitute the background cells of Hodgkin's disease.

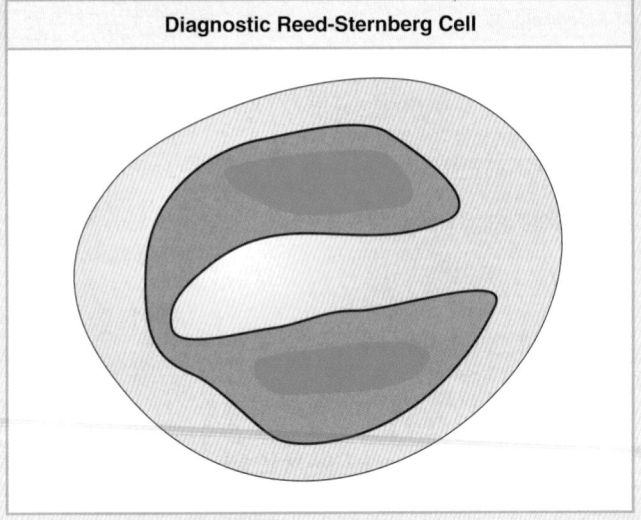

Diagnostic Reed-Sternberg Cell

with a low-grade B-cell NHL. This uncommon tumor has a characteristic morphologic appearance and a different immunophenotype from classical Hodgkin's disease. Reed-Sternberg cells are rare but usually show monoclonal immunoglobulin heavy chain gene rearrangement.

Lymphocyte-depleted Hodgkin's disease (LDHD) is a rare, highly aggressive lymphoma that tends to occur in older patients. Hodgkin's cells are numerous in LPHD and usually outnumber background cells. Fibrosis is usually extensive, and tumor cells may show bizarre cytologic features.

Plasma Cell Myeloma

Plasma cell myeloma is a tumor of differentiated plasma cells that usually express large amounts of monoclonal immunoglobulin or immunoglobulin light chain. The incidence of plasma cell myeloma increases markedly with age and is rare

before age 30. Most patients have focal or diffuse infiltration of the bone marrow with plasma cells, and they may have pathologic bone fractures or hypercalcemia owing to bone resorption (Figs. 11-20A and 11-20B). Younger patients sometimes have so-called plasmacytomas in bone or at extramedullary sites. Plasmacytomas are solid tumors composed almost exclusively of plasma cells. Some patients with plasmacytomas have isolated disease (without evidence of diffuse bone marrow involvement) that may be cured by localized radiation therapy or surgery, but many patients eventually develop myeloma.

Myeloma can usually be diagnosed with a bone marrow biopsy specimen showing more than 30% plasma cells. The

many organs, but renal and cardiac involvement usually cause the most serious complications. The heavy load of filtered paraprotein can also cause renal dysfunction by distending and blocking renal tubules with proteinaceous material (so-called thyroidization of the kidney).

Myeloma produces lytic bone lesions by activating bone resorption and often results in symptomatic hypercalcemia, which may further exacerbate renal dysfunction (Fig. 11-21). Myeloma cells produce RANKL (receptor activator of NFκB ligand), which binds to receptors on osteoclasts, causing their activation. Another plasma cell–derived protein, DKK1 (Dickkopf1), inhibits canonical Wnt signaling in osteoblasts to inhibit new bone formation. In this manner, the balance of osteoblastic and osteoclastic activity in normal bone remodeling is shifted to produce lytic bone lesions. The prognosis for myeloma in older individuals is poor although new agents that inhibit the proteosome (inducing apoptosis by causing degradation of NFκB in neoplastic plasma cells) have shown some promise in myeloma that is refractory to other forms of chemotherapy. Recently, younger myeloma patients have been treated with various bone marrow transplantation protocols.

Myeloma must be distinguished from so-called MUGUS (monoclonal gammopathy of undetermined significance), which is common in older individuals. This corresponds to a presence of a low-level paraprotein on serum protein electrophoresis. Most patients with MUGUS do not develop signs and symptoms of myeloma in their lifetime.

●●● SPLEEN

The spleen is a relatively common site for metastatic carcinoma. Splenic infarcts may mimic metastatic carcinoma. Primary solid tumors of the spleen are rare and include angiosarcoma. Patients lacking a functional spleen may also develop severe disease from RBC parasites (e.g., malaria and babesiosis) and are at greatly increased risk for *Streptococcus pneumoniae* sepsis.

Most Hodgkin's and non-Hodgkin's lymphomas can involve the spleen secondarily, but primary splenic lymphomas are uncommon. Primary marginal zone lymphoma of the spleen shows expansion of the marginal zone about white pulps and is usually associated with peripheral blood involvement (Fig. 11-22). Hairy cell leukemia is a low-grade B-cell neoplasm involving the spleen and bone marrow. Tumor cells have villous cytoplasmic membrane projections, giving cell borders an indistinct appearance. Hairy cells characteristically express tartrate-resistant acid phosphatase (TRAP), which can be identified cytochemically on cytologic smears.

●●● THYMUS

The thymus is the primary organ in which T-cell progenitors from the bone marrow mature and autoreactive T cells are eliminated. Specialized thymic epithelial cells with intricate processes provide a microenvironment suitable for this

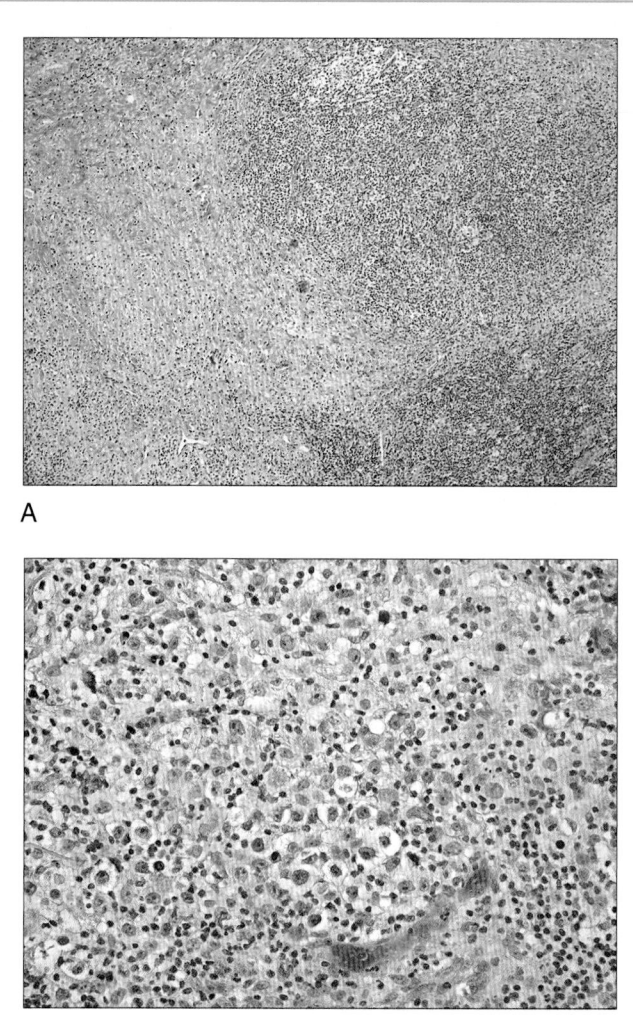

Figure 11-18. A, Nodular sclerosis Hodgkin's disease (NSHD). Microscopic section of a lymph node effaced by Hodgkin's disease. There is prominent fibrosis with well-developed extracellular collagen-forming nodules. Hodgkin's cells are barely visible at this magnification. **B**, Lacunar cells. Microscopic section from a case of NSHD with abundant lacunar cells that show cytoplasmic retraction, creating the impression of haloes about tumor cell nuclei.

presence of other diagnostic features (e.g., demonstration of monoclonality by either PCR or light chain restriction by flow cytometry or immunohistochemistry) or the presence of a monoclonal paraprotein can aid in establishing the diagnosis if the bone marrow findings are inconclusive (see Fig. 11-20C). Some cases of myeloma are poorly differentiated, making them difficult to recognize as plasma cell tumors.

Patients with myeloma are at greatly increased risk for the development of amyloidosis as a result of their paraprotein assuming a β-pleated sheet configuration to form amyloid. Lambda (λ) light chains are particularly prone to amyloid formation. Amyloid deposition can cause dysfunction in

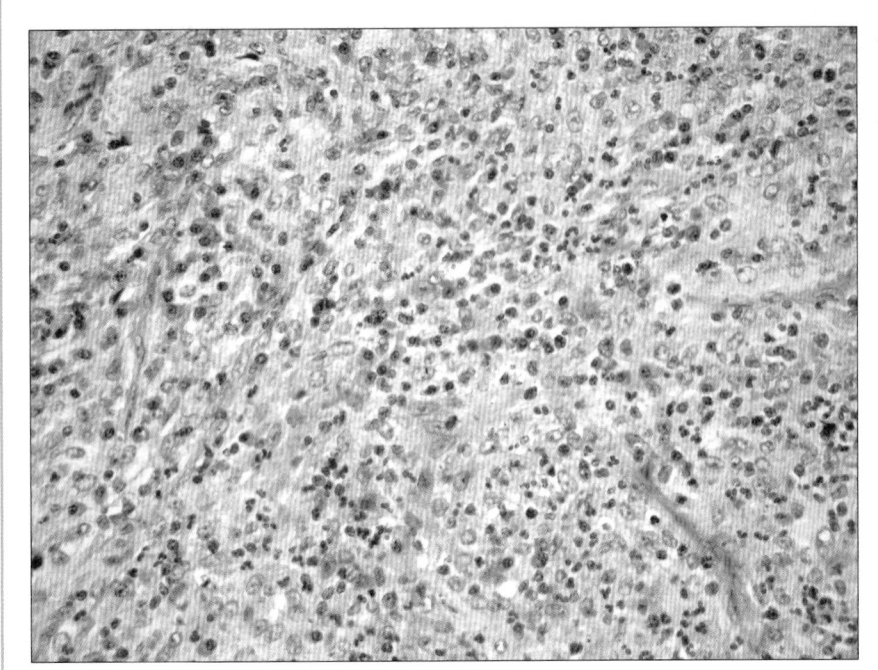

Figure 11-19. Mixed cellularity Hodgkin's disease (MCHD). Microscopic section of a lymph node effaced by Hodgkin's disease with little fibrosis, abundant Hodgkin's cells, and a prominent infiltrate of eosinophils.

maturation and selection process in the cortex and medulla. The thymus is the most common site for lymphoblastic lymphoma (see Acute Lymphoblastic Leukemia and Lymphoblastic Lymphoma section).

Thymoma

Thymoma is a primary tumor of the thymus composed of a mixture of small T cells and thymic epithelial cells (Fig. 11-23). Some thymomas contain large numbers of lymphocytes, obscuring the epithelial component of the neoplasm, while other tumors are largely epithelial and may mimic metastatic carcinoma. Most thymomas are benign and are cured by local excision. Invasive thymomas show either pathologic or surgical evidence of invasion into other organs.

Thymic carcinomas are extremely rare and show differing patterns of differentiation including squamous cell carcinoma.

Myasthenia Gravis

Most patients with myasthenia gravis have thymic hyperplasia with infiltration of the thymus by B cells with germinal center formation. A subset of these patients develop thymomas, and surgical excision of the tumor may result in remission of muscle weakness. Some patients with pure RBC aplasia (isolated failure of erythropoiesis) also have thymomas, and thymectomy may result in restoration of normal erythropoiesis. The pathophysiologic mechanisms that result in thymic involvement in these diseases are unknown.

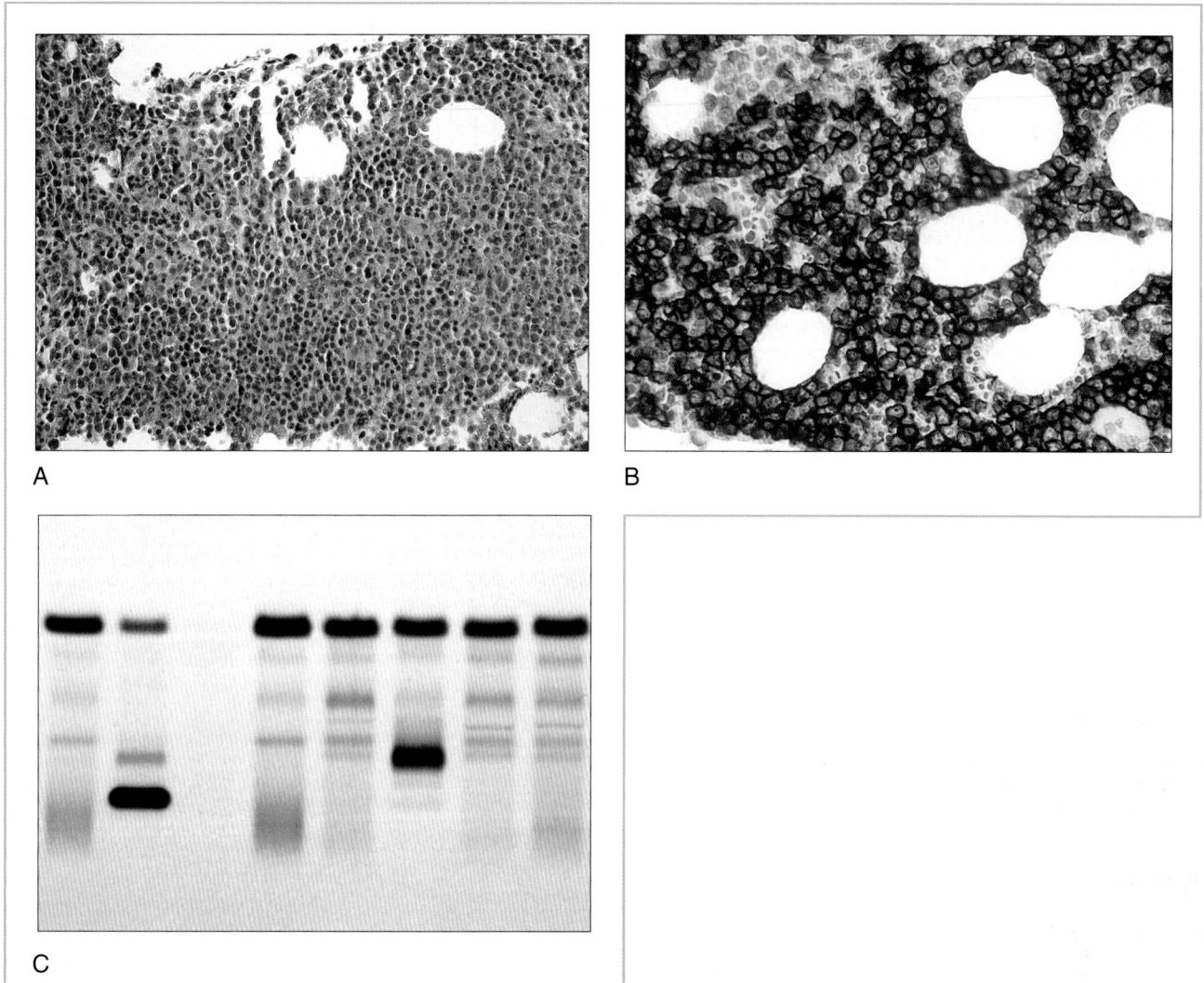

Figure 11-20. A, Multiple myeloma. Microscopic section of bone marrow partially replaced by poorly differentiated plasma cells. Plasmacytoid differentiation of tumor cells is minimal in this high-grade tumor. **B,** Immunohistochemical stain for CD138 in multiple myeloma. Microscopic section of the same tumor shown in **A** stained for the plasma cell marker CD138. There is extensive infiltration by poorly differentiated plasma cells, with effacement of normal bone marrow elements. **C,** Serum protein electrophoresis. Gel electrophoresis of serum protein components showing a prominent IgA paraprotein (*fifth sample from the right*).

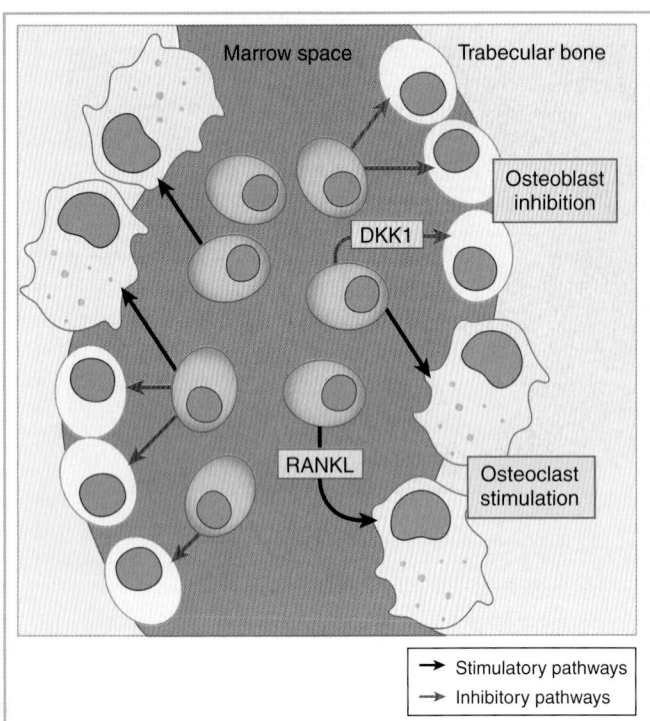

Figure 11-21. Bone resorption in multiple myeloma.

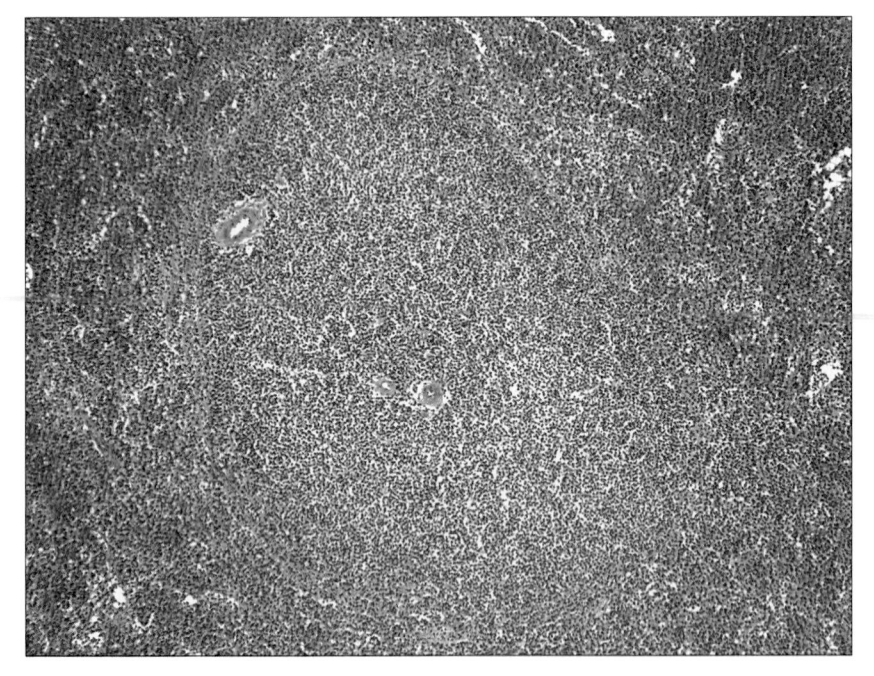

Figure 11-22. Marginal zone lymphoma. Section of spleen showing expansion of the marginal zone around white pulp characteristic of marginal cell lymphoma.

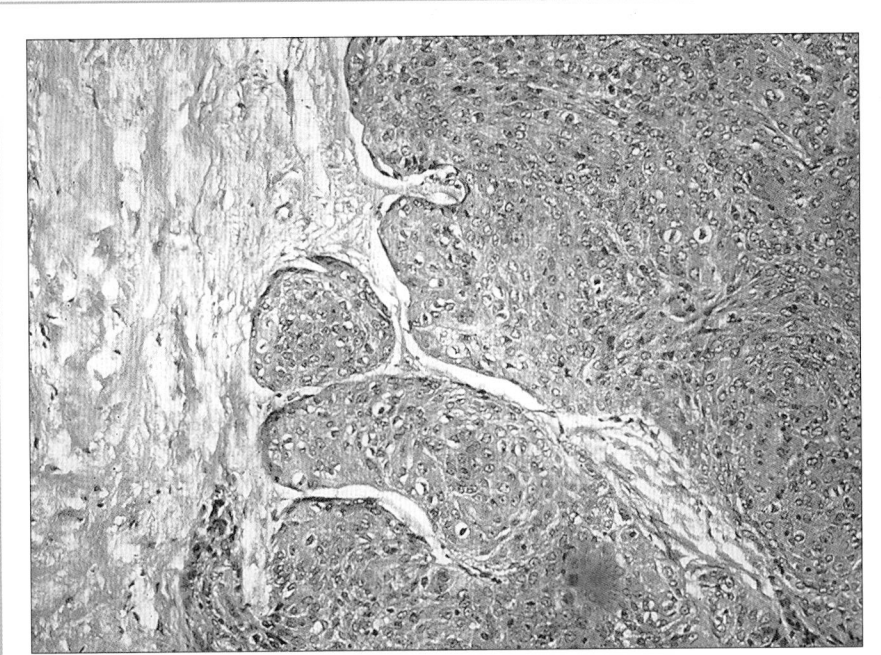

Figure 11-23. Invasive thymoma. Neoplastic thymic epithelium invades dense connective tissue. T lymphocytes are scant in this largely epithelioid thymoma.

Renal and Urinary Tract 12

CONTENTS

The kidney and lower urinary tract are functionally connected so that abnormalities in one component can profoundly affect the function of other components of the system. The bladder, urethra, ureters, and renal pelvis are lined by transitional epithelium (urothelium), which is subject to similar types of disease processes in each of these locations.

●●● INFLAMMATORY DISEASES AND INFECTION

Infections and other inflammatory conditions of urinary tract are the most common pathologic processes that affect the renal-urinary system. Obstruction of urine flow (e.g., secondary to stones (lithiasis) can markedly exacerbate the effects of inflammation and infection. Urinary tract infections typically begin in the bladder and are most frequently caused by gram-negative organisms from the gastrointestinal tract. The shorter female urethra puts women at much higher risk for urinary tract infection than men. Prostatic hypertrophy can result in a large postvoid residual volume of urine predisposing to infection in older males. Normal bladder anatomy includes functional valves in the trigone that prevent reflux of urine into the ureters. If this anatomic mechanism is not functional, increased hydrostatic pressure during micturition (urination) can cause reflux of urine into the ureters; ascending infection of the urinary tract can result and lead to acute pyelonephritis (bacterial infection of the kidney).

Several noninfectious inflammatory conditions of the bladder also occur. Interstitial cystitis causes pain and urgency and is associated with an increased number of mast cells in the lamina propria. Hemorrhagic cystitis is a distinctive complication of chemotherapy (usually cyclophosphamide) with diffuse ulceration and hemorrhage of bladder mucosa (Fig. 12-1). In endemic areas, schistosomes are a common cause of chronic hematuria and may predispose to the formation of bladder tumors.

Ascending infection of the ureters is the most common cause of acute pyelonephritis (bacterial infection of the renal parenchyma) although hematogenous seeding of renal tissue can occur in septic patients. Acute pyelonephritis typically involves the upper and lower poles of the kidney owing to the anatomy of the renal papillae that drain these portions of the collecting system. Acute pyelonephritis causes acute renal dysfunction because of direct damage to tubules. If obstruction (e.g., due to ureteropelvic junction abnormality or pelvic or ureteral stones) is present in conjunction with acute pyelonephritis, rapid and irreversible destruction of renal parenchyma can result (i.e., destruction of the extracellular matrix precludes regeneration of tubular epithelium).

Chronic pyelonephritis results from repeated episodes of acute pyelonephritis. Kidneys with severe chronic pyelonephritis have a dense chronic inflammatory cell infiltrate in the interstitium with prominent periglomerular fibrosis (Fig. 12-2). Tubules may show "thyroidization" similar to that seen in patients with multiple myeloma with dense proteinaceous deposits that distend dilated, atrophic tubules. Before the advent of antibiotics, chronic pyelonephritis was a common cause of renal failure (particularly in women) but is now rarely the sole cause of chronic renal failure. Patients with uncorrected ureteropelvic junction abnormalities (causing functional obstruction) are at risk for chronic renal insufficiency as a complication of chronic pyelonephritis. Infection with some organisms may predispose to the development of stones in the renal pelvis (e.g., struvite stones are usually a consequence of *Proteus* infection).

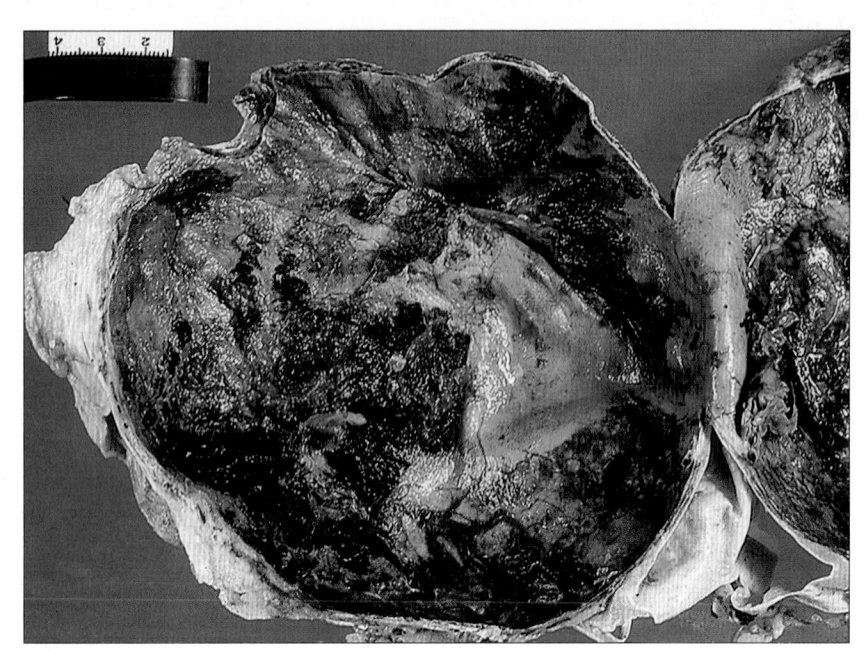

Figure 12-1. Hemorrhagic cystitis. Gross photograph of an opened urinary bladder showing extensive mucosal ulceration and marked hemorrhage.

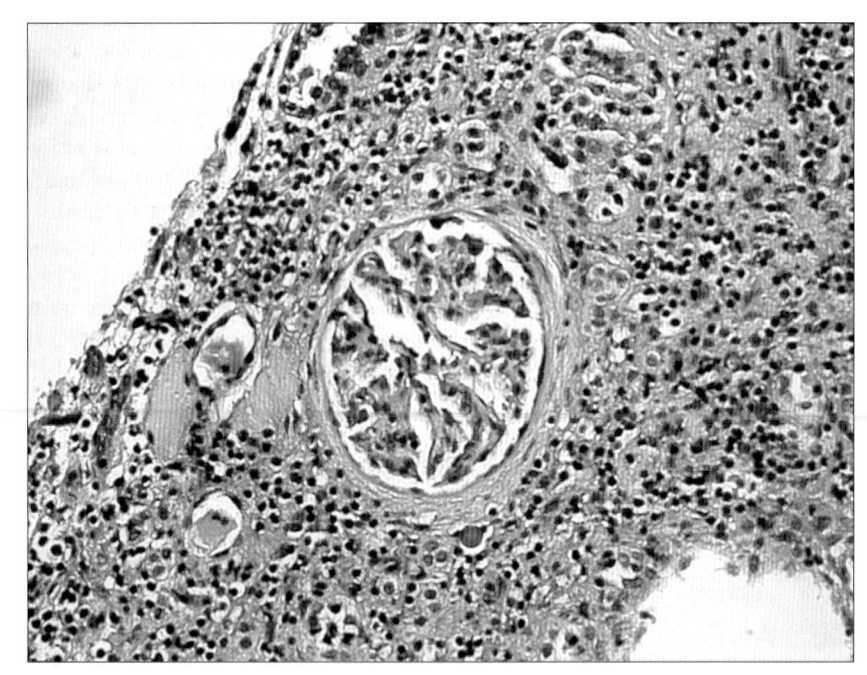

Figure 12-2. Chronic pyelonephritis. Microscopic section of kidney showing prominent periglomerular fibrosis and a dense interstitial chronic inflammatory cell infiltrate between residual tubules.

Glomerular Diseases

The main function of glomeruli is production of an ultra-filtrate from blood that is processed into urine by the actions of the tubules and collecting ducts. Conditions that alter the glomerular basement membrane (GBM) frequently result in significant renal dysfunction. In particular, diseases that cause glomerular basement membrane thickening result in decreased and abnormal glomerular filtration. There is a slow, incremental decrease in renal function with increasing age that results from the dropout of individual glomeruli. This process can be greatly accelerated by comorbid diseases including hypertension and diabetes mellitus. Normal kidneys have a large functional reserve so that loss of 50% of renal function (e.g., one kidney) in a normal individual does not result in increased serum creatinine or blood urea nitrogen (BUN).

Both acute and chronic inflammatory processes of the glomeruli can interfere with glomerular function. Deposition

MICROBIOLOGY

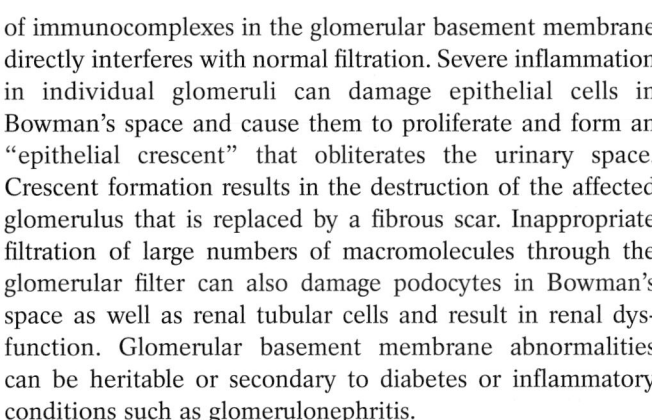

Proteus mirabilis

Proteus mirabilis is a gram-negative bacterium that is a member of the Enterobacteriaceae. *P. mirabilis* is a normal component of gastrointestinal flora but unlike most other such organisms is motile and may show swarming of colonies when cultured on agar plates, which facilitates its identification.

P. mirabilis is the second most common cause of community-acquired urinary tract infection after *Escherichia coli,* but infection of other sites is uncommon. *P. mirabilis* is a common cause of infection in chronically catheterized patients.

P. mirabilis produces urease, which cleaves urea to form ammonia and bicarbonate to alkalinize infected urine and predispose to stone formation. Struvite stones are composed of ammonium magnesium phosphate and can take on a "staghorn" shape when they fill the renal pelvis. *P. mirabilis* can persist in struvite stones despite antibiotic therapy, and microbiologic clearance of infection usually requires stone removal.

PHYSIOLOGY

Creatinine Clearance as a Measure of Renal Function

Creatinine is produced predominantly from muscle cells at a relatively steady rate and is filtered through the glomerulus and excreted in the urine. The clearance rate of creatinine is therefore essentially the same as the glomerular filtration rate.

The endogenous creatinine clearance test is a reliable measure of renal function in most individuals and depends on the collection of a 24-hour urine specimen and the measurement of its volume and creatinine concentration. The normal range for creatinine clearance is 90–110 mL/min. Individuals with differing muscle mass release different amounts of creatinine into their serum daily. A somewhat more accurate measure of renal function can be obtained by adjusting the measured creatinine clearance for the patient's calculated surface area. Adjusted creatinine clearance is obtained by dividing the measured creatinine clearance by the patient's surface area in meters squared and has a normal range of 70–140 mL/min.

In older individuals who have diminished muscle mass, creatinine clearance may overestimate residual renal function and other measures may be more predictive of ensuing renal failure or death. The use of exogenous substances (e.g., inulin) or other endogenous substances (e.g., cystatin) may allow more reliable measurement of renal function in selected patients.

Blood urea nitrogen (BUN) also is a measure of renal function and is dependent on protein intake (the main precursor of urea). BUN does not become significantly elevated until >70% of renal function is lost, making it a much less sensitive measure of renal dysfunction than creatinine clearance is.

of immunocomplexes in the glomerular basement membrane directly interferes with normal filtration. Severe inflammation in individual glomeruli can damage epithelial cells in Bowman's space and cause them to proliferate and form an "epithelial crescent" that obliterates the urinary space. Crescent formation results in the destruction of the affected glomerulus that is replaced by a fibrous scar. Inappropriate filtration of large numbers of macromolecules through the glomerular filter can also damage podocytes in Bowman's space as well as renal tubular cells and result in renal dysfunction. Glomerular basement membrane abnormalities can be heritable or secondary to diabetes or inflammatory conditions such as glomerulonephritis.

Glomerulonephritis

Glomerulonephritis is an inflammatory condition of the glomeruli that can present with two different clinicopathologic patterns on urinalysis: nephrotic or nephritic. Patients with nephrotic syndrome inappropriately filter large amounts of plasma proteins into the glomerular ultrafiltrate as a result of abnormalities of the basement membrane. *Nephrotic syndrome* is defined as the renal excretion of more than 3.5 g of protein during a 24-hour period and is assessed by the collection of a cumulative 24-hour urine specimen. By definition, nephrotic syndrome is not associated with significant glomerular inflammation and red blood cell casts or other signs of glomerular inflammation are present. Low-level proteinuria can result from heavy exercise (skeletal muscle damage) or minor abnormalities of the kidney that may be of little functional consequence. Patients with diabetes mellitus frequently have proteinuria but usually not in the nephrotic range (>3.5 g/d) unless additional renal pathology is present.

The loss of nephrotic quantities of proteins for prolonged periods can result in hypoproteinemia, and nephrotic patients may have peripheral edema because of loss of plasma oncotic pressure. Nephrotic syndrome may be an early manifestation of some types of chronic glomerulonephritis, but in many cases it is attributed to so-called minimal change disease. Renal biopsy specimens in patients with minimal change disease show podocyte foot process fusion, but no other morphologic abnormalities are observed by light or electron microscopy or by immunofluorescence. Fusion of foot processes results from toxicity of the high protein concentration in the ultrafiltrate and so is a consequence rather than the cause of the nephrotic syndrome. Many cases of minimal change disease respond to low-dose corticosteroid therapy with resolution of proteinuria, but the underlying cause of the glomerular basement membrane abnormality is not known.

The *nephritic syndrome* is characterized by variable amounts of proteinuria with the presence of red blood cell casts (linear aggregates of red blood cells formed in tubules as a consequence of glomerular hemorrhage) and/or other inflammatory features (e.g., white blood cell and tubular cell casts) on urinalysis. Nephritic syndrome is usually associated with glomerulonephritis, and nephritic findings on urinalysis should initiate a rapid evaluation of renal function, since some forms

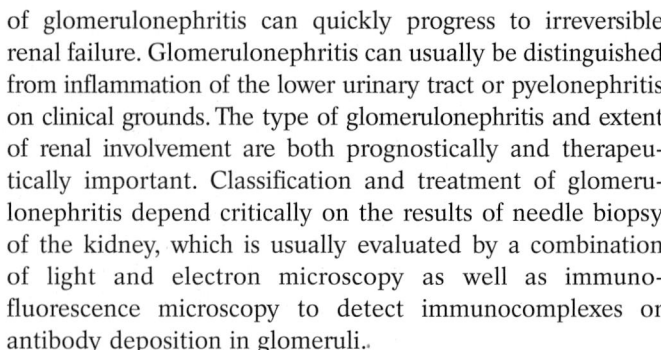

Urinalysis

Urinalysis consists of a number of standard measurements and assays that are best performed on midstream-voided urine. Urinalysis is more informative and accurate if testing is performed soon after collection (e.g., bacteria grow and crystals can form as urine incubates in vitro). Abnormalities on urinalysis may prompt microbiologic culture or more detailed testing.

Urine specific gravity is normally between 1.003 and 1.035 g/mL and is usually measured with a refractometer. Increased specific gravity most frequently results from dehydration.

Chemical examination of urine is typically accomplished with a dipstick, which can be read manually or quantitated by machine. Dipsticks usually provide semiquantitative measurements of pH and of protein, glucose, ketone, bilirubin, blood, urobilinogen, nitrite (presence of bacteria), and esterase (presence of neutrophils) concentrations.

Microscopic examination of urine sediment (centrifuged urine) is usually performed by means of a phase-contrast microscope to detect crystals, bacteria, and red and white blood cells. The identification of cellular casts (molded by formation in renal tubules) is one of the most important potential observations from urinalysis and can be a clue to serious renal disease (e.g., glomerulonephritis). Casts are labile and may dissociate as urine incubates in vitro.

Urine cytology is a more specialized assay in which Papanicolaou staining is used to detect tumor cells in patients at risk for urothelial cancer or to detect polyomavirus infection in renal transplant patients.

HISTOLOGY

Glomerular Basement Membrane (GBM)

The glomerular basement membrane (GBM) is a trilaminar structure composed principally of type IV collagen with laminin, heparan sulfate, and enactin as well as smaller components of other proteins and proteoglycans. The normal adult GBM varies between 310 and 380 nm in thickness and has an inner dense zone (lamina densa) surrounded by two laminae rarae. The GBM is synthesized by the endothelial cells of the glomerulus as well as by specialized epithelial cells lining Bowman's space, known as podocytes, which have foot processes that make contact with the GBM in the urinary space. There are 25- to 60-nm filtration slits (spaces) between foot processes, which are bridged by a slit-like diaphragm that is approximately 6 nm in thickness.

Glomerular capillaries are lined by fenestrated endothelium that is attenuated, allowing extensive contact between the GBM and plasma.

The GBM provides the main filter function in the creation of the initial urinary ultrafiltrate. The role of foot processes in ultrafiltration is less clear but appears to be important.

of glomerulonephritis can quickly progress to irreversible renal failure. Glomerulonephritis can usually be distinguished from inflammation of the lower urinary tract or pyelonephritis on clinical grounds. The type of glomerulonephritis and extent of renal involvement are both prognostically and therapeutically important. Classification and treatment of glomerulonephritis depend critically on the results of needle biopsy of the kidney, which is usually evaluated by a combination of light and electron microscopy as well as immunofluorescence microscopy to detect immunocomplexes or antibody deposition in glomeruli.

Anti–Glomerular Basement Membrane Glomerulonephritis

Goodpasture's syndrome and Henoch-Schönlein purpura are rare autoimmune diseases that result from autoantibodies directed against basement membrane components. These autoantibodies can bind directly to basement membrane materials in glomeruli and alveolar capillaries, resulting in acute glomerulonephritis or pulmonary hemorrhage (or both). Both syndromes can cause fulminant glomerulonephritis with rapid loss of renal function. Kidney biopsy shows glomerular inflammation (hypercellularity) and hemorrhage by light microscopy. Immunofluorescence reveals linear deposits of immunoglobulin along glomerular capillary basement membranes indicative of a type II hypersensitivity reaction. Treatment with immunosuppressive agents may induce remission.

Poststreptococcal Glomerulonephritis

Poststreptococcal glomerulonephritis is a transient antibody-mediated inflammatory reaction caused by certain strains of group A streptococci. Nephritogenic strains of streptococci are distinct from those that produce rheumatic heart disease (see Chapter 7). Glomerulonephritis develops during or immediately after infection, and nephritic features are evident on urinalysis. Immune complexes formed by host antibodies and bacterial antigens are deposited in the glomerular basement membrane, inducing a strong inflammatory reaction that causes acute injury to glomeruli. Antigen-antibody complexes disappear from serum as the bacterial infection is cleared, and most glomeruli resolve the inflammatory process with restoration of normal renal function. If renal biopsy is performed, it shows hypercellularity of involved glomeruli with acute and chronic inflammatory cells infiltrating the glomerular tuft and proliferation of glomerular endothelial cells. These changes in the glomerular basement membrane (so-called proliferative glomerulonephritis) are caused by inflammatory mediator release as a consequence of immune complex deposition (Fig. 12-3A). Immunofluorescence shows a granular pattern of immunoglobulin and complement deposition in glomerular basement membranes corresponding to the type III hypersensitivity reaction that underlies this disease process (see Fig. 12-3B).

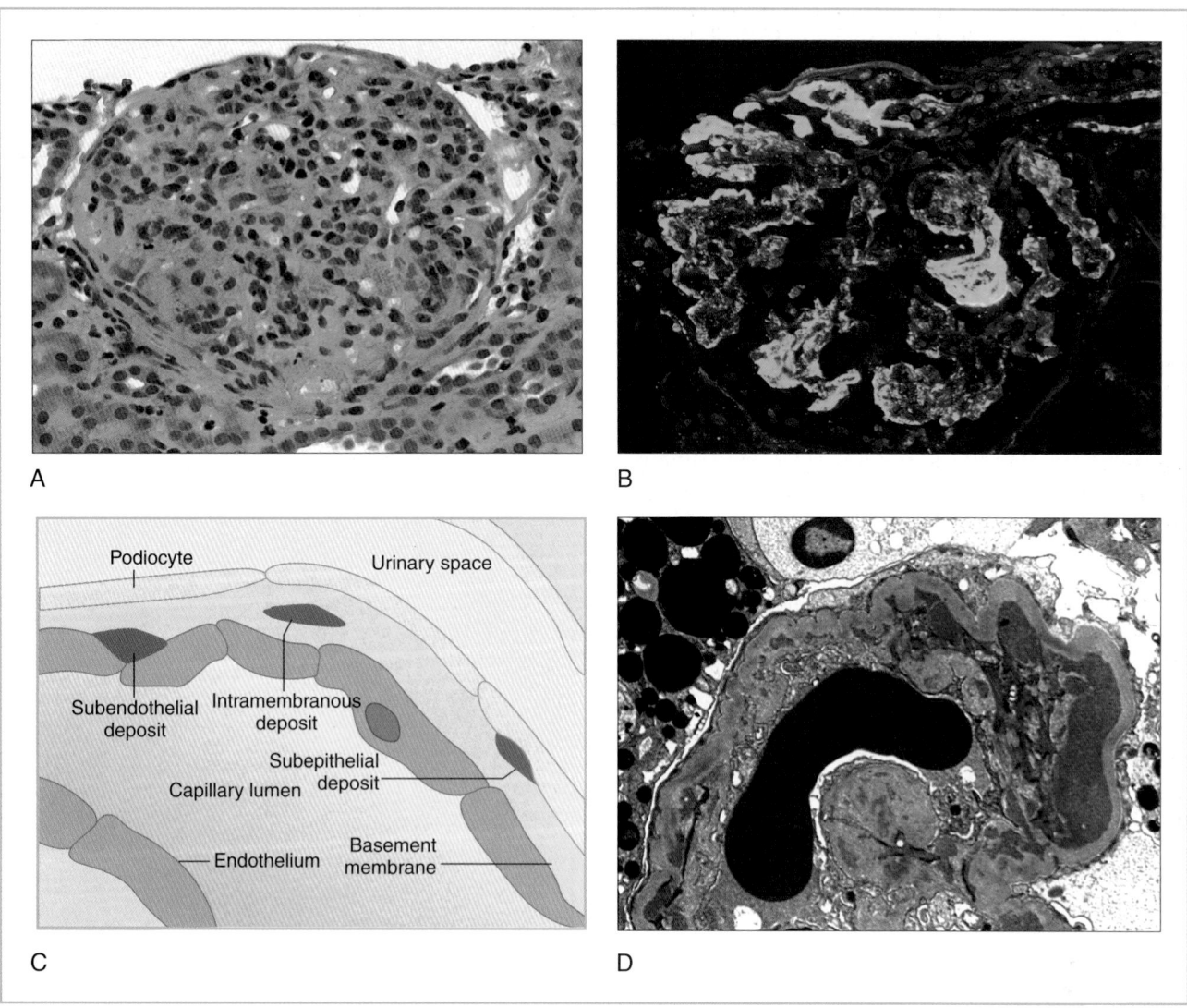

Figure 12-3. A, Proliferative glomerulonephritis. Microscopic section showing a single hypercellular glomerulus with acute and chronic inflammatory cells in the glomerular tuft with proliferation of injured endothelial and epithelial cells. **B,** Immunocomplex glomerulonephritis. Immunofluorescence of a frozen section of kidney stained for IgG. Granular green fluorescence is present in the basement membrane of the glomerular tuft, indicative of immune complex deposition. **C,** Immune complex deposits in glomerulonephritis. **D,** Subendothelial immune complex deposits in glomerulonephritis. Electron micrograph of a glomerular capillary loop with subendothelial dense deposits (electron-dense clumps of material that appear darker than the basement membrane in which they are embedded). A red blood cell occupies most of the center of the field, marking the vascular space. A podocyte in the urinary space is visible near the top of the figure.

Systemic Lupus Erythematosus

Renal failure secondary to glomerulonephritis is the most common cause of serious morbidity and mortality in patients with systemic lupus erythematosus (SLE). Glomerulonephritis is almost always mediated by immunocomplex deposition in glomerular basement membranes (type III hypersensitivity), similarly to poststreptococcal glomerulonephritis. The persistent nature of glomerular injury in SLE prevents restoration of normal glomerular function and can ultimately result in renal failure as more and more glomeruli are destroyed. The size and chemical properties of different immunocomplexes formed in lupus patients determine their site of deposition in glomeruli (subendothelial, intramembranous, or subepithelial) and the type of pathologic changes produced (see Figs. 12-3C and 12-3D).

Patients with lupus glomerulonephritis can have a number of different patterns of glomerulonephritis, which can also be observed in cases of sporadic glomerulonephritis that are not associated with SLE. The World Health Organization (WHO) classification of lupus nephritis classifies renal biopsy results in five categories of disease type and activity, although individual specimens may show more than one pattern. Class I means that no demonstrable glomerulonephritis is identified on renal biopsy. Class II is mesangial glomerulonephritis in which immunocomplex deposition and inflammation are predominantly localized in the mesangial region. This is the mildest form of lupus nephritis and tends to progress slowly. Class III is focal proliferative glomerulonephritis in which there is proliferative glomerulonephritis (similar to post-streptococcal glomerulonephritis) that involves a subset of glomeruli while other glomeruli appear normal. Class V is membranous glomerulonephritis in which immunocomplexes are deposited within the glomerular basement membrane (intramembranous deposits). Membranous glomerulonephritis tends to result in a slower loss of renal function than diffuse proliferative glomerulonephritis.

Class IV lupus nephritis is diffuse proliferative glomerulonephritis in which all glomeruli are involved. Class IV is the most destructive form of glomerulonephritis and is the most common pattern observed in patients with lupus nephritis. Class IV is usually associated with subendothelial immunocomplex deposits, and immunofluorescence shows evidence of immunoglobulin and complement in a granular pattern in glomerular basement membranes. Intense glomerular inflammation in diffuse proliferative glomerulonephritis frequently results in the formation of epithelial crescents with destruction of involved glomeruli. Long-term accumulation of immunocomplexes in SLE often results in marked thickening of the glomerular basement membrane, producing a "wire loop" pattern histologically (the basement membrane is thick and rigid, making it resemble a rigid wire that has been bent into a loop). Persistent and recurrent immune-mediated injury over years frequently results in chronic renal insufficiency in SLE patients.

Crescentic Glomerulonephritis

Glomerular crescents result from proliferation of epithelial cells in Bowman's space and signal the demise of glomeruli (Fig. 12-4A). Crescentic glomerulonephritis can result from severe immunocomplex-mediated injury (e.g., more severe proliferative glomerulonephritis) or may develop as a primary disease (sometimes called rapidly progressive glomerulonephritis, or RPGN). Patients with RPGN frequently do not show evidence of immunocomplex deposition in glomeruli (so-called pauci-immune glomerulonephritis) but often have other manifestations of autoimmune disease. RPGN is the typical pattern of renal involvement in patients with Wegener's granulomatosis who frequently are ANCA-positive and may have coexisting granulomatous inflammation and vasculitis in the upper and lower respiratory tracts.

IgA Nephropathy

IgA nephropathy results from the deposition of IgA immunocomplexes in glomeruli that usually results in focal segmental glomerulonephritis (proliferative glomerulonephritis that involves a portion of the glomerular tuft, in a subset of glomeruli). IgA nephropathy usually is less destructive than other forms of proliferative glomerulonephritis and in some cases may be associated with celiac disease, suggesting that luminal antigen in the intestine (gliadin) that stimulates IgA

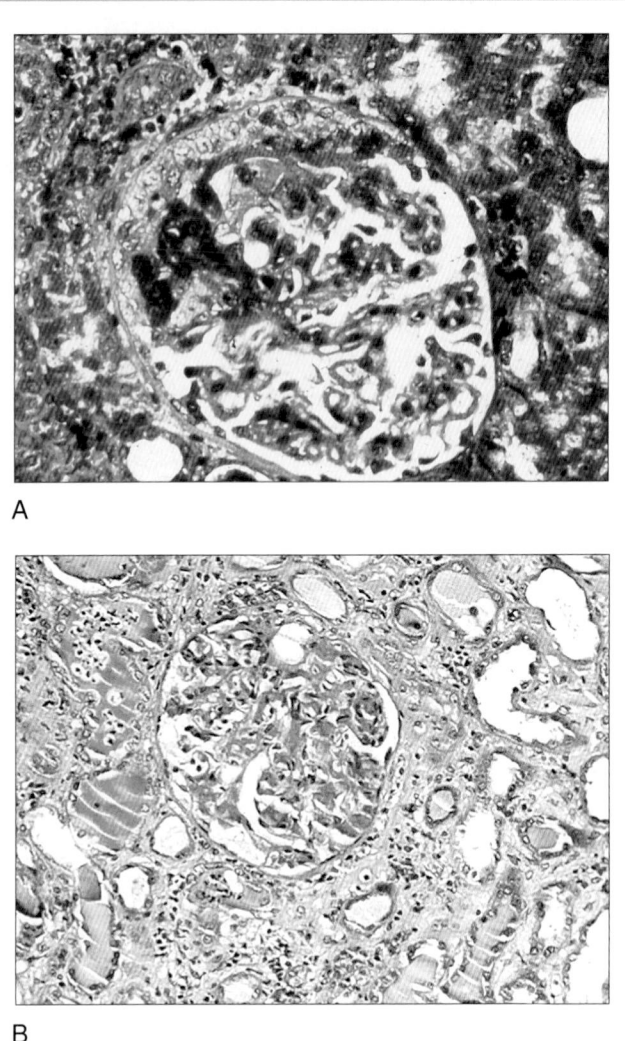

A

B

Figure 12-4. A, Crescentic glomerulonephritis. Microscopic section of a renal glomerulus showing a partial epithelial crescent in Bowman's capsule (*upper left*). **B**, Amyloid glomerulopathy. Microscopic section of kidney showing basement membrane thickening resulting from amyloid deposition in the glomerular tuft.

production may underlie the pathophysiology of this form of glomerulonephritis (see Chapter 9).

Amyloidosis

Some patients with systemic amyloidosis have amyloid deposits in glomerular basement membranes that result in loss of normal filtration function. Amyloid deposits do not usually incite an inflammatory reaction so that involved glomerular tufts are not hypercellular but show prominent basement membrane thickening with Congo red–positive material (see Fig. 12-4B) resulting in decreased glomerular filtration rate (GFR) and proteinuria. Amyloid deposits are often present in renal blood vessels as well. Patients with myeloma are at risk for amyloid glomerulopathy but may also develop plugging of renal tubules by monoclonal immunoglobulin or light chain proteins that can also result in significant renal dysfunction.

Alport's Syndrome

Alport's syndrome is the most common heritable form of hereditary nephritis and is caused by mutations in type IV collagen, which is the main component of the glomerular basement membrane. Alport's syndrome may present with hematuria and usually progresses to renal failure at a relatively young age. Most cases show X-linked dominant inheritance, and patients may have associated sensorineural deafness.

Tubulointerstitial Nephritis

Inflammatory and infectious processes of the renal tubules can cause acute renal dysfunction by damaging tubular cells. If the insult is removed, regeneration of tubular epithelial cells usually results in complete restoration of normal renal function. If the injury is sufficient to damage or destroy tubular basement membranes, regeneration is not possible, and irreversible renal failure may develop. Immunologic reactions to various drugs are a relatively common cause of intersitial nephritis that may be severe and cause acute renal failure. Drug-induced interstitial nephritis typically resolves after cessation of drug therapy and usually responds rapidly to a short course of corticosteroid therapy. If renal biopsy is performed, the specimen typically shows a dense chronic inflammatory cell infiltrate in the interstitium with evidence of tubular cell injury but without significant glomerular inflammation.

●●● LITHIASIS AND HYDRONEPHROSIS

Most cases of lithiasis (stone formation) in the urinary tract are sporadic and are not associated with obvious predisposing factors. Some forms of lithiasis are related to transient or permanent metabolic abnormalities (e.g., gout) or to specific genetic diseases that result in abnormal concentrations of some metabolites (e.g., cystinuria). Transient hyperuricemia can result from tumor lysis syndrome and can lead to diffuse precipitation of uric acid crystals in the urinary tract, causing acute renal failure. Stone analysis may be helpful in identifying the cause of lithiasis in some cases. Calcium phosphate stones are by far the most common type, and their formation is facilitated by acidic or highly concentrated urine. Stones can form in the renal pelvis, ureter, or bladder.

Stones can act as a nidus for bacterial infection, but their major consequence is blockage of the urinary tract. Obstruction may occur at any point in the urinary tract but is most common in anatomically narrow areas in the ureter near the bladder trigone and at the ureteropelvic junction. Stone impaction usually results in severe, colicky pain that is often referred to the flank (ureteral stones). Long-term urinary obstruction results in hydronephrosis, which can cause renal failure unless decompressed (Fig. 12-5). Hydronephrosis combined with bacterial infection can destroy renal parenchyma very quickly.

Therapy for stones initially involves hydration to allow the urine stream to facilitate stone passage. Alkalinization of the urine and good hydration may prevent repeated episodes of lithiasis. Intractable stones may be managed by fracturing by means of lithotripsy or by surgical or endoscopic removal. Patients with lithiasis as a consequence of genetic disease may benefit from therapies targeted at abnormal metabolites.

●●● CONGENITAL ABNORMALITIES

Many different congenital abnormalities of the urinary tract can occur, and most are identified in the perinatal or pediatric

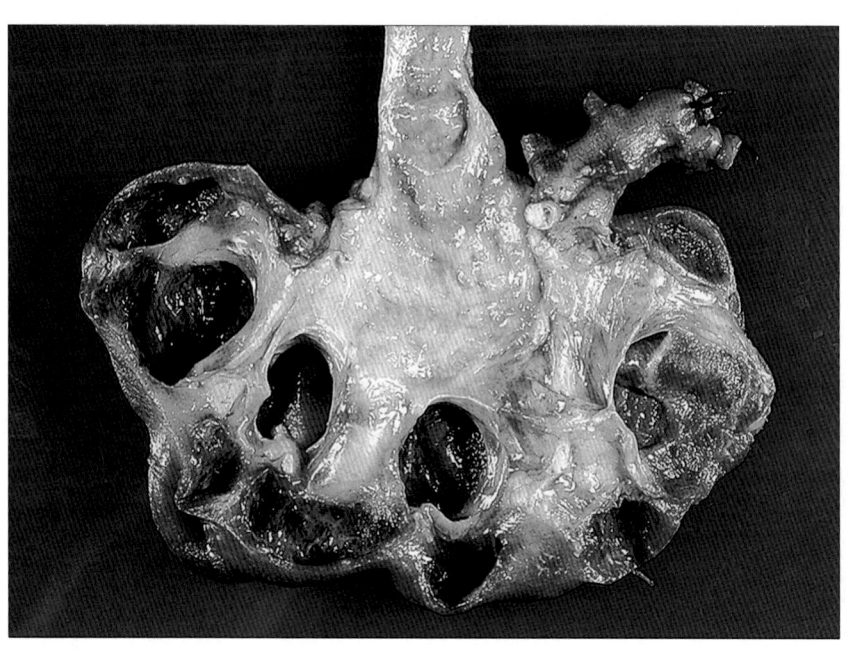

Figure 12-5. Hydronephrosis. Gross cross-section of a kidney with marked dilatation of the ureter (*top*) and balloon-like dilatations of the pelvis with marked atrophy of renal parenchyma.

period (see Chapter 4) with only a few conditions initially presenting in adults.

Ureteropelvic Junction Obstruction

Ureteropelvic junction (UPJ) abnormalities can result in functional kinking of the ureter at its junction with the renal pelvis to produce transient obstruction of urine flow out of the renal pelvis. UPJ abnormalities can result in colicky pain or may be asymptomatic. In combination with infection, UPJ obstruction can lead to rapid loss of kidney function, and some patients may have a nonfunctioning kidney as a result of chronic pyelonephritis. UPJ abnormalities may be unilateral or bilateral and can usually be surgically corrected.

Polycystic Kidney Disease

Two forms of polycystic kidney disease are recognized. The infantile form is a recessive genetic disease whereby homozygotes develop progressive dilatation of the cortical collecting ducts that leads to renal failure in childhood. Adult-type polycystic kidney disease is inherited as an autosomal dominant disease and is caused by mutations in the PKD-1 or PKD-2 gene. These genetic alterations result in the formation of cysts at all levels of the kidney, including Bowman's space. Patients with adult polycystic kidney disease tend have slowly enlarging cysts that compress and destroy renal parenchyma over many years. Renal failure typically develops between the fifth and seventh decades in affected individuals (Fig. 12-6). Cysts of the pancreas and liver also occur and may produce additional clinical symptoms.

● ● ● DEGENERATIVE AND VASCULAR DISEASES

Acute Tubular Necrosis

Acute tubular necrosis (ATN) can be caused by transient ischemia, since the high metabolic rate of proximal tubules makes them unusually susceptible to interruptions in energy or oxygen delivery. Clinically, ATN most often occurs following transient hypotension. If the whole kidney is involved by ATN, acute renal failure develops that is usually corrected over the course of days as precursor cells proliferate and reepithelialize tubules. Recovery is typically preceded by a marked diuresis and is usually complete if the patient survives because the extracellular matrix and tubular basement membranes are not damaged.

Hypertension and Nephrosclerosis

Chronic hypertension results in arterial nephrosclerosis with thickening of large and small blood vessels in the kidney by atherosclerosis. Disease of larger blood vessels can result in segmental infarcts of the kidney (small or large), which produce the typical pattern of arterial nephrosclerosis with small indentations in the renal cortex that are visible on gross examination (Fig. 12-7). These indentations result from the loss of parenchymal tissue owing to small, discrete infarcts and the contraction of fibrous scar tissue, producing a football-like appearance. The thickening of afferent arterioles to glomeruli can ultimately result in loss of glomerular function and devascularization of glomeruli.

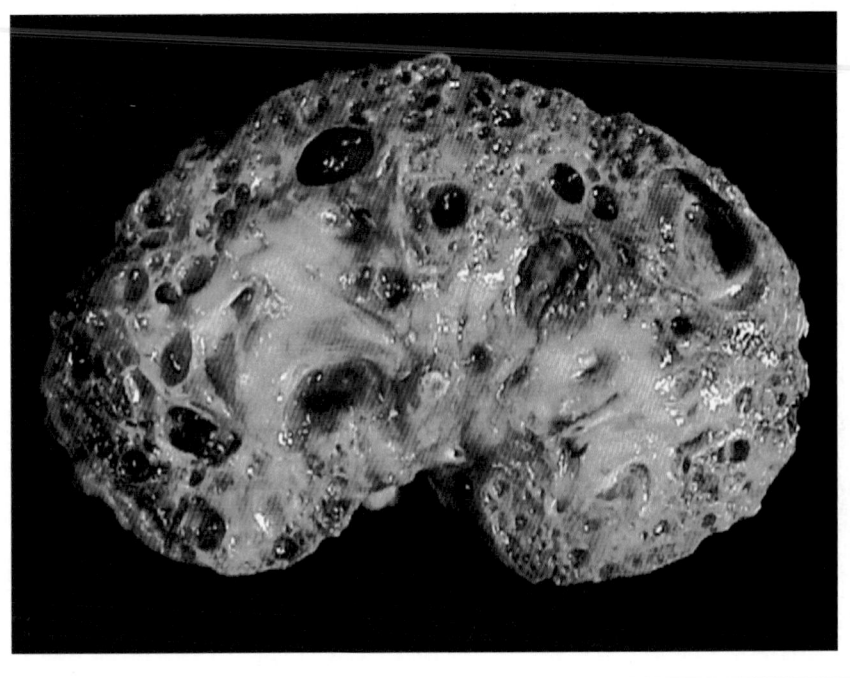

Figure 12-6. Adult-type polycystic kidney disease. Gross cross-section of a kidney with innumerable cysts replacing renal parenchyma.

BIOCHEMISTRY

Polycystic Kidney Disease

Autosomal dominant polycystic kidney disease can be caused by missense mutations in either the PKD-1 or the PKD-2 gene.

PKD-1 (polycystin-1) is a transmembrane protein with collagen-, fibronectin-, and laminin-binding domains. PKD-1 is normally expressed on the lateral surfaces of renal epithelial cells and transduces signals from focal adhesion complexes with the extracellular matrix and adjacent cells.

PKD-2 (polycystin-2) is a member of a family of transient receptor potential calcium and sodium transmembrane channels that normally functions as a membrane calcium channel.

The normal nephron has 15 distinct segments having different epithelial polarity that is established during embryogenesis by selective alterations in gene expression. Renal epithelial cells from patients with polycystic kidney disease show a persistent fetal pattern of polarization with abnormal locations of the sodium/potassium-ATPase as well as hormone receptors and other proteins. These findings suggest that the PKD-1 and -2 mutations result in faulty control of cell polarization. Knockout mice with defective apoptosis also develop polycystic kidneys, suggesting that the balance between proliferation and apoptosis in renal epithelial cells is also important in cyst formation.

Patients with autosomal recessive polycystic kidney disease usually have protein-truncating mutations (nonsense mutations) in a large protein of unknown function, PKHD1 (fibrocystin).

Severe hypertension can produce the syndrome of malignant hypertension, which can result in rapid loss of renal function. Patients with malignant hypertension show hyperplastic arteriolosclerosis with an "onionskin" pattern (concentric rings of fibrosis) around afferent arterioles. Fibrinoid necrosis of blood vessel walls may develop in very severe hypertension, resulting in loss of individual glomeruli or in renal infarcts.

Diabetes Melllitus

Diabetes mellitus is an important cause of chronic renal insufficiency and renal failure. Abnormal glycosylation of macromolecules in small blood vessels (including afferent arterioles and the capillaries of the glomerular tuft) results in wall thickening with luminal compromise that blocks blood supply to glomeruli and decreases glomerular blood flow. Deposition of glycosylated materials in the glomerular basement membrane results in thickening and charge abnormalities of the basement membrane filter that impair filtration, causing proteinuria and decreased GFR. Lobular deposition of glycosylated materials in the glomerular tuft results in the typical segmental pattern of diabetic glomerulosclerosis called Kimmelstiel-Wilson nodules. PAS stains of glomeruli highlight these glycosylated materials (Fig. 12-8) and emphasize the lobular pattern of disease. Patients with diabetes mellitus typically have a combination of proteinuria and decreased renal function as a consequence of GBM abnormalities, microvascular disease, and associated macrovascular

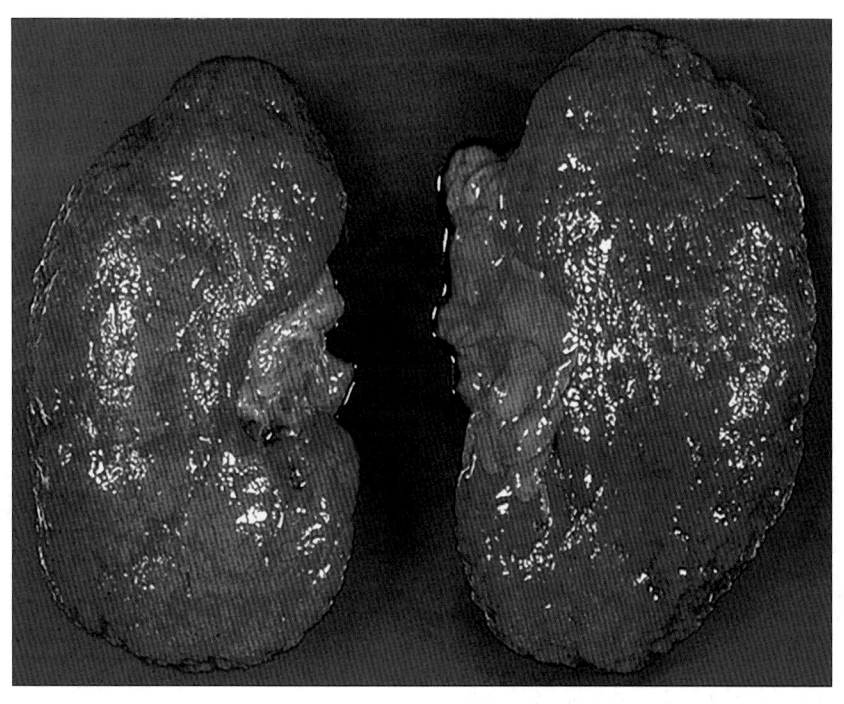

Figure 12-7. Nephrosclerosis. Gross image of renal cortical surface after the renal capsule has been stripped away showing punctate depressions resulting from small infarcts.

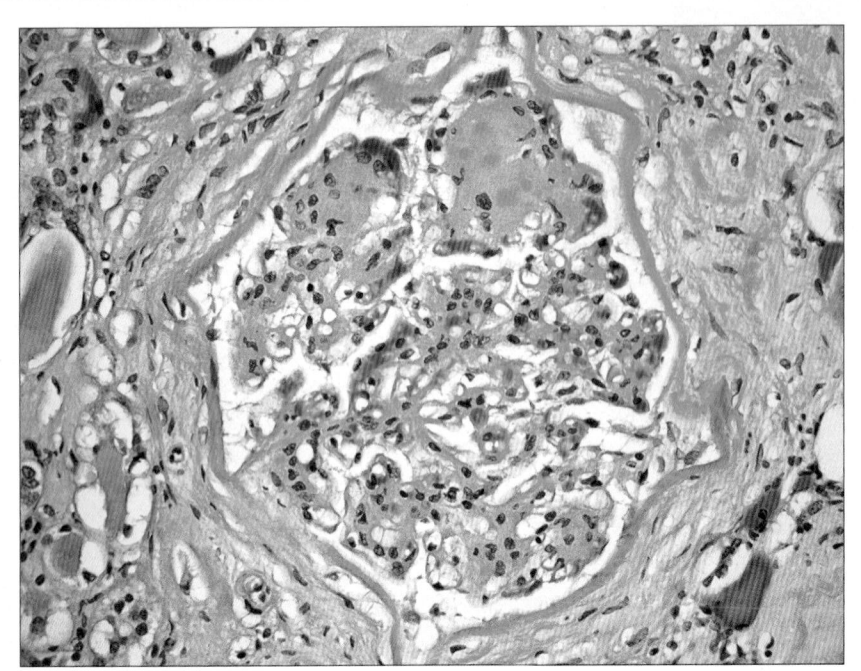

Figure 12-8. Diabetic glomerulo-sclerosis. Microscopic section of a renal glomerulus showing lobular accentuation of the glomerular basement membrane.

disease resulting from accelerated atherosclerosis. As for other complications of diabetes, the severity of diabetic renal complications is primarily related to the effectiveness of blood glucose control. Hypertension exacerbates the loss of renal function in diabetes mellitus, and the two conditions frequently coexist.

Chronic Renal Insufficiency

Chronic renal insufficiency and renal failure are the end results of a number of different types of kidney disease including hypertension, diabetes mellitus, infection, and glomerulonephritis. Chronic renal insufficiency corresponds to a state in which glomerular filtration rate is not adequate to effectively manage waste removal from the bloodstream. End-stage renal disease is always associated with significant elevations in serum creatinine and blood urea nitrogen. The kidneys in chronic renal insufficiency typically have a shrunken appearance with sclerosis of most glomeruli regardless of the primary cause of renal failure (Fig. 12-9A). Patients treated with long-term renal dialysis can develop numerous cysts in their nonfunctional kidneys (so-called dialysis kidney) (see Fig. 12-9B) and are at increased risk for the development of renal carcinoma (usually papillary carcinoma).

●●● RENAL TRANSPLANTATION

Renal transplantation is the most functionally effective treatment for chronic renal insufficiency. Renal transplants can develop the same primary disease that resulted in renal insufficiency, and transplant rejection is another major cause of morbidity and graft loss (see Chapter 2). Immunosuppression to prevent rejection may result in graft infection with a ubiquitous polyomavirus (BK virus) that can cause graft failure. Urine cytology can be used to monitor for BK virus infection. Transplant patients are also at risk for other types of opportunistic infection and posttransplant lymphoproliferative disorder (PTLD).

●●● TUMORS

The two major neoplasms of the kidney and urinary tract are transitional cell carcinoma (which can involve the urothelium at any level of the urinary tract) and renal cell carcinoma. Wilms' tumor is the most common renal pediatric tumor (see Chapter 4). Adult Wilms' tumor is rare but shares many morphologic features with its pediatric counterpart.

Transitional Cell Carcinoma

Transitional cell carcinoma can develop in the urothelium of the renal pelvis, ureter, or bladder. There is often a field effect change in the urothelium that results in multifocal tumors developing at different levels of the urinary tract. Cigarette smoking is a major risk factor for transitional cell carcinoma while specific industrial exposures (e.g., aniline dyes) were an important risk factor in the past. Transitional cell carcinomas of the bladder usually present with hematuria, whereas tumors of the ureter and renal pelvis may produce obstruction. Tumors can develop as exophytic papillary lesions (common pathway) or via flat urothelial dysplasia (relatively uncommon pathway).

Papillary tumors of the bladder often develop as papillomas lined by urothelium with low-grade cytologic features similar to normal urothelium. As papillary lesions grow, they often develop increased cytologic atypia with thickening

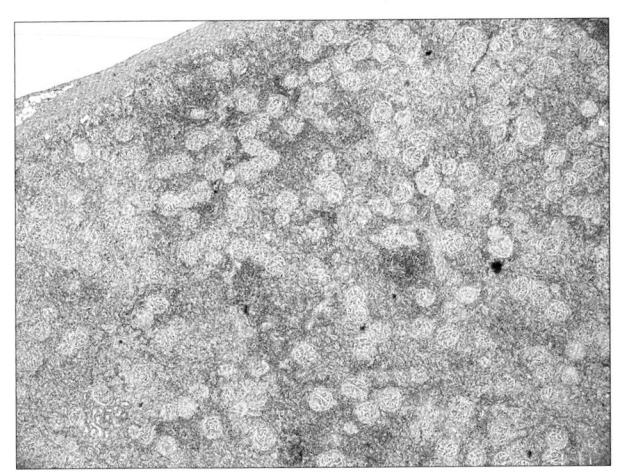

A

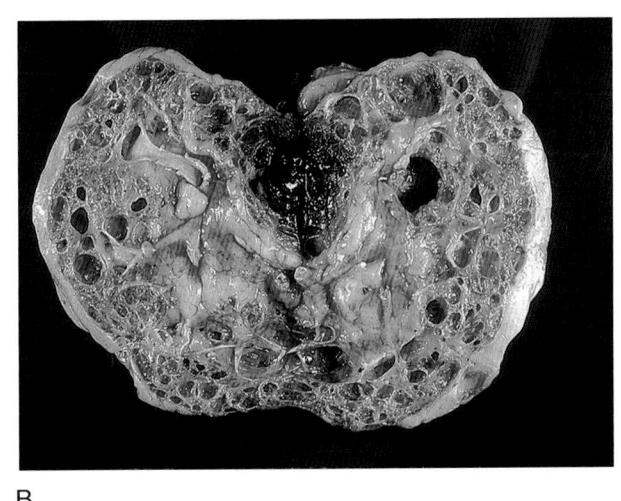

B

Figure 12-9. A, End-stage kidney disease. Microscopic section of kidney showing numerous globally sclerotic glomeruli in a background of chronic inflammation. **B**, Dialysis kidney. Gross cross-section of kidney from a chronic dialysis patient showing extensive cyst formation. The hemorrhagic area (*top*) is a small papillary renal cell carcinoma.

and disorganization of the urothelium lining the fibrovascular cores. Eventually, some papillary tumors invade the submucosa and may extend into the muscularis propria (Fig. 12-10A). Papillary transitional cell carcinomas are typically slow growing and often produce hematuria, which may lead to their clinical detection. Cystoscopy is an excellent screening test for papillary neoplasms, most of which can be removed by snaring with an electrocautery and fulgurating the tumor base (see Fig. 12-10B). In many patients, recurrent tumors develop over time, and these may be of progressively higher histologic grade (due to the field effect in the urothelium).

Grade 3/3 tumors show significant mitotic activity with full-thickness atypia and disorganization of the urothelial cells lining the fibrovascular cores. Grade 3 tumors frequently invade the muscular wall of the bladder and gain access to

vascular spaces, with potential for metastatic spread. Papillary transitional cell carcinomas that have invaded the muscular wall of the bladder are often treated by radical cystectomy and replacement of the bladder with a segment of ileum (ileal loop). Low-grade and superficial tumors are often treated with simple excision or localized chemotherapy (installation of chemotherapeutic agents directly into the bladder, called intravesical chemotherapy). Bladder tumors may also be treated with intravesical installation of attenuated *Mycobacterium tuberculosis* called bacille Calmette-Guérin (BCG), which incites a granulomatous inflammatory response that can be effective in eradicating some tumors. Papillary tumors of the ureter and renal pelvis are usually low grade at diagnosis, since they often produce obstruction, but their location usually necessitates more radical surgery (see Fig. 12-10C).

Transitional cell carcinoma in situ is a flat dysplasia of the urothelium that can develop into invasive carcinoma (Fig. 12-11A). Unlike papillary tumors, transitional carcinoma in situ is difficult to identify endoscopically and usually appears as reddish mucosa that can closely resemble inflammatory lesions of the bladder. Transitional cell carcinoma in situ shows full thickness cytologic atypia and disorganization histologically. Urothelial cytology can be useful in identifying dysplastic and malignant cells (see Fig. 12-11B). Treatment with installation of chemotherapeutic or immunotherapeutic agents may be helpful, but it can progress rapidly to invasive carcinoma and require radical cystectomy.

Renal Cell Carcinoma

Renal cell carcinoma is typically a tumor of adults. Clear-cell renal cell carcinoma is the most common and the most aggressive type (this tumor is now referred to as "conventional clear-cell carcinoma" (Fig. 12-12A). Clear-cell carcinomas are almost invariably associated with genetic lesions in chromosome 3p, encompassing the von Hippel–Lindau gene. As a consequence, these tumors generally are highly vascular. Clear-cell carcinomas arise from proximal tubular cells, and tumor cells characteristically have abundant clear cytoplasm that contains abundant glycogen and lipid (see Fig. 12-12B). Demonstration of glycogen by special stains can be helpful in confirming the diagnosis of conventional clear-cell carcinoma as well. Tumor grade and stage are both helpful in predicting the likelihood of metastatic disease, which often is to the lungs or to bone. Sarcomatoid renal cell carcinoma is a rare, high-grade variant of clear-cell carcinoma that morphologically mimics retroperitoneal sarcoma. Sarcomatoid carcinomas are metaplastic carcinomas that retain a cytokeratin expression pattern typical of clear-cell carcinoma.

On gross examination, clear-cell carcinomas are typically golden yellow and often develop hemorrhage and infarction with the formation of cysts within the tumor. A contrast-enhanced computed tomography (CT) scan usually demonstrates the high vascularity of these tumors and is helpful in preoperative diagnosis. Clear-cell carcinomas are usually sharply circumscribed from renal parenchyma and appear

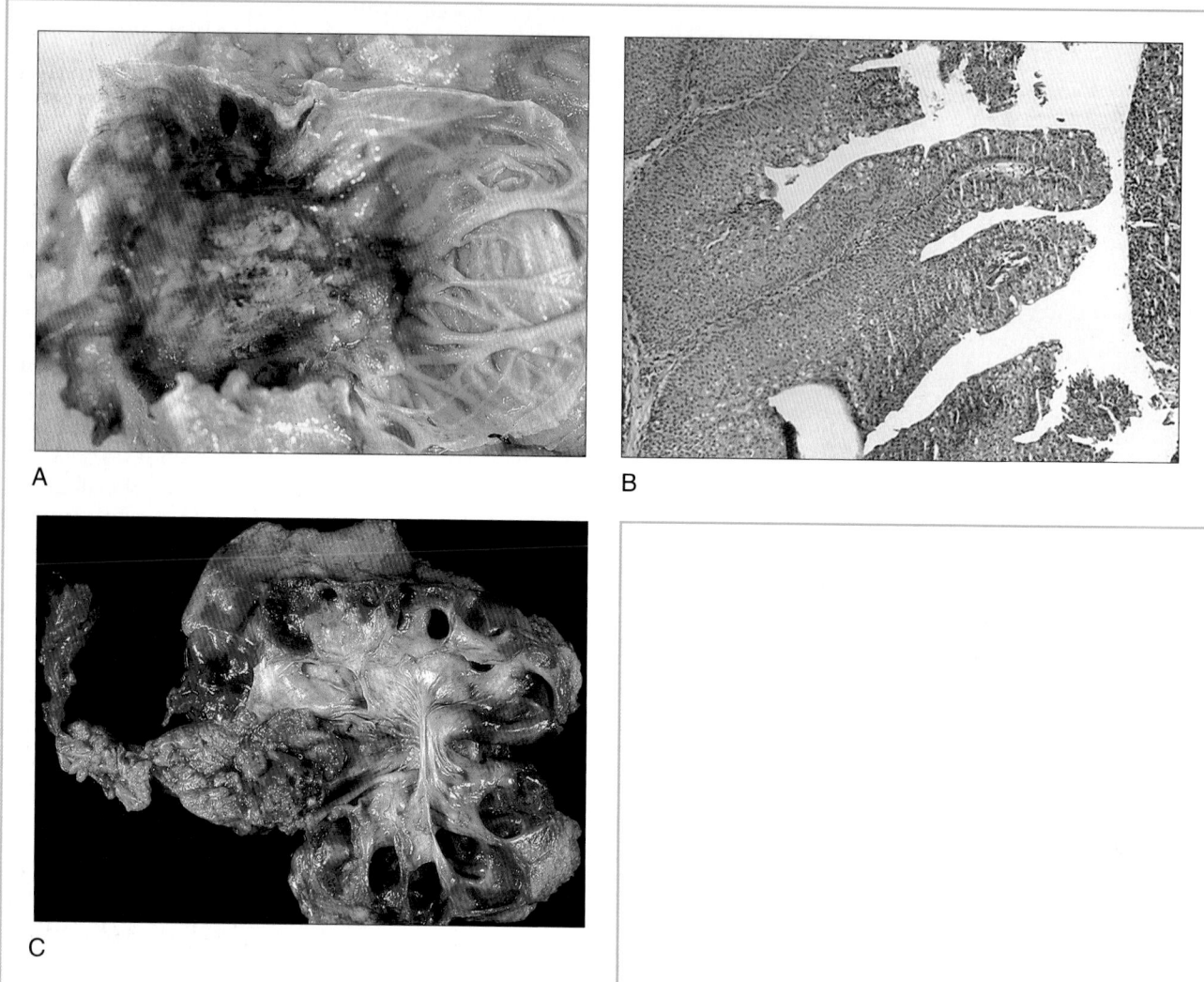

Figure 12-10. A, Invasive transitional cell carcinoma. Gross photograph of an opened bladder with an ulcerated hemorrhagic tumor mass (*bottom*). Uninvolved bladder mucosa (*top*) shows marked trabeculation secondary to prostatic obstruction. **B**, Papillary transitional cell carcinoma. Microscopic section showing fibrovascular cores lined by moderately atypical urothelial cells. **C**, Transitional cell carcinoma of the renal pelvis. Gross photograph of bisected kidney showing papillary transitional cell carcinoma filling the renal pelvis and ureter (*bottom*).

encapsulated. Tumors tend to bulge the renal capsule outward into perinephric adipose tissue. Evidence of capsular invasion or extrarenal extension is a grim prognostic factor. Clear-cell carcinomas show a strong tendency to invade vascular spaces. Tumors with large vessel space invasion evident on gross examination are considered of higher pathologic stage. Vascular invasion may extend into the renal vein, and tumors may grow as insular extensions all the way up the vena cava into the right side of the heart.

Two other classes of renal cell carcinoma are less frequent and less aggressive than clear-cell carcinoma. *Papillary renal cell carcinomas* show well-developed papillary architecture with tumor cells lining fibrovascular stromal cores. The epithelial tumor cells do not demonstrate features typical of clear-cell carcinoma (occasional papillary tumors that have focal cytologic features of clear-cell carcinoma should be classified as conventional clear-cell carcinomas). Papillary

carcinomas typically have a large number of foamy histiocytes within fibrovascular papillae (Fig. 12-13A) and are the most common type of renal tumor occurring in patients receiving long-term renal dialysis. *Chromophobe carcinomas* are low-grade malignant tumors having a characteristic morphologic appearance with prominent cell borders between individual tumor cells that usually have eosinophilic cytoplasm (see Fig. 12-13B). Hale's colloidal iron stain is classically positive in these tumors.

Other Renal Tumors

Oncocytomas are characteristic benign renal neoplasms that are mahogany brown in color and typically have a prominent stellate central scar, which may suggest the diagnosis radiographically. Oncocytomas are usually spherical and are well circumscribed from renal parenchyma. Tumor cells are cyto-

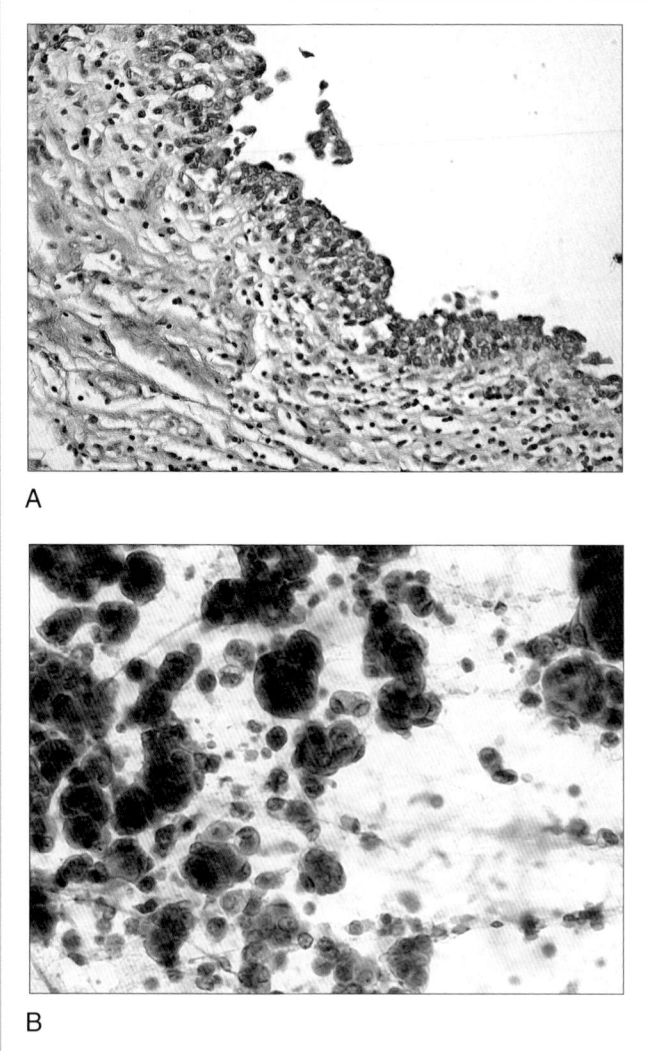

A

B

Figure 12-11. Transitional cell carcinoma in situ. **A**, Microscopic section showing flat urothelial dysplasia with full-thickness cytologic atypia and disorganization. **B**, Urine cytology preparation showing clusters of malignant transitional cells.

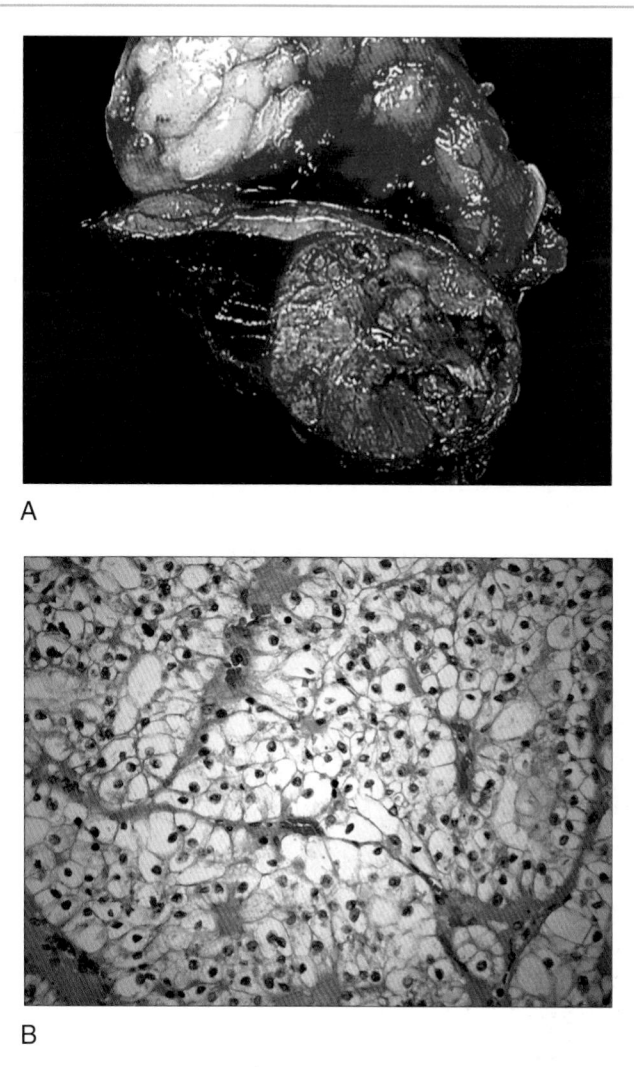

A

B

Figure 12-12. Conventional clear-cell renal carcinoma. **A**, Gross cross-section of a kidney with a golden yellow hemorrhagic tumor (*bottom*). Residual normal kidney is visible (*middle left*) as well as perirenal adipose tissue (*top*). **B**, Microscopic section showing tumor cells with abundant clear cytoplasm and intermediate-sized nuclei.

logically bland epithelial cells with abundant granular eosinophilic cytoplasm (see Fig. 12-13C). This granular cytoplasmic appearance results from the presence of numerous mitochondria within tumor cells, similarly to oncocytic tumors in other tissues.

Angiomyolipoma is an unusual tumor of the kidney or perirenal soft tissue that is composed of varying amounts of blood vessels with adipose and muscle tissue. When all three components are present, angiomyolipomas are easily recognized, but in some cases one component predominates, raising the possibility of a retroperitoneal sarcoma. Angio-

myolipoma is relatively common in patients with tuberous sclerosis and should be suspected in patients with an apparently solitary angiomyolipoma. Angiomyolipomas typically express HMB45 protein (which can be detected immunohistochemically) as do most other tumors and tumor-like lesions in patients with tuberous sclerosis.

Medullary carcinoma is a rare malignant tumor that occurs exclusively in patients with sickle cell anemia. *Collecting duct carcinoma* is a rare malignant renal tumor that arises in the medulla and may be difficult to distinguish from high-grade transitional cell carcinoma of the renal pelvis.

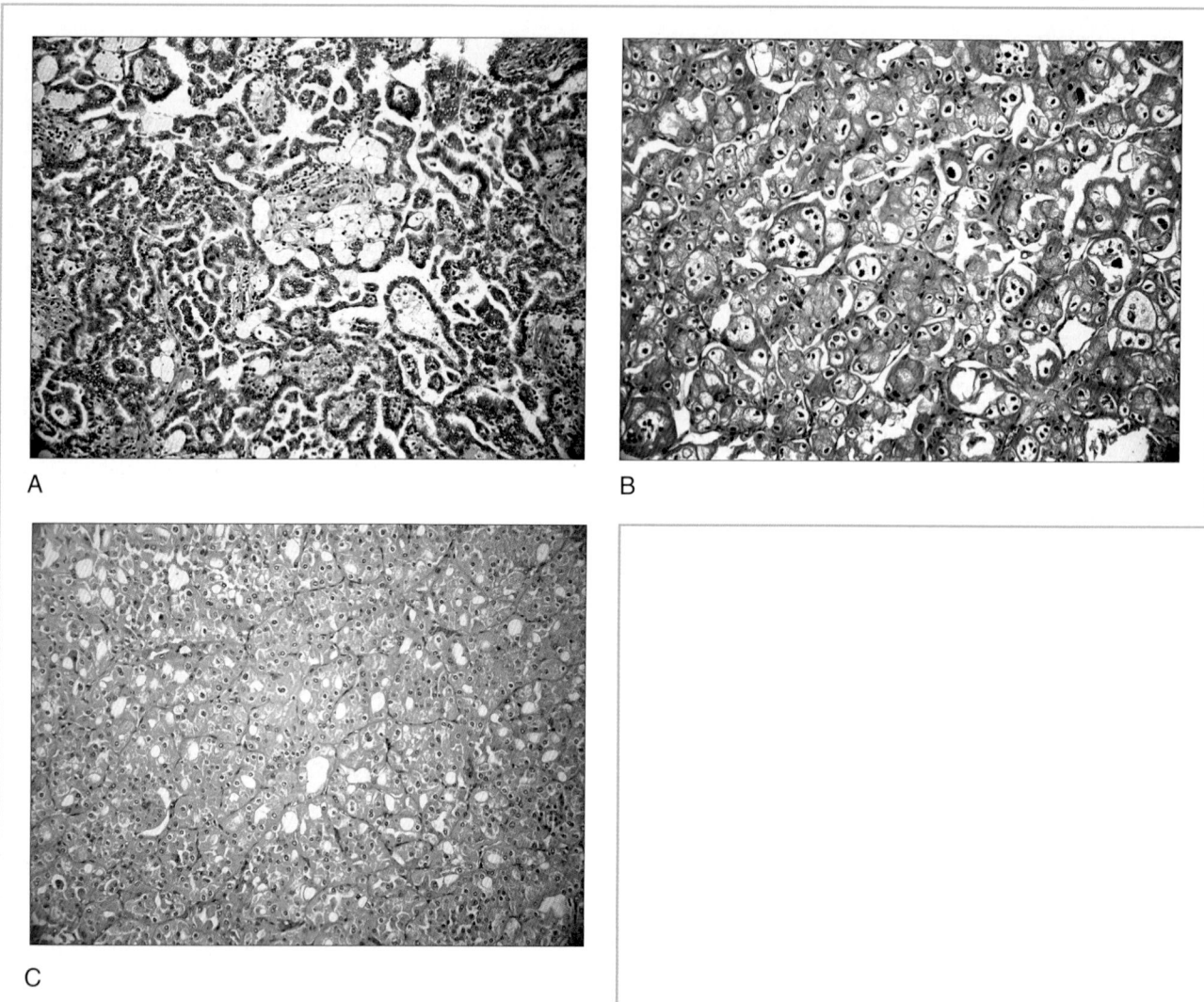

Figure 12-13. A, Papillary renal cell carcinoma. Microscopic section showing numerous papillae lined by bland epithelial cells with eosinophilic cytoplasm. Clusters of histiocytes with clear foamy cytoplasm are present within the fibrovascular cores. **B**, Chromophobe renal cell carcinoma. Microscopic section showing tumor cells with hyperchromatic but otherwise bland nuclei and prominent cell borders between tumor cells. **C**, Renal oncocytoma. Microscopic section showing bland tumor cells with abundant granular eosinophilic cytoplasm.

Male and Female Genital Tracts and Breast Pathology

13

CONTENTS

●●● TESTIS AND EPIDIDYMIS

The testis is composed predominantly of seminiferous tubules and interstitial Leydig cells. Sertoli cells in the tubules provide nourishment for germ cells and direct their maturation. Primitive germ cells (spermatogonia) reside at the periphery of tubules and migrate toward the lumen as they divide, undergo meiosis, and mature into spermatids. The testis is originally an abdominal organ that migrates to the scrotum during embryogenesis. Therefore, the vasculature and lymphatic drainage of the testis are to the periaortic region. The testis is covered by a tunica albuginea, which is composed of dense connective tissue covered by mesothelium. The tunica vaginalis surrounds the testis and is similarly covered by mesothelium. The epididymis is composed of tubules lined by ciliated columnar epithelium similar to that of the vas deferens.

Congenital Anomalies

Congenital abnormalities of the testis can result from chromosomal and intersex syndromes. The most common congenital abnormality is failure of the testis to normally descend from its abdominal location to the scrotum (cryptorchidism). Normal spermatogenesis requires a temperature lower than body core temperature so that cryptorchidism results in infertility. If cryptorchidism is not corrected early in life, patients develop testicular atrophy with infertility and are markedly predisposed to germ cell tumors.

Inflammatory Conditions of the Testis

Bacterial infection of the testis and epididymis can results from venereal transmission of gonorrhea. Torsion of the testis (twisting of the spermatic cord that contains the blood vessels supplying the testis) results in congestion and ischemia of the testis, which may lead to infarction. Prompt decompression of torsion may prevent infarction. In some individuals, the testis is not normally anchored to the scrotum, resulting in an increased risk of testicular torsion.

Testicular Tumors

Germ cell tumors are the most important testicular neoplasms. Other types of tumors can arise in the testis and epididymis, but their major importance is in simulating a malignant germ cell tumor. All germ cell tumors of the testis are malignant, whereas most other primary tumors of the testis (e.g., Leydig cell tumors) are benign.

Germ Cell Tumors

Germ cell tumors of the testis arise from germ cells within testicular tubules (Fig. 13-1) and broadly are either seminomas or nonseminomatous germ cell tumors. Most testicular germ cell tumors present in young men, and most are unilateral. The usual therapy for lesions suspected to be germ cell tumors is high inguinal orchiectomy in which the spermatic cord is ligated in the inguinal canal prior to removal of the testis (Fig. 13-2A). Needle or incisional biopsy of testicular germ cell tumors is contraindicated because of possible contamination of the space between the tunica albuginea and tunica vaginalis. Germ cell tumors are quite uncommon after the age of 40 years with the exception of an unusual tumor called spermatocytic seminoma, which is morphologically and clinically distinct from a typical seminoma. Spermatocytic seminomas characteristically occur in older men and are usually cured by surgery. Typical seminomas are composed of tumor cells having a "fried egg" configuration with moderately abundant, clear cytoplasm and vesicular nuclei (see Fig. 13-2B). Seminomas are usually infiltrated by small lymphocytes, and in some cases the lymphocytic infiltrate may obscure tumor cells. In situ germ cell neoplasia (so-called intratubular germ cell neoplasia, or IGCN) frequently precedes the development of an invasive seminoma (see Fig. 13-2C). IGCN is present in up to 5% of testicular biopsies performed to evaluate infertility, reflecting a much higher incidence of germ cell neoplasia in this selected population (i.e., patients with cryptorchidism or other genitourinary anomalies).

Most seminomas are cured by radical orchiectomy alone. Patients are usually evaluated for possible metastatic disease by CT scan of the retroperitoneum, since the lymphatic drainage of the testis is to periaortic lymph nodes. Even in patients with widely metastatic seminoma, cure rates are very high with conventional chemotherapy, since most seminomas are exquisitely sensitive to radiation therapy or chemotherapy. Seminomas tend to produce placental alkaline phosphatase, and staining for this marker can be useful in identifying tumor deposits.

Seminoma is the precursor of other, more differentiated forms of testicular germ cell tumors including teratoma, yolk sac tumor, embryonal carcinoma, and choriocarcinoma. All of these nonseminomatous germ cell tumors are more differentiated and tend to be more biologically aggressive than seminoma. In contrast, most other better differentiated types of tumors tend to have a more favorable prognosis. Nonseminomatous germ cell tumors recapitulate different embryonic and postembryonic structures, with yolk sac tumor corresponding to primitive blood-forming organs in the embryo, choriocarcinoma to placental trophoblast, and teratoma to mature tissues derived from all three embryonic layers.

Embryonal carcinoma is a primitive tumor that shows morphologic features similar to many high-grade carcinomas in adults and usually expresses cytokeratins, similarly to conventional carcinomas (see Fig. 13-2D). Choriocarcinoma is composed of cytotrophoblast and syncytiotrophoblast, as is normal placenta, but organized villous structures are not formed. Choriocarcinoma is aggressive and is prone to systemic metastasis and can cause prominent hemorrhage. Choriocarcinomas invariably produce human chorionic gonadotropin (hCG), which is a highly specific and sensitive tumor marker. Pure yolk sac tumors rarely develop in the testis and are more common in extragonadal germ cell tumors in pediatric patients. Yolk sac tumor does occur as a component of some mixed nonseminomatous germ cell tumors and has a characteristic architectural pattern, with the formation of Schiller-Duvall bodies (see Fig. 13-2E).

Yolk sac tumors and embryonal carcinomas frequently produce α-fetoprotein (AFP), which is a useful cellular and serum marker for these tumors. A high serum level of hCG or AFP is an indication that a testicular mass is almost certainly a nonseminomatous germ cell tumor. Preoperative measurement of serum tumor marker levels is important for managing patients postoperatively. After orchiectomy, tumor marker levels should fall to zero if no metastatic disease is present. Subsequent monitoring of tumor markers is useful to detect early recurrence of tumor that may still be treated effectively with chemotherapy.

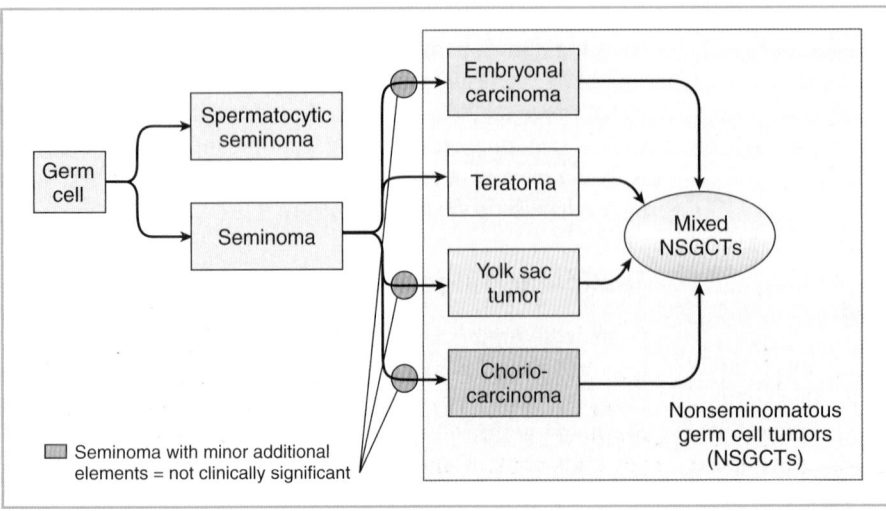

Figure 13-1. Testicular germ cell tumor development.

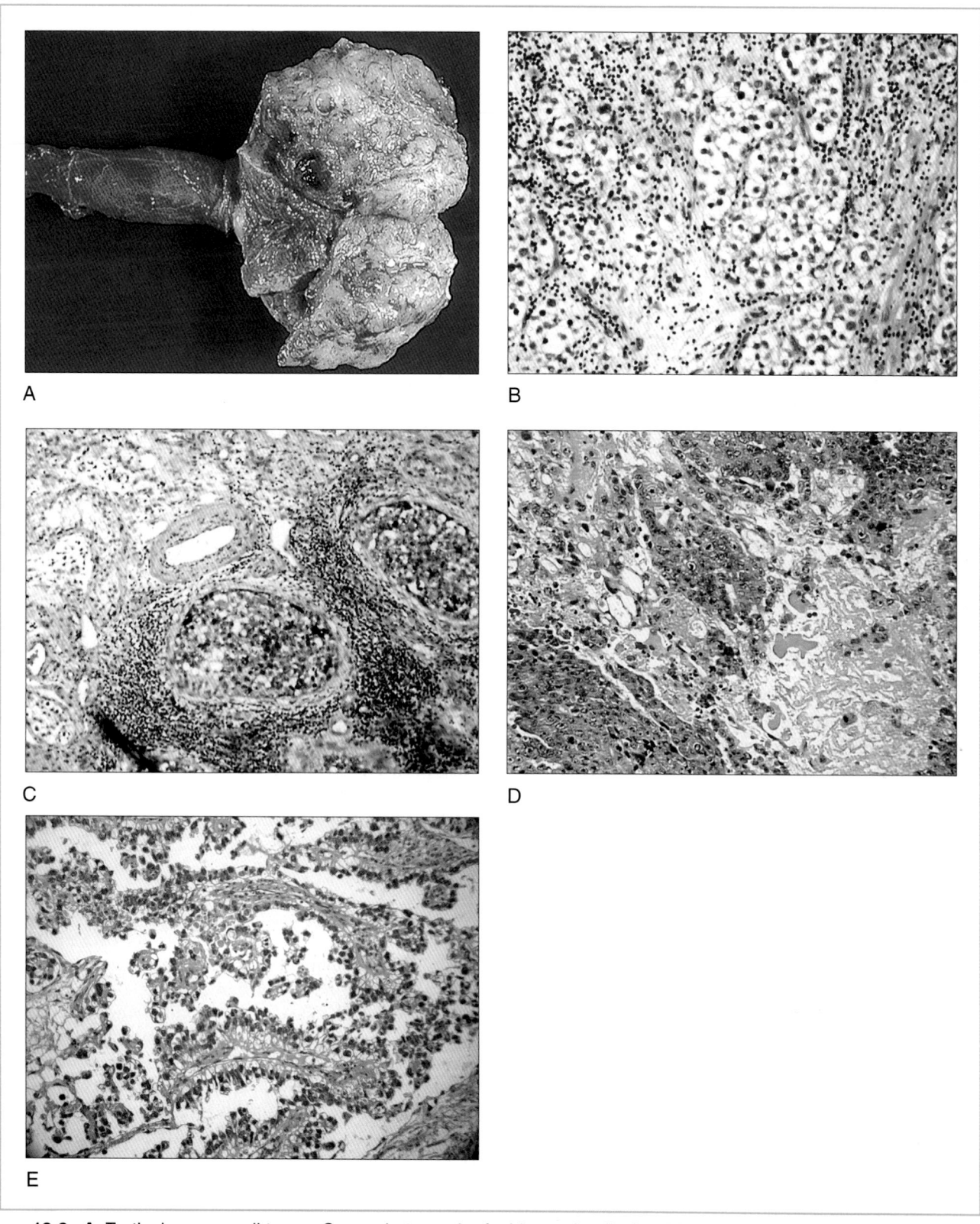

Figure 13-2. **A,** Testicular germ cell tumor. Gross photograph of a bisected radical orchiectomy specimen with a large, mixed germ cell tumor with extensive hemorrhage and tumor necrosis. The spermatic cord is visible at left. **B,** Classic seminoma. Microscopic section showing tumor cells with relatively abundant clear cytoplasm with scattered lymphocytes in the background. **C,** Intratubular germ cell neoplasia. Microscopic section of testis showing several seminiferous tubules filled with neoplastic cells similar to invasive seminoma. A dense lymphoid infiltrate is present in the interstitium. **D,** Embryonal carcinoma. Microscopic section showing pleomorphic tumor cells forming irregular epithelium-like structures. **E,** Yolk sac tumor. Microscopic section showing fibrovascular cores surrounded by tumor cells with clear cytoplasm and pleomorphic nuclei.

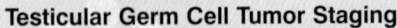

BIOCHEMISTRY

Testicular Germ Cell Tumor Staging

Staging of testicular germ cell tumors involves standard pathologic characterization of the extent of local tumor growth as well as evaluation of nodal and distant metastasis. In addition, the preoperative levels of serum tumor markers α-fetoprotein (AFP) and human chorionic gonadotropin (hCG) can directly affect tumor staging. Serum tumor marker levels provide a measure of systemic tumor burden.

If the serum hCG or AFP level is markedly elevated (stage S2 or S3; see table below), patients are more likely to be treated with systemic chemotherapy regardless of the TMN stage. Postoperative levels of these tumor markers and of lactate dehydrogenase (LDH) are important therapy guides in all patients with nonseminomatous germ cell tumors (NSGCTs).

| | Serum Level | | |
Stage	hCG (mIU/mL)	AFP (ng/mL)	LDH
SX	Unknown	Unknown	Unknown
S0	Within normal limits	Within normal limits	Within normal limits
S1	<5000	<1000	<1.5 × Normal
S2	5000–50,000	1000–10,000	1.5–10 × Normal
S3	>50,000	>10,000	>10 × Normal

Many seminomas contain scattered syncytiotrophoblast cells and show immunohistochemical evidence of individual hCG-positive cells. These findings are not clinically significant in the absence of discrete areas of pure nonseminomatous germ cell tumor and do not affect prognosis. Some patients with seminomas may have mild serum elevations of hCG as a result of these scattered trophoblastic cells. Higher levels of serum tumor markers should prompt a search for a small, discrete nonseminomatous component in an otherwise typical seminoma, which would be prognostically significant.

Lymphoma and Leukemia

Testicular masses in older men (>50 years) are more likely to be lymphomas (usually large-cell lymphomas) than germ cell tumors. The testis is a "sanctuary" for leukemia and lymphoma cells that may allow them to escape the effects of systemic chemotherapy, and some patients treated successfully for acute lymphoblastic leukemia may have a testicular relapse. Myeloid leukemia occasionally presents as an extramedullary myeloid cell tumor in the testis.

●●● PROSTATE

The prostate is composed of acinar glands that drain into larger ducts and ultimately into the urethra, and prostatic secretions are a large component of normal semen. Prostatic glandular cells produce prostate-specific antigen (PSA), which is a useful tumor marker, and serum levels of PSA provide an important screening test for prostate cancer. Acini and ducts are surrounded by a specialized fibromuscular stroma. The prostate gland surrounds the urethra so that hypertrophy can

result in significant urethral obstruction. The seminal vesicles are located at the proximal pole of the prostate.

Inflammatory Conditions of the Prostate

Most prostate glands in older men show some degree of chronic inflammation that is related to ductal obstruction, infection, or small infarcts, all of which are relatively common. Bacterial infection of the prostate is usually retrograde through its ducts and may be venereal in origin (e.g., gonorrhea). Bacterial infection of the prostate usually results in severe pain on digital rectal exam. Granulomatous prostatitis is an unusual condition that may simulate cancer on digital rectal exam because of the hard nodularity produced by granulomas. Some cases result from mycobacterial infection but often a causative organism cannot be demonstrated.

Prostatic Hyperplasia

Prostatic hypertrophy and hyperplasia is almost universally present in older men and usually increases with age. Hyperplasia involves predominantly the mid zone of the prostate and can produce marked obstruction to urinary outflow, resulting in bladder trabeculation and urinary tract infection (Fig. 13-3). Hyperplastic glands are usually nodular as a result of lobular expansion of acini and proliferation of both epithelial and stromal cells. Some patients show predominance of hyperplastic glandular or stromal components. Nodular hyperplasia is usually associated with a moderate-to-marked chronic inflammatory cell infiltrate. Hormonal treatment can block hyperplasia in many patients and may help reverse urinary tract obstruction. Transurethral resection of prostate tissue using electrocautery can also decompress urethral stenosis.

Tumors of the Prostate

Almost all prostate cancers develop from glandular epithelial cells in prostatic acini. Prostate cancer is extremely common in older men, and autopsy series identify microscopic foci of prostate cancers in more than 80% of men over 80 years of age. Many of these minute tumors are indolent and do not result in morbidity during the patient's lifetime although a subset of these tumors is clinically aggressive and can result in cancer death. Many invasive prostate cancers are associated with prostatic intraepithelial neoplasia (PIN), which is an intraluminal proliferation of atypical cells with prominent nucleoli surrounded by a normal layer of basal cells. Basal cells do not express PSA but do express high-molecular-weight cytokeratin. Invasive prostate cancer cell nests and glands lack a basal cell layer, and staining for high-molecular-weight cytokeratin can be clinically useful in differentiating adenocarcinoma from other lesions in the prostate (e.g., PIN or adenosis). The association between PIN and prostate cancer is less strong than that between intraductal and invasive breast cancer. Prostate cancer is often multifocal and frequently involves both left and right

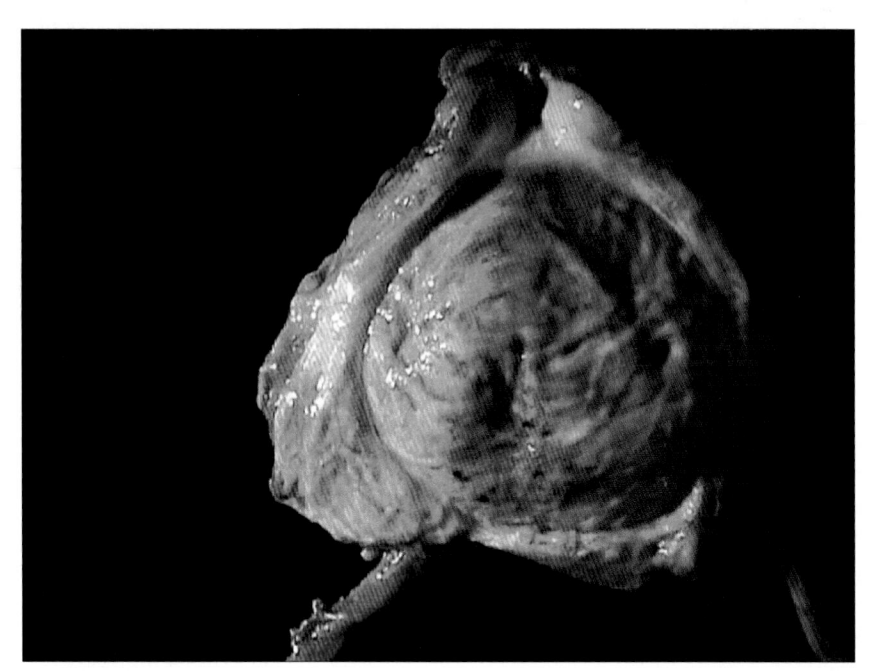

Figure 13-3. Bladder trabeculation. Gross photograph of an opened bladder showing prominent bands of hypertrophic smooth muscle that elevate the urothelium.

lobes of the prostate gland. Almost all prostate cancers arise in the peripheral zone of the prostate (adjacent to the rectum) so that digital rectal examination and transrectal needle biopsy are useful diagnostic tools.

Older men are usually screened for prostate cancer by measurement of serum PSA levels. PSA levels greater than 4.0 ng/dL are considered abnormal, and patients may be further screened by transrectal ultrasound (TRUS)–guided needle biopsy. Six biopsies (three from each of the right and left lobes) are typical. While PSA level is a useful screening test, its specificity is low, since prostatic inflammation can also increase serum PSA levels. Patients with localized prostate cancer (without evidence of systemic metastases) are often treated by radical prostatectomy. Alternatively, external beam radiation therapy or cryoablation of the prostate gland may be performed. Prostate cancer can invade through the capsule of the prostate into the rectum or bladder neck or involve the seminal vesicles. The presence of any of these features makes tumors technically unresectable, and these patients are considered incurable by radical prostatectomy.

Patients with metastatic disease are usually treated with hormonal therapy with antiandrogens, since most tumors are androgen responsive. Prostate cancers typically metastasize to vertebral bone via the venous plexus in the pelvis. Most tumors are initially responsive to hormonal therapy but may become unresponsive after prolonged treatment. Very poorly differentiated prostate cancers may metastasize to solid organs such as lung.

Most prostatic adenocarcinomas are moderately differentiated and composed of small glands made up of cells with prominent eosinophilic nucleoli that lack a normal basal cell layer at their periphery. In needle biopsy specimens, moder-

BIOCHEMISTRY

Prostate-specific Antigen (PSA)

PSA is produced by prostatic epithelial cells and by most prostate adenocarcinomas. A small amount of PSA is produced by salivary gland epithelium, but other cell types do not normally produce PSA, making it a highly lineage specific tumor marker. When prostate cells undergo apoptosis or necrosis, some PSA is released into the serum, resulting in a low but detectable serum level in normal men. PSA is a kallikrein-like serine protease whose normal function is to liquefy seminal fluid after ejaculation. It circulates in blood complexed with protease inhibitors and has a serum half-life of 2 to 3 days.

Serum PSA has been used as a screening test for prostate cancer for many years. A serum PSA level of 4 ng/mL measured by a monoclonal antibody assay is the current upper limit for the normal range; however, some authors advocate lowering this threshold, since some men with significant prostate cancer have serum PSA levels below 4 ng/mL. Using a cutoff of 4 ng/mL, a positive test has sensitivity and specificity of approximately 60%, depending on the population evaluated.

PSA velocity is the rate of change in serum PSA levels over time in one individual, and a velocity greater than 0.75 ng/mL per year is suspicious for carcinoma.

Free PSA (not complexed with plasma proteins) level is usually lower in cancer than in benign prostatic disease, and assessing the ratio of free to total PSA may enhance test specificity.

PSA is currently the only serum tumor marker used for screening the general population.

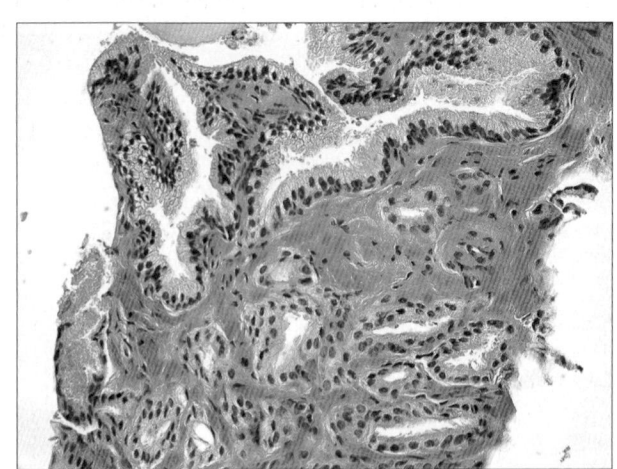

A

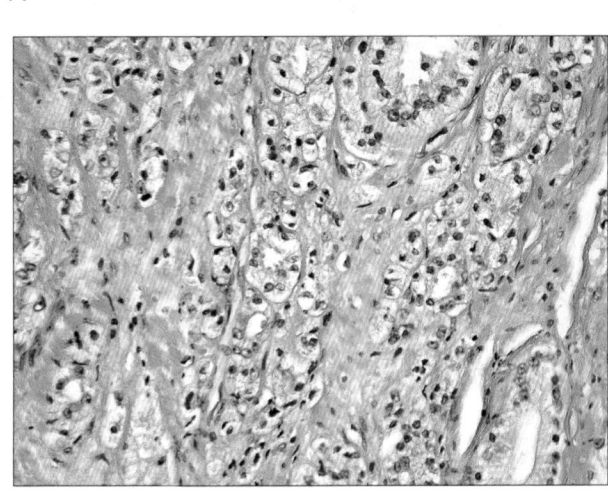

B

Figure 13-4. **A**, Prostatic adenocarcinoma (Gleason grade 3). Microscopic section showing small- to intermediate-sized, well-formed neoplastic glands with prominent nucleoli infiltrating between benign prostatic glands (*top*). **B**, Prostatic adenocarcinoma (Gleason grade 4). Microscopic section showing irregular, poorly formed glands that fuse together to form a syncytium of tumor cells.

ately differentiated tumors characteristically invade between normal glands (Fig. 13-4A). Prostate cancer is graded according to the Gleason score, which has been in use for more than 50 years. The Gleason score is the sum of two numeric grades corresponding to the major architectural patterns in the tumor (Gleason grades 1–5 summing to possible Gleason scores of 2–10). Gleason grading is purely architectural (i.e., tumor necrosis, mitotic activity, and cytologic atypia are not considered) but is a powerful prognostic indicator. Tumors corresponding to Gleason grades 4 and 5 almost always behave aggressively and are frequently associated with lymph node and bone metastases (see Fig. 13-4B). Gleason grades 1 and 2 tumors are usually indolent and rarely cause death.

Grade 3 tumors are the most common and are clinically heterogeneous in behavior. Since prostate cancer generally is a disease of older men, most men with low- and intermediate-grade prostate cancer will not die as a result of their cancers. For older men with low-grade prostate cancer on needle biopsy, many clinicians favor a "watchful waiting" strategy, measuring PSA levels and sampling tumor by needle biopsy to assess possible progression to a higher grade tumor. Conversely, patients with high-grade tumors usually receive some form of therapy. Patients under 70 years of age with predominantly grade 3 tumors are problematic, and the likelihood of aggressive or indolent disease is uncertain in individual patients. There is an urgent need for biologic markers that better predict clinical behavior in these prostate cancers. Racemase gene expression has emerged as a possible candidate biomarker of tumor aggressiveness, but its clinical utility has not yet been demonstrated.

Rarely, adenocarcinomas can develop from large ducts of the prostate, and these neoplasms have a different morphologic appearance and clinical behavior. Rhabdomyosarcoma can arise in the prostate in pediatric patients.

●●● PENIS

The penis is composed of corpora cavernosa and corpora spongiosa that surround the urethra. Fibrosis can develop within the cavernosa that interferes with erectile function and may lead to progressive distortion of the penis (Peyronie's

disease). Radical prostatectomy and external beam radiation frequently destroy the neurovascular bundles that supply autonomic information necessary for erection. Drug therapy can also cause erectile dysfunction.

The squamous mucosa of the penis can be infected by sexually transmitted diseases including syphilis and human papillomavirus (HPV). Syphilitic infection typically results in a visible chancre, but HPV infection may be asymptomatic. Some patients may develop condylomas on the penis as a result of HPV but much less commonly than in the uterine cervix. Gonorrhea can involve the periurethral glands and prostate.

Uncircumcised men frequently have persistent inflammation of the foreskin that may eventually cause it to contract and painfully compress the glans (phimosis) or predispose to cancer development. Squamous cell carcinoma of the penis is a rare tumor that occurs much more commonly in uncircumcised men. HPV plays a role in the development of some squamous cell carcinomas of the penis. Metastatic spread is usually to lymph nodes in the inguinal region. Tumor invasion of erectile tissue is a grim prognostic sign and is frequently associated with metastatic disease.

●●● UTERINE CERVIX

The uterine cervix comprises an ectocervix and an endocervix with a transition zone that undergoes squamous and glandular metaplasia during the menstrual cycle (Fig. 13-5). The inward and outward migration of the squamocolumnar junction is important to pathologic changes in the cervix related to HPV infection and cancer (see below). During gestation, the cervix must act as an effective valve preventing extrusion of the pregnancy, and cervical incompetence can result in gestational loss.

Before the advent of Papanicolaou (Pap) smears to screen for cervical dysplasia, carcinoma of the cervix was a major cause of cancer death in women in the United States. The effective implementation of screening with Pap smears has greatly reduced cervical cancer deaths although it remains a major killer of women in countries in which routine Pap smear screening is not performed. Infection with HPV is responsible for virtually all cases of squamous cell carcinoma of the cervix as well as many cases of cervical adenocarcinoma. Chronic infection with high-risk HPV can transform epithelial cells in the transition zone of the cervix that can ultimately result in invasive carcinoma. Squamous and glandular metaplasia in the transition zone predisposes to

infection with HPV by venereal spread. Male partners are usually unaware of infection.

So-called high-risk viral subtypes of HPV are more likely to progress to high-grade dysplasia and carcinoma than are other viral strains. In the United States, serotypes 16 and 18 are most frequently associated with the development of cervical cancer. Cytologic evaluation of brushings from the cervix and endocervix allows the identification of HPV-infected cells as well as cytologic changes indicative of dysplasia or carcinoma. Cells infected with HPV tend to show nuclear irregularity and enlargement with associated perinuclear clearing (so-called koilocytes) (Fig. 13-6A). If infection with high-risk virus is not cleared by the immune system, dysplastic cells may progress with an increase in the nuclear:cytoplasmic ratio and the development of hyperchromatic chromatin, which are features of high-grade dysplasia (i.e., high-grade squamous intraepithelial lesion, or HGSIL) (see Fig. 13-6B). The identification of persistent dysplasia by Pap smear usually leads to colposcopic examination and cervical biopsy to further evaluate the extent of dysplasia. Women with high-grade dysplasia and some women with persistent low-grade dysplasia are typically treated by electrocautery removal of dysplastic epithelium (Figs. 13-7A and 13-7B). Dysplasia usually involves the transition zone, and this area (around the cervical os) is targeted for excision. Since dysplasia is limited to the surface epithelium and endocervical glands, superficial excision has the potential to remove all dysplastic epithelium and prevent further progression to invasive carcinoma. A minority of patients have wider field effect changes or extension of dysplasia to the peripheral ectocervix or vaginal mucosa, making conservative management more difficult. Patients with micro-

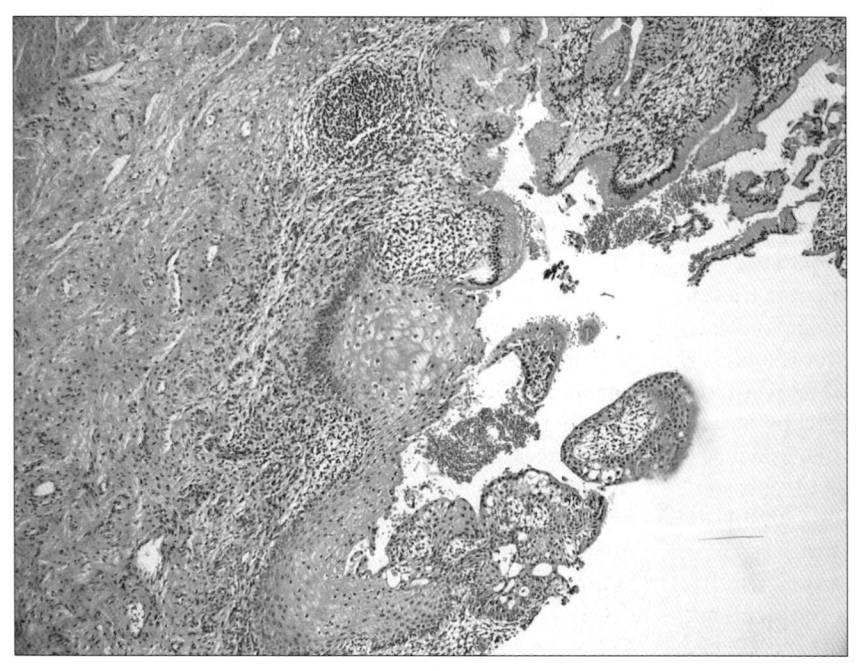

Figure 13-5. Squamous metaplasia of the cervical transformation zone. Microscopic section of uterine cervix with abutting squamous and glandular mucosa.

MICROBIOLOGY

Human Papillomavirus (HPV)

HPV is a double-stranded DNA virus that replicates as an episome in productively infected epithelial cells.

HPV can also transition to a latent stage in which provirus integrates into the host cell's genome at random sites. Latent virus produces relatively low-level expression of most viral genes. However, viral integration frequently interrupts the E2 gene, resulting in de-repression of E6 and E7 gene expression. If E6 and E7 proteins are effective in abrogating P53 and Rb control of cell cycle progression and apoptosis, these proteins can cause cell transformation and dysplasia or cancer.

Different viral serotypes code for E6 and E7 proteins that are more or less effective in transforming cells. HPV serotypes 16 and 18 are the most important causes of high-grade dysplasia and cancer in the United States by virtue of their highly oncogenic E6 and E7 proteins.

Different HPV serotypes have relatively specific affinity for different types of epithelia. Some serotypes preferentially infect the skin and other sites and produce warts but are only occasionally associated with neoplasia.

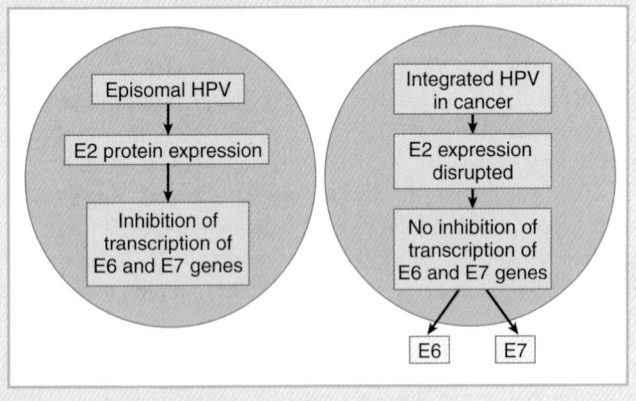

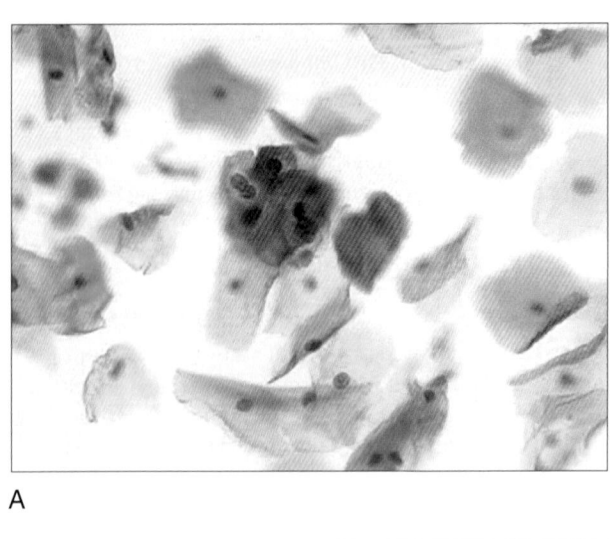

A

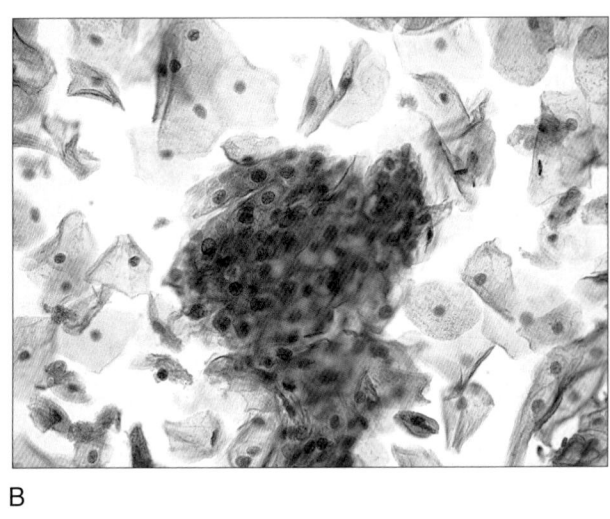

B

Figure 13-6. A, Low-grade squamous intraepithelial lesion (LGSIL). Liquid-based monolayer cytologic preparation showing a central cluster of LGSIL cells with perinuclear clearing, increased nuclear size, irregular nuclear contours, and nuclear hyperchromasia. Benign squamous superficial (pink cytoplasm) and intermediate (blue cytoplasm) cells are visible. **B,** High-grade squamous intraepithelial lesion (HGSIL). Liquid-based monolayer cytologic preparation showing a central cluster of HGSIL cells with markedly increased nuclear:cytoplasmic ratio and nuclear hyperchromasia.

invasive carcinomas are usually treated by radical hysterectomy (see Fig. 13-7C). Patients with more deeply invasive squamous cell carcinomas are often treated primarily with radiation therapy because their risk of tumor spread to lymph nodes is high (see Fig. 13-7D).

High-risk HPV strains can transform cervical epithelial cells by expressing proteins that interfere with normal cell cycle control functions. Expression of E6 and E7 proteins typically occur after viral integration into the human chromosome. E6 and E7 proteins can inactivate the P53 and retinoblastoma proteins, respectively, to bypass the G_1S checkpoint and initiate DNA synthesis. This two-hit attack on the G_1S checkpoint results in abnormal cell proliferation, and persistent infection promotes genetic instability, allowing dysplastic cells to acquire additional genetic changes that may result in the formation of an invasive carcinoma (see Chapter 5).

Most high-grade dysplasia does not progress to carcinoma, even in the absence of therapy, since HPV infection is cleared by an effective immune response. Most low-grade dysplasia

does not progress to high-grade dysplasia because of an effective immune response. A recent vaccine trial that immunized female college students against HPV-16 was effective in reducing the frequency of persistent HPV infections, at least over the limited time span of the study. Effective immunotherapy may have the potential to prevent the development of cervical dysplasia in the future.

●●● VULVA

The vulva is composed of specialized skin with underlying glands that can be infected with bacteria, resulting in abscess

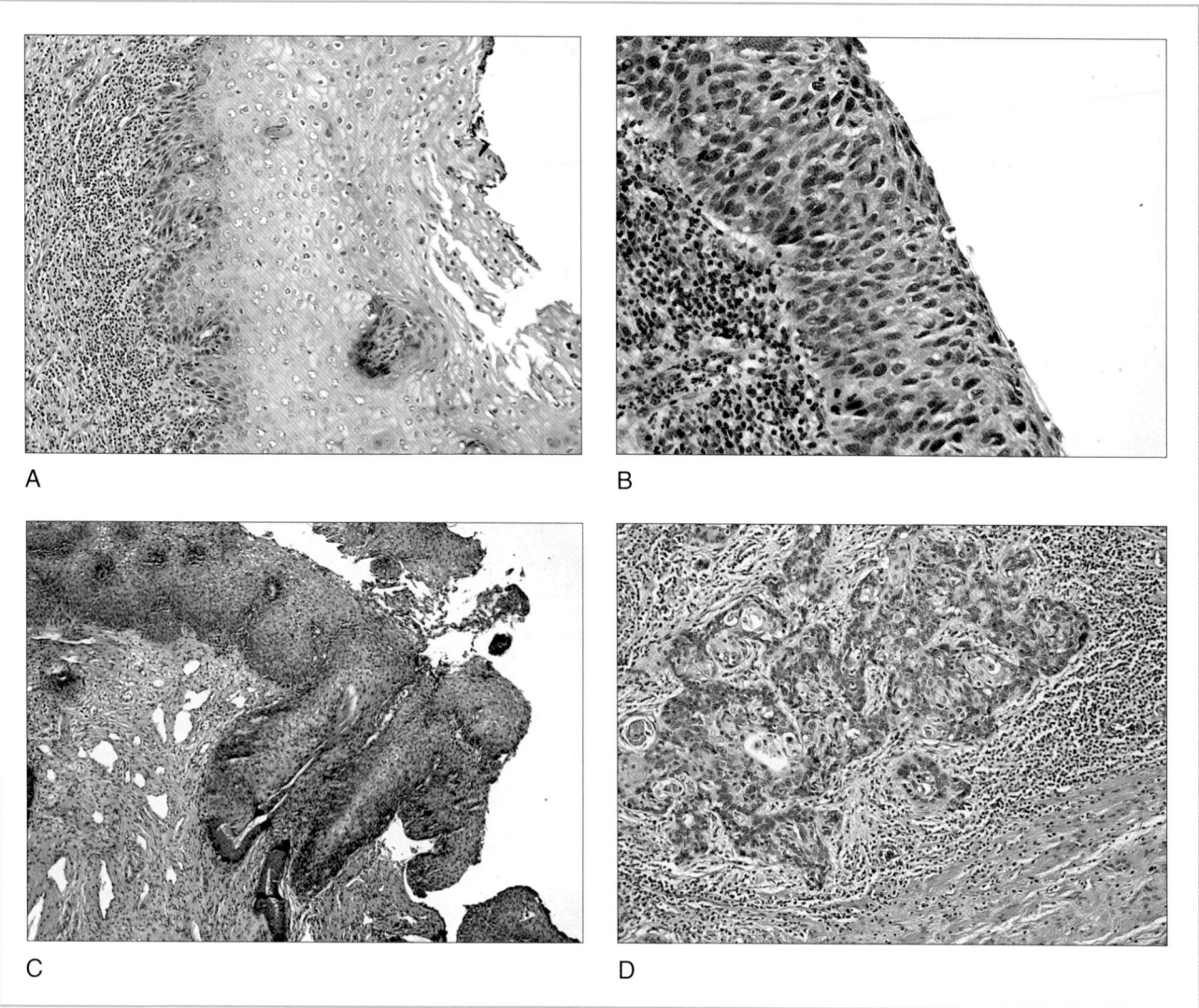

Figure 13-7. A, Low-grade squamous dysplasia (cervical intraepithelial neoplasia [CIN] I). Microscopic section of the cervical transformation zone showing koilocytosis (nuclear irregularity, perinuclear vacuolization, and occasional binucleation) with dysplastic squamous cells occupying the bottom third of the epithelium. **B,** High-grade squamous dysplasia (CIN II–III). Microscopic section of the cervical transformation zone showing replacement of the normal epithelium by dysplastic cells with markedly increased nuclear:cytoplasmic ratios and almost complete loss of surface maturation. The underlying basement membrane has a smooth, regular contour consistent with an in situ lesion. **C,** Squamous dysplasia involving endocervical glands. Microscopic section of the cervical transformation zone showing dysplastic squamous cells replacing the normal epithelial lining of endocervical glands. The underlying basement membrane has a smooth, regular contour that helps distinguish this in situ lesion from microinvasive squamous cell carcinoma. **D,** Microinvasive squamous cell carcinoma. Microscopic section of the cervical transformation zone showing invasive nests of squamous cell carcinoma. The contours of these nests are irregular and angulated (in contrast with in situ lesions). The depth of invasion in this case is less than 0.5 cm from the surface mucosa (which defines microinvasive carcinoma).

formation (e.g., Bartholin gland abscess). Postmenopausal atrophy of the hormonally responsive vulvar mucosa can result in bleeding and inflammation. Two forms of vulvar dystrophy are usually distinguished. Hyperplastic dystrophy corresponds to a thickening of the squamous mucosa with increased layers of keratinocytes. Lichen sclerosis is an inflammatory dystrophy that causes fibrosis of dermal collagen and atrophy and flattening of the squamous mucosa (loss of normal rete ridges) (Fig. 13-8A). Both of these conditions are responsive to estrogen. Vulvar dystrophy usually does not evolve into dysplasia or carcinoma, but some patients may have combined features of dystrophy and dysplasia.

Dysplasia and Carcinoma

Vulvar dysplasia is usually a disease of older women and is usually not associated with HPV infection. Vulvar intraepithelial neoplasia (VIN) is similar to cervical intraepithelial neoplasia, and high-grade VIN corresponds to squamous cell carcinoma in situ. There is often a field effect with

HISTOLOGY

Cervical-Vaginal Cytology

The Papanicolaou (Pap) smear was originally performed using a smooth stick to sample the ectocervix, endocervix, and transformation zone. Exfoliated cells were smeared on a glass slide and spray-fixed to prevent air-drying artifact. This procedure is technically difficult and can result in suboptimal preparations because of inadequate sampling of the transformation zone or air-drying artifact (particularly in postmenopausal women).

The use of a cytobrush allows more complete and reliable sampling of the endocervix and transformation zone, and the advent of liquid-based cytology in which the cytobrush is immersed in a fixative solution has greatly enhanced the analytical reproducibility of Pap smears.

Specialized equipment can utilize liquid-based Pap smears to produce a cell monolayer on glass slides. These monolayer smears are more readily interpreted by humans and can be assessed morphometrically by computer-based image analysis. Since the major cytologic features of dysplasia and carcinoma correspond to morphometric abnormalities (e.g., changes in nuclear:cytoplasmic ratio, nuclear staining intensity, dispersion pattern of nuclear chromatin), these new techniques have enhanced the quality and reproducibility of cervical-vaginal screening.

More recently, the addition of a hybridization assay to detect high-risk HPV DNA in cytologically equivocal cervical-vaginal specimens has further improved risk stratification and streamlined patient management.

Cytology (Bethesda System)	Histology	Cervical Intraepithelial Neoplasia (CIN)
NILM	Negative for dysplasia	—
ASCUS	(Variable)	—
LGSIL	Koilocytosis	—
	Mild dysplasia	CIN I
HGSIL	Moderate dysplasia	CIN II
	Severe dysplasia	CIN III
Carcinoma	Carcinoma	—

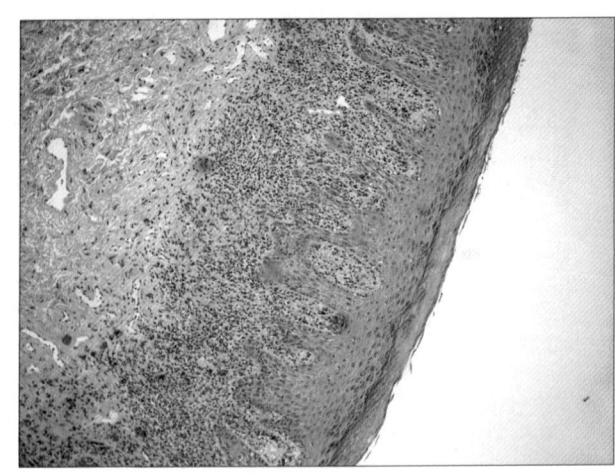

A

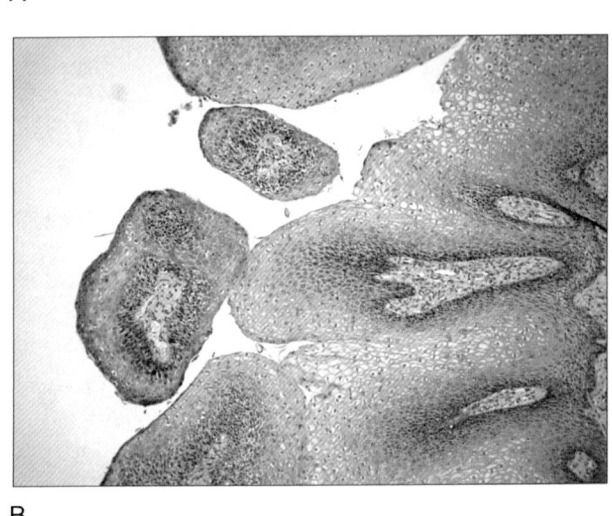

B

Figure 13-8. A, Lichen sclerosis. Microscopic section of vulvar mucosa showing hyperkeratosis and loss of rete ridges with flattening of the mucosa and a mild chronic inflammatory cell infiltrate. **B,** Vaginal condyloma. Microscopic section of a condyloma acuminatum with papillary growth pattern and prominent koilocytic change in squamous cells.

dysplastic changes that can involve the entire vulva and may require a skinning vulvectomy (excision of the entire epidermis). Invasive squamous cell carcinoma can quickly result in inguinal lymph node metastases. Vulvar and perianal condylomas are more common in younger women and also are caused by HPV infection and may progress to carcinoma (see Fig. 13-8B).

Melanoma

The vulva is a pigmented squamous mucosa with melanocytes from which melanomas can arise. Vulvar melanomas are usually polyploid and nodular and differ substantially from cutaneous melanomas that are strongly associated with sun exposure. Vulvar melanoma is often deeply invasive when it is discovered, and lymph node and systemic metastases are frequently present.

Paget's Disease

Paget's disease can develop in the vulva as well as in perianal skin and the nipple of the breast (see In situ Carcinoma in the Breast section). Paget's disease corresponds to the migration of individual tumor cells between keratinocytes in the skin. Paget's disease of the vulva is usually associated with an underlying adenocarcinoma, but in some cases no underlying tumor is discovered and excision of the involved mucosa may be curative.

●●● VAGINA

HPV-related squamous dysplasia of the vagina occurs but much less commonly than cervical dysplasia (probably as a result of viral affinity for the epithelium at the transformation zone of the cervix). Patients treated with hysterectomy for cervical dysplasia or cervical cancer may have recurrence of dysplasia in the vagina. Rhabdomyosarcoma of the vagina can occur in the pediatric age group and produces nodular tumor masses protruding into the vagina (so-called sarcoma botryoides).

Adenosis of the vagina means the development of glands beneath the squamous mucosa. Vaginal adenosis is almost completely restricted to patients who were exposed to diethylstilbestrol (DES) during gestation. This drug has not been used in pregnant women for more than 30 years so the affected cohort is currently over 30 years of age. Patients with adenosis are at risk for the development of adenocarcinoma of the vagina that has distinctive clear-cell morphology (Fig. 13-9). Patients treated with DES may also have cervical incompetence that predisposes to pregnancy loss.

●●● UTERINE CORPUS

The uterus is a dynamic organ that changes markedly during the menstrual cycle and undergoes massive change during normal pregnancy. Endometrial biopsy or endometrial curettage is often performed for the evaluation of abnormal uterine bleeding, which may result from endometrial hyperplasia or adenocarcinoma. Endometrial biopsy is also used to assess possible causes of infertility and to establish the precise time of ovulation for in vitro fertilization procedures.

The menstrual cycle begins after the completion of menses when there is a transition to the proliferative phase with active cell division in small endometrial glands and stromal cells. Just before ovulation, endometrial glands acquire subnuclear vacuoles in their cytoplasm, and the presence of well-developed subnuclear vacuoles in more than half the glands in a biopsy specimen is diagnostic of ovulation. Following ovulation, vacuoles disappear and glands expand, becoming tortuous and producing luminal secretions. Endometrial stroma becomes edematous and then undergoes pseudo-decidual change as progesterone dominates the latter portions of the menstrual cycle. This pseudodecidual change begins as a swelling of stromal cells beneath the endometrial lining epithelium and around blood vessels and eventually involves all the stroma just before menses. Decidualized stromal cells have abundant eosinophilic cytoplasm and reactive-appearing nuclei. At menses, acute inflammatory cells infiltrate the endometrium, and there is ischemic necrosis of endometrium with exodus of degenerating endometrial tissue fragments. If pregnancy occurs, hormonal changes cause the endometrium to maintain a so-called hypersecretory pattern.

In perimenopausal women, diminished hormonal signaling often results in anovulatory cycles in which endometrial sloughing is incomplete, and the endometrium may build up in thickness from cycle to cycle. This buildup may result in the formation of endometrial polyps, which typically have large, thick-walled blood vessels at their core (Figs. 13-10A and 13-10B). Endometrial polyps are common causes of abnormal intramenstrual bleeding. Since polyps persist from cycle to cycle, long-term exposure to estrogen stimulation can result in hyperplasia and neoplasia.

Endometriosis and Adenomyosis

Endometriosis is the presence of endometrial glands with endometrial stroma and hemosiderin-containing macrophages

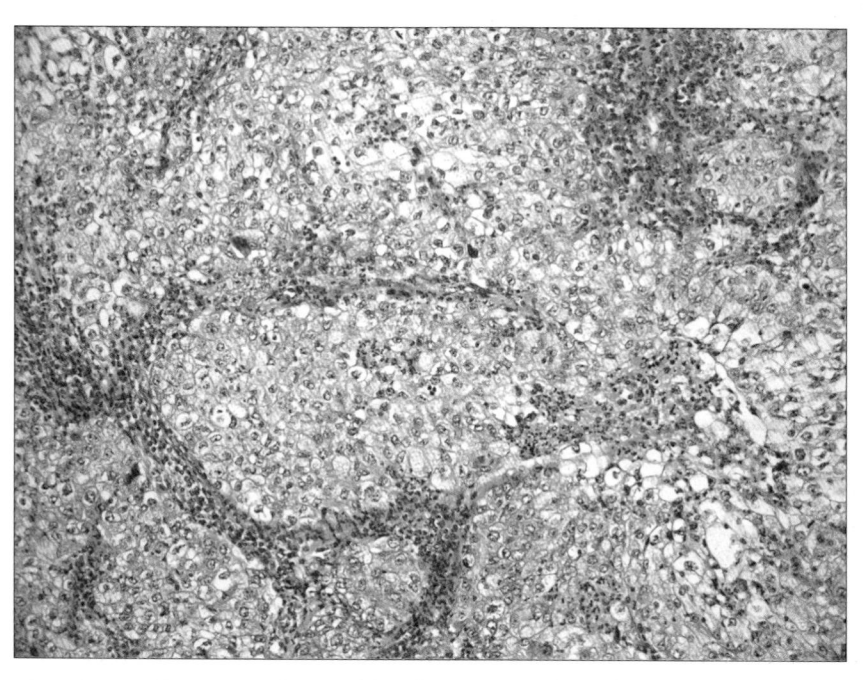

Figure 13-9. Clear-cell carcinoma of the vagina. Microscopic section from a vaginal tumor showing invasive nests of tumor cells with abundant, clear cytoplasm. Lymphocytes are abundant in the intervening stroma.

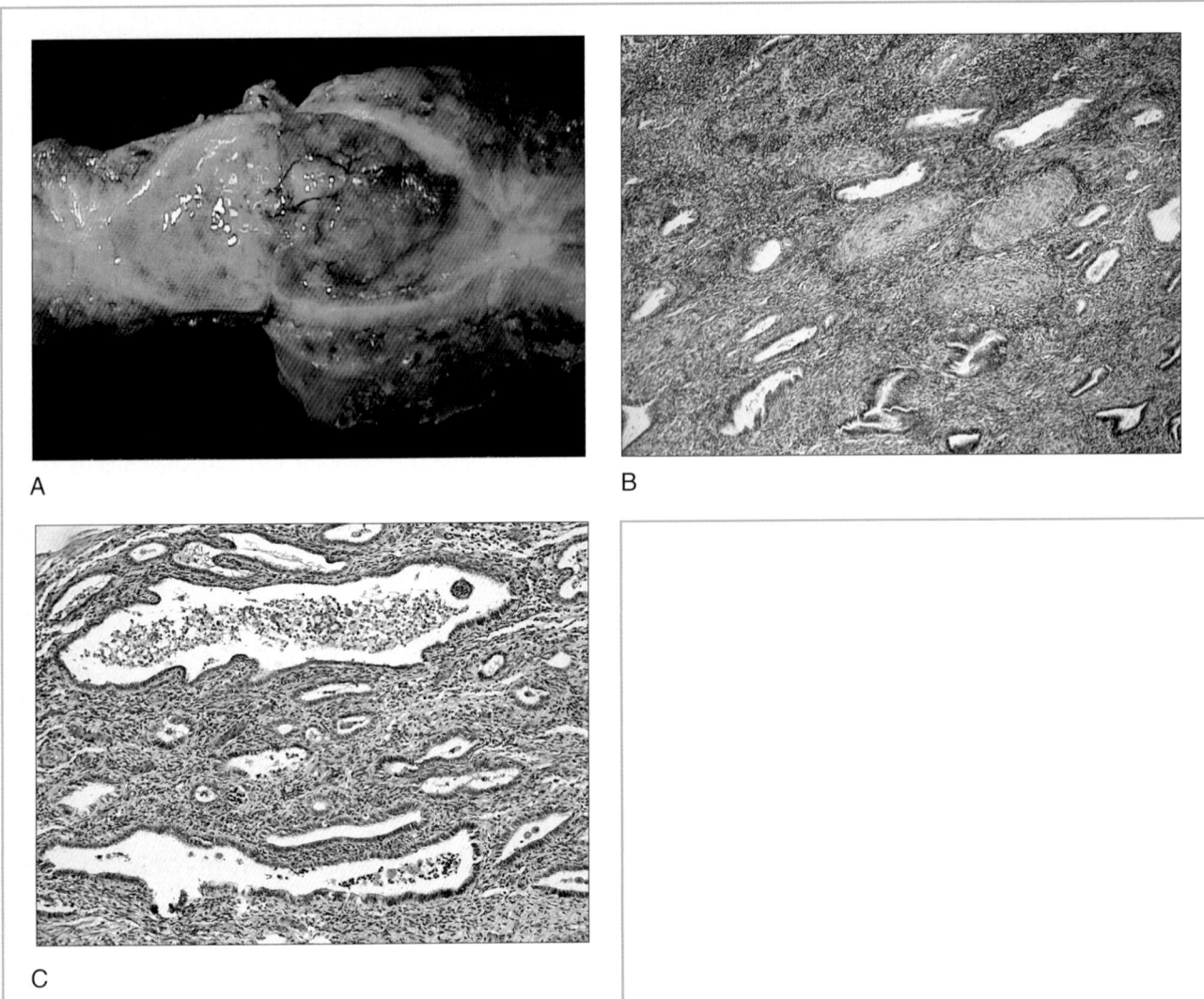

Figure 13-10. A, Endometrial polyp. Gross photograph of an opened endometrial cavity showing a large polyp in the uterine fundus. **B**, Microscopic section of endometrial polyp showing benign endometrial glands and prominent, thick-walled blood vessels. **C**, Endometriosis. Microscopic section from a focus of endometriosis showing endometrial glands and stroma with scattered histiocytes containing hemosiderin.

at a site outside the uterine myometrium (see Fig. 13-10C). Endometriosis may involve any location throughout the abdominal cavity (or occasionally beyond) but is more common in the pelvis and uterine adnexa. The cause of endometriosis is controversial. For many years it was thought that reflux of endometrial contents through the fallopian tubes into the abdominal cavity resulted in implants of endometriosis that then grew and responded to hormonal stimulation during the menstrual cycle. Other investigators believe that endometriosis results from metaplasia of müllerian-derived peritoneal epithelium in response to hormonal stimulation. Regardless of its cause, endometriosis causes pain and occasionally significant intra-abdominal bleeding that is menstrual cycle dependent. Endometriosis may involve the appendix and simulate acute appendicitis as well as an acute abdomen. The presence of endometriotic implants at various sites throughout the pelvis and

associated inflammation is a significant cause of infertility. Endometriosis is also a risk factor for endometrial clear-cell carcinoma, which can develop in foci of endometriosis and has similar or identical features to ovarian clear-cell carcinoma.

Adenomyosis is essentially endometriosis within the myometrium. Since the myometrium and endometrial stroma interdigitate at their junction, adenomyosis is operationally defined as the presence of endometrial glands and stroma more than one low-power microscope field deep to the endometrial cavity.

Uterine Tumors

Endometrial Hyperplasia and Endometrial Adenocarcinoma

Endometrial hyperplasia means an abnormal increase in the ratio of glands to endometrial stroma. Endometrial hyperplasia usually results from prolonged or unopposed estrogen stimulation without the effects of progesterone to cause sloughing of the endometrium. The development of endometrial polyps facilitates the development of hyperplasia. Anovulatory cycles in perimenopausal women may predispose to hyperplasia (similar to the effects of unopposed estrogen stimulation in postmenopausal women). Endometrial hyperplasia is usually categorized as simple or complex. Complex hyperplasia corresponds to branched and tortuous glands, whereas simple hyperplasia corresponds to regularly shaped glands that are too numerous and may become tightly packed together.

Atypical hyperplasia is the direct precursor of endometrial adenocarcinoma and shows significant cytologic atypia in hyperplastic endometrial glands. Endometrial adenocarcinoma is usually diagnosed on the basis of endometrial biopsy or curettage and back-to-back glands, cytologic atypia, and the presence of cribriforming (punched-out spaces in the neoplastic epithelium caused by apoptosis). Most endometrial adenocarcinomas are of the endometrioid type and resemble normal endometrial glands (Fig. 13-11A). FIGO (Fédération Internationale de Gynécologie et d'Obstétrique) tumor grade is based on the amount of solid (non-gland-forming) tumor present, with higher grade tumors being composed predominantly of solid sheets of neoplastic cells. High-grade nuclear features can increase the FIGO tumor grade, which is predictive of the likelihood of extrauterine tumor extension.

Squamous metaplasia is common in well to moderately differentiated endometrioid adenocarcinomas but does not affect the prognosis or clinical behavior (see Fig. 13-11B). Patients with either FIGO grade 3/3 tumors or invasion of more than 50% of the myometrium are usually treated with radical hysterectomy and lymph node dissection because of their substantially higher risk of metastatic disease. Patients with lower grade tumors and more superficial myometrial invasion are usually treated with radical hysterectomy alone. Precise tumor staging is important for assessing prognosis, with invasion of the parametrium or involvement of the endocervix upstaging tumors.

Other morphologic types of adenocarcinoma can develop in the endometrium including clear-cell carcinoma and papillary serous adenocarcinoma, which share many features with their more common ovarian counterparts.

Tumors of the ovary or fallopian tube can secondarily involve the endometrium by extension through the lumen of the fallopian tube. In some cases, it may be difficult or impossible to distinguish metastatic ovarian carcinoma from synchronous adenocarcinomas in the endometrium and ovary.

Leiomyoma

Leiomyomas are smooth muscle tumors that are extraordinarily common in the myometrium (Fig. 13-12). In premenopausal women, submucosal leiomyomas are an important cause of infertility and abnormal uterine bleeding and may present as adnexal or abdominal masses. Uterine leiomyomas can become quite large, are often hyalinized

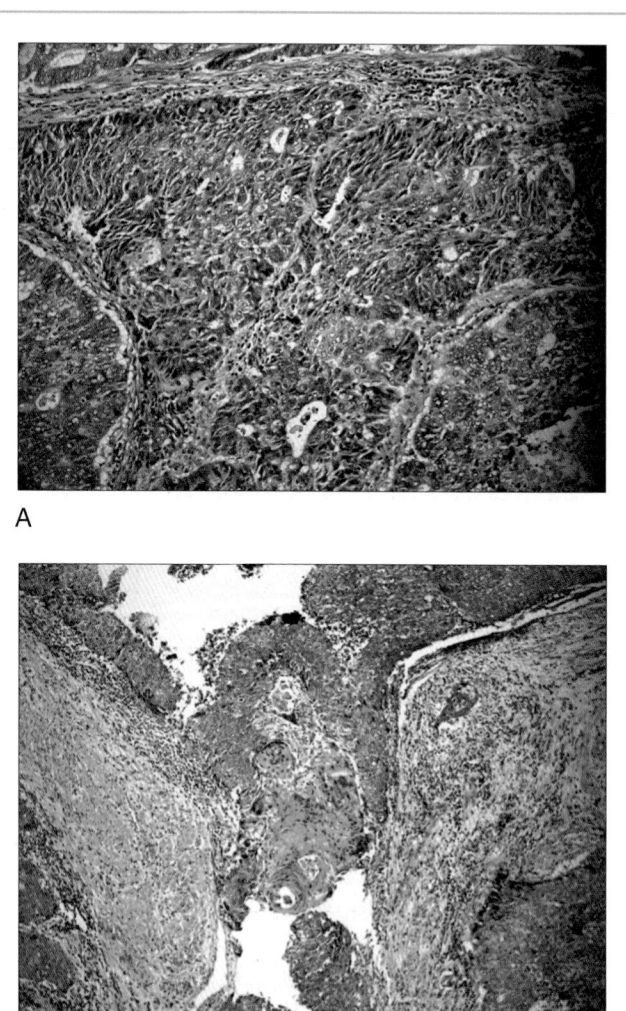

Figure 13-11. A, Uterine endometrioid adenocarcinoma. Microscopic section from a moderately differentiated adenocarcinoma of the endometrium. Irregular nests of tumor cells invade myometrial tissue. **B**, Uterine endometrioid adenocarcinoma with squamous metaplasia. Microscopic section of an endometrioid adenocarcinoma with prominent squamous metaplasia.

(hypocellular fibrosis), and may undergo dystrophic calcification.

Leiomyosarcomas are rare, malignant smooth muscle tumors that can develop from leiomyomas in the uterus. Tumor necrosis and mitotic rate are important predictors of malignancy in smooth muscle tumors, and gross evaluation for necrosis is a useful screening tool in hysterectomy specimens. Tumors with more than ten mitotic figures per ten high-power fields are usually diagnosed as leiomyosarcomas while tumors with an intermediate number of mitotic figures are provisionally classified as smooth muscle tumors of uncertain malignant potential. Leiomyomas with significant cytologic atypia may be classified as leiomyosarcomas with a lower proliferative rate than cytologically bland tumors. If metastatic disease develops, hematogenous spread to the lungs is typical.

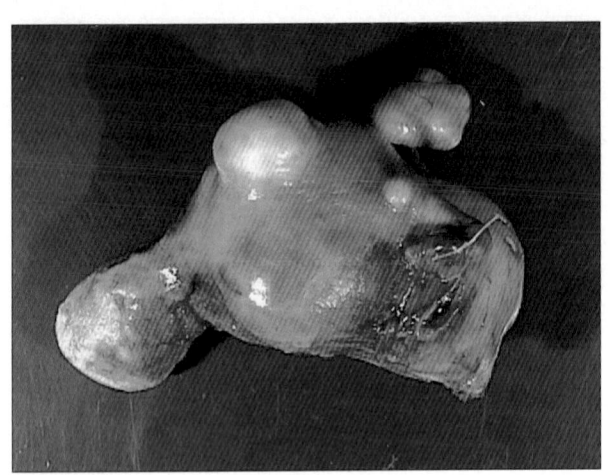

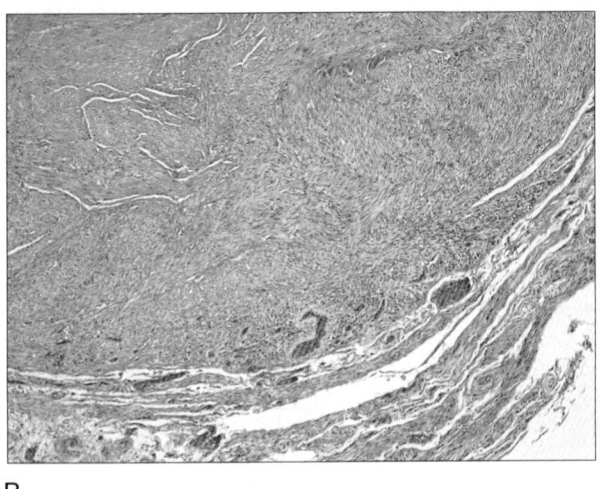

Figure 13-12. Uterine leiomyomas. **A**, Gross image of excised uterus (cervix at bottom left) with multiple leiomyomas bulging and distorting the serosal surface. **B**, Microscopic section of a leiomyoma with central hyalinization (*top*). A small amount of normal myometrium is visible (*bottom*).

Intravenous leiomyomatosis is an unusual condition that corresponds to a cytologically benign smooth muscle tumor in an intravascular location possibly involving large vessels in the pelvis. A so-called benign metastasizing leiomyoma is a cytologically bland smooth muscle tumor (a very low grade leiomyosarcoma) that typically presents as lung metastasis with a histologically benign appearance (i.e., no pleomorphism, necrosis, or demonstrable mitotic activity).

Other Tumors

Endometrial stromal sarcoma is a neoplasm of variable aggressiveness that arises from endometrial stromal cells and typically expresses estrogen and progesterone receptors. A *malignant mixed müllerian tumor* (MMMT) is a highly malignant tumor in older women that may arise in the uterus or the ovary. MMMT shows both epithelial and sarcomatous differentiation, and components of rhabdomyosarcoma and osteosarcoma may be present. There is now compelling evidence that MMMT is a metaplastic carcinoma (i.e., a carcinoma with mesenchymal metaplasia) rather than a truly biphasic neoplasm. Most MMMTs have spread beyond the uterus at the time of diagnosis and are incurable.

●●● COMPLICATIONS OF PREGNANCY

Hypertension can develop as a complication of normal pregnancy with maternal blood pressure increasing during the third trimester (preeclampsia) that usually responds to bed rest. Some patients with preeclampsia develop more severe hypertension, which may progress to eclampsia with seizure activity if blood pressure is not reduced. Delivery is curative, but severe maternal complications can develop (permanent renal damage and hemorrhagic stroke).

Gestational diabetes is the development of diabetic blood glucose levels during pregnancy in patients who were previously normoglycemic. Additional demand for insulin because of the stress of pregnancy or increased insulin resistance underlies gestational diabetes. Some affected patients may have borderline type 2 diabetes prior to pregnancy. Gestational diabetes can result in macrosomia of neonates (abnormally large babies), which can complicate vaginal delivery.

Placental Disease

Diseases of the placenta can result in intrauterine growth retardation or fetal death. Maternal hypertension during pregnancy (preeclampsia and eclampsia) predisposes to placental infarction. A few small infarcts are common in term placentas; however, infarction of a larger amount of placental tissue can compromise fetal nutrition and may result in intrauterine growth retardation or death in utero. Placental abruption (separation of the placenta from the myometrium by the formation of a large hematoma) can occur at or before delivery and may result in loss of fetal nutrition and oxygen supply. Placental location over the cervical os (placenta previa) precludes normal delivery. Premature rupture of placental membranes usually results in an ascending bacterial infection that can cause chorioamnionitis if delivery is significantly delayed, resulting in fetal stress or demise.

Gestational Trophoblastic Disease

Gestational trophoblastic disease is the abnormal persistence of placental tissue after a normal pregnancy or any type of molar pregnancy. Placental site trophoblastic tumor is a rare complication of normal pregnancy in which the placental implantation site in the myometrium persists after delivery and continues to grow as a tumor. Hysterectomy is usually curative, but metastatic disease can develop (Fig. 13-13A).

Hydatidiform mole is in abnormal placental proliferation that is usually not associated with the presence of a viable fetus. Hydatidiform moles consist of markedly dilated chorionic villi lined by hyperplastic trophoblast that can fill

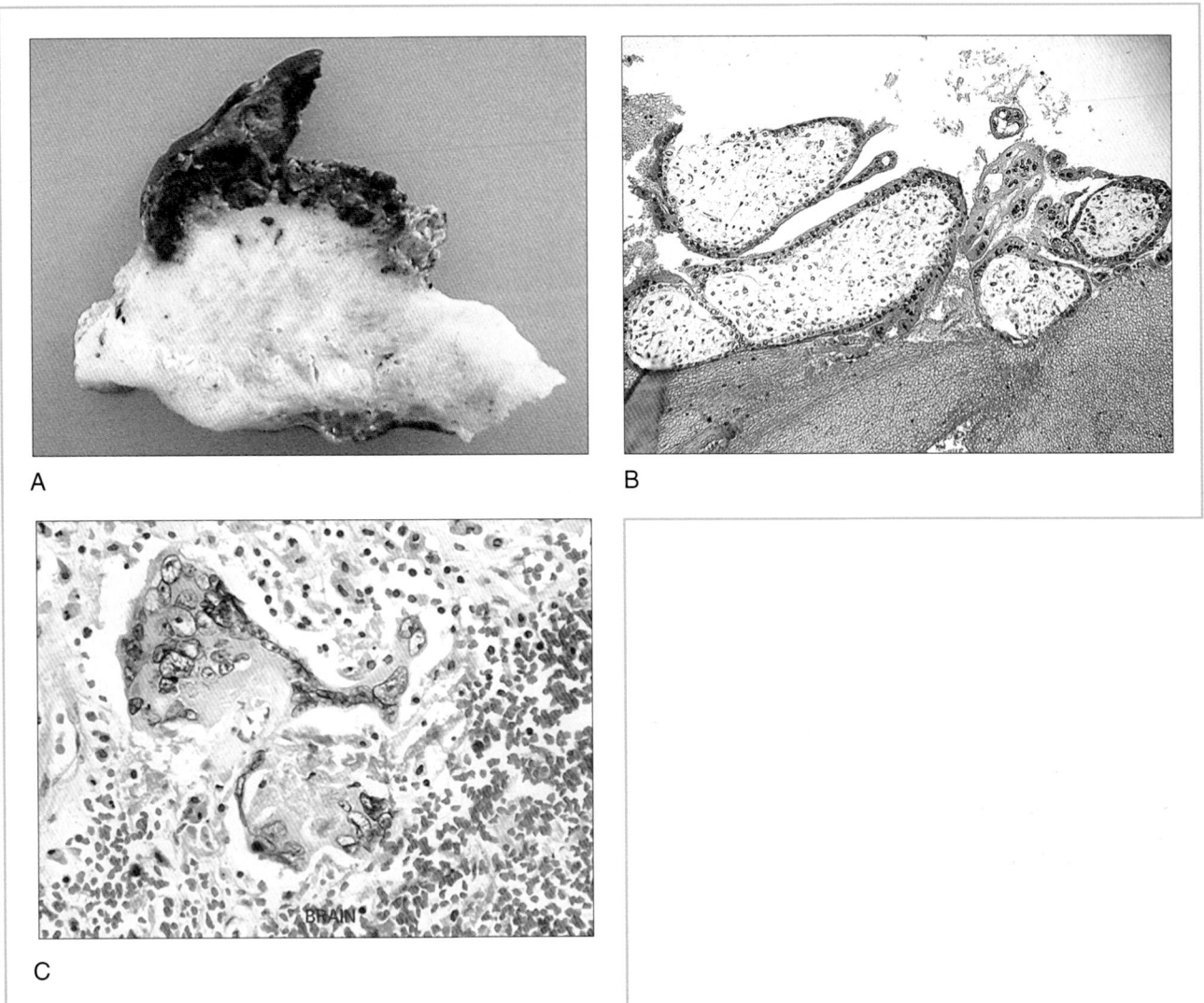

Figure 13-13. A, Placental site trophoblastic tumor. Gross cross-section of uterine wall showing invasive trophoblastic disease (reddish-brown tissue) infiltrating the myometrium (tan-white tissue). **B,** Hydatidiform mole. Microscopic section showing markedly edematous chorionic villi with central spaces (cisterns). The abnormal villi are lined by hyperplastic trophoblast. **C,** Choriocarcinoma. Microscopic section showing neoplastic syncytiotrophoblast (multinucleated tumor giant cells) mixed with neoplastic cytotrophoblast (single nuclei).

the endometrial cavity, resulting in the typical ultrasound and gross appearance of multiple fluid-filled cysts (see Fig. 13-13B). Hydatidiform mole produces larger amounts of hCG than a normal gestation, and increased serum hCG levels may be the first clue to the diagnosis. Endometrial curettage is usually curative although some moles invade the myometrium (invasive moles) and may persist after curettage. Persistent moles can be eliminated with a brief course of methotrexate therapy. Moles are classified as partial or complete. Partial moles usually have triploid chromosome content and may be associated with a fetus, whereas complete moles are usually diploid. Since hydatidiform moles secrete large amounts of hCG, patients can be followed by serial serum hCG measurements to exclude recurrent or persistent disease.

Choriocarcinoma is a fully malignant tumor composed of cytotrophoblast and syncytiotrophoblast that can derive from a molar pregnancy or from a germ cell tumor (see Fig. 13-13C). Choriocarcinoma often metastasizes widely, producing hemorrhagic metastatic deposits. Even patients with extensive metastatic disease are potentially curable by conventional chemotherapy.

●●● FALLOPIAN TUBE

The fallopian tube is lined with ciliated columnar epithelium. Blockage of the fallopian tube may cause infertility and predispose to the development of ectopic pregnancy. Mesonephric and wolffian embryonic remnants commonly form small cysts about the fallopian tubes, which generally are not of clinical significance. Venereal spread of gonorrhea and *Chlamydia* can both produce ascending infection that results in abscess formation within the fallopian tube or in the formation of a tubo-ovarian abscess involving the entire adnexa (Fig. 13-14). Infection can result in sepsis and scarring with secondary infertility.

Ectopic pregnancy most often occurs in the fallopian tube but can occur in the peritoneal cavity as a result of an abnormal implantation event. As the gestational sac grows, the tube is stretched and usually ruptures if the pregnancy is not removed. Tubal obstruction is a significant predisposing factor to ectopic pregnancy.

Primary adenocarcinomas of the fallopian tube are rarely diagnosed although advanced tumors of the fallopian tube may present clinically as more common ovarian adenocarcinomas.

●●● OVARY

The ovary is composed of characteristic stroma with embedded germ cells. A few germ cells are activated during each menstrual cycle and induce the differentiation of granulosa cells to form follicles that eventually rupture at the time of ovulation, causing the ovum to pass to the fallopian tube where fertilization may occur. The ovary is supplied by a neurovascular bundle with the potential to undergo torsion similarly to the testis. The ovary (as well as the remainder of the adnexa and pelvic peritoneum) is lined by müllerian-derived mesothelium that has the potential to form epithelial ovarian tumors (see below).

Polycystic Ovary Syndrome

Polycystic ovary syndrome typically occurs in obese young women and is often associated with hirsutism and evidence of androgen access. Patients usually have primary infertility, and their ovaries appear polycystic on ultrasound examination.

Ovarian Tumors

Tumors of the ovary are divided into three categories based on their origin from the surface epithelium, stroma, or germ cells. Epithelial tumors are the most frequent and clinically serious type of ovarian tumor and correspond to a number of different subtypes of ovarian carcinoma and epithelial tumors of low malignant potential (frequently called borderline tumors).

EMBRYOLOGY

Wolffian and Mesonephric Duct Remnants

Wolffian and müllerian ducts form sequentially in the embryonic pronephros that will become the kidney.

The wolffian duct is an extension of the mesonephric ducts that will become the tubular portion of the epididymis, vas deferens, and ejaculatory duct in males. In females, the wolffian duct atrophies but remains as blind tubules and cysts in the mesosalpinx and para-ovarian and parametrial soft tissue.

In females, the müllerian ducts develop into the fallopian tubes and fuse to form the uterus and vagina. In males, the müllerian ducts atrophy, and traces remain in the appendix testis and the prostatic utricle.

Any of these residual epithelial inclusions can enlarge and undergo metaplasia, which may mimic cysts and tumors of the urogenital organs.

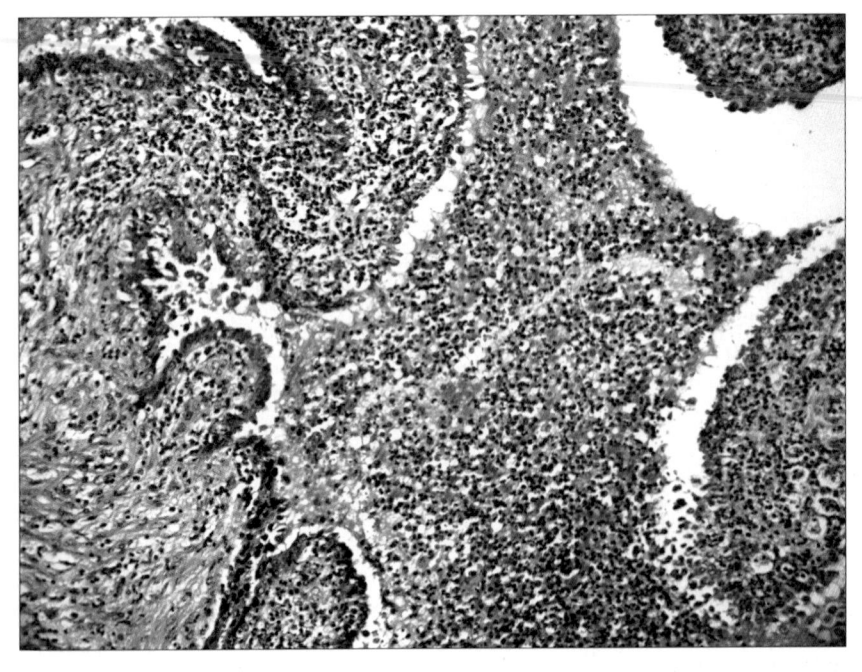

Figure 13-14. Acute salpingitis. Microscopic section of fallopian tube showing marked acute inflammation in the lumen and lining mucosa.

Epithelial Tumors

Epithelial tumors of the ovary derive from the mesothelium that covers the adnexa and pelvic peritoneum. Tumors that are identical to ovarian tumors can arise from multipotential müllerian-derived mesothelium at any of these sites although a primary ovarian surface location is most common.

Cystadenoma

Cystadenomas and cystadenofibromas are benign proliferative cysts lined by a bland layer of epithelium that is usually cuboidal or columnar. Most are unicystic, but multicystic cystadenomas may occur. Cystadenomas usually have a few blunt papillations; however, complicated papillary architecture and significant cytologic atypia are not present. Cystadenomas have stroma that is similar to ovarian stroma, and their epithelial lining is usually serous or mucinous. Cystadenomas can become very large and contain huge amounts (liters) of mucinous or serous fluid. Cystadenofibromas have a more prominent stromal component than cystadenomas and tend to form more prominent blunt papillae that can extend into the lumen of the cyst or outward from its wall. Simple adenofibromas are benign, but borderline forms also occur.

Borderline Tumors

Borderline tumors (also called tumors of low malignant potential) merge some features of cystadenoma (or adenofibroma) with those of ovarian carcinoma. Most borderline tumors are serous and are multicystic with prominent papillations on their internal and external surfaces (Fig. 13-15A). Borderline tumors show cytologic atypia with characteristic tufting of epithelial cells forming a pseudostratified epithelium (see Fig. 13-15B). Borderline tumors may be large, and many serous borderline tumors are bilateral at presentation.

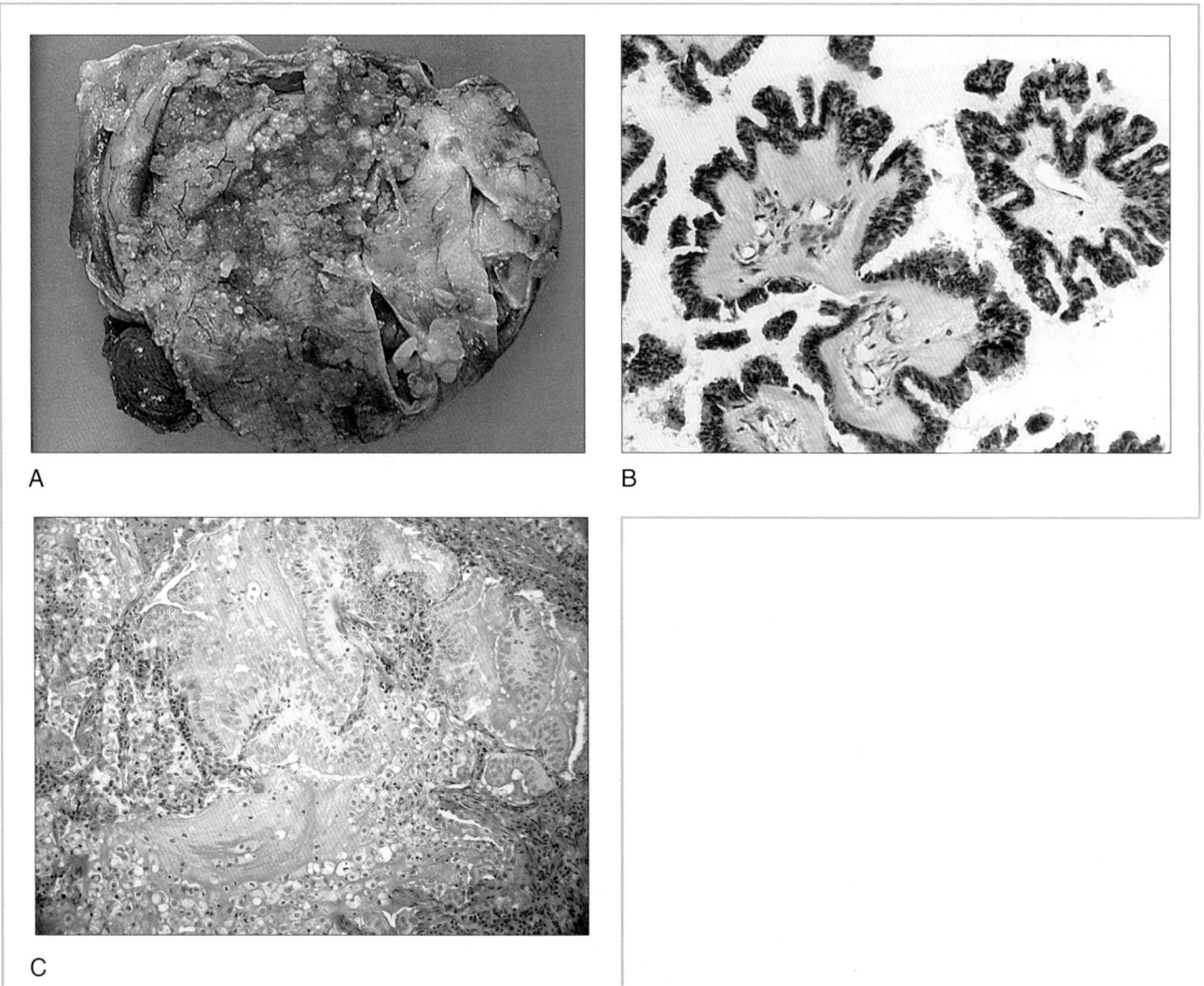

A

B

C

Figure 13-15. Ovarian serous borderline tumor. **A**, Gross photograph of a cystic tumor mass with papillations on its external and internal surfaces. **B**, Microscopic section showing stromal papillae lined by serous epithelium with prominent tufting. No destructive stromal invasion is present. **C**, Ovarian mucinous borderline tumor. Microscopic section showing abundant mucin produced by cytologically bland tumor cells that line stromal cores.

Borderline tumors can develop outside the ovary (in müllerian-derived mesothelium) although most are confined to the ovary at the time of diagnosis. Borderline tumors are distinguished from carcinomas by the lack of destructive stromal invasion. Since these tumors are multicystic and contain complex populations, usual histologic criteria cannot be used to assess stromal invasion. Destructive stromal invasion is a relatively subtle pathologic concept that distinguishes tumor-induced stromal overgrowth from destructive invasion of stroma by tumor cells (a feature of carcinomas). Mucinous borderline tumors are less common (see Fig. 13-15C) than serous tumors and are often more heterogeneous with a greater likelihood that a focal invasive carcinoma may be present.

Borderline tumors may result in "noninvasive" tumor implants throughout the peritoneal cavity and omentum. These implants are not called metastases, and it is not clear whether they represent synchronous tumor foci or actual spread from the primary tumor. Implants that show destructive stromal invasion are classified as invasive implants and have a less favorable prognosis that is still far superior to the prognosis for most ovarian carcinomas. Although borderline tumors are not fully malignant neoplasms, borderline tumors with widespread peritoneal implants are usually treated with chemotherapy. The response is usually excellent, and they are often cured. This markedly favorable prognosis compared with ovarian carcinoma justifies their clinical categorization as borderline tumors. Some borderline tumors (particularly mucinous tumors) likely represent a transitional stage in the development of a fully malignant carcinoma, whereas others (particularly serous borderline tumors) probably are not precursors of carcinoma (Fig. 13-16). Borderline tumors can also have endometrioid

or clear-cell morphology and are thought to arise in foci of endometriosis similarly to their malignant counterparts.

Carcinoma

The most common ovarian carcinoma is papillary serous adenocarcinoma, which usually shows prominent papillary architecture, often with psammoma bodies (Fig. 13-17). Tumor cells are pleomorphic and show prominent tufting with malignant cytologic features and destructive stromal invasion. Serous tumors are usually widely disseminated throughout the abdominal cavity at the time of diagnosis, and peritoneal fluid cytologic specimens may be diagnostic. Tumors tend to spread along peritoneal surfaces and may encase abdominal organs. Lymph node metastases and solid intraparenchymal metastases occur with ovarian carcinomas but are less common and less characteristic than surface spread and involvement of ascites fluid. Tumors are frequently bilateral, and extensive omental disease (so-called omental caking) is typical.

Patients with ovarian carcinoma typically have markedly elevated CA125 levels. Standard therapy for ovarian cancer is to maximally debulk the tumor surgically (i.e., remove primary tumor and secondary metastatic foci within the abdominal cavity in a piecemeal fashion to the maximum extent possible). Patients who can be "debulked" to a point where no remaining individual tumor foci are greater than 1 cm in diameter have a better outcome than patients who cannot be debulked to this extent. Many patients with ovarian cancer have a good response to paclitaxel (Taxol) and platinum-based chemotherapy, although recurrence is common.

Mucinous ovarian carcinomas often develop in the setting of mucinous borderline tumors with transformation of these tumors to invasive adenocarcinomas. Mucinous ovarian tumors tend to be heterogeneous so that extensive sampling

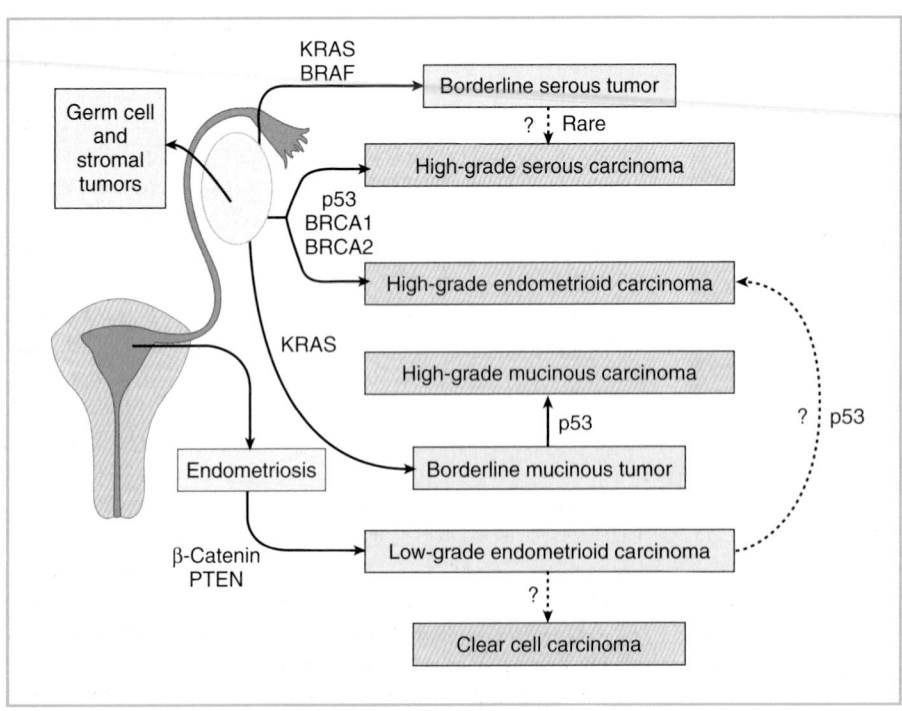

Figure 13-16. Epithelial ovarian tumor development.

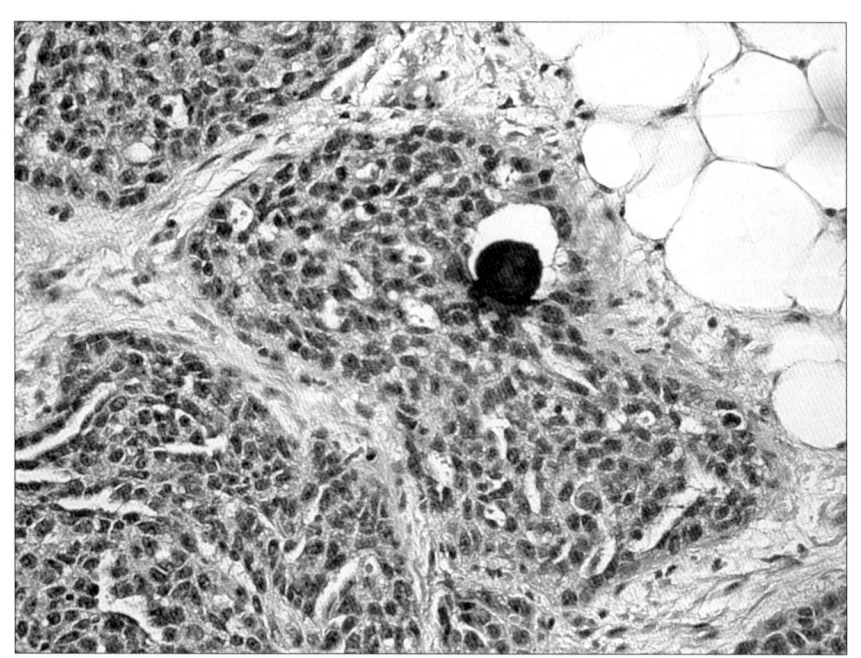

Figure 13-17. Ovarian papillary serous carcinoma. Microscopic section showing pleomorphic tumor cells with a micropapillary growth pattern. A characteristic psammoma body is visible (laminated calcification that appears purple-blue).

BIOCHEMISTRY

CA125 Tumor Marker

CA125 is a heavily glycosylated protein that is elevated in the serum of more than 80% of women with epithelial ovarian cancer. The first antibody directed against CA125 was produced using an ovarian tumor cell line as an immunogen, and more than 25 different antibodies against CA125 have been produced.

Immunohistochemical stains for CA125 show a membrane pattern of expression in ovarian tumor cells as well as in normal peritoneal and pleural mesothelium. Its expression in normal mesothelium limits the utility of CA125 as a screening biomarker because mesothelial inflammation (e.g., endometriosis or benign ascites) can cause elevations of serum CA125.

Secretion of CA125 from the luminal surface of cells can be triggered by protein phosphorylation. CA125 levels are also elevated after successful embryo implantation in normal pregnancy or after in vitro fertilization procedures.

Surprisingly, the gene encoding CA125 protein has not been definitively identified. The sugar components of CA125 are mucin-like and consist of a heterogeneous mixture of *O*-linked oligosaccharides with a core of two Galβ1,3(GlcNAcβ1,6)GalNAc moieties.

of mucinous borderline tumors is essential to exclude the possibility of occult invasive adenocarcinoma. Clear-cell and endometrioid adenocarcinomas of the ovary are thought to develop in prior foci of endometriosis. These tumors tend to be somewhat less aggressive than papillary serious adenocarcinoma.

The frequent bilaterality and multicentricity of ovarian tumors are not fully explained. Genetic studies have shown that multiple tumor foci in one patient share the same genetic changes, suggesting that they arise from a common precursor cell or that genetic abnormalities are disseminated throughout the pelvic peritoneum prior to tumor development.

Sex Cord Stromal Tumors

Sex cord stromal tumors comprise a morphologically diverse group of lesions that can be diagnostically confusing. Many of these tumors are quite uncommon and have descriptive names (e.g., "sex cord stromal tumor with annular tubules" and "steroid cell tumor"). Many sex cord stromal tumors produce hormones (estrogens or androgens), which can cause secondary changes in the endometrium and ovary.

Fibromas are the most common type of ovarian stromal tumor and are almost invariably benign although they can reach very large size. Fibromas are composed of bland spindle cells similarly to ovarian stroma. Fibromas often have areas with decidual change (thecoma cells) as a consequence of progesterone stimulation and are typically referred to as fibroma-thecomas. Estrogen production by fibromas in postmenopausal women may produce endometrial hyperplasia and lead to the development of endometrial adenocarcinoma.

Granulosa cell tumors are characteristic lesions that arise from granulosa cells in primary ovarian follicles. Tumor cells have coffee bean–shaped nuclei with prominent nuclear grooves (Fig. 13-18A). Both juvenile and adult types of granulosa cell tumors occur, with somewhat different morphologic patterns and a different clinical course. Most granulosa cell tumors behave in a benign fashion, but late tumor

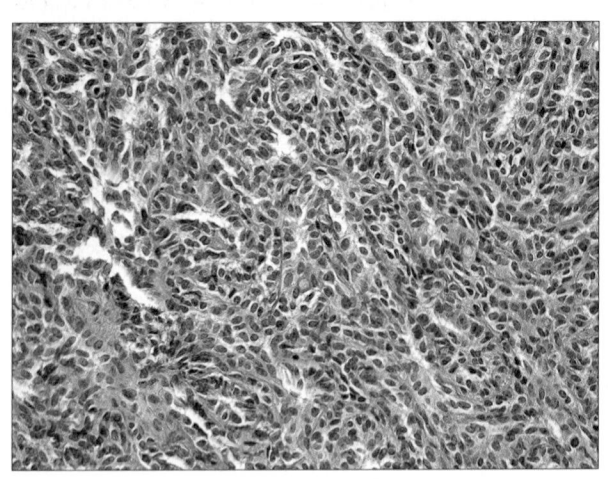

A

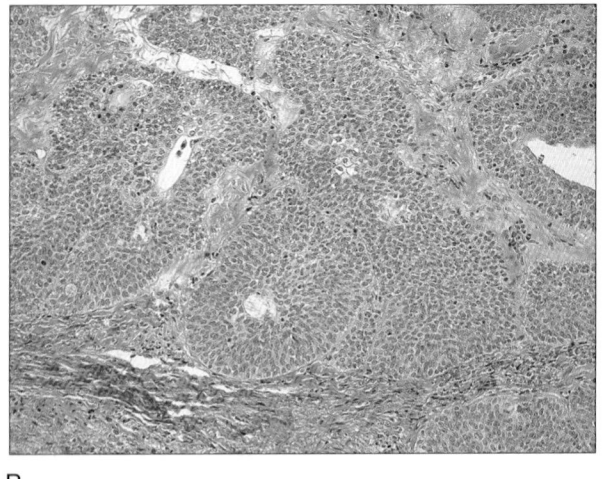

B

Figure 13-18. A, Ovarian granulosa cell tumor. Microscopic section showing cytologically bland tumor cells with prominent nuclear grooves growing in a trabecular pattern. **B**, Ovarian Brenner tumor. Microscopic section showing nests of bland-appearing transitional cells in stromal tissue.

recurrence or metastasis based on morphologic features of the primary tumor is not reliably predictable.

Brenner tumors consist of nests of bland transitional epithelium that morphologically resemble transitional cells of the urinary bladder. These nests are surrounded by ovarian type stromal cells (see Fig. 13-18B). Brenner tumors are frequently associated with mucinous ovarian tumors and generally are benign although a small number behave aggressively.

Germ Cell Tumors

The vast majority of ovarian germ cell tumors are benign (in sharp contrast to testicular germ cell tumors, which are all malignant or potentially malignant). By far the most common germ cell tumor of the ovary is the benign cystic teratoma (so-called dermoid cyst) (Fig. 13-19). Dermoid

cysts are usually composed predominantly of squamous epithelium and skin adnexa (including hair) but can contain all types of mature tissue derived from endoderm, mesoderm, and ectoderm. Dermoid cysts frequently present as adnexal masses, often with calcifications corresponding to formed teeth. Larger tumors may completely replace the ovary. Immature teratomas contain incompletely differentiated structures, which usually correspond to immature brain tissue with neuroblasts. Tumors with a small percentage of immature components have an excellent prognosis. More immature teratomas can give rise to peritoneal implants and behave aggressively. Immature teratomas are rare (<10% of ovarian teratomas) and are usually encountered in the pediatric and adolescent age group.

Dysgerminomas are malignant ovarian germ cell tumors that are morphologically similar to seminomas of the testis. Dysgerminomas express placental alkaline phosphatase and tend to occur in younger patients. Other forms of nonseminomatous germ cell tumor can develop in the ovary but are much less common.

Metastatic Tumors

The ovary is a relatively common site for metastatic deposits from tumors of the gastrointestinal tract as well as other primary sites. Metastatic adenocarcinoma may simulate the clinical presentation of primary ovarian adenocarcinoma with adnexal masses. Metastatic tumors are usually bilateral although many primary ovarian epithelial neoplasms can be bilateral as well. From a clinical point of view, differentiation of ovarian cancer from metastatic tumors is extremely important because ovarian carcinoma is substantially responsive to appropriate chemotherapy (even when it is widely metastatic throughout the abdomen). In contrast, metastatic gastrointestinal carcinomas to the ovary are not curable and are usually poorly responsive to chemotherapy. Immunohistochemical stains are usually helpful in distinguishing primary from metastatic tumors in the ovary, since ovarian carcinomas are almost invariably positive for cytokeratin CK7 and negative for CK20, whereas most gastrointestinal adenocarcinomas show the opposite pattern of reactivity.

Krukenberg's tumors are bilateral ovarian metastases from a signet ring cell adenocarcinoma of the stomach (Fig. 13-20). Krukenberg's tumors have a relatively characteristic morphologic appearance with signet ring cells interdigitating between ovarian stromal cells. Signet ring cell tumors of the pancreas and colon can produce a similar morphologic pattern. Carcinoid tumors can also metastasize to the ovary, and bilateral carcinoid tumors are considered metastatic until proved otherwise.

Small-Cell Carcinoma

Small-cell carcinoma of the ovary is a highly malignant tumor occurring in young women that is usually associated with hypercalcemia. Unlike small-cell carcinomas at other sites, these tumors do not usually show evidence of neuroendocrine differentiation.

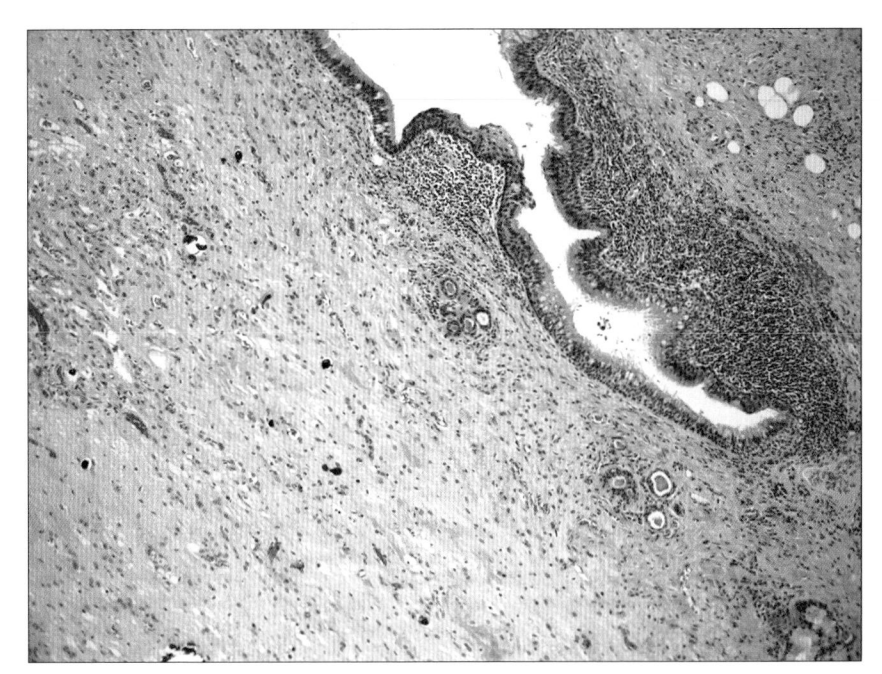

Figure 13-19. Mature ovarian teratoma (dermoid cyst). Microscopic section showing benign mature squamous and columnar mucosa of different types.

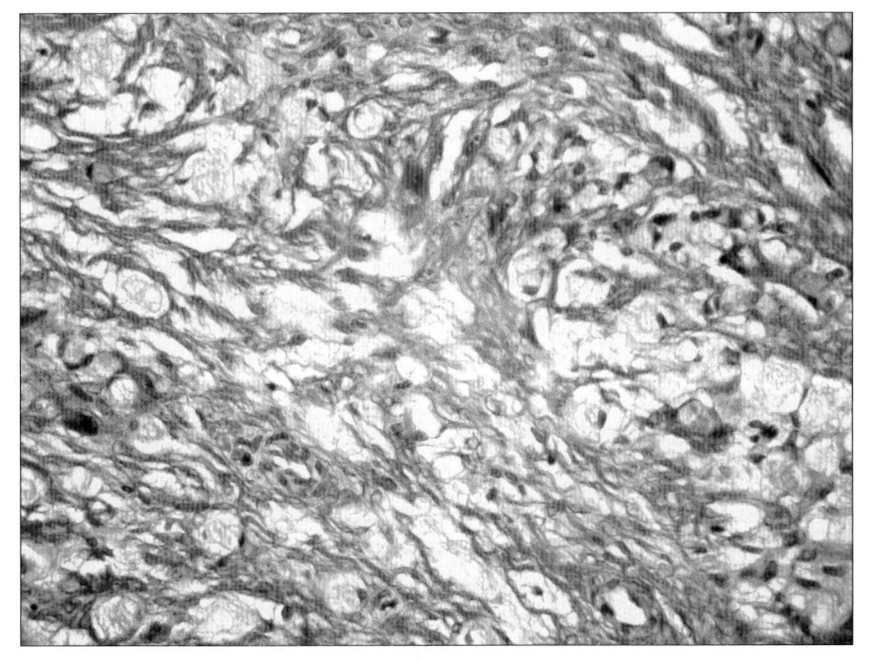

Figure 13-20. Metastatic adenocarcinoma to the ovary (Krukenberg's tumor). Microscopic section showing signet ring cells and mucin infiltrating between residual ovarian stromal cells.

●●● BREAST

The breast is a modified sweat gland that develops under hormonal stimulation in women. The functional unit of the female breast is the terminal duct–lobular unit. The male breast also contains ducts but does not develop lobules. The breast epithelium is hormonally responsive and undergoes changes during the menstrual cycle. Much more extensive secretory change develops in the lobules during pregnancy and in the postpartum period. Lobules contain secretory cells (which are modified to produce milk after pregnancy) surrounded by a layer of myoepithelial cells, which are stimulated to contract during lactation and breast-feeding. Lobules drain into small terminal ducts, which then connect with the larger duct system within the breast that terminates in the

HISTOLOGY

Breast Microscopic and Ductal Anatomy

A myoepithelial layer extends throughout the duct system, and its presence or absence is important in distinguishing invasive from in situ carcinoma as well as from other benign conditions (e.g., sclerosing adenosis). The ductal system has a complex branching pattern that arborizes inward from the lactiferous sinuses. Adjacent ducts in a tissue section may connect with different lactiferous sinuses in the nipple (see Figure A, below) making it difficult or impossible to trace the spread of intraductal carcinoma through the ductal system.

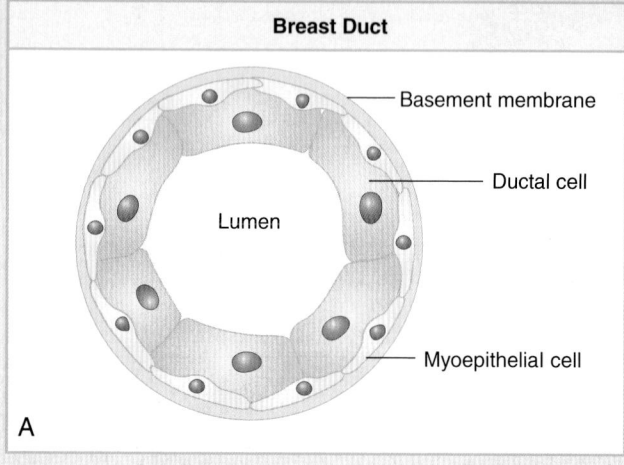

Breast Duct

Basement membrane

Ductal cell

Lumen

Myoepithelial cell

A

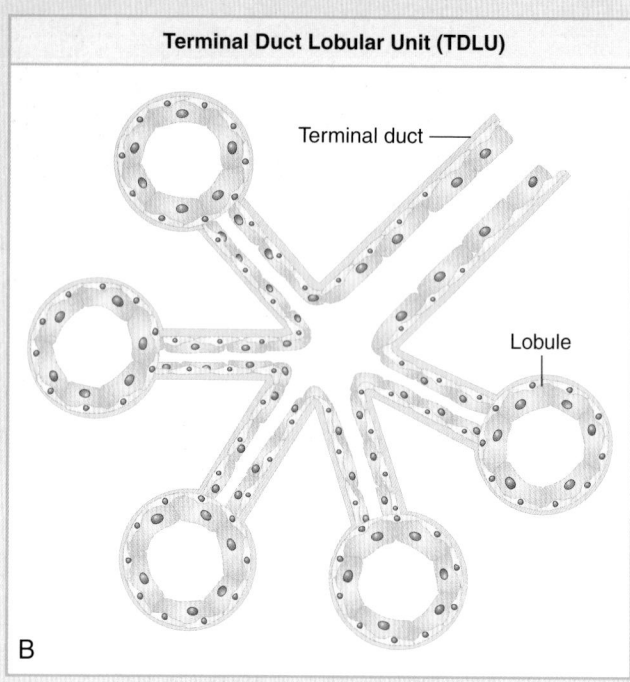

Terminal Duct Lobular Unit (TDLU)

Terminal duct

Lobule

B

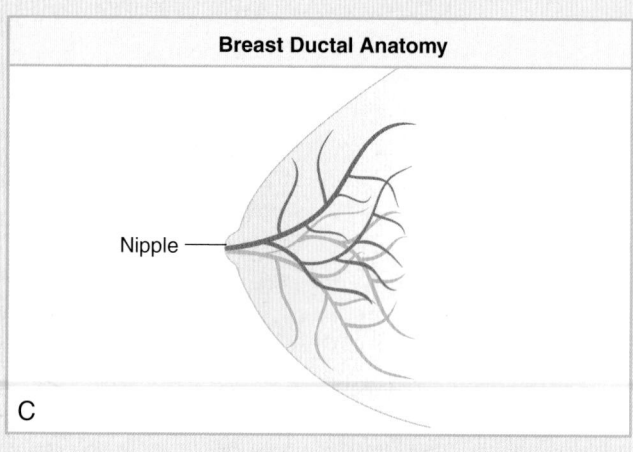

Breast Ductal Anatomy

Nipple

C

lactiferous sinuses at the nipple. The breast stroma in young women is composed predominantly of dense extracellular matrix with abundant collagen. Gradual replacement of this fibrous tissue by adipose tissue begins around the time of menopause with adipose tissue predominating in older postmenopausal women. This physiologic change is important for breast cancer detection by mammography, which depends on the contrasting density of adipose and tumor tissue.

Fibrocystic Change and Epithelial Hyperplasia

Fibrocystic changes are a constellation of epithelial changes within breast tissue that are extremely common and may produce palpable or mammographic lesions as well as cause

discomfort that varies with the menstrual cycle. Some fibrocystic lesions are clinically suspicious for cancer and prompt sampling by fine-needle aspiration or tissue biopsy.

Apocrine metaplasia is a common form of fibrocystic disease in which ductal epithelium undergoes metaplasia to apocrine cells having abundant eosinophilic cytoplasm and vesicular nuclei with prominent nucleoli (Fig. 13-21A). These cells also have apocrine snouts that undergo decapitation secretion and may form large fluid-filled cysts. Cysts can also develop by dilatation (ectasia) of small- and medium-sized ducts or as a consequence of ductal obstruction. Cysts can rupture, causing inflammation and a fibrotic tissue reaction that is often painful and may produce a palpable mass. None of these fibrocystic changes is associated with an increased cancer risk.

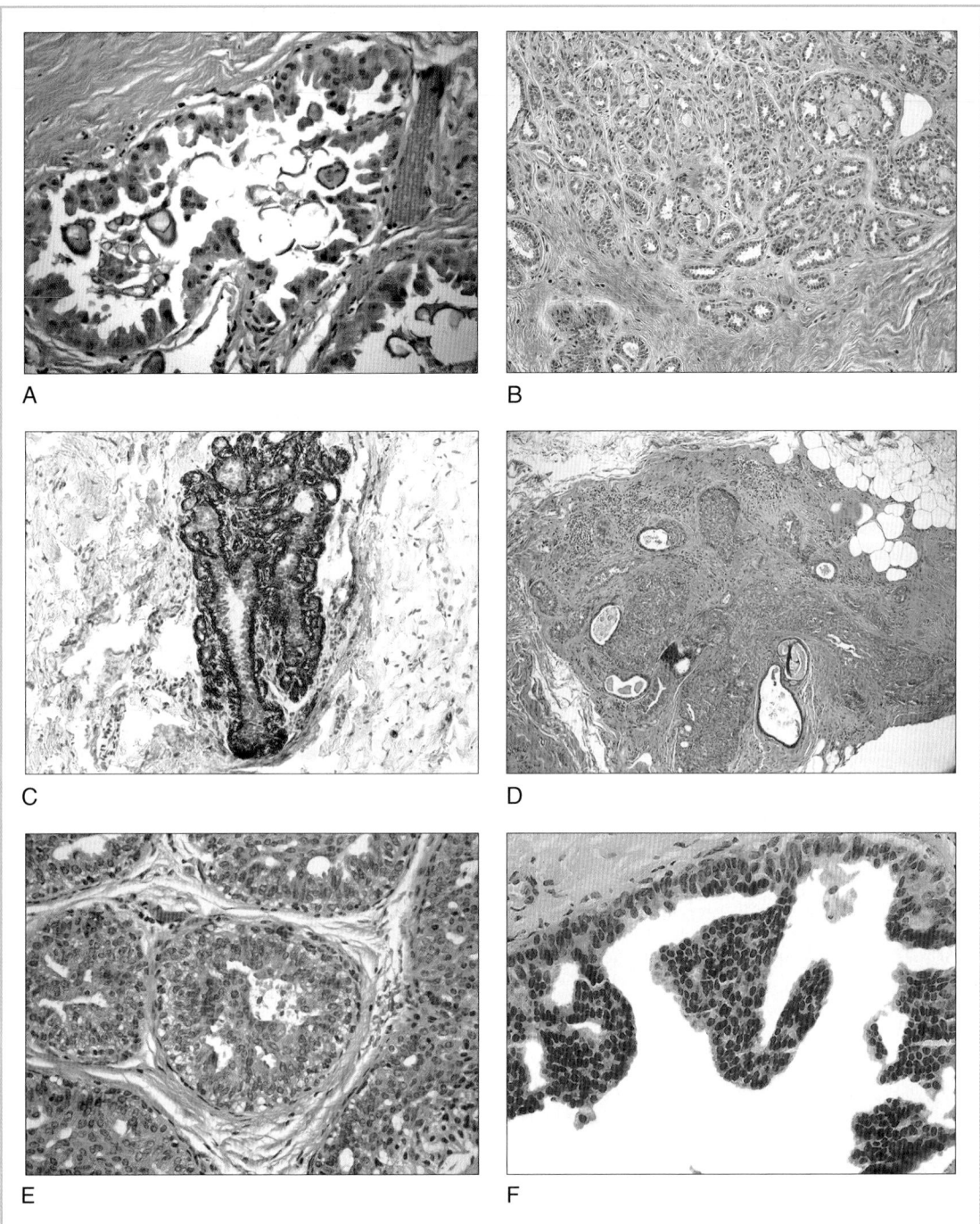

A

B

C

D

E

F

Figure 13-21. A, Fibrocystic change, apocrine metaplasia. Microscopic section of breast tissue showing cysts lined by a single layer of apocrine epithelium with densely eosinophilic cytoplasm, vesicular nuclei, moderately prominent nucleoli, and luminal secretory snouts. **B,** Fibrocystic change, sclerosing adenosis. Microscopic section of breast tissue showing small benign glands and cell nests invading stroma. No desmoplastic stromal response is present, and interface between adenosis and uninvolved breast tissue is smooth and conforms to the anatomic distribution of breast lobules. Myoepithelial cells are clearly visible in only a few areas, but they are present around all epithelial nests in sclerosing adenosis. **C,** Myoepithelial cells. Microscopic section of breast tissue with an immunoperoxidase stain for CD10 to highlight myoepithelial cells. Myoepithelial cells surrounding terminal ducts and lobules appear dark brown in this section while ductal epithelial cells are not stained. **D,** Radial scar. Microscopic section of breast tissue showing a focal area of elastotic fibrosis with embedded glands and cell nests composed of ductal epithelium. The overall lesion has a stellate configuration. Myoepithelial cells are present about all epithelial nests although they are difficult to recognize in some areas. **E,** Usual type ductal hyperplasia. Microscopic section of breast ducts showing prominent epithelial hyperplasia composed of polymorphous ductal cells that nearly fill the duct lumens. The epithelial cells have a streaming quality, and residual spaces between ductal cells are irregular and slit-like with angulated contours. **F,** Atypical ductal hyperplasia. Microscopic section of a breast duct showing unsupported epithelial cell growth forming small micropapillae that do not have fibrovascular cores. These ductal cells have increased nuclear:cytoplasmic ratios and are somewhat polymorphous (i.e., they do not closely resemble one another).

Sclerosing adenosis is an invasive process in which small benign glands infiltrate breast stroma (see Fig. 13-21B). Sclerosing adenosis mimics invasive adenocarcinoma in some aspects of its pattern of growth, but the glands in sclerosing adenosis retain a myoepithelial layer that absolutely distinguish it from invasive carcinoma (which lacks surrounding myoepithelial cells). Myoepithelial cells may be inconspicuous morphologically but can be highlighted by several immunohistochemical stains (see Fig. 13-21C). Sclerosing adenosis retains a lobular distribution so that the small glands remain confined to an area corresponding to a terminal duct–lobular unit and the edges of these lesions have smooth contours (in contrast to the randomness of invasive carcinoma).

Radial scars are small lesions (almost never larger than 1 cm) with a stellate shape formed by stromal elastosis around entrapped glands (see Fig. 13-21D). Radial scars are often associated with ductal hyperplasia and confer a slightly increased risk of carcinoma. Radial scars must be distinguished from tubular carcinomas, which are small, well-differentiated invasive carcinomas with a stellate configuration. Tubular carcinomas lack the myoepithelial cell layer that is retained in radial scars.

Proliferative fibrocystic disease means hyperplasia of ductal epithelial cells that usually causes epithelial ingrowth into duct lumens that is not supported by fibrovascular stromal core. Ductal hyperplasia of the usual type is associated with a small increased risk for the development of carcinoma. The usual type of hyperplasia is composed of polymorphous epithelial cells that tend to have a flowing growth pattern and tend to form compressed, slit-like spaces at the periphery of involved ducts (see Fig. 13-21E).

Atypical ductal hyperplasia is associated with a more significant risk of carcinoma (approximately five times that of

the general population) and shows some features of intraductal carcinoma but lacks some critical diagnostic features of intraductal carcinoma (see Fig. 13-21F). Epithelial proliferation is usually more exuberant (larger foci of unsupported epithelial growth) than in the usual hyperplasia, and cytologic atypia is more pronounced. Atypical hyperplasia may be associated with necrosis, but the presence of necrosis or of significant cytologic atypia increases the likelihood that an intraductal lesion is malignant. Since fairly rigid and complex criteria must be met to make a diagnosis of intraductal carcinoma, atypical hyperplasia can be operationally defined as a hyperplastic lesion that falls short of the diagnosis of intraductal carcinoma in one or more ways (see below).

Intraductal Papilloma

Papillomas are benign lesions composed of fibrovascular cores lined by ductal epithelium forming a characteristic papillary architecture (Fig. 13-22A). The fibrovascular cores in most papillomas are blunt and sclerotic. A complete myoepithelial layer is usually present between epithelial cells and the underlying basement membrane in the stromal cores. Intraductal papillomas in larger ducts can cause ductal obstruction and may present with nipple discharge as a consequence of obstruction. Ductal obstruction can result in the sclerosis around papillomas, creating a "pseudoinvasive" pattern in which benign epithelial nests are entrapped by fibrous stroma. Pseudoinvasion must be distinguished from invasive carcinoma. This distinction is usually not difficult for an experienced pathologist, and stains for myoepithelial cells are helpful in more difficult cases.

Intraductal papilloma must also be distinguished from papillary carcinoma, which is a rare form of invasive breast cancer. Papillary carcinomas lack a myoepithelial cell layer and are composed of extremely monomorphic epithelial cells lining stromal cores that usually are thin and delicate (see Fig. 13-22B). These features generally allow reliable distinction between the benign and the malignant papillary lesions.

Gynecomastia

Gynecomastia develops in some men and adolescent boys with enlargement of breast tissue that may be unilateral or bilateral. Morphologically, gynecomastia shows marked intraductal hyperplasia with associated periductal chronic inflammation and edema.

Breast Tumors

Breast lesions that produce palpable or mammographic masses must be distinguished from invasive and intraductal carcinoma, which is the most common type of cancer in women (the lifetime risk of developing breast cancer for a woman in the United States is one in nine). The prognosis for breast cancer is substantially better if tumors are detected when they are low stage. Early cancer detection is critical from both the clinical and the medicolegal points of view.

HISTOLOGY

Myoepithelial Cells

Myoepithelial cells are true epithelial cells that form desmosomes and hemidesmosomes with cadherin-mediated cell junctions. They also contain large amounts of microfilaments and contractile proteins characteristic of smooth muscle cells, and they form dense plaques (cell-matrix adherence junctions) typical of smooth muscle cells.

Myoepithelial cells are attached to the basement membrane and form a basket-like layer around breast lobules so that their contraction results in the extrusion of lobular contents (milk in lactation) into terminal ducts. Myoepithelial cells in ducts form a more complete layer that almost completely separates ductal epithelial cells from the basement membrane.

Myoepithelial cells are present in organs other than the breast (e.g., salivary gland) and can subserve similar contractile functions in these organs.

Tumors of myoepithelial cells do occur in the breast but are much less common and usually less aggressive than tumors of ductal or lobular epithelial cells.

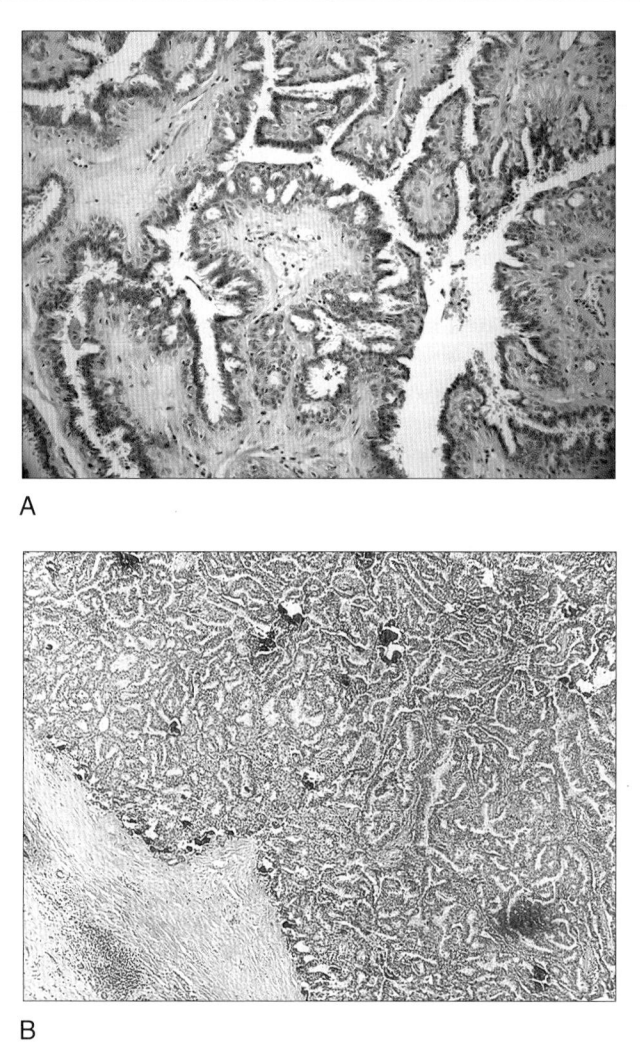

A

B

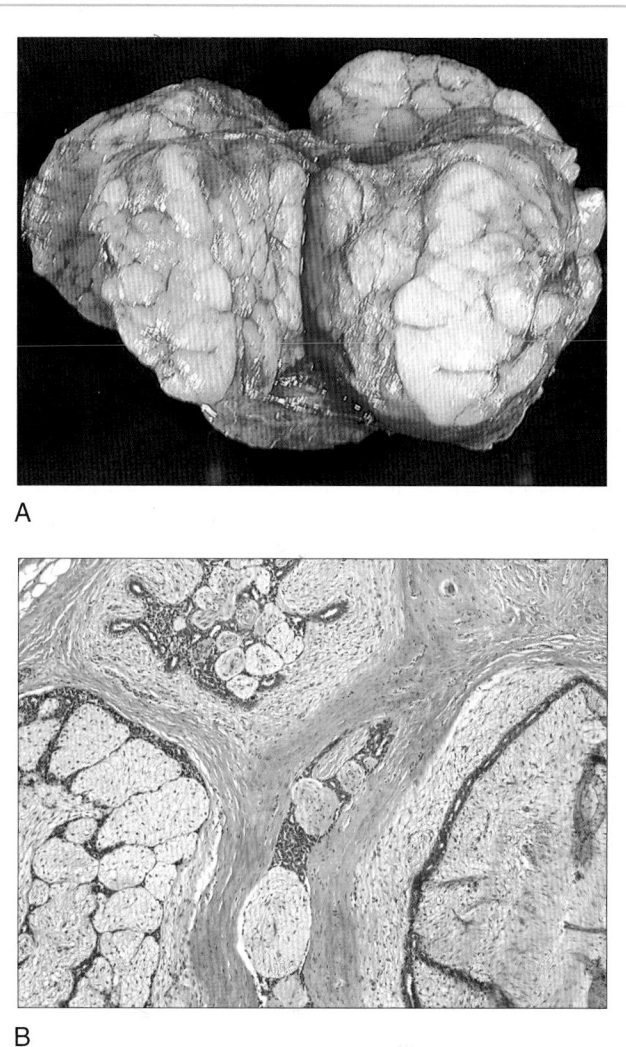

A

B

Figure 13-22. A, Intraductal papilloma. Microscopic section showing a sclerotic intraductal papilloma. Fibrovascular cores containing abundant collagen are lined by polymorphous ductal cells. Myoepithelial cells are evident between the ductal cells and the stromal papillae. **B**, Papillary carcinoma. Microscopic section showing a papillary tumor with delicate fibrovascular cores lined by extremely monomorphous epithelial cells. No myoepithelial cells are present.

Figure 13-23. A, Fibroadenoma. Gross cross-section of breast tissue showing a circumscribed fibroadenoma with cleft-like spaces in white-tan fibrous stroma. **B**, Microscopic section of a fibroadenoma showing lobules of myxoid stroma (pale blue) with strands of bland epithelial cells forming cleft-like spaces. This is the more common intracannilicular pattern. Pericannilicucar fibroadenomas consist of gland-like structures in similar stroma.

Fibroadenoma

Fibroadenomas are benign tumors having both stromal and epithelial components that occur more often in younger than in older women (Fig. 13-23A). Fibroadenomas can attain a large size but usually have sharply circumscribed borders and a characteristic appearance on ultrasound examination. The epithelium in fibroadenomas typically has an intracanalicular growth pattern (see Fig. 13-23B). Fibroadenomas can be secondarily involved by fibrocystic change (e.g., apocrine metaplasia and sclerosing adenosis). Atypical epithelial hyperplasia in a fibroadenoma usually is not considered a significant risk factor for the development of ductal carcinoma. Rarely, invasive lobular carcinomas may arise within a fibroadenoma.

Phyllodes Tumor

Phyllodes tumors share many morphologic features with fibroadenomas but lack their gross circumscription and show disproportionate stromal growth in relation to their epithelial component. The stroma typically splits apart residual breast ducts, and stromal cells usually show cytologic atypia. Most phyllodes tumors are benign although they may be locally aggressive. Rare malignant phyllodes tumors have cytologically malignant stromal cells and behave as low-grade sarcomas.

Carcinoma

The incidence of breast cancer increases with age and increased estrogen stimulation. Two major forms of invasive breast cancer exist: ductal and lobular. Both have unique features and in situ precursor lesions. Ductal carcinomas account for the majority of invasive and in situ carcinomas, and lobular carcinomas correspond to most remaining types. A few less common variants of ductal carcinoma are distinguished because of their unusual and relatively characteristic clinical and morphologic features. Ductal breast cancer can occur in men, but male breast cancer accounts for only 1% of all breast cancers. Since male breasts lack lobules, lobular carcinomas do not occur.

All invasive breast cancers are thought to arise from in situ carcinomas although the in situ carcinoma may no longer be identifiable at the time of diagnosis. Invasive breast cancer usually spreads to regional lymph nodes before (or concurrent with) systemic metastasis so that lymph node metastasis is an important prognostic marker. Breast cancers tend to metastasize early in their clinical course compared with neoplasms of similar size in other organs.

In situ Carcinoma

Several different morphologic variants of carcinoma in situ are recognized in the breast. Most in situ carcinomas are composed of relatively monomorphic cell populations (i.e., one tumor cell looks similar to all other tumor cells). Monomorphism is present even in lesions that are composed of cytologically malignant cells (even though the tumor cells show pleomorphism, all are pleomorphic in a similar manner). In contrast, hyperplasia and atypical hyperplasia tend to be polymorphous with significant variation in size and appearance of different epithelial cells. Application of these concepts to the interpretation of biopsy specimens can be difficult and requires considerable skill. In addition to monomorphism, lesions qualifying as in situ carcinoma in the breast must meet diagnostic criteria for a specific type of in situ carcinoma, as described below.

One of the most easily recognized types of ductal carcinoma in situ is comedo type intraductal carcinoma (comedocarcinoma), in which a solid epithelial proliferation fills and distends breast ducts and develops prominent central coagulation necrosis (Fig. 13-24A). Most comedocarcinomas are composed of cytologically malignant epithelial cells (nuclear grade 3/3).

Cribriform type intraductal carcinoma is made up of a solid epithelial proliferation that usually fills and distends a duct. Prominent apoptosis of tumor cells results in the formation of sharply circumscribed (i.e., "punched-out") empty spaces that are scattered through the neoplastic epithelium (as though a cookie cutter had removed a portion of the epithelium) (see Fig. 13-24B). The cytologic features of tumor cells in cribriform carcinoma may be of high grade, but most are of intermediate grade (nuclear grade 2/2), and it is the architectural pattern rather than the cytologic features that justifies a diagnosis of intraductal carcinoma.

Other morphologic variants of intraductal carcinoma include micropapillary carcinoma, in which small intraductal invaginations composed exclusively of epithelium (no stromal component) with malignant cytologic features extend into ducts.

Distinction of atypical hyperplasia from intraductal carcinoma may be difficult in marginal cases. Some clinicians use the lesion size criterion of 2 mm as a minimum for the diagnosis of intraductal carcinoma. Intraductal carcinoma is often associated with microcalcifications, which may lead to its mammographic detection (see Fig. 13-24C). Microcalcifications can also occur in many invasive tumors, atypical hyperplasia, and benign fibrocystic disease.

Clinically, intraductal carcinoma is managed as a malignant tumor; complete surgical excision of intraductal carcinoma is undertaken even in the absence of invasive disease. Because of the complex connections of the ductal system, even patients with negative surgical margins may be at risk for residual intraductal carcinoma. Patients with completely excised intraductal carcinoma typically receive breast irradiation as an adjunctive therapy to sterilize possible residual foci of in situ carcinoma.

Intraductal carcinoma may involve breast ducts extensively and extend intraluminally to the lactiferous sinuses. Intraductal carcinoma may present as Paget's disease of the nipple, giving a crusted appearance to the nipple. Nipple biopsy shows individual tumor cells within the epidermis (see Fig. 13-24D). Paget's disease is almost always associated with underlying intraductal or invasive carcinoma.

Rupture and sclerosis around ducts involved by intraductal carcinoma can produce a "pseudoinvasive" appearance that must be distinguished from true invasive carcinoma. Intraductal carcinoma retains a normal layer of myoepithelial cells at its periphery, and detection of myoepithelial cells immunohistochemically can be useful in distinguishing invasive from intraductal carcinoma (see Fig. 13-24E). Distinction of invasive from in situ carcinoma is clinically important because patients with invasive disease will typically undergo sentinel lymph node biopsy to assess the possibility of metastatic disease.

Lobular carcinoma in situ is a proliferation of epithelial cells in breast lobules (rather than in ducts). In lobular carcinoma, discohesive cells with monomorphous nuclei and abundant cytoplasm fill and distend lobules (see Fig. 13-24F). Tumor cells appear to fall apart from one another in histologic sections, and this poorly cohesive pattern results from loss of E-cadherin expression in tumor cells. The clinical significance of lobular carcinoma in situ is more similar to that of atypical ductal hyperplasia than ductal carcinoma in situ. Patients with lobular carcinoma in situ have a significantly increased risk for invasive carcinoma, but the risk applies equally to both breasts. For this reason, a diagnosis of lobular carcinoma in situ results in increased clinical surveillance but does not usually initiate wider local excision of the affected area.

Invasive Carcinoma

Invasive breast carcinoma can give rise to nodal and systemic metastases and constitutes the most serious form of breast cancer. Ductal and lobular carcinomas are usually distinct from one another, but some tumors (e.g., terminal duct carcinomas) may merge their morphologic features. Invasive

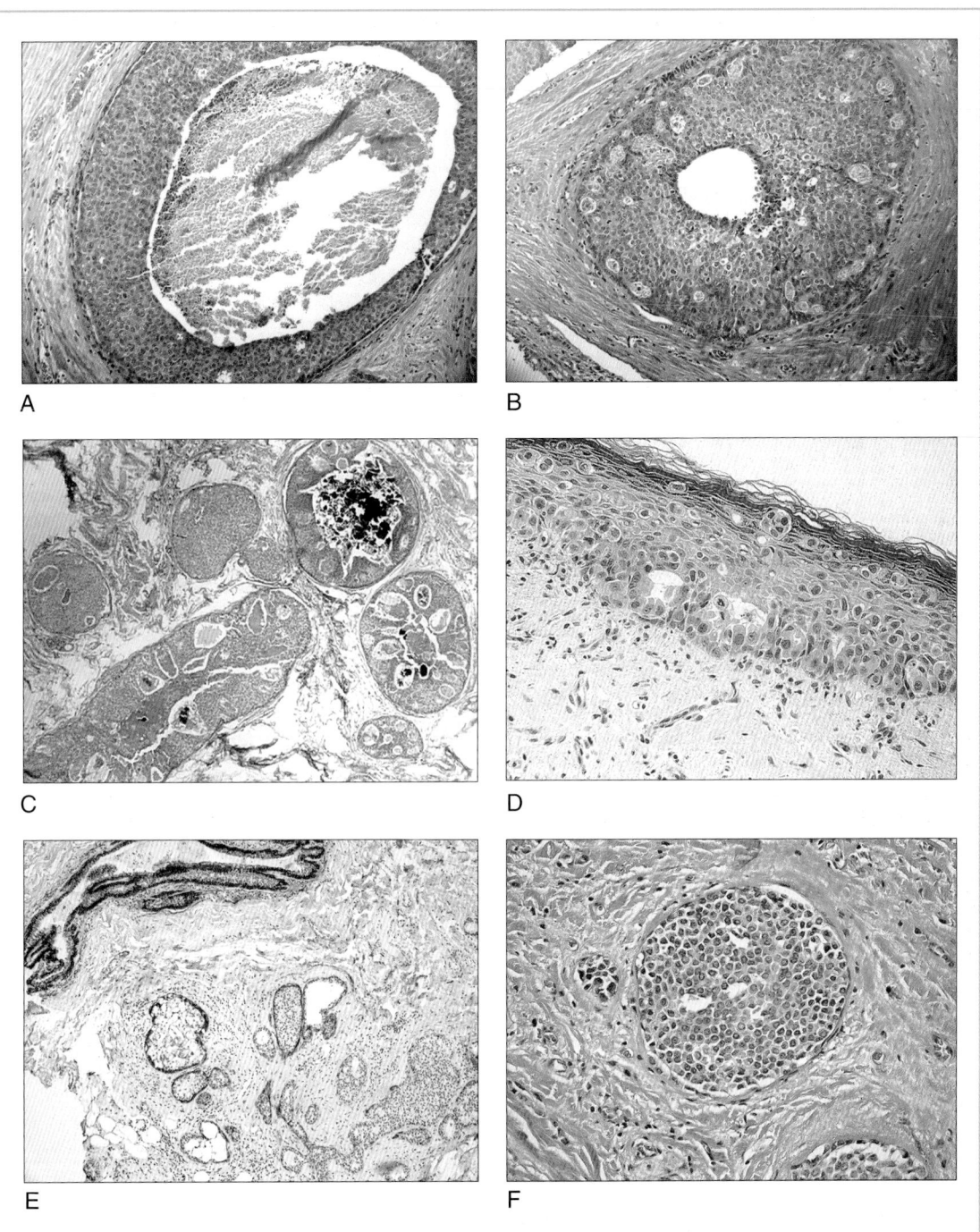

Figure 13-24. **A**, Comedo type intraductal carcinoma. Microscopic section of a breast duct with prominent central coagulation necrosis. Multilayered neoplastic epithelium fills the remainder of the duct. These tumor cells are cytologically high grade. **B**, Cribriform intraductal carcinoma. Microscopic section of a breast duct showing monomorphous (the cells closely resemble one another) proliferation of ductal cells that nearly fills the duct. A small residual lumen is visible at the center. The round spaces within the solid epithelial proliferation appear sharply defined as though they had been "punched out." These spaces result from apoptosis of tumor cells, which creates the cribriform architecture in this intraductal carcinoma. **C**, Intraductal carcinoma with microcalcifications. Microscopic section showing multiple ducts involved by intraductal carcinoma with central necrosis and dystrophic calcification. **D**, Paget's disease of the nipple. Microscopic section of skin from the nipple showing pleomorphic tumor cells interdigitating between keratinocytes in the squamous epithelium. **E**, Intraductal carcinoma with pseudoinvasion versus early invasive carcinoma. Microscopic section of breast tissue stained for myoepithelial markers. A benign duct with prominent myoepithelial cells (stained dark brown) is visible (*top*). Irregular epithelial nests (bottom half of the figure) are composed of intraductal carcinoma. Myoepithelial cells are decreased around many of these nests (compared with the benign duct at the top), but a few myoepithelial cells are still present. This may be a transitional lesion with early microinvasion by intraductal carcinoma. **F**, Lobular carcinoma in situ (LCIS). Microscopic section of a breast lobule filled and distended (enlarged) by a monomorphous epithelial cell proliferation. Individual tumor cells appear discohesive (i.e., they tend to fall apart from one another in this histologic section).

ductal carcinomas are substantially more common than lobular carcinomas (approximately four to one) and although there are some differences in tumor behavior, the two are managed in essentially the same manner clinically.

Invasive Ductal Carcinoma

Invasive ductal carcinoma usually presents as a discrete mass within breast tissue that infiltrates stroma and or surrounding adipose tissue, creating a stellate, scar-like appearance (scirrhous carcinoma) (Fig. 13-25A). Fat necrosis may simulate the gross appearance of invasive ductal carcinoma. Most tumors produce a marked desmoplastic response and are much firmer than surrounding breast tissue (see Figs. 13-25B and 13-25C). Invasive tumor cells are not surrounded by a myoepithelial layer and are usually associated with some degree of gland formation. These morphologic features are used in the modified Bloom-Richardson grading system for breast carcinomas, which provides an important prognostic index for individual tumors. Obvious lymphatic or vascular space invasion within or adjacent to the tumor is an adverse prognostic factor. Careful pathologic staging and grading of the primary breast tumors and axillary lymph nodes are essential to arrive at an appropriate therapeutic strategy. Evaluation of resection margins is important, and positive or close (approximately 2 mm) margins are often re-excised in an attempt to assure tumor-free surgical margins. Most patients with invasive carcinoma are treated with localized surgery (lumpectomy) followed by

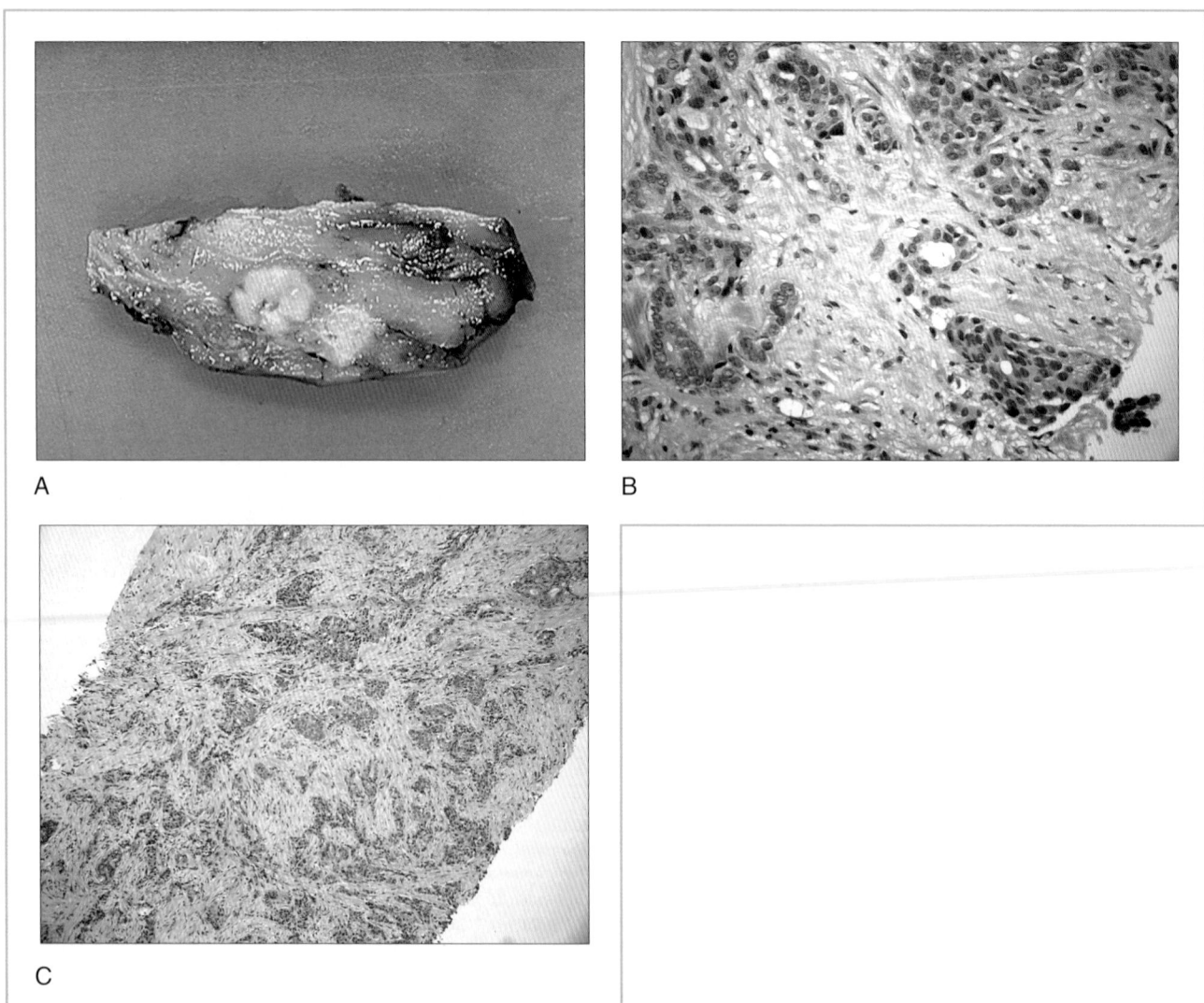

A

B

C

Figure 13-25. A, Infiltrating ductal carcinoma (IDC). Gross cross-section of breast tissue with a central invasive carcinoma having irregular but well-defined margins. Some ink is present on the surface of the biopsy specimen to mark the resection margins. Breast stroma has largely been replaced by adipose tissue in this postmenopausal patient. **B**, IDC (modified Bloom-Richardson [MBR] grade 2/3). Microscopic section showing a moderately differentiated infiltrating ductal carcinoma with occasional gland formation. Tumor cell nests are surrounded by desmoplastic stroma. **C**, Poorly differentiated IDC (MBR grade 3/3). Microscopic section showing nests of pleomorphic infiltrating tumor cells infiltrating desmoplastic stroma without evidence of gland formation.

adjuvant radiation therapy to the breast. This adjuvant therapy is predominantly aimed at sterilizing possible residual intraductal carcinoma. Lumpectomy with irradiation has been shown to be as effective as radical mastectomy for small tumors.

Invasive Lobular Carcinoma

Invasive lobular carcinoma forms a much less well-defined mass than ductal carcinoma and may be difficult to localize with radiologic techniques. Tumor cells tend to infiltrate in a single-file manner (with no gland formation) and often form target-like patterns around benign breast ducts (like the rings around a bull's eye in an archery target). Lobular carcinomas do not express E-cadherin (Fig. 13-26), and this molecular abnormality results in their characteristic loss of normal cellular adhesion and diffuse growth pattern. Invasive lobular carcinoma may be associated with in situ lobular carcinoma but may also coexist with intraductal carcinoma and invasive ductal carcinoma. Some tumors arising from terminal ducts share morphologic features of lobular and ductal carcinoma. Initial metastatic spread is usually to axillary lymph nodes, but invasive lobular carcinomas frequently produce a relatively characteristic and unusual pattern of systemic metastases and can involve sites (e.g., the uterine cervix) that are not usually targeted by metastatic disease.

Unusual Invasive Ductal Carcinomas

Several morphologic variants of invasive ductal carcinoma have individual clinical significance and are usually diagnosed as distinct entities. Mucinous carcinomas (also called colloid carcinomas) occur in older women and are composed predominantly of acellular mucin with only occasional tumor cell nests (Fig. 13-27A). Colloid carcinomas tend to have an excellent prognosis if they do not contain foci of usual type invasive ductal carcinoma. Tubular carcinomas are thought to be early invasive ductal carcinomas that have a cruciform shape and are often associated with intraductal carcinoma. Tubular carcinomas are almost always small (often <0.5 cm) and are only rarely associated with lymph node metastases. Tubular carcinomas must be distinguished from radial scars (see above), which are frequently encountered benign lesions.

Metaplastic carcinoma is an unusual high-grade variant of ductal carcinoma in which tumor cells undergo metaplasia to take on a mesenchymal (spindle cell) appearance and may show features suggestive of chondrosarcoma or osteosarcoma. Inflammatory carcinoma is a clinical variant of breast cancer that presents with dermal edema over the

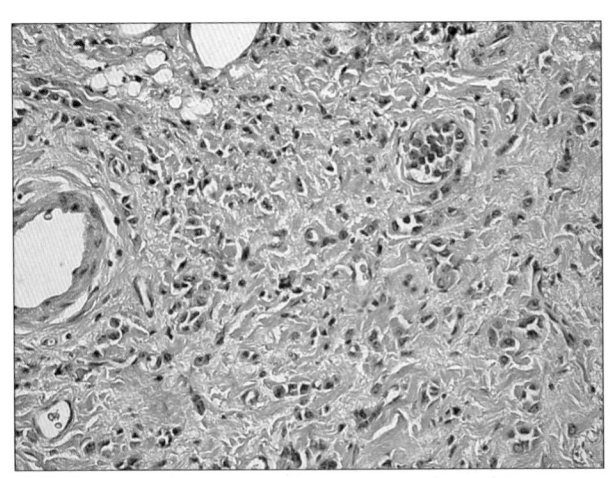

A

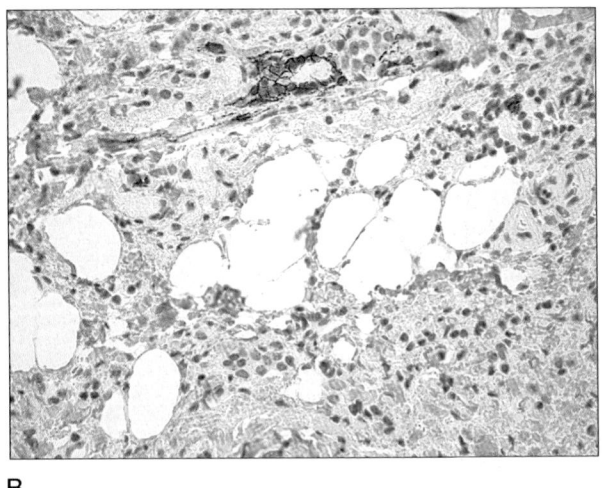

B

Figure 13-26. Infiltrating lobular carcinoma (ILC). **A**, Microscopic section of breast tissue showing haphazard infiltration of breast stroma by single tumor cells. Tumor cells are cytologically bland compared to most ductal carcinomas. **B**, Microscopic section of ILC stained for E-cadherin. Single tumor cells infiltrate breast stroma and do not show staining for E-cadherin. A residual benign breast duct (*upper center*) shows positive staining for E-cadherin.

breast creating the so-called peau d'orange appearance. Pathologically, inflammatory carcinoma usually corresponds to extensive dermal lymphatic invasion by tumor cells that cause extensive lymphatic obstruction to produce the characteristic edema of breast skin (see Fig. 13-27B).

Most patients with inflammatory carcinoma and other patients with locally advanced breast cancer (tumors > 5 cm in diameter) are treated with neoadjuvant chemotherapy prior to surgical excision of their breast tumor. This therapeutic choice recognizes that these patients are at risk of dying of metastatic breast cancer and that this risk will not be significantly altered by removal of the primary tumor. Many of these patients undergo mastectomy following neoadjuvant chemotherapy. Some patients have complete or near-complete pathologic responses while others show no response or rapid regrowth of tumor in the mastectomy specimen.

Tumor Biomarkers

Evaluation of estrogen and progesterone receptor expression in breast carcinomas is important prognostically (Fig. 13-28A). Most breast carcinomas in postmenopausal women express estrogen and progesterone receptor and are responsive to tamoxifen and other therapies that decrease endogenous estrogen levels (e.g., aromatase inhibitors). More breast cancers in premenopausal women are hormone receptor negative, and these patients may not benefit from hormonal manipulation.

Evaluation of HER2/neu expression and gene amplification in tumors is important in choosing appropriate therapy (see

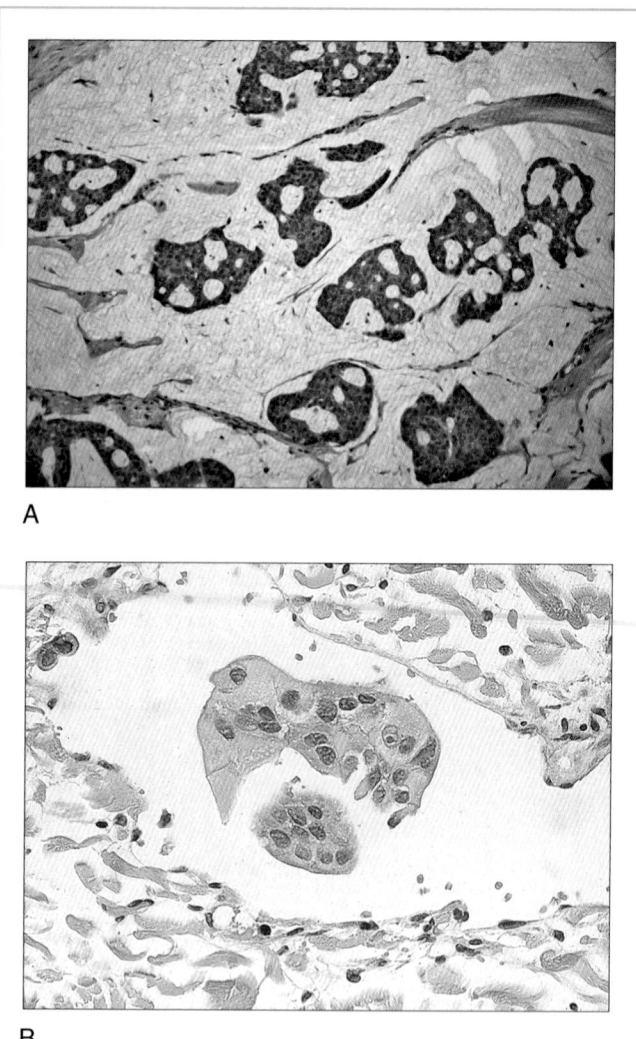

Figure 13-27. A, Colloid breast carcinoma. Microscopic section of breast tissue showing nests of bland tumor cells floating in lakes of acellular mucin. **B**, Inflammatory breast cancer. Microscopic section of breast skin with extensive lymphatic invasion by nests of ductal carcinoma cells.

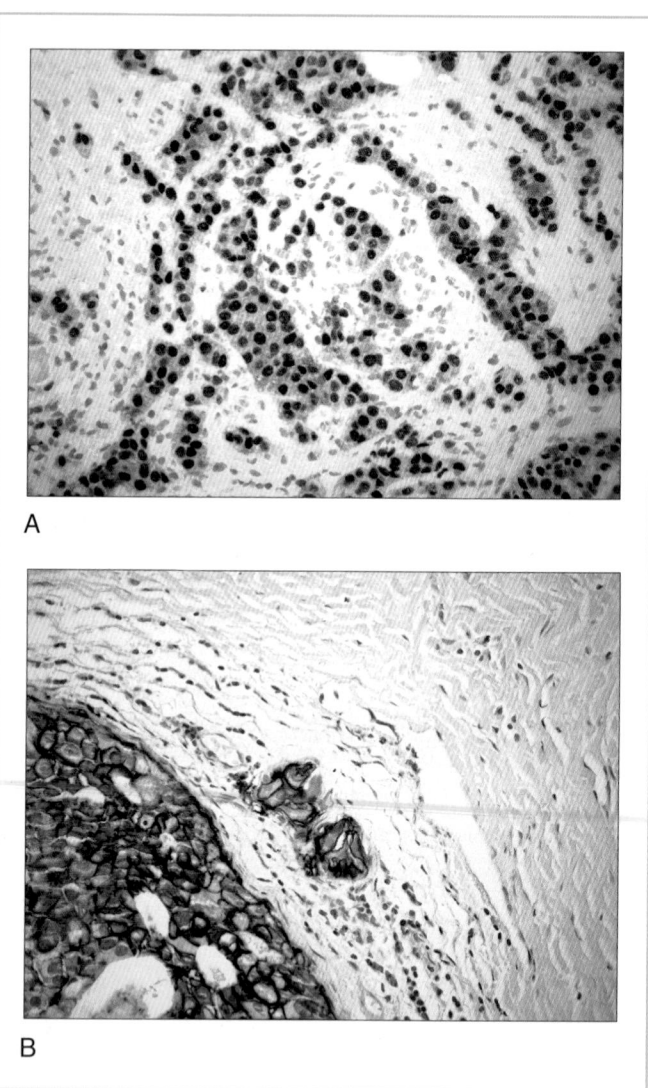

Figure 13-28. A, Estrogen receptor expression in breast cancer. Microscopic section of infiltrating ductal carcinoma stained for estrogen receptor by immunoperoxidase. Most tumor cells show strong nuclear staining (brown) in this neoplasm. **B**, HER2/neu expression in breast cancer. Microscopic section of invasive (*center*) and intraductal (*lower left*) carcinoma stained for Her2/neu protein by immunoperoxidase. Strong, continuous cytoplasmic membrane staining (brown) is present in both the invasive and the in situ carcinoma.

PHYSIOLOGY

Hormonal Therapies in Breast Cancer

Estrogen is the main hormone involved in the development of breast cancer, and oophorectomy was shown to be of therapeutic benefit in patients with advanced breast cancer many years ago.

Tamoxifen has been a mainstay of breast cancer treatment and chemoprevention. Tamoxifen is an estrogen antagonist in many tissues but also is a partial estrogen agonist that can cause undesirable estrogenic effects (e.g., there is an increased risk for endometrial cancer in postmenopausal women treated with estrogen).

Aromatase inhibitors block the action of a member of the cytochrome P-450 family (CYP19) that is normally expressed in ovarian tissue as well as extraovarian tissues including adipose tissue, muscle, brain, and breast cancers. After menopause, estrogen production derives solely from CYP19 activity in these nonovarian tissues. Effective inhibition of CYP19 by aromatase inhibitors can then completely block estrogen synthesis in postmenopausal women without the agonist side effects of tamoxifen. Aromatase inhibitors are not used in premenopausal women because the induced estrogen deficiency would drive gonadotropin production by the pituitary, resulting in compensatory ovarian hypertrophy.

BIOCHEMISTRY

PTEN Mutations and Treatment Response in Breast Cancer

Overexpression of HER2/neu receptor in a subset of breast cancer patients is associated with adverse prognosis because high-level receptor expression favors receptor dimerization, autophosphorylation, and constitutive signaling by HER2/neu, which then activates signaling through PI3 kinase and Akt to enhance tumor proliferation and cause resistance to apoptosis.

The PTEN gene product normally down-regulates PI3 kinase-Akt signaling. Constitutive HER2/neu activation (in breast tumors with gene amplification) results in Src kinase activation, which inactivates PTEN (by phosphorylation) and prevents it from inhibiting PI3 kinase-Akt signaling.

Binding of the trastuzumab monoclonal antibody to HER2/neu appears to interfere with Src activation, allowing PTEN to block Akt signaling to favor cell cycle arrest and increase tumor cell sensitivity to apoptosis. Some breast cancers with HER2/neu gene amplification also have genetic alterations in the PTEN gene that tend to render these tumors resistant to trastuzumab therapy. PTEN mutations now appear to be the major cause of resistance to trastuzumab in HER2/neu-overexpressing breast cancers.

A similar paradigm may apply to brain tumors in which PTEN mutations can abrogate response to treatment with EGFR inhibitors.

Fig. 13-28B). The availability of trastuzumab (Herceptin) monoclonal antibody therapy has made HER2/neu over-expression an important predictive biomarker. Tumors that overexpress HER2/neu usually do not express hormone receptors and have a somewhat worse prognosis than HER2/neu-negative tumors although they have an enhanced response to anthracycline-based chemotherapy. Immunohistochemical evaluation of HER2/neu overexpression is technically difficult and can be unreliable. Many laboratories have turned to FISH analysis to directly assess for HER2/neu gene amplification in these tumors. This technique is more analytically reproducible and provides a clinically reliable indication of the likelihood of response to trastuzumab therapy. Emerging tumor biomarkers such as PTEN gene mutations may become important in selecting optimal therapy in the future.

Sentinel Lymph Node

Sentinel lymph node biopsy is an important technical advance in breast cancer therapy that has come into clinical practice over the last 15 years. Sentinel lymph node biopsy is performed by instilling a radioactive tracer in the primary breast tumor (or in the cavity left by surgical excision of the breast tumor). Radionuclide then migrates through lymphatic spaces to localize in the primary lymph nodes draining the breast tumor site. Detection of the radioactive lymph nodes by means of a sensitive detection probe allows the targeted removal of one or a few lymph nodes that are the most likely to contain initial tumor metastasis. If thorough pathologic analysis of sentinel lymph nodes does not show evidence of

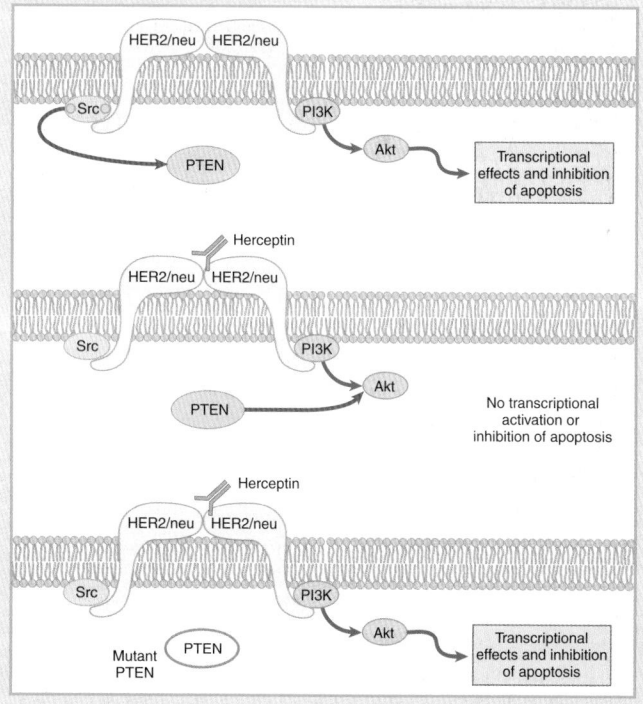

metastatic disease, the likelihood of metastasis in residual axillary lymph nodes is low. The application of sentinel lymph node biopsy has spared many women the morbidity associated with full axillary dissection, which can result in crippling lymphedema of the involved arm. Sentinel lymph node biopsy is also applied in other selected clinical situations including high-risk cutaneous melanomas.

Extensive pathologic sampling of sentinel lymph nodes (often serial sections are evaluated with immunohisto-chemical stains for cytokeratin to detect minute tumor cell deposits) has raised an important issue in breast cancer concerning the clinical significance of very small tumor deposits within axillary lymph nodes. Micrometastatic disease is defined as tumor deposits that are larger than 0.2 mm and smaller than 2 mm. Patients with micrometastases have a much lower risk of systemic metastasis or of metastasis to additional axillary lymph nodes than do patients with larger lymph node metastases. The clinical implications of micrometastases in terms of the need for a full axillary dissection and the potential benefit of adjuvant chemotherapy are not clearly defined.

Even more controversial is the detection of even smaller deposits of tumor cells (<0.2 mm) by immunohistochemical analysis. Patients with these very small foci of tumor cells are currently classified as lymph node negative in pathologic staging. It is important to remember that lymph node metastasis requires not only the deposition of tumor cells in a lymph node but their successful engraftment and growth in this location. The identification of the small clusters of tumor cells does not prove that these cells are clonagenic. In some laboratories, even more sensitive means of breast cancer detection are employed using reverse transcriptase PCR (RT-PCR) analysis to assess expression of cytokeratin messenger RNA in nucleic acid isolated from sentinel lymph nodes.

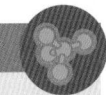

BIOCHEMISTRY

Reverse Transcriptase–Polymerase Chain Reaction (RT-PCR)

RT-PCR is usually accomplished by converting mRNA to cDNA by means of RT followed by standard PCR using fluorophores for signal detection in a real-time PCR instrument. RT requires a primer to initiate DNA synthesis, which can be provided as oligo(dT) (to prime polyA at the 3′ end of mRNAs), a sequence-specific primer, or random hexamers (all possible combinations of six nucleotides).

DNA contamination of mRNA can lead to false-positive signals if primers can bind to and amplify chromosomal DNA (either the native gene or pseudogenes [mutated inactive copies of normal genes that remain in the genome]). Designing primers that span introns or effectively treating RNA preparations with DNAase prior to cDNA synthesis can lessen these potential artifacts.

Nested PCR reactions can potentially detect a single mRNA molecule so that the sensitivity of the assay must be considered in interpreting results, since some cells may express many genes at very low levels (so-called illegitimate transcription) that could be detected by this type of assay.

Nervous System   14

CONTENTS

●●● CONGENITAL MALFORMATIONS

Many different types of congenital anomalies of the central nervous system (CNS) can occur. Many of these are related to neural tube closure, but others can initiate later during intrauterine development or during postnatal brain development. A few chromosomal syndromes result in relatively specific CNS anomalies. Abnormalities in the in utero environment can affect the development of the CNS and result in many different defects of varying severity. Hydranencephaly is an extreme from of porencephaly in which a cyst filled with cerebrospinal fluid (CSF) replaces some or all of the cerebral hemispheres. Hydranencephaly is thought to result from injury at week 12 in gestation, and infants appear normal at birth but lack higher cognitive function and usually die by the end of their first year (Fig. 14-1A). Birth injury or injury in the perinatal period can interfere with postnatal development, particularly in premature infants.

Neural Tube Defects

Neural tube defects are one of the most common causes of congenital anomalies in the CNS. Closure of the neural tube normally begins at about 22 days' gestation and is completed within 4 to 6 days. This narrow time window is a period of significant vulnerability in which abnormalities leading to major and minor birth defects may be initiated. All levels of the neural tube can be affected and, depending on the extent of the abnormality, may result in cystic dilatation of the coverings of the brain (encephaloceles) or spinal cord (meningomyeloceles) (see Fig. 14-1B). In more severe cases, neural tissue is herniated outward though large defects in the vertebrae or cranium. The most severe neural tube defect is anencephaly, in which the brain fails to form because of defective closure of the rostral neural tube (see Fig. 14-1C). Anencephaly is not compatible with life but is a relatively common defect that occurs in up to 1 in 500 pregnancies. Neural tube defects are more common in older mothers, and folate deficiency predisposes to their development. Prenatal screening by measuring α-fetoprotein (AFP) concentration in amniotic fluid can detect neural tube abnormalities in high-risk pregnancies.

Hydrocephalus

Chronic increases in CSF pressure produce hydrocephalus with enlargement of the ventricles and pressure atrophy of both gray and white matter. Obstruction of CNS outflow of any cause (e.g., tumor) can produce hydrocephalus. Congenital

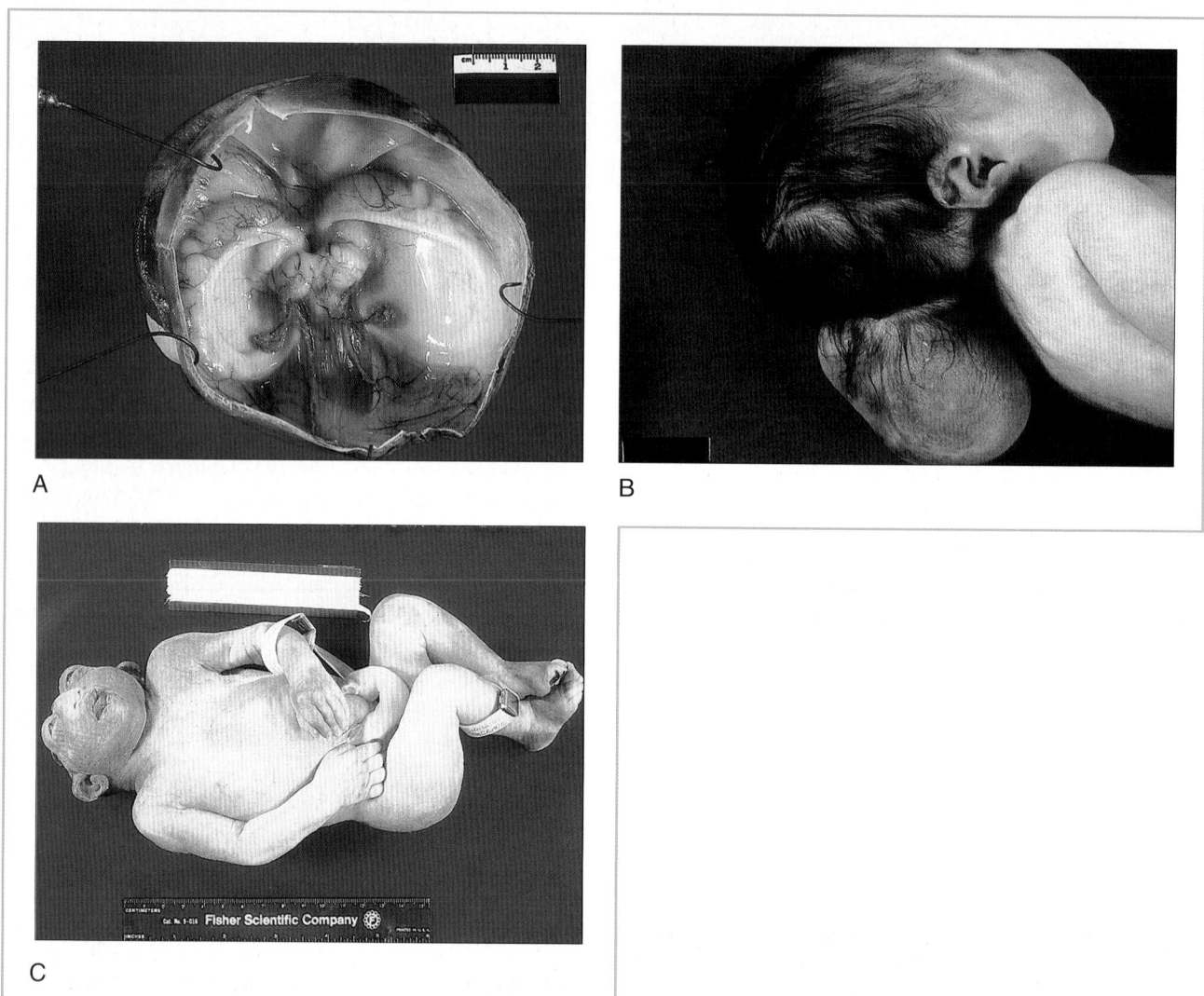

Figure 14-1. A, Hydranencephaly. Gross photograph of brain in situ from a perinatal autopsy (the calvarium has been removed). Brain parenchyma has been compressed into a thin rim by a large CSF filled cyst. **B**, Meningomyelocele. Gross photograph of a neonate with a large cyst (meningomyelocele) arising from the cervical spine that contains neural and meningeal tissue. **C**, Anencephaly. Gross photograph of a neonate with complete absence of upper cranial development.

anomalies such as the Arnold-Chiari and the Dandy-Walker malformations anatomically restrict CSF flow, resulting in hydrocephalus.

Perinatal Injury

The brain is immature even in full-term infants, and the early stage of brain development in premature infants puts them at risk for a number of specific complications in the perinatal period. The germinal matrix adjacent to the cerebral ventricles is predisposed to spontaneous hemorrhage that dissects into the ventricles, producing obstruction to CSF flow and secondary hydrocephalus as well as parenchymal inflammation and destruction (Fig. 14-2). Digestion of extravasated red blood cells by macrophages releases bilirubin, which is neurotoxic.

The blood-brain barrier is immature in both premature and term infants and is not capable of excluding bilirubin from the CNS. Deposition of bilirubin (formed either in situ or from hyperbilirubinemia) results in kernicterus (deposition of bilirubin in the brain parenchyma causing severe, permanent neurologic dysfunction). Hypoxic or mechanical injury during or around the time of birth can result in cerebral palsy with heterogeneous neural and neuromuscular deficits.

●●● CEREBRAL EDEMA AND HERNIATION

Cerebral edema develops in response to any brain injury, infection, or tumor but also can be idiopathic or related to environmental factors (e.g., high altitude or drug exposure).

EMBRYOLOGY

Embryology of the Central Nervous System

Early segmentation of the neural tube forms the major divisions of the CNS including the telencephalon (cerebral hemispheres), diencephalon (thalamus and hypothalamus), mesencephalon (midbrain), metencephalon (pons and cerebellum), and myelencephalon (medulla). Following this segmentation, there is extensive proliferation and migration of neurons between 8 and 16 weeks' gestation. Abnormalities of neuronal proliferation (microcephaly) or migration at these stages result in severe developmental abnormalities.

After 16 weeks' gestation, neural proliferation diminishes but neural migration continues with prominent synapse formation and proliferation of glial cells that begin to myelinate axons. Many aspects of CNS development, particularly neuronal migration and polarity, are controlled by paired homeobox genes. Genes (such as Notch) determine cell lineage. Cell division is regulated predominantly by protein kinases.

Neuronal differentiation is orchestrated by neuronal precursor selector genes (of the helix-loop-helix family). Programmed neuronal death (apoptosis) is also critical for normal CNS development.

PHYSIOLOGY

Blood-Brain Barrier

The blood-brain barrier was discovered in the 19th century by Paul Ehrlich, who injected aniline dyes into the vasculature of animals and observed that dye did not penetrate the CNS as it did other tissues. The blood-brain barrier allows the same signaling molecules (e.g., hormones, cytokines) to be utilized in the CNS and peripheral tissues without cross-talk between the two systems. Blood vessels in the hypothalamus lack a blood-brain barrier so that hypothalamic neurons can respond to hormone levels in the circulation (e.g., leptin).

Structurally, the blood-brain barrier is formed by tightly packed endothelial cells along all blood vessels in the CNS. This arrangement prevents movement of molecules between endothelial cells. Capillary networks outside the CNS permit variable amounts of solute flow between endothelial cells. The fenestrated endothelium of renal glomeruli allows the most extensive periendothelial solute flow in normal physiology.

The blood-brain barrier effectively blocks movement of molecules into the CNS unless they are lipid soluble or utilize specific transporters on endothelial cells. Enzyme systems in endothelial cells inactivate some lipid soluble compounds (e.g., L-dopa) to prevent their entry into the CNS.

Monoclonal antibodies reactive with by $\alpha_4\beta_1$-integrin (a treatment for multiple sclerosis that blocks T-cell access to the CNS) can directly damage the blood-brain barrier, which expresses this adhesion molecule.

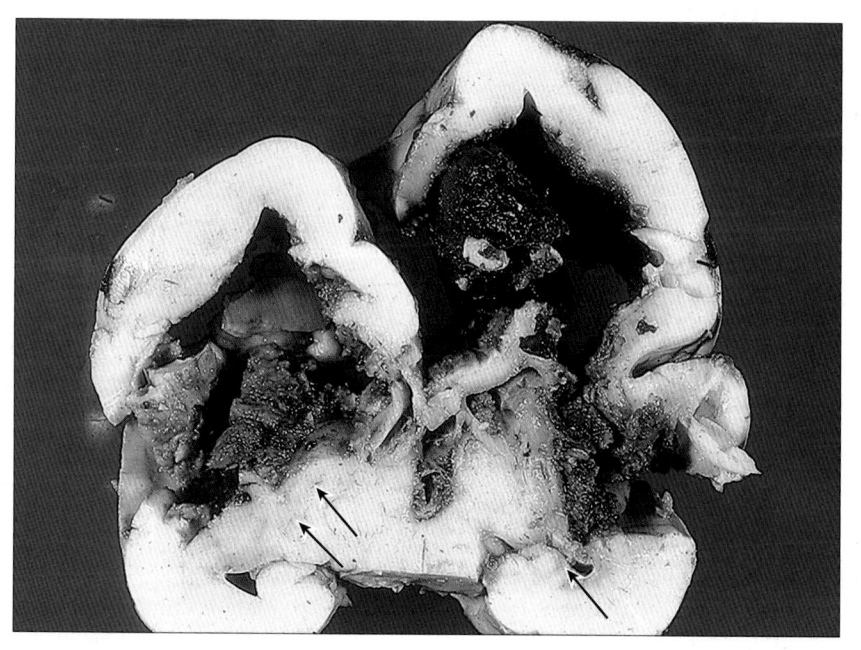

Figure 14-2. Perinatal intraventricular hemorrhage. Gross cross-section of brain from a severely premature neonate with extensive hemorrhage filling and distending the ventricles. The yellowish-green discoloration in brain tissue adjacent to the hematoma (*arrows*) results from bilirubin deposition (kernicterus).

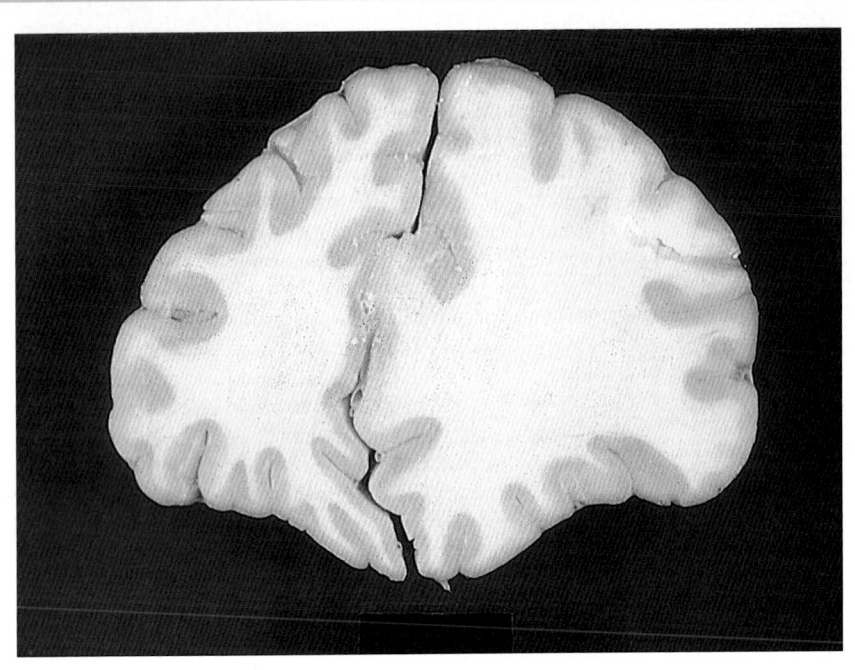

Figure 14-3. Cerebral edema. Gross cross-section of adult brain showing extensive edema of the left hemisphere causing a midline shift.

Since the cranial vault is a closed space, increased brain volume can displace portions of the brain stem into the foramen magnum and result in herniation. As herniation progresses, the cerebral vasculature is compressed, causing ischemia and hemorrhage that is rapidly fatal. Cerebral edema can be decreased by treatment with corticosteroids and by lowering blood CO_2 levels to induce cerebral vasoconstriction and decrease the effective blood volume in the brain. Localized cerebral edema around tumor or infarcts can cause midline shift and may result in additional neurologic abnormalities (Fig. 14-3).

●●● VASCULAR DISEASES

Vascular diseases are an important cause of CNS pathology and are a major cause of morbidity and mortality in the United States. The most common cause of cerebral ischemia is atherosclerosis of the vasculature supplying the brain, leading to cerebral infarction.

Hemorrhage and Hematoma

Subarachnoid hemorrhage can result from the rupture of berry aneurysms around the circle of Willis (congenital out-pouchings at the junctions between cerebral blood vessels) or from the rupture of damaged (e.g., vasculitis, atherosclerosis) or abnormal (e.g., arteriovenous malformation or congophilic angiopathy) blood vessels. Subarachnoid hemorrhage initially results in severe headache (blood provokes a marked inflammatory reaction) and can progress to death quickly depending on the volume of blood released in the intracranial space (Fig. 14-4). Localizing symptoms

may be present if hematoma or an expanding aneurysm compresses cranial nerves.

Mechanical trauma can result in rupture of blood vessels in meninges or dura that produces a subdural hematoma. The accumulation of blood in the subdural space compresses brain tissue, and large hematomas can cause herniation. Hematomas may enlarge or slowly resolve by organization of the blood clot (chronic subdural hematoma). Chronic subdural hematomas are at increased risk for recurrent hemorrhage.

Arteriovenous Malformation

Arteriovenous malformations (AVMs) are abnormal connections between the arterial and venous circulation and can occur in the brain as well as other sites. The abnormal blood vessels in AVMs are prone to spontaneous hemorrhage, and expansion and contraction of AVMs may produce seizure foci within the brain. Hemorrhage can cause intra-parenchymal hematomas or subarachnoid hemorrhage. Some patients have multiple AVMs as part of genetic syndromes (e.g., Sturge-Weber syndrome).

Cerebral Infarct

The location of a cerebral infarct is directly related to the anatomy of the cerebral vasculature. Since all cerebral arteries are essentially end arteries, their vascular occlusion results in infarction of distal brain tissue. Watershed areas at the junction of the distribution of different arteries may be damaged but not infarcted when a vessel is occluded. Conversely, hypotension may cause dysfunction or infarction preferentially in watershed areas, since they correspond to

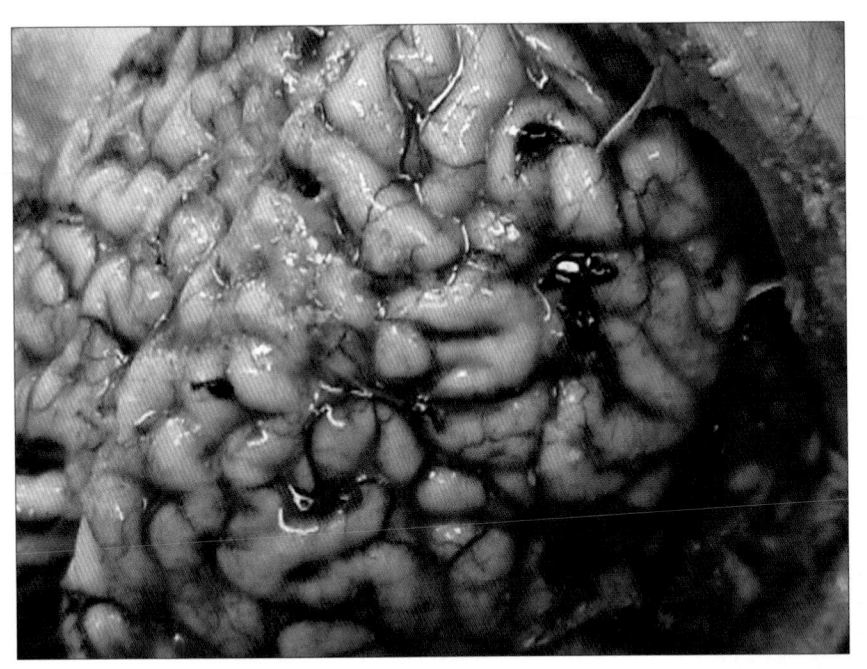

Figure 14-4. Subarachnoid hemorrhage. Gross photograph of the external surface of adult brain showing focal subarachnoid hemorrhage that elevates the arachnoid membrane.

the most distal penetration of each artery. Most cerebral infarcts are thrombotic, and most of these do not result in hemorrhage (Fig. 14-5A). Some patients have transient ischemic attacks (TIAs) before a cerebral infarct, which result from the release of microemboli from thrombi or ruptured atherosclerotic plaques.

Aside from thrombotic events, emboli are the next most common cause of cerebral infarcts, and embolic infarcts are frequently hemorrhagic. Most embolic infarcts are caused by fragments of atherosclerotic plaque, but arterial thrombi or mural thrombi of the left side of the heart and cardiac valves can also produce embolic infarcts. Rarely, paradoxical emboli that pass from the right to the left circulation through a patent foramen ovale or septal defect cause embolic cerebral infarcts. Anticoagulation and antiplatelet agents may diminish the size of some nonhemorrhagic infarcts if they can be administered soon after the onset of ischemia, but these agents are usually contradicted in patients with hemorrhagic infarcts.

Infarcts that are associated with hemorrhage produce more inflammation and a greater amount of brain edema than nonhemorrhagic infarcts of similar size. Hemorrhagic infarcts can also dissect brain tissue and extend into the cerebral ventricles or the subarachnoid space, producing additional complications (see Fig. 14-5B).

Cerebral infarcts undergo liquefactive necrosis because of the limited supporting extracellular matrix in the CNS. Infarcts liquefy and resolve over very long time intervals as necrotic debris is slowly removed by the action of microglial cells and recruited inflammatory cells. Conversion of a cerebral infarct to a cystic space filled with CSF may require

many months. Lacunar infarcts are small cerebral infarcts (less than 1 cm in maximal dimension) that typically develop in hypertensive patients. Lacunar infarcts tend to occur in the basal ganglia and are often clinically asymptomatic but may be visible on magnetic resonance imaging (MRI).

Retinopathy

Diabetic retinopathy is caused by ischemia of retinal tissue secondary to microvascular disease in diabetes. Hypoxia induces the neovascularization of the retina, and these new blood vessels interfere with vision directly and are prone to hemorrhage, which can result in retinal detachment (separation of the retina from the choroid), causing retinal necrosis and blindness.

Macular degeneration is a relatively common condition of older adults and can occur in wet and dry forms. Both begin with the accumulation of drusen (yellowish amorphous material) within Bruch's membrane in the macula that displace retinal cells from their underlying vascular supply. The slow accumulation of material eventually decreases visual acuity. The less common wet form of macular degeneration results from vascular proliferation in association with drusen that can cause rapid visual loss.

●●● INFECTIOUS DISEASES

Bacterial infections of the blood do not usually result in CNS infection in adults owing to the blood-brain barrier. In neonates, the blood-brain barrier is not effective in excluding bacteria so that all bacterial infections of blood

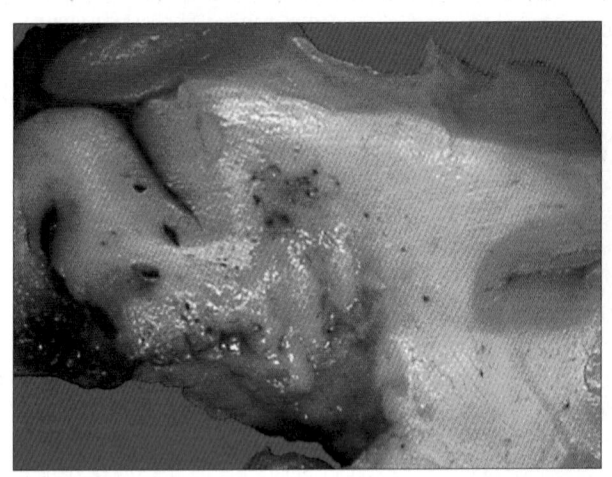

A

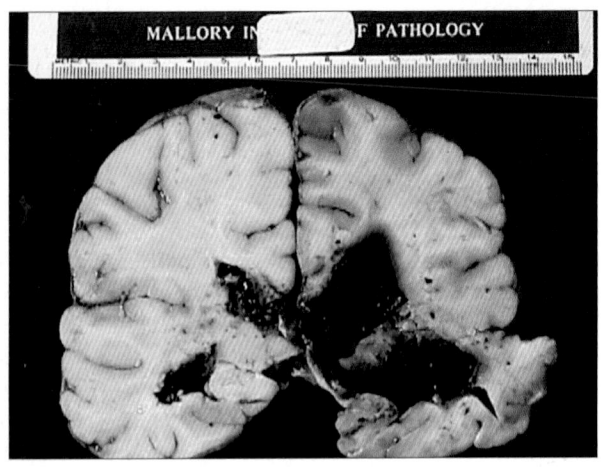

MALLORY IN   F PATHOLOGY

B

Figure 14-5. A, Subacute cerebral infarct. Gross cross-section of cerebral cortex and white matter with a discrete area of softening and degeneration with early liquefaction. **B,** Cerebral infarct with intraventricular hemorrhage. Gross cross-section of brain with a right cerebral infarct complicated by dissection of blood into the ventricular system with massive hemorrhage.

ANATOMY

Central Nervous System Vascular Anatomy

Eighty percent of cerebral infarcts involve the distribution of the carotid arteries while the remaining 20% occur in the distribution of the vertebrobasilar artery.

Thrombotic infarcts predominate in the anterior (carotid) circulation, and most large infarcts produce readily identifiable cognitive or motor dysfunction. Embolic infarcts are more common in the vertebrobasilar circulation and often present with more ambiguous symptoms (e.g., gait disturbance due to cerebellar infarcts) and may be underdiagnosed. The communicating arteries are usually too small to provide useful collateral circulation in the event of a proximal occlusion or carotid artery disease. Most berry aneurysms develop at the connections between the anterior communicating and carotid arteries.

IMMUNOLOGY

Macular Degeneration

Macular degeneration is strongly associated with advanced age and affects up to 10% of individuals by age 70 years and 30% by age 80 years. Exudative (wet) macular degeneration develops in a minority of affected patients (10%) and can rapidly destroy useful vision. Wet macular degeneration results from neovascularization of the macula with leakage of plasma proteins that elevate the retina.

Some cases of macular degeneration show a familial pattern of inheritance with a fourfold higher lifetime risk in patients' primary relatives. Evidence of ongoing systemic inflammation (elevated serum C-reactive protein) is associated with a two-fold increased risk of developing macular degeneration.

There is a strong association between polymorphisms in the complement factor H (CFH) gene and the development of macular degeneration (e.g., CFH gene variants may explain up to 50% of cases). Some familial cases of macular degeneration are associated with mutations in the fibulin genes, which are extracellular matrix components of Bruch's membrane.

have the potential to progress to meningitis. Many viral infections produce transient encephalitis that is subclinical and unrecognized, but a few viruses have an affinity for brain tissue and can produce severe encephalitis, resulting in serious long-term complications or death.

Meningitis

Meningitis means inflammation of the meningeal coverings of the brain that can result from bacterial or viral infection or, less commonly, parasites. Viral meningitis is the most common and least damaging form of meningitis and can be produced by a variety of viruses, many of which are transmitted by insect vectors. Inflammation of the meninges results in severe

headache with other symptoms and signs related to increased intracranial pressure. Examination of CSF may show a mild polymorphonuclear leukocytosis early in infection that rapidly converts to lymphocytosis. CSF protein is also increased, and patients typically show meningeal signs on physical examination, with prominent neck stiffness and rigidity (any traction on the inflamed meninges causes severe pain). Most cases of viral meningitis are self-limited although the symptoms may be severe and protracted.

Bacterial meningitis is much less common than viral meningitis, and most cases are caused by a limited number of specific organisms. Different bacteria can cause meningitis that is more likely to develop in compromised hosts, for example, individuals with comorbid disease or neonates with an ineffective blood-brain barrier. CSF examination in patients with bacterial meningitis typically shows a marked increase in cell count with neutrophils predominating. Intracellular and extracellular bacteria may be visible on Gram's stain of CSF sediment. Rapid diagnosis may allow immediate initiation of antibiotic therapy that may be life-saving.

Neisseria meningitidis is the prototypical agent of infectious bacterial meningitis. Its classic presentation is as an epidemic infection in the setting of a college dormitory or among military recruits. Most adolescents do not have protective antibodies against *N. meningitidis*, so there is a high probability of person-to-person transmission in this population. *N. meningitidis* causes fulminant septicemia and meningitis in naïve patients and can be rapidly fatal. Older adults tend to have protective antibodies so that epidemic infection in the general population does not occur.

Streptococcus pneumoniae can produce meningitis in susceptible individuals although most patients with *S. pneumoniae* pneumonia do not develop meningitis, because of an effective blood-brain barrier. Meningitis tends to develop in debilitated and elderly individuals with impaired host defenses and comorbid disease or in young children. Patients with *S. pneumoniae* meningitis accumulate acute inflammatory cells in their meninges, resulting in whitish opacification of the sulci (Fig. 14-6A). Untreated cases are usually fatal.

In the past, *Haemophilus influenzae* was a very important cause of meningitis in children, but widespread vaccination has greatly reduced the incidence of *H. influenzae meningitis* in the United States. Bacterial meningitis often results in permanent neurologic complications (e.g., hydrocephalus), particularly in children.

Encephalitis

Encephalitis means direct microbial infection of the brain and is almost always caused by viruses. Subclinical encephalitis occurs in many viral illnesses, but only a limited number of viruses produce clinically significant encephalitis. Most encephalitis viruses are mosquito-borne viruses that can produce a range of effects in humans. Some of these viruses are zoonoses, with various animals being the definitive host (e.g., eastern equine encephalitis). Microscopic examination of brain tissue from patients with encephalitis often shows microglial nodules, which are accumulations of proliferating glial cells at sites of inflammation and infection in the brain (see Fig. 14-6B). Some types of viral encephalitis target specific areas of the brain. St. Louis encephalitis (which occurred in epidemic form in 1919) preferentially destroyed neurons in the substantia nigra, producing permanent Parkinson's disease in a significant percentage of patients.

Herpes simplex can cause severe encephalitis with neuronal necrosis that predominantly affects the frontal lobes. While latent herpes simplex infection is common in the general population, herpes encephalitis is rare. The host factors that predispose to herpes encephalitis in adults are not well understood. Neonatal herpes simplex infection results in a fatal disseminated infection (herpes neonatorum) with encephalitis.

Brain Abscess and Epidural Abscess

Brain abscess is usually caused by bacterial infection although it can also result from parasitic infection. Brain abscesses are similar to abscesses at other sites and consist of a cavity filled with neutrophils, microorganisms, and scattered macrophages. The limited ability of the CNS to respond to infection often results in a failure to effectively wall off the abscess, and progressive infection of brain tissue is common. Abscesses can initiate seizures and typically show a ring-enhancing pattern on contrast-enhanced computed tomography (CT) scan. Abscess formation in the epidural space usually occurs along

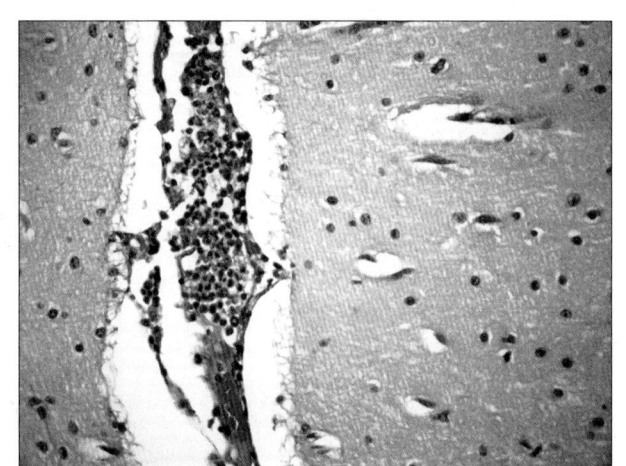

A

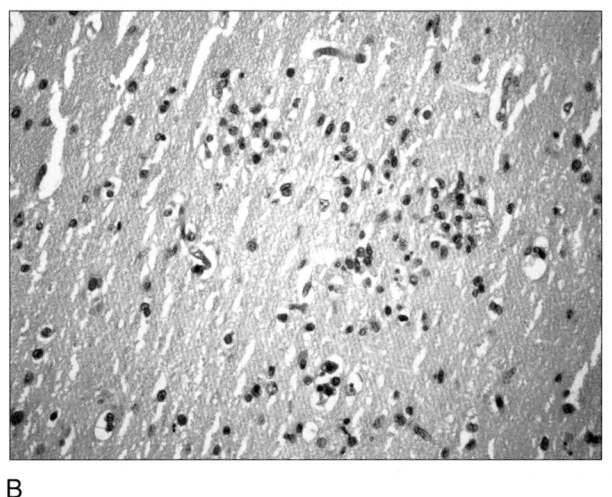

B

Figure 14-6. A, Bacterial meningitis. Microscopic section of cerebral cortex with overlying arachnoid membrane (*center*) containing a dense neutrophilic infiltrate. **B**, Microglial nodule. Microscopic section of cerebral cortex showing a focal area of increased cellularity (proliferating microglial cells) caused by viral encephalitis.

the vertebral column and can result in leukocytosis in the CSF. Epidural abscess may put pressure on the spinal cord and nerve roots, leading to localizing neurologic symptoms.

Other Diseases

Tuberculosis can directly infect the CNS to cause meningitis or brain abscess (tuberculoma), which may obstruct CSF flow, resulting in hydrocephalus. Tuberculous osteomyelitis of the vertebral bodies (Pott's disease) causes inflammation and dysfunction of spinal nerve roots.

Human immunodeficiency virus (HIV) can directly infect neurons and result in CNS dysfunction (HIV dementia). Immunodeficiency associated with HIV also predisposes to a number of different infectious complications in the CNS that can occur in patients who are immunosuppressed for other reasons. Progressive multifocal leukoencephalopathy (PML) is caused by a papovavirus (JC virus) that is not capable of producing disease in immunocompetent individuals. PML results in demyelination of the deep white matter, which can be rapidly fatal. Treatment of multiple sclerosis or Crohn's disease with monoclonal antibodies directed against integrins involved in transporting T cells to the CNS can cause PML. Toxoplasmosis can produce abscesses within the CNS in immunosuppressed patients, and cytomegalovirus (CMV) can cause encephalitis in immunosuppressed patients.

●●● DEMYELINATING DISEASES

Demyelinating diseases result in damage to or destruction of the myelin sheaths of axons and thereby block neuronal conduction. Neurons are usually left intact, and subsequent remyelination usually restores normal function (in contrast, diseases that target and kill neurons are largely irreversible).

Multiple Sclerosis

Multiple sclerosis is an autoimmune disease in which T cells attack oligodendroglial cells in the CNS causing demyelination of neurons and failure of normal axonal conduction. Multiple sclerosis tends to be a relapsing and remitting disease in which localized areas in the brain are targeted at different times, resulting in demyelinated white matter plaques that can be visualized radiographically (Fig. 14-7A). Cranial nerve involvement is common and may suggest the diagnosis of multiple sclerosis. Since multiple sclerosis does not usually result in axonal necrosis, remyelination of axons can occur after inflammation diminishes, with partial or complete restoration of neuronal function. Demyelinated plaques cause the characteristic clinical presentation of multiple sclerosis in which patients develop neurologic lesions that vary both over time and in the location of CNS involvement. Although T cells target oligodendroglial cells in multiple sclerosis, repeated attacks can eventually result in neuron loss and permanent neurologic deficit (see Fig. 14-7B).

Multiple sclerosis is more common in some geographic areas (northern latitudes), and many cases show a strong

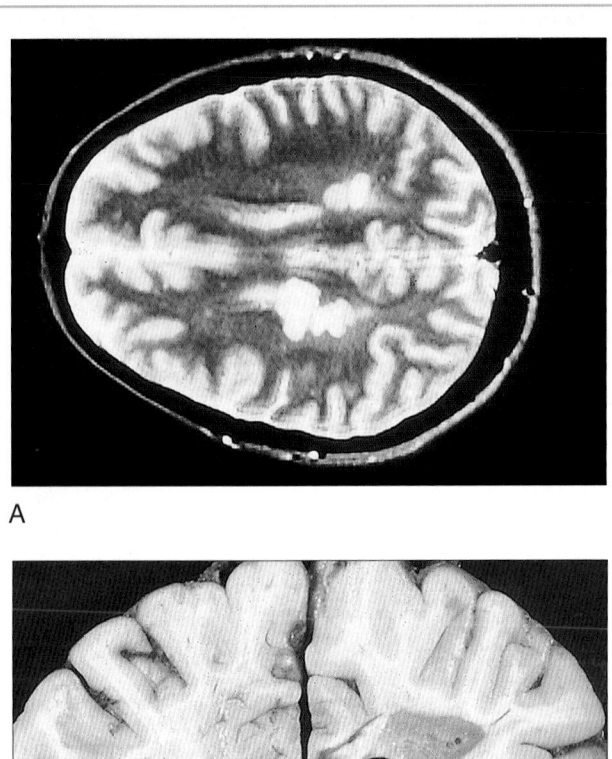

A

B

Figure 14-7. A, Multiple sclerosis. CT scan with contrast showing irregular plaques of demyelination in the central white matter (note the loss of normal symmetry between the left and right hemispheres). **B,** Gross cross-section of brain showing plaques (yellowish variegated areas) in the cortical white matter (most prominent on the left).

genetic predisposition. The cause or trigger of the autoimmune reaction in multiple sclerosis is not known. Viruses have been suspected as triggers (e.g., canine distemper virus), but none have been convincingly implicated. Some patients may have one attack of multiple sclerosis in their lifetime and no subsequent recurrences. Most patients have a waxing and waning course that eventually results in permanent neurologic deficit. Cognitive function is usually preserved until late in disease. A minority of patients have a clinical course characterized by unremitting disease that progresses to death over a few years.

Many patients with multiple sclerosis develop oligoclonal bands of immunoglobulin in their CSF at some point during their illness. Oligoclonal bands are produced by the clonal expansion of a limited number of B cells in the CNS. Since the immunoglobulins produced by each clone are identical, they comigrate to form a band on protein electrophoresis. By definition, oligoclonal bands are not present in patient serum and so must derive from B cells in the CNS. While oligoclonal bands seem to suggest a significant role for B cells in the pathogenesis of multiple sclerosis, other evidence does not support this view, and oligoclonal bands are thought to be an epiphenomenon related to inflammation and tissue destruction in the CNS.

Antibody-based therapy that eliminates the subclass of T cells that would normally migrate to the CNS (via specific integrins expressed on their surface) has been shown to decrease the appearance of new lesions in multiple sclerosis patients, but the resulting CNS-specific immunodeficiency can cause complications (e.g., PML; see above) and the safety of this form of therapy is uncertain.

Guillain-Barré Syndrome

Guillain-Barré syndrome is an acute to subacute demyelinating neuropathy that affects both the central and peripheral nervous systems and most often develops as an idiosyncratic reaction to vaccination. By definition, the symptoms and signs of demyelination must evolve in less than 1 month. Since myelin sheaths rather than neurons are damaged, many patients make a complete, although protracted, recovery (remyelination of long tracts may require months).

● ● ● NUTRITIONAL AND METABOLIC DISEASES

Some specific nutritional deficiencies can damage neurons in the CNS and cause specific neurologic deficits. Maternal folate deficiency during early pregnancy predisposes to neural tube closure defects. Severe deficiency of vitamin B_{12} (usually in persons with alcoholism) can cause Wernicke-Korsakoff syndrome, in which a loss of neurons in the hippocampus results in an almost complete failure to process information into long-term memory. Affected patients can hold new memories for only a few minutes before they are lost.

A number of different genetic diseases manifest predominantly as CNS pathology. Most of these diseases show autosomal or X-linked recessive inheritance. Since neurons are long-lived cells, even minor accumulations of abnormal metabolites (or the inability to degrade normal metabolites) can eventually result in neuronal dysfunction and death as a result of relatively mild abnormalities in enzyme function. Tay-Sachs disease (hexosaminidase α-subunit deficiency) is a lysosomal storage disease that results in the accumulation of G_{M2} gangliosides in the lysozomes of neurons that causes swelling and dysfunction. Many individual mutations have been characterized in Tay-Sachs disease, and the frequency of heterozygotes is high in some populations (1 in 30 in Ashkenazi Jews). Other genetic deficiency diseases disrupt myelination (so-called leukodystrophies) and include Krabbe's disease (galactocerebrosidase deficiency) and meta-

chromatic leukodystrophy (arylsulfatase A deficiency). These diseases usually cause death in early childhood with symmetric loss of myelin throughout the white matter.

● ● ● DEGENERATIVE DISEASES

Degenerative diseases of the central and peripheral nervous systems are a heterogeneous group of disease processes. Some degenerative diseases are genetic or have significant genetic risk factors, others are infectious, and in still others the pathophysiology is unclear.

Alzheimer's Disease

Alzheimer's disease is by far the most common cause of dementia in United States. Alzheimer's disease usually does not affect patients before their sixth decade but can occur earlier, particularly in familial and genetic cases. Alzheimer's disease is a slowly progressive dementia that results in the gradual loss of higher level cognitive functions over the course of years or decades. Patients with Alzheimer's disease show progressive brain atrophy and loss of cortical volume. Examination of Alzheimer's brains at autopsy typically shows marked hydrocephalus secondary to loss of brain tissue (lost brain volume is replaced with CSF because of the closed cranial vault). The external surface of the brain typically shows deep sulci and thin, razor-like gyri owing to the extensive loss of gray matter.

Known risk factors for Alzheimer's disease include a history of a relative with dementia (particularly early-onset dementia) or inheritance of the ApoE4 lipoprotein allele (which increases the rate of dementia progression by unknown mechanisms). Cases with a strong familial inheritance pattern of Alzheimer's disease are uncommon compared with sporadic cases, and disease often develops at an earlier age in familial cases. Patients with familial Alzheimer's disease usually have abnormalities in one of several genes that are now thought to be related to the pathogenesis of Alzheimer's disease in sporadic cases.

Amyloid precursor protein (APP) is a normal cellular protein that can be abnormally processed (cleaved by a novel protease) into a peptide ($A\beta_{42}$) that tends to form amyloid deposits within the CNS. As amyloid deposits grow, they produce plaques, which are one of the characteristic lesions of Alzheimer's disease. Amyloid plaques form outside neurons in the neuropil (space containing axons and dendrites) and are usually surrounded by a proliferation neurites, which can be seen in silver-stained sections of brain tissue (Fig. 14-8A). These plaques cause disruption of the brain substance and death of neurons. Inheritance of point mutations in the APP gene in some cases of familial Alzheimer's disease results in a protein that is much more likely to be abnormally processed and by γ-secretase to form $A\beta_{42}$ amyloid plaques. Patients with Down syndrome (trisomy 21) have an extra copy of the APP gene and tend to develop Alzheimer's disease at an early age as a result of increased APP gene dosage. Other cases of familial

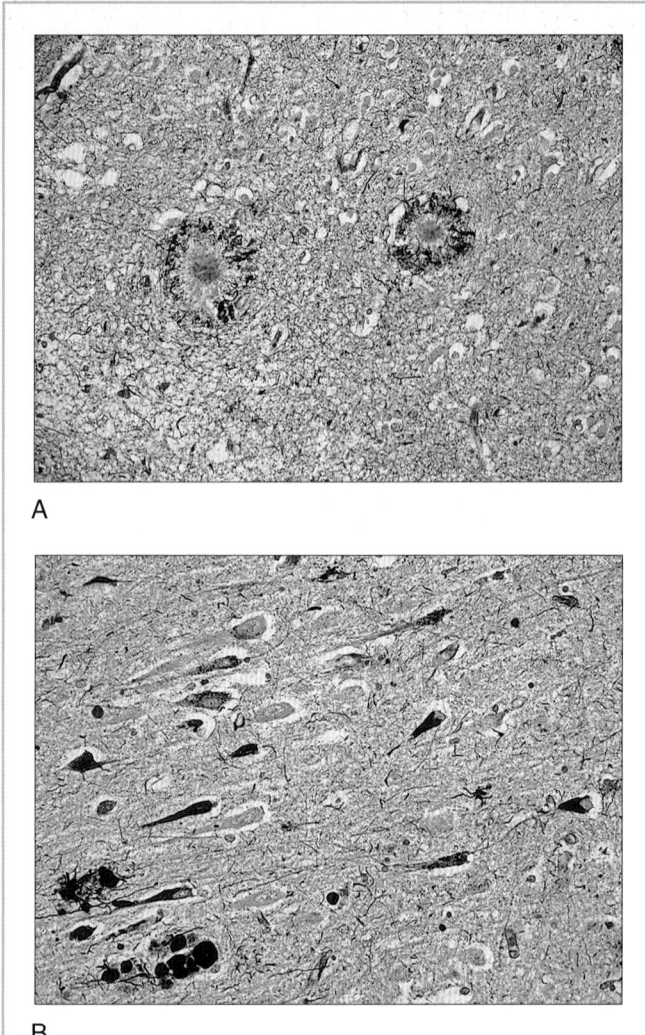

A

B

Figure 14-8. Alzheimer's disease. **A**, Microscopic section of cerebral cortex showing two amyloid plaques in a silver-stained section. Amyloid appears as a brownish-red dot surrounded by proliferating neurites (stained black) creating a "bull's-eye" pattern. **B**, Microscopic, silver-stained section of cerebral cortex showing neurofibrillary tangles (black fibers in neuron cell bodies).

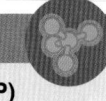

BIOCHEMISTRY

γ-Secretase and Amyloid Precursor Protein (APP) Processing

γ-Secretase is an unusual aspartyl protease that cleaves proteins within the membrane lipid bilayer. γ-Secretase activity depends on the presence of multiple protein components including presenilin 1, which is mutated in some familial cases of Alzheimer's disease.

APP is normally processed by α- and γ-secretase to produce three peptide fragments. Occasionally, APP is cleaved by β-secretase rather than α-secretase. This rare cleavage product can be cleaved again by γ-secretase to release the $A\beta_{40}$ peptide into the extracellular space. $A\beta_{40}$ peptide has the potential to form amyloid but does so with low efficiency.

Aberrant cleavage by γ-secretase (two amino acids away from its normal cleavage site) creates the $A\beta_{42}$ peptide, which forms amyloid with high efficiency. Mutations in the APP gene in some cases of familial Alzheimer's disease favor β-secretase cleavage and aberrant cleavage by γ-secretase to preferentially generate the $A\beta_{42}$ peptide. Presenilin 1 mutations in familial Alzheimer's disease may also modify γ-secretase to favor $A\beta_{42}$ peptide production.

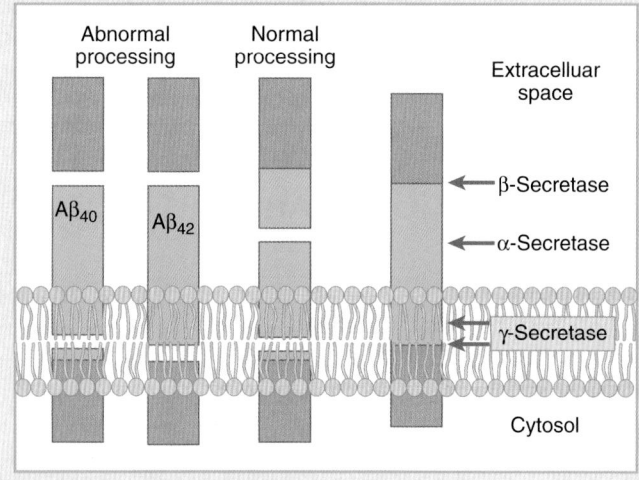

Alzheimer's disease have mutation in the presenilin 1 gene, which appears to be a component of the γ-secretase complex and which may modify its function to favor the creation of $A\beta_{42}$ peptides.

Many patients with Alzheimer's disease also have amyloid deposition in the blood vessels of the brain (so-called congophilic angiopathy), which may cause vascular narrowing with ischemia or predispose to hemorrhage. Some demented patients who do not have clinical features of Alzheimer's disease also have congophilic angiopathy. Patients with Alzheimer's disease characteristically develop neurofibrillary tangles in addition to amyloid plaques. Abnormal tau proteins accumulate in the axons and cell bodies of neurons to form neurofibrillary tangles (see Fig. 14-8B).

Amyloid plaques and neurofibrillary tangles accumulate in all individuals as they age but are much more frequent in patients with Alzheimer's disease. Lesions tend to be more extensive in the hippocampus (so-called paleocortex), which is involved in memory function, and Alzheimer's patients initially have a prominent and characteristic loss of recent memory with minimal effects on long-term memory.

Creutzfeldt-Jakob Disease and New Variant CJD

Creutzfeldt-Jakob disease (CJD) is caused by the accumulation of an abnormal protein derivative (prion) within neurons that results in neuronal dysfunction and death. CJD

NEUROANATOMY

Hippocampus

The hippocampus is a portion of the inferior temporal lobe that is part of the limbic system, which mediates emotion. Hippocampus means seahorse, which describes the shape of this portion of the brain that is evolutionarily conserved but is proportionately increased in size in humans and other higher primates.

The hippocampus is required for making new memories about personally experienced events and is more severely affected in patients with Alzheimer's disease than are other cortical regions. Hippocampal dysfunction does not usually affect memories that have already formed or the ability to learn new skills. Some hippocampal neurons are involved in spatial memory and navigation, which are also affected early in most Alzheimer's patients.

MICROBIOLOGY

Prions

Prions are proteinaceous infectious particles that can recruit specific host proteins or peptides to mimic their abnormal conformation. The human protein that can be converted into prions is called PrP (prion-related protein), and it is designated PrPSc when it takes on prion conformation.

Prions are present in many plants and animals and may have beneficial functions in some contexts. Yeast prions have been studied extensively and contain numerous repeats of the amino acids glutamine and asparagine (Q/N-rich domains), which are not present in mammalian prions.

Prions tend to have rigid three-dimensional structures in contrast to the normal proteins from which they derive. This rigidity may favor the assembly of prion monomers into filaments that cause cellular dysfunction.

Prions cause disease similar to Creutzfeldt-Jakob disease in sheep and goats (scrapie), mink (transmissible mink encephalopathy), deer (chronic wasting disease), and other species. The amino acid sequences of prion proteins are strongly conserved across different species, enabling some animal prions to produce disease in humans.

occurs in both familial and sporadic (infectious) forms. Most familial cases have a point mutation in the prion precursor protein (PPP) gene that results in its abnormal processing by cellular proteases and the formation of a prion peptide. In infectious cases, exposure to infected individuals may transfer sufficient numbers of prions to cause infection (e.g., transmission has been documented to occur via contaminated neurosurgical instruments). Prion infection is not nucleic acid based and so is markedly different from other types of infectious disease. Infectious prions are thought to recruit cellular proteins and cause conformational changes that convert these proteins into functional prions. Prions are highly resistant to most means of decontamination (e.g., autoclaving, formalin fixation, hypochlorite) so that infection control in hospital and autopsy settings is problematic.

CJD causes rapidly progressive dementia, and patients tend to lose cognitive function over the course of days to weeks (in Alzheimer's disease functional loss is measured in month to years). Gross examination of the brain in patients with CJD usually does not show prominent atrophy because of the extremely rapid progression to death (there is insufficient time for damaged neural tissue to be removed by microglial cells). Microscopic sections of CJD brains show spongiform changes with a "Swiss cheese"–like pattern in cortical brain tissue. Rare amyloid plaques composed of prions are present predominantly in the molecular layer of the cerebellum.

New variant CJD results from infection of humans with the prion that causes bovine spongiform encephalopathy (BSE). Ingestion of large quantities of infected bovine tissue can result in a similar illness in human beings. Most prions in affected animals are present in neural tissue so that meat contaminated with brain tissue likely confers a much higher risk of infection. An epidemic of BSE occurred in England during the late 1980s as a result of recycling residual bovine tissues from slaughterhouses (largely neural and bone tissue) as feed products for other cattle. This practice resulted in the concentration of prions in the bovine food chain and in the

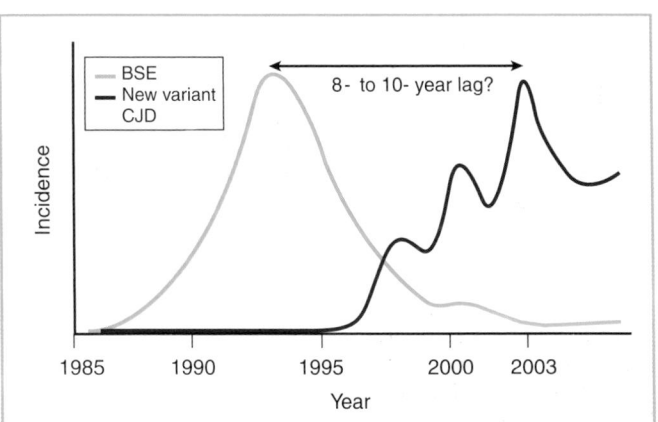

Figure 14-9. Epidemiology of bovine spongiform encephalopathy (BSE) and new variant CJD.

appearance of cases of new variant CJD in a few young adults during the 1990s and early in this century (Fig. 14-9). The number of cases of new variant CJD is very small with less than 300 cases known to have occurred worldwide. Patients with new variant CJD usually have prominent neuropsychiatric symptoms and progress rapidly to death, usually within a year of diagnosis. Examination of brain reveals prominent spongiform change at the microscopic level as well as prominent amyloid plaques throughout the CNS. In contrast, amyloid plaques are scant or absent in CJD. Public health measures have largely eliminated BSE, and cases of new variant CJD are trending downward. Since the incubation period for new variant CJD is not precisely known, it is not certain whether this disease has been eradicated.

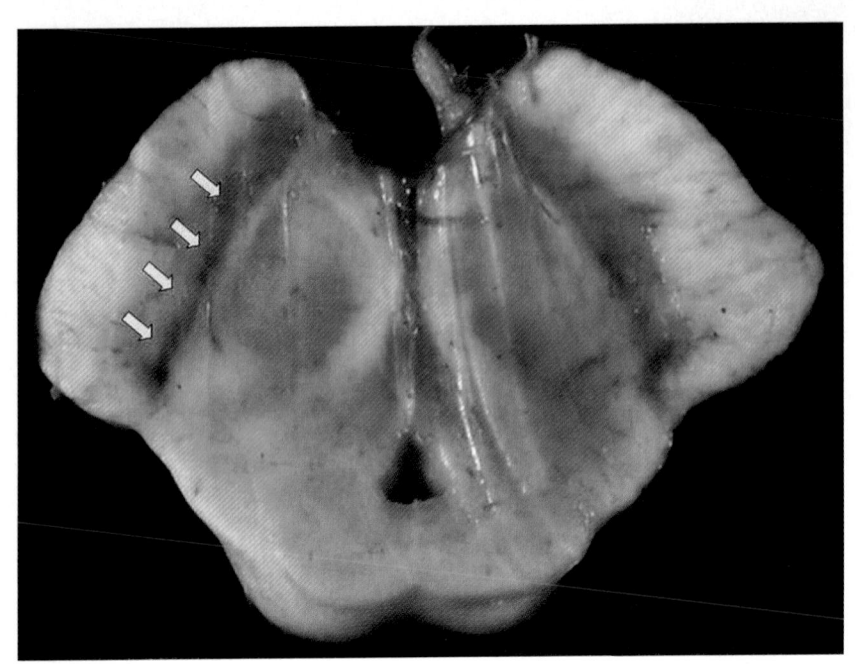

Figure 14-10. Parkinson's disease. Gross cross-section of midbrain in a patient with long-standing Parkinson's disease. The substantia nigra (*arrows*) is markedly pale compared with a normal midbrain in which it would appear as a distinct black stripe.

Parkinson's Disease

Parkinson's disease results from loss of dopaminergic neurons in the substantia nigra and locus caeruleus. These neurons normally contain melanin pigment (neuromelanin), and loss of these neurons results in pallor of the substantia nigra that can be appreciated grossly in cross-sections of the midbrain (Fig. 14-10). Most patients with Parkinson's disease have Lewy bodies (intracytoplasmic inclusions of eosinophilic material containing aggregates of α-synuclein) in residual dopaminergic neurons. Lewy bodies are not specific for Parkinson's disease and may be observed in other types of neurons in some demented patients (i.e., dementia with Lewy bodies).

Loss of dopaminergic neurons results in the characteristic symptoms of Parkinson's disease of increased rigidity, halting gait, and intention tremor. As Parkinson's disease progresses, cognitive dysfunction often develops as well. A substantial number of patients develop both Parkinson's and Alzheimer's diseases. Infection with some encephalitis viruses has resulted in a Parkinson's disease–like syndrome in surviving patients who show loss of dopaminergic neurons.

The cause of Parkinson's disease is not known. Genetic mutations in a number of different genes appear to be involved in cases of familial Parkinson's disease (which account for a very small percentage of cases of Parkinson's disease). The gene defects in these families suggest that abnormalities in protein folding or in targeting of misfolded proteins (e.g., α-synuclein) to the proteasome (mutations have been identified in ubiquitin ligase gene) may be involved in neuronal toxicity and loss in sporadic cases.

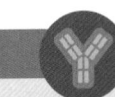

NEUROANATOMY

Dopaminergic Neurons

Parkinson's disease results from dysfunction of the extrapyramidal motor system owing to loss of dopaminergic neurons in the substantial nigra of the midbrain. Dopamine normally inhibits extrapyramidal neurons, and the loss of this inhibition results in their hyperactivity. The symptoms of Parkinsonism result from excess extrapyramidal motor activity and include bradykinesia (decreased movement), tremor at rest, and rigidity.

The substantia nigra in patients with Parkinson's disease has increased levels of free radicals and decreased amounts of antioxidants compared with normal brain, suggesting a possible mechanism for neuron loss. Parkinsonism (with symptoms similar to those in patients with Parkinson's disease) can be caused by drugs including narcoleptics, reserpine, and lithium or by toxins such as carbon monoxide, mercury, and MPTP.

Huntington's Disease

Huntington's disease is a genetic disease caused by an abnormally large number of triplet repeats in the Huntington gene. This genetic lesion results in a protein that is abnormally processed by secretase in the plasma membrane to produce a toxic protein fragment. These toxic peptides accumulate as aggregates in the cytoplasm of neural cells and after many years (average clinical age of onset is 40 years) results in the

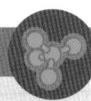

α-Synuclein and Parkinson's Disease

α-Synuclein is a small, presynaptic protein of unknown function that is a component of Lewy bodies in both Parkinson's disease and other neurodegenerative diseases including dementia with Lewy bodies.

Point mutations in α-synuclein have been identified in some cases of familial Parkinson's disease, and these amino acid changes may lead to protein misfolding, aggregation, and Lewy body formation. Patients with sporadic Parkinson's disease do not have mutations in α-synuclein, but most do have Lewy bodies containing α-synuclein.

Other cases of familial Parkinson's disease have abnormalities in proteins that control protein targeting to the proteasome. Defective proteasome mediated degradation of abnormally folded α-synuclein may lead to Lewy body formation and neuronal toxicity in these patients. Mutations in ubiquitin ligase or ubiquitin hydrolase have been identified in these families.

Other studies suggest that increased oxidative stress in dopaminergic neurons may result in protein denaturation and contribute to protein misfolding and Lewy body formation. Since concordance for Parkinson's disease in identical twins is relatively low, environmental factors must also be important in producing disease.

dysfunction and death of neurons, predominantly in the basal ganglia. Loss of basal ganglia neurons causes the characteristic symptom of ataxia (difficulty walking) followed by loss of higher functions. The genetics of Huntington's disease is discussed in more detail in Chapter 4.

Amyotrophic Lateral Sclerosis

Amyotrophic lateral sclerosis (Lou Gehrig disease) targets upper and lower motor neurons (cranial nerves and spinal cord) and results in neuronal cell death and progressive loss of motor function. Patients usually have lower extremity weakness that progresses to complete paralysis over the course of years. Genetic abnormalities in superoxide dismutase (SOD) 1 have been identified in rare cases of familial amyotrophic lateral sclerosis, suggesting that O_2-derived free radical damage may be responsible for neuronal damage. A mouse model system also implicates superoxide dismutase. Deficient glutamate uptake in synapses (with persistent neuronal stimulation and hyperreactivity) may also contribute to neuron damage and may be a therapeutic target. Hyperexcitation could enhance oxygen-mediated damage, resulting in a synergistic effect.

Diabetic Neuropathy

Diabetic neuropathy is a peripheral neuropathy in which sensory and motor nerves are damaged or destroyed as a result of ischemic microvascular disease and nonenzymatic glycosylation of neuronal component.

●●● TUMORS OF THE CENTRAL NERVOUS SYSTEM

Most primary tumors of the CNS derive from glial cells, and tumors of neurons are very uncommon. Adults and children develop a different spectrum of brain tumors with posterior fossa tumors (cerebellum) being common in children but rare in adults. Many brain tumors, whether benign are malignant, initially present with seizure activity. Localizing symptoms relating to specific brain areas or cranial nerve compression may be a clue to the diagnosis. Radiologic imaging (particularly MRI) is quite sensitive for detecting tumors and characterizing their location and extent.

Astrocytoma

Astrocytomas (also called gliomas) are neoplasms of the supporting cells of the CNS (astrocytes) and usually arise in the gray matter. Astrocytomas vary from extremely low-grade tumors to high-grade neoplasms with extensive necrosis. Low-grade gliomas (grade I) may be difficult to distinguish from reactive astrocytosis (a reactive proliferation of astrocytes in response to brain injury or infarcts) on brain biopsy. Low-grade astrocytomas are compatible with prolonged survival although they may cause seizures or blockage of CSF flow, leading to hydrocephalus. Most low-grade gliomas diffusely infiltrate brain tissue, and their margins are difficult to define grossly or microscopically. As a result, complete local excision of low-grade gliomas is uncommon (because of the severe neurologic deficits that would result from a large resection).

Intermediate-grade astrocytomas (grades II and III) are more cellular and show some pleomorphism but usually lack necrosis (Fig. 14-11A). Grade IV astrocytomas (so-called glioblastoma multiforme) is a high-grade neoplasm that characteristically shows prominent vascular proliferation and palisading of tumor cells about foci of tumor necrosis (see Figs. 14-11B and 14-11C). Glioblastoma multiforme often crosses the midline to involve the contralateral cerebral hemisphere and usually results in death within months to a few years (see Fig. 14-11D).

Pilocytic astrocytoma is a glial tumor that is more common in children and has a markedly better prognosis than other forms of astrocytoma. Pilocytic astrocytomas are composed predominantly of elongated cell processes (pilocytes), often with so-called Rosenthal fibers, which are eosinophilic glial cells. Pilocytic astrocytomas usually occur in the cerebellum and tend to be sharply circumscribed (in contrast with other gliomas), and they are often resectable.

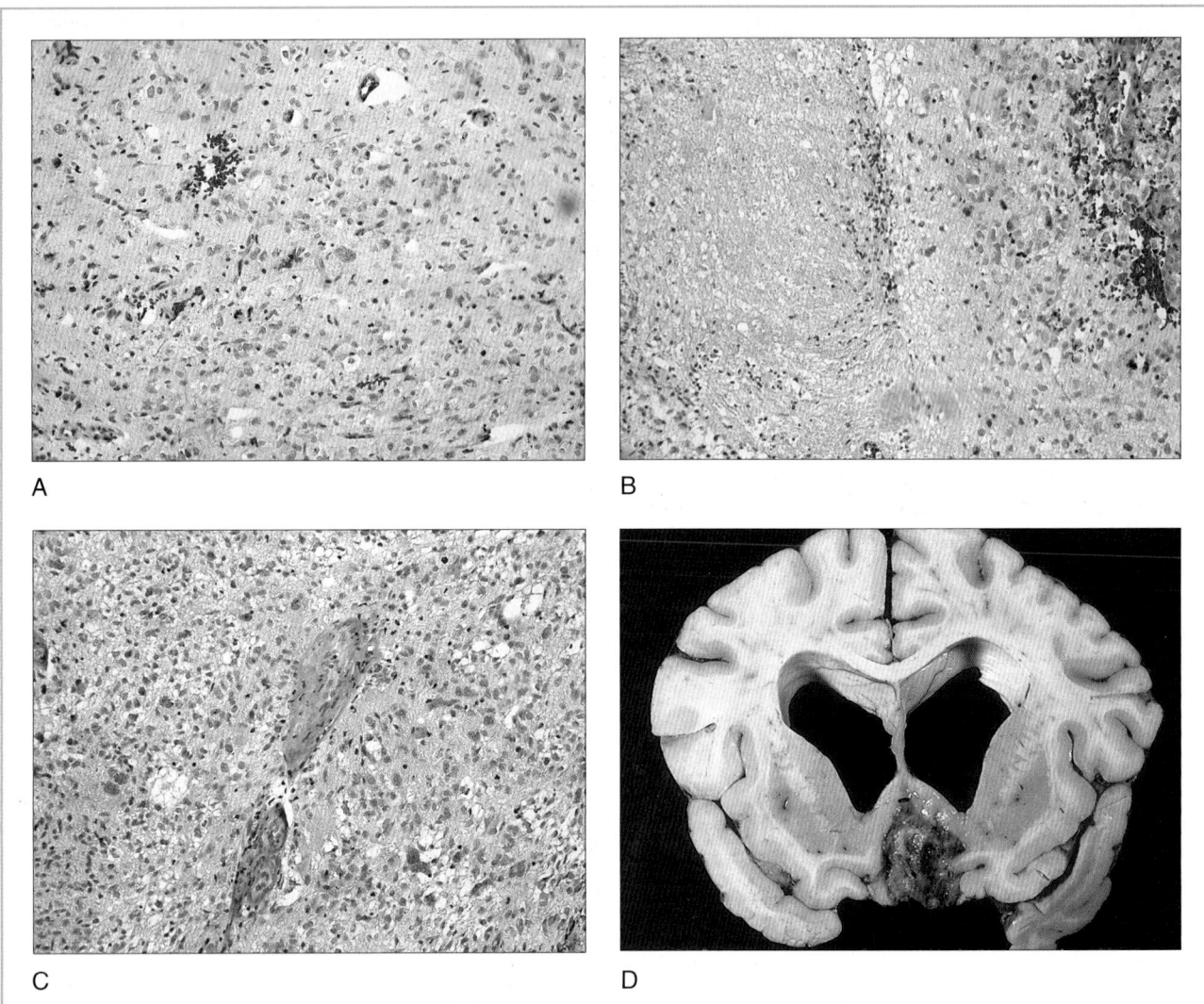

Figure 14-11. A, Astrocytoma. Microscopic section of a grade 2–3 astrocytoma. The tumor has infiltrative margins and is a moderately cellular neoplasm composed of pleomorphic glial cells. No necrosis is present, and vascular proliferation is not observed. **B,** Glioblastoma multiforme. Microscopic section showing extensive tumor necrosis with palisading (alignment) of tumor cells around the area of necrosis. **C,** Glioblastoma multiforme. Microscopic section showing prominent vascular proliferation and pleomorphic glial tumor cells. **D,** Glioblastoma multiforme. Gross cross-section of brain showing a hemorrhagic necrotic tumor in the hypothalamus (midline) that caused obstruction of CSF flow resulting in secondary hydrocephalus (prominent ventricular dilatation).

Oligodendroglioma

Oligodendrogliomas derive from oligodendroglial cells (which provide myelin sheaths for axons in the CNS) and usually arise in the white matter. Tumor cells usually have a typical "fried egg" appearance with clear cytoplasm resembling normal oligodendroglial cells (Fig. 14-12). Oligodendrogliomas have a substantially better prognosis than astrocytomas and often demonstrate chromosome 1p and/or 19q deletions, which confer a favorable prognosis. Occasional tumors show combined features of astrocytoma and oligodendroglioma and have a somewhat better prognosis than pure astrocytic tumors.

Ependymoma

Ependymomas arise from the ependymal cells that line the ventricles and central canal of the spinal cord. These tumors typically show rosette formation and have a more epithelial appearance than glial tumors (Fig. 14-13). Ependymomas are usually less aggressive than astrocytomas and often present with signs of CSF obstruction. A unique variant of ependymoma, myxopapillary ependymoma, occurs in the distal spinal cord (filum terminale) and has a distinctive morphologic appearance and excellent prognosis. Myxopapillary ependymomas must be distinguished from chordomas (tumors of notochord remnants), which also occur at this location.

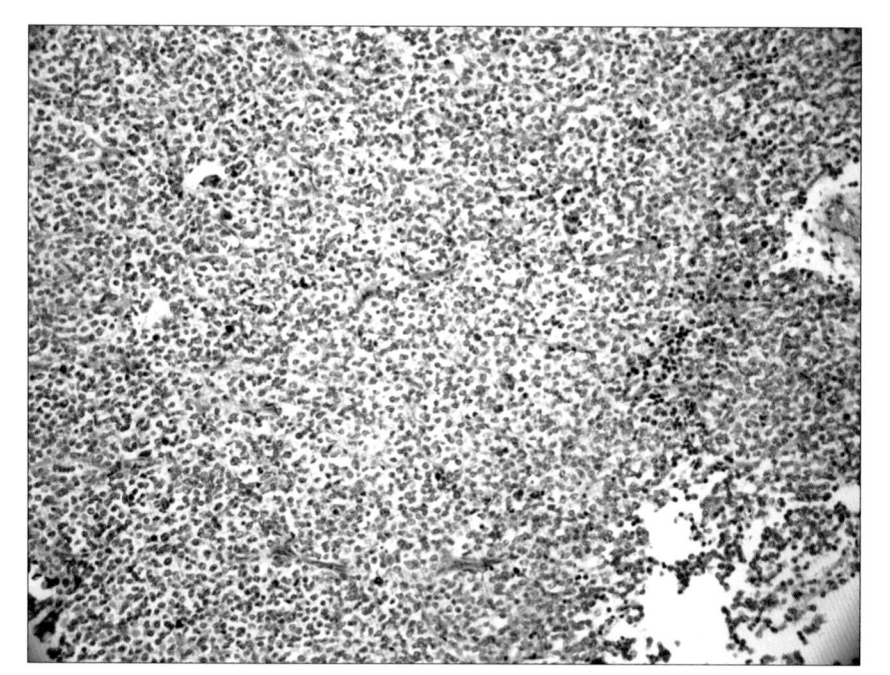

Figure 14-12. Oligodendroglioma. Microscopic section showing the typical "fried egg" appearance of tumor cells in this grade 2–3 oligodendroglioma.

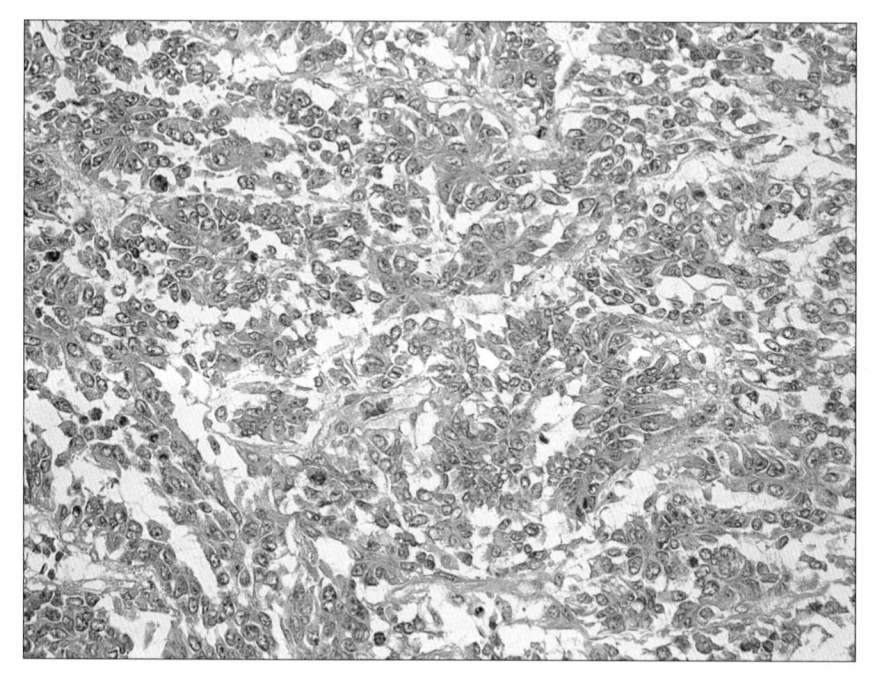

Figure 14-13. Ependymoma. Microscopic section showing cytologically bland, epithelium-like tumor cells forming prominent rosettes.

Meningioma

Meningiomas are tumors of the meningeal coverings of the brain. Meningiomas can have a variety of different microscopic patterns including fibrillary, psammomatous (numerous psammoma bodies are present with spindled tumor cells), and meningotheliomatous (Fig. 14-14). None of these patterns is prognostically significant. Most meningiomas are low grade, and mitotic activity is somewhat predictive of clinical behavior. Meningiomas tend to be circumscribed and are almost always clearly separate from brain parenchyma, making it possible to completely resect these tumors with minimal loss of neurologic function. Meningiomas grow slowly, displacing brain tissue, and many present with seizures.

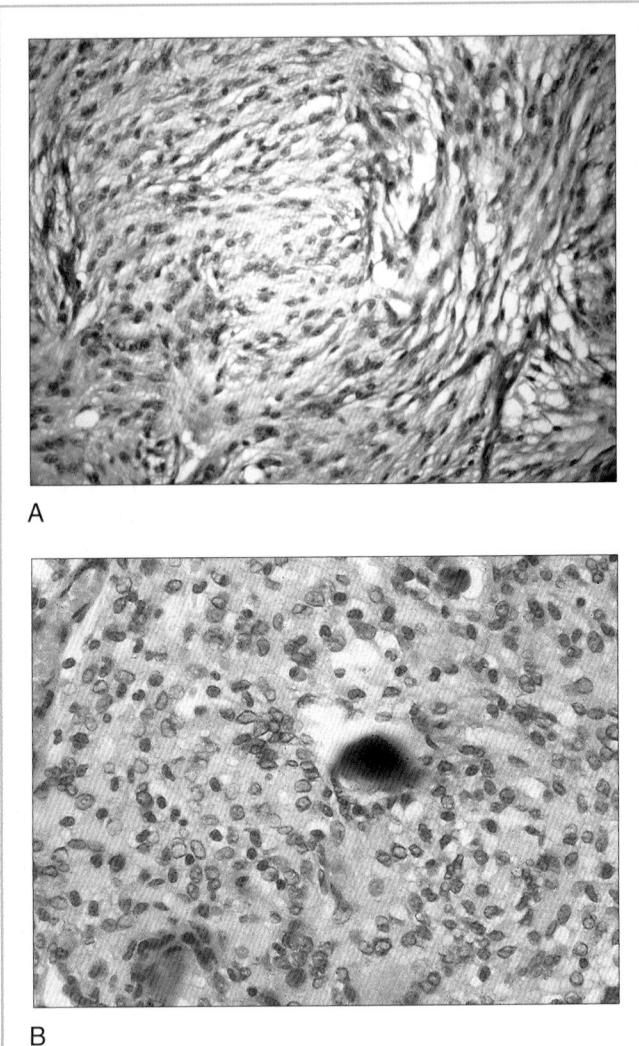

Figure 14-14. A, Meningioma. Microscopic section showing typical whorled pattern formed by cytologically bland tumor spindle cells. **B,** Microscopic section of a meningioma showing a typical psammoma body.

Some meningiomas may induce bone formation in overlying skull, resulting in a characteristic radiographic presentation.

Retinoblastoma and Medulloblastoma

Both retinoblastoma and medulloblastoma are rare, small, blue round-cell tumors of childhood. Retinoblastoma is a rare tumor of retinal epithelial cells that almost always occurs in early childhood and usually presents with unilateral visual loss and leukocoria (white reflex to light shined on the retina). Patients with retinoblastoma confined to the orbit are often cured by radical surgery (orbital exenteration). Familial cases with bilateral tumors may be treated with irradiation to salvage useful vision in one eye. Patients with extension beyond the orbit or with distant metastases usually have a poor response to conventional therapy. Retinoblastoma has played an important role in understanding the role of tumor

suppressor genes in tumor development (see Chapter 5). Medulloblastomas are malignant tumors of the midline cerebellum in children that are aggressive neoplasms and may metastasize outside the CNS.

Metastatic Tumors

In adults, metastatic tumors to the CNS greatly outnumber primary brain tumors. The presence of a solitary brain metastasis can be confused with a primary brain tumor, and distinction is critical for selecting appropriate therapy. Brain biopsy (either open or stereotactic needle biopsy) is often required to establish a specific diagnosis. Non–small cell lung cancer is a particularly common cause of brain metastasis.

Other Tumors

Hemangioblastoma is a tumor of the cerebellum that characteristically occurs in patients with von Hippel–Lindau disease and is related to genetic alterations in this tumor suppressor gene. Hemangioblastomas are benign tumors but often result in hemorrhagic complications that may be fatal. Patients with tuberous sclerosis develop tumor-like masses in the CNS (called tubers) that may produce seizure foci.

Severely immunosuppressed individuals are at increased risk for CNS lymphomas (usually large-cell B-cell lymphomas). Some lymphoproliferative diseases and leukemias can also secondarily involve the CNS. Hematopoietic tumor cells tend to fill Virchow-Robin spaces around cerebral blood vessels before invading brain parenchyma. The CNS is an important sanctuary site for leukemia cells in childhood acute lymphoblastic leukemia, and direct treatment of the CNS with intrathecal chemotherapy can decrease the likelihood of CNS relapse.

●●● TUMORS OF THE PERIPHERAL NERVOUS SYSTEM

Peripheral nerve tumors often present as mass lesions rather than with symptoms related to neuronal dysfunction. When neural tumors occur in parenchymal organs, they may be confused with more common primary tumors of that organ, or with sarcomas when they arise in soft tissue. Anatomic attachment to a nerve is a diagnostic clue. Most neural tumors express S100 protein, which is a useful immunohistochemical marker although it is expressed in other tumors (e.g., melanoma) as well.

Schwannoma

Schwannomas are tumors of the Schwann cells that produce the myelin sheaths about peripheral nerves. Schwannomas usually have a characteristic morphologic appearance with fibrillary tumor cells palisading in parallel arrays (so-called Antoni A and Antoni B areas) (Fig. 14-15A). Most schwannomas are benign and are sharply circumscribed from surrounding tissue. Schwannomas can cause neural dysfunc-

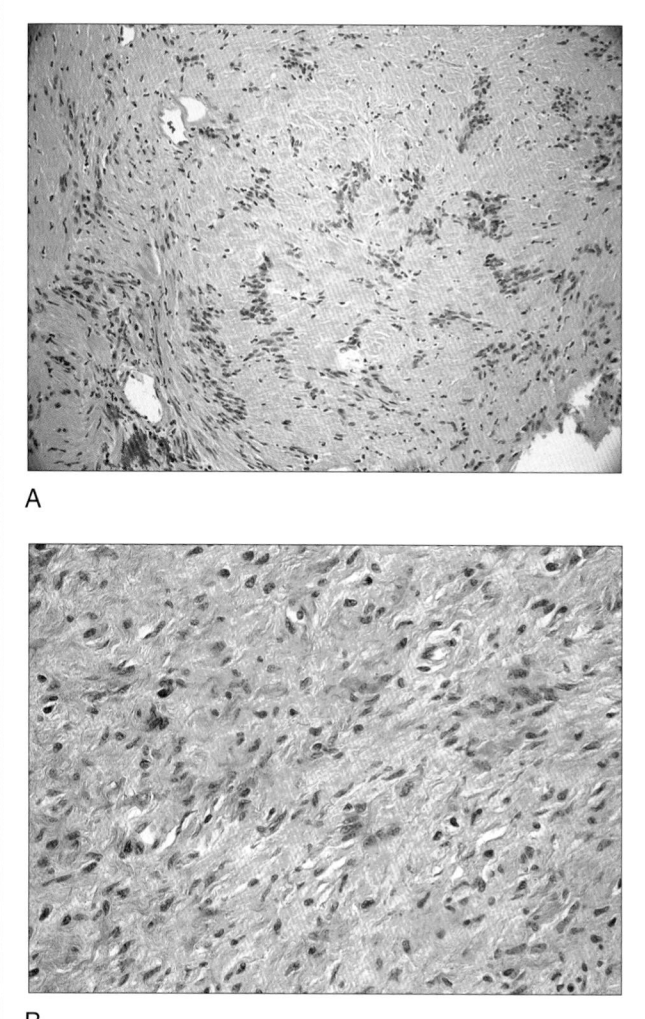

A

B

tion, and schwannomas of the eighth nerve (acoustic neuromas) typically present with hearing loss. Acoustic neuromas may be sporadic or associated with type II neurofibromatosis. Deep-seated schwannomas in patients with genetic neurofibromatosis (see below) are more likely to undergo malignant degeneration than are sporadic schwannomas.

Neurofibroma

Neurofibromas can occur sporadically, but patients with multiple neurofibromas often have genetic neurofibromatosis. Most sporadic neurofibromas occur in the skin and mucous membranes, where they are poorly circumscribed lesions composed of spindle cells with elongated wavy nuclei (see Fig. 14-15B). Mast cells are usually prominent in neurofibromas and can be helpful diagnostically. Most sporadic neurofibromas are small and do not produce significant clinical symptoms. Patients with genetic neurofibromatosis tend to develop many neurofibromas, which often grow to large size and cause significant dysfunction and deformity.

Patients with neurofibromatosis type 1 have mutations in the NF1 tumor suppressor gene that normally down-regulates RAS signaling. These patients tend to develop numerous plexiform neurofibromas and schwannomas that have an increased risk for malignant degeneration (particularly in deep-seated tumors). Affected patients often have café-au-lait spots (flat pigmented lesions of the skin), which may suggest the diagnosis. Patients with neurofibromatosis type II have mutations of the merlin gene and have a much different constellation of findings, with acoustic neuromas, meningiomas, and characteristic spinal neurofibromas.

Figure 14-15. **A**, Schwannoma. Microscopic section showing prominent palisading of tumor cell nuclei that have elongated, slightly wavy contours. **B**, Neurofibroma. Microscopic section showing plexiform neurofibroma with thin, wavy tumor cell nuclei. Palisading of tumor cell nuclei is not present.

Case Studies

Chapter 1: Acetaminophen Poisoning

A 47-year-old nurse is brought to the emergency room by ambulance after her landlord found her unconscious in her apartment. On physical examination, she is comatose with obvious scleral icterus. Her blood pressure is 100/60 with a hematocrit of 38%. Chemical examination of her serum shows a bilirubin level that is three times normal and aspartate transaminase (AST) and alanine transaminase (ALT) levels that are more than 50 times normal. On questioning, the patient's co-workers indicate that she seemed despondent and withdrawn for the past week and had not come in for a scheduled work shift 2 days go. Examination of the patient's apartment identified a large (300 tablet), open, empty container labeled acetaminophen in the patient's bedroom.

Despite maximum supportive measures including intubation, mechanical ventilation, and hemodialysis, the patient's condition continued to deteriorate, with increasing serum ammonia and bilirubin levels. She died on the fifth hospital day, and an autopsy was performed.

1. What is the most likely diagnosis?

2. What is the mechanism of acetaminophen toxicity, and why is the liver targeted?

3. What findings would you expect at autopsy?

Chapter 2: Toxic Shock Syndrome

A 27-year-old woman comes to the emergency room with hypotension and decreased mental status. She was brought to the ED by her husband, who said that she had been well during the morning but had become rapidly ill over the past 2 hours. Physical examination shows a normally-developed woman with a rapid pulse and dry warm skin. Her temperature is 38.5°C, and respiratory rate is 42/min. Blood pressure is 80 systolic, and hematocrit is 43%. A urine toxicology screen is negative for drugs of abuse.

Intravenous (IV) fluids are started, and additional history is obtained from the patient's husband. The patient had had severe menstrual bleeding during the last week when they were visiting relatives in another state. She had used super-absorbent tampons during the last few days to manage bleeding. They had driven home during the previous day and a half. The patient may or may not have changed her tampon during the last 36 hours. On pelvic examination, the tampon has a foul odor, and bacterial culture shows a pure population of *Staphylococcus aureus*.

Antibiotic therapy was started immediately with vancomycin, and the patient's blood pressure was supported with IV fluids, crystalloid, and fresh-frozen plasma. She improved on this therapy and became oriented to place and time, with a blood pressure of 120/75 mm Hg. Eighteen hours after admission, her urine output abruptly diminished and she became anuric but otherwise appeared to be improving. She was managed expectantly, and diuresis occurred on the third hospital day with restoration of normal renal function.

1. Were this patient's symptoms caused by sepsis?

2. What other complications might have developed in this patient?

3. Why did acute renal failure develop?

Chapter 3: Cardiomyopathy

A 79-year-old man was admitted to the hospital because of increasingly severe shortness of breath and prominent edema in his legs. The patient was known to have had proteinuria for at least 6 months, and urine protein electrophoresis showed free lambda light chains (Bence Jones protein). The same monoclonal immunoglobulin protein was also detected on serum protein electrophoresis. A 24-hour urine collection demonstrated more than 3.2 g of protein excreted in 24 hours (normal, <150 mg). On physical examination, the patient had pitting pedal and lower leg edema. A few rales were heard on auscultation of the chest, but no cardiac murmurs were appreciated. The temperature was 36.5°C, heart rate was 73 beats/min, and respiratory rate was 24. The blood pressure was 80/40 mm Hg, and marked jugular venous distention was present.

Troponin I and creatine kinase isoenzymes were both in the normal range, and the electrocardiogram (ECG) showed normal sinus rhythm with no acute changes. Voltage amplitude on ECG was decreased in all leads. The chest radiograph demonstrated bilateral pleural effusions, and diffuse irregular densities were noted in both lung fields. A cardiac ultrasound study showed left atrial dilatation but no valvular abnormalities. The left ventricular wall was symmetrically thickened, with diminished motion. The estimated ejection fraction was 42% (normal range, 55% to 75%). A therapeutic thoracentesis removed 1200 mL of transudate fluid (specific gravity, 1.010 g/mL) from the right side of the chest, and the cytologic study was negative for tumor cells. The patient was treated with a diuretic (furosemide), but his shortness of breath and peripheral edema continued to worsen. Repeat troponin I and creatinine kinase levels were in the normal range. An endomyocardial biopsy was performed.

1. **What are the significant symptoms and physical signs in this patient?**

2. **What is the most likely cause of this patient's condition?**

3. **What is the endomyocardial biopsy likely to show?**

Chapter 4: Krabbe's Disease

A 7-month-old girl is brought to your office because of failure to thrive. The child was the product of an uncomplicated 38-week gestation and was normal at birth. She was at or near the median for height and weight at her 3- and 6-month examinations. Recently she has shown less interest in breast-feeding and is now somnolent most of the time. Physical examination shows a minimally arousable infant in no distress. She shows minimal response to visual and auditory stimuli but responds to noxious stimuli. She appears to move all extremities equally, and funduscopic examination is unremarkable. There is no history of unusual food ingestion, and no one else in the household is ill. On further questioning, her mother describes a similar illness in one of her sister's children. This infant was diagnosed with Krabbe's disease at 18 months and died at 3 years of age. Your patient's father and mother are both of Syrian descent and share a number of second- and third-degree relatives.

On the basis of this family history, you suspect that the child may have Krabbe's disease and send a blood sample for genetic testing of the galactocerebrosidase gene, which is altered in patients with Krabbe's disease. The diagnosis is confirmed by the findings of mutations in both alleles of the patient's galactocerebrosidase gene. You refer the child for evaluation for possible stem cell transplantation using cord blood from an HLA-matched unrelated donor. After myeloablative therapy and stem cell transplantation, the child

has partial engraftment in her bone marrow (confirmed by genetic testing) and has subjective improvement in neurologic function (more response to visual and auditory stimuli). Over the next 2 years, her neurologic function declined and she fell behind all developmental milestones and eventually died at 6 years of age.

1. **What pathologic changes would you expect to find in the child's brain?**

2. **Can bone marrow transplantation cure this disease?**

3. **What are cord blood stem cells?**

Chapter 5: Non–Small Cell Lung Cancer with EGFR Mutation

A 60-year-old man visits a private medical doctor with complaints of shortness of breath and coughing up blood. The chest radiograph shows a large left lower lobe mass, and needle biopsy confirms the diagnosis of non–small cell carcinoma. Computed tomographic (CT) scan of the chest shows bilateral mediastinal lymphadenopathy and mediastinoscopy, and biopsy of contralateral mediastinal lymph nodes shows metastatic squamous cell carcinoma. On the basis of these staging findings (AJCC stage IIIB (pT3, pN3, pMX), the patient's tumor is not curable by surgery, and he is treated with radiation and chemotherapy. The patient has an objective response to combined modality therapy with 15% shrinkage of the tumor mass, but symptomatic liver metastases develop 5 months later.

Immunohistochemical staining of the patient's tumor shows strong membrane expression of the epidermal growth factor receptor (EGFR). Sequencing analysis of tumor cell DNA isolated from the diagnostic needle biopsy by laser capture microdissection shows an activating point mutation in one copy of the EGFR gene. This mutation has been associated with response to gefitinib (a small-molecule EGFR inhibitor) in some clinical trials. The patient is treated with combination chemotherapy including gefitinib and has an objective response with marked shrinkage of liver metastases. He continues to respond to therapy but ultimately succumbs to lung cancer 3 years after the initial diagnosis.

1. **What is immunohistochemistry?**

2. **What is the role of pathologic staging in selecting therapy?**

3. **Is EGFR expression a prognostic, diagnostic, or predictive tumor biomarker in this case?**

Chapter 6: Sickle Cell Anemia and Osteomyelitis

A 15-year-old African American girl presents to the emergency room with difficulty walking. The patient is known to be homozygous for hemoglobin S. She is well known in the emergency room because of frequent pain crises, usually managed with hydration and pain medications. The patient has not been transfusion dependent and has had no other major complications related to her sickle cell disease. She denies illicit drug use and sexual activity. On physical examination, she appears in acute distress with a temperature of 38.3°C, heart rate of 85 beats/min, and respiratory rate of 32. She gives no history of trauma, but says that pain has been increasing in her right leg over the last 5 to 6 days and that she now has trouble walking.

Examination of her right leg shows marked point tenderness over the distal right femur. The knee joint appears unremarkable on examination with intact ligaments and no palpable joint effusion. The skin overlying the area of point tenderness is slightly warm to touch. Laboratory examination shows a white blood cell count of 13,000/mm^3 including 80% neutrophils and 5% band forms. Her hematocrit is 25% with 1% reticulocytes. Hemoglobin electrophoresis shows 70% hemoglobin S and 30% hemoglobin F with no detectable hemoglobin A.

Three sets of blood cultures are drawn, and the patient is empirically started on a cephalosporin antibiotic. She is admitted to the hospital and transfused with two units packed red blood cells. On the second hospital day, two of three blood cultures are reported to show gram-negative rods, which are subsequently classified as *Salmonella typhi*. These findings confirm the clinical impression of bacterial osteomyelitis. The patient is started on intravenous antibiotics chosen on the basis of in vitro antibiotic susceptibility testing of the cultured organism for a planned 6-week course. After 2 weeks of antibiotic therapy, radiographic evaluation of the femur shows enlargement of the lesion with extension into the epiphysis and a new central area of opacity. A focus of necrotic bone (sequestrum) is suspected to be present within the bone infection, and the patient is taken to surgery on the 23rd hospital day for en bloc resection of the distal femur and repair with a cadaveric bone graft.

1. What are the likely morphologic findings in the bone resection specimen?

2. Why did the initial antibiotic therapy fail?

3. What factors predisposed this patient to osteomyelitis?

Chapter 7: Hypertrophic Cardiomyopathy

A 29-year-old white man presented to the emergency room with a 2-month history of fatigue with decreased exercise tolerance. He was always active in numerous team sports but had recently experienced difficulty with base running during softball games because of severe shortness of breath. During the past 2 nights he has had difficulty sleeping, and he propped himself up in bed to make himself more comfortable. On questioning, he recalls two fainting spells over the past 3 years, both related to physical exertion. He denies recreational drug use and takes no medications. He has not sought medical attention in the past 12 years and has never experienced chest pain. He is a moderate drinker but admits to occasional binge drinking.

The patient's father died of "heart disease" at 42 years of age. One paternal aunt and one uncle also died of "heart disease" in their 40s or 50s. One 37-year-old male cousin is being treated by a "heart doctor" in another state. His mother and two younger siblings are alive and well. His older sister died at 35 because of a "complicated pregnancy."

The patient is a well-developed young male who appears uncomfortable. He has mild pedal edema with a normal neurologic examination. Chest auscultation reveals fine crackles at the lung bases. Cardiac examination shows a mild systolic ejection murmur, and minimal jugular venous distention is noted. His blood pressure is 145/95 mm Hg with a pulse of 90 beats per minute. Chest radiograph shows small bilateral pleural effusions and patchy infiltrates in the lower lobes. The cardiac shadow is 1.5 times the normal width. ECG shows normal rate and rhythm with increased peak voltage in all leads. Doppler echocardiography shows marked thickening and dilatation of the left ventricle with disproportionate septal thickening. The ejection fraction is 30% with symmetrically diminished wall motion. A diagnostic procedure is performed.

1. The primary pathologic abnormality is in which organ system?

2. What is the most likely pathologic diagnosis?

3. Are the patient's illness and family history consistent with a genetic disease?

4. Why is the patient's ejection fraction reduced?

Chapter 8: Familial Asthma

A 10-year-old boy comes to your office with difficulty breathing and marked wheezing. He has a history of atopy with severe allergy to ragweed and other environmental allergens. He has not shown evidence of restrictive airway disease in the past but now has definite wheezing. Treatment with bronchodilators reverses the bronchoconstriction and produces symptomatic improvement. Over the next 2 years, the child has increasing respiratory symptoms and is seen multiple times in local emergency rooms with shortness of breath and prominent wheezing. Attempts to limit home and school environmental exposure to allergens are not effective. Three days ago, he had status asthmaticus that required hospitalization for 1 day.

On further investigation, the mother also had asthma in childhood, which diminished in severity after age 25. Two of her brothers and one sister also have asthma. Based on the strong family history of asthma, you meet with the parents and discuss the possibility of performing genetic testing for abnormalities in the IL-13 gene in affected family members. The parents agree and provide informed consent to participate in a national study evaluating the role of IL-13 gene polymorphisms in asthma. Analysis of the child's and mother's DNA shows polymorphisms in the coding sequence of the IL-13 gene that result in a nonconservative substitution of glutamine for arginine at position 2044.

1. **What is the role of IL-13 in the development of asthma?**

2. **What other therapeutic options would you consider for this patient?**

3. **What pathologic changes would you expect to find in a lung biopsy specimen?**

Chapter 9: Gastric Malt Lymphoma

A 50-year-old woman visits your gastroenterology practice with complaints of heartburn. The symptoms have been severe and unremitting for the past 3 months and have responded poorly to over-the-counter H_2 blockers. You schedule the patient for upper endoscopy and find erosions of the gastroesophageal junction as well as diffuse thickening of the gastric mucosa with partial disappearance of rugal folds. The gastric mucosa appears markedly edematous and hyperemic, and you take multiple biopsy specimens from the antrum and fundus.

Pathologic examination of the endoscopic specimens shows a dense infiltrate composed of small lymphocytes and plasma cells in the lamina propria with lymphoid nodules. Prominent lymphoepithelial lesions (small aggregates of lymphocytes within the gastric epithelium) are present. Special stains show numerous *Helicobacter pylori* organisms in gastric mucus. Because of the extensive lymphoplasmacytic infiltrate, immunohistochemical stains are performed that show most of the lymphocytes to be small B cells with a scattering of T cells. PCR analysis of DNA isolated from both fundic and antral biopsy specimens to assess possible clonal immunoglobulin heavy chain gene rearrangement shows monoclonal bands of identical size in both.

1. **What is the most likely diagnosis based on these findings?**

2. **What further studies would you undertake?**

3. **What is the most appropriate treatment for this patient?**

Chapter 10: Diabetes Mellitus

You are consulted about a 12-year-old girl who enjoys playing video games and watching television but has avoided sports and other types of physical activity. Her height is at the 55th percentile for age, and her weight is at the 98th percentile with a calculated body mass index (BMI) of 30. In prior years, her schoolwork was in the B+ range, but her school performance has declined recently, leading to several parent-teacher conferences. The patient is the result of a normal pregnancy and weighed 8 lb 7 oz at birth. She had been at the 60th to 70th percentile for weight and near the median for height throughout early childhood but began to gain weight rapidly after her ninth birthday. She now weighs 160 lb and is 5 ft 1 in. tall.

Because of concern about her school performance, her parents consult their pediatrician, who finds a positive urine dipstick test for glucose. A random serum glucose is 250 mg/dL. Urinalysis does not show evidence of ketones. A subsequent fasting serum glucose level is 150 mg/dL with elevated serum insulin levels. A diagnosis of diabetes mellitus is made, and oral hypoglycemic agents are prescribed as well as a weight management diet and increased exercise. The child loses 5 lb over the next 3 weeks but regains this weight and increases her BMI to 32 over the next 6 months. Reevaluation at this time shows a random serum glucose of 220 mg/dL.

1. **Does this patient have type 1 or type 2 diabetes mellitus?**

2. **How does increased central adipose tissue affect insulin action?**

3. **What other diseases is this child at increased risk for?**

4. **Is this child likely to have a mutation in her leptin gene?**

Chapter 11: Hodgkin's Disease

A 28-year-old woman noticed a nodule in her right axilla while performing routine self-examination for breast cancer. She immediately went to her family practitioner, who identified a 3-cm, firm, mobile ovoid mass in the right axilla consistent with an enlarged, firm lymph node. No breast masses were palpated. The patient had been in good health with no prior malignancies or serious diseases. She did not have night sweats and felt well. Chest radiograph showed prominent mediastinal widening, and subsequent CT scan of the thorax and abdomen showed multiple enlarged right axillary lymph nodes as well as multiple lymph nodes in the mediastinum measuring up to 5 cm.

On the basis of these findings, the patient was referred to a general surgeon, who performed an excisional lymph node biopsy. On pathologic examination, the axillary lymph node measures 2.5 cm in maximal dimension and appears fibrous on cut section. A portion of lymph node is submitted for flow cytometry, and analysis shows a mixture of polytypical B and T cells, with T cells predominating. Histologic study of the lymph node shows effacement of the normal lymph node architecture by a polymorphic infiltrate composed of lymphocytes, plasma cells, eosinophils, and atypical mononuclear cells. Substantial collagenous fibrosis is also present in the lymph node, dividing it into nodules. Immunohistochemical stains show the large atypical mononuclear cells to be positive for CD30, CD15, and Epstein-Barr virus latent membrane protein (LMP-1). These cells are negative for leukocyte common antigen as well as B- and T-cell differentiation antigens. PCR assays for monoclonal immunoglobulin and T-cell receptor gene rearrangement in DNA isolated from lymph node tissue do not show evidence of a monoclonal tumor cell population.

A bone marrow biopsy is performed on the basis of these findings. The bone marrow biopsy shows normocellular bone marrow with no focal lesions and no evidence of metastatic tumor. CT scans of the abdomen and pelvis are within normal limits. The patient is begun on a course of radiation therapy using a mantle port (targeting the mediastinum) with a boost to the right axilla.

1. **What causes prominent tumor fibrosis in this disease?**

2. **Is the pathologic stage important in choosing therapy for this patient?**

3. **Is this patient likely to be cured by radiation therapy?**

4. **What is the role of Epstein-Barr virus and chromosomal translocations in this tumor?**

Chapter 12: Transitional Cell Carcinoma of the Bladder

A 75-year-old man comes to your office with complaints of hematuria for the past 4 months. On physical examination, he is a well-nourished elderly man with a persistent cough and a 40-pack-year smoking history. Urinalysis shows numerous red blood cells (but no red cell casts) with a few white cells. Urine culture is negative, but urine cytologic study shows a few atypical papillary clusters of urothelial cells. The postvoid residual urine volume is 100 mL, consistent with moderate prostatic obstruction. Digital rectal examination shows an enlarged, boggy prostate without nodularity. Creatinine and blood urea nitrogen are within the normal range, and serum PSA is 3.1 ng/mL. Chest radiograph shows mild-to-moderate emphysema, but no mass lesions are identified.

On the basis of these findings, you refer the patient for cystoscopy, which shows three large papillary tumors in the region of the trigone, dome, and right lateral wall. Each of these tumors is excised by means of electrocautery, and the excised material is sent for pathologic examination. The lesion from the trigone and dome each shows grade 1/3 papillary transitional cell carcinoma with focal submucosal invasion but no evidence of deep muscle or vascular space invasion. The right lateral wall tumor shows a grade 3/3 transitional cell carcinoma with deep muscle invasion.

1. **What additional studies should be performed at this time, and what are the most likely sites for metastatic tumor spread?**

2. **If the patient's metastatic disease workup is negative, what is the most appropriate therapeutic approach?**

3. **What is the most important risk factor for the development of transitional cell carcinoma in this patient?**

Chapter 13: Breast Cancer

A 40-year-old G_1P_1 woman goes to her primary care doctor because she has noticed a slight asymmetry in her left breast during the last month. The patient is otherwise in good health and has no other physical complaints. Breast examination shows a subtle fullness in the lower outer quadrant of her left breast. There is no skin change or nipple retraction, and no axillary adenopathy is palpable. The patient is referred for a mammogram, which is completed during the next week. The radiology report describes a 1.3-cm area of spiculation in the lower outer quadrant of the left breast with associated microcalcifications. This lesion had not been present on her baseline mammogram 2 years ago.

The patient is scheduled for ultrasound-guided needle biopsy of the mass. Ultrasound demonstrates a 1.0-cm irregular mass in the same location as identified by mammography. The needle biopsy shows an invasive ductal carcinoma, modified Bloom-Richardson grade 3/3. Immunohistochemical stains show tumor cells to be negative for estrogen and progesterone receptors and equivocally positive for HER2/neu protein (2+ cytoplasmic membrane staining). Subsequent FISH analysis shows high-level HER2/neu gene amplification with approximately six HER2/neu hybridization signals per tumor cell. The patient is scheduled for local excision of the mass (lumpectomy) with sentinel lymph node biopsy. At the time of surgery, a cocktail of radioactive tracer is injected into the tumor site several hours prior to its excision. Following lumpectomy, a radiation detector is used to identify the most radioactive lymph nodes in the axilla for excisional biopsy.

Pathologic examination of the breast mass shows an invasive ductal carcinoma measuring 1.2 cm in greatest dimension with an associated high-grade intraductal carcinoma of the comedo type with 3 mm clear margins. Examination of the sentinel lymph node shows a single focus of metastatic adenocarcinoma (measuring 3 mm in diameter) in a subcapsular sinus. A bone scan is negative for metastatic disease as are CT scans of the chest and abdomen.

On the basis of these findings, an axillary lymph node dissection is performed 3 weeks later. The 15 axillary lymph nodes removed are pathologically negative for tumor. The patient is treated with radiation therapy to the breast followed by standard adjuvant chemotherapy. The patient makes a full recovery with good cosmesis, but 18 months later she is found to have a left pleural effusion. Cytologic examination of the effusion shows metastatic adenocarcinoma consistent with breast cancer. The patient is treated with trastuzumab (Herceptin) with concurrent chemotherapy and has an objective response with resolution of the pleural effusion.

1. What is the significance of HER2/neu gene amplification in this cancer?

2. What is the role of HER2/neu in tumorigenesis?

3. What is the significance of a 3-mm metastasis in the sentinel lymph node?

4. Why was an axillary dissection performed, what are its possible complications?

Chapter 14: New Variant Creutzfeldt-Jakob Disease

A 32-year-old man is brought to the emergency room by the police. He was involved in a dispute with his roommate that led to physical violence. On questioning by the police, the patient indicates that his roommate and several neighbors were plotting against him and that his father had convinced them to do this. On examination, his recent memory is only partially intact and he is oriented to person but not to place or time. Physical examination is otherwise unremarkable aside for a few minor abrasions. A urine toxicology screen does not show evidence of drugs of abuse, and his blood alcohol level is undetectable. According to family members, the patient appeared to be in good health until approximately 1 month ago, when his personality seemed to change abruptly and he began having trouble remembering day-to-day events. He was fired from his job as a video store clerk 1 week ago. The patient has lived in the United States since 2002, having lived in England throughout his childhood.

A trial of phenothiazine therapy results in mild improvement in mental status, but the patient's psychiatric symptoms continue to intensify, requiring hospitalization. Four weeks later the patient develops myoclonic jerks and is somnolent much of the time. He dies 4 months after the initial presentation. At autopsy his brain is of normal size and weight. Microscopic examination of brain tissue shows numerous amyloid plaques in the cerebral cortex and cerebellum and extensive spongiform changes in the cortex.

1. What is the most likely diagnosis?

2. What type of precautions should be taken in performing an autopsy on this patient?

3. Why doesn't his brain show evidence of atrophy?

4. What is the chemical nature of the amyloid plaques in this patient?

Case Study Answers

Chapter 1: Acetaminophen Poisoning

1. Self-induced acetaminophen poisoning resulting in massive hepatic necrosis.

2. Metabolism of acetaminophen by the liver produces free radicals, which rapidly consume intracellular glutathione in hepatocytes and then oxidize macromolecules, causing cell injury and death.

3. The liver is shrunken and weighs one third of the expected amount. Histologic examination shows diffuse coagulative necrosis. Most organs show extensive staining with bilirubin.

Chapter 2: Toxic Shock Syndrome

1. This patient probably did not have sepsis but developed staphylococcal toxic shock syndrome as a result of bacterial proteins (superantigens) released from bacteria growing in the contaminated tampon.

2. Staphylococcal sepsis and secondary infection are possible complications, since the patient's immune system is compromised by shock. Disseminated intravascular coagulation (DIC) could also cause in widespread hemorrhage.

3. The patient developed acute renal failure because of hypotension secondary to toxic shock syndrome. Decreased renal perfusion resulted in ischemic necrosis of metabolically active renal proximal tubular cells. Because the underlying extracellular matrix is not damaged, proliferation of tubular cell precursors resulted in complete recovery of renal function.

Chapter 3: Cardiomyopathy

1. This patient shows prominent signs of congestive heart failure but does not show evidence of an acute coronary syndrome. The finding of an enlarged heart with decreased electrocardiographic potentials suggests an infiltrative process in the myocardium. This is also consistent with the decreased ventricular motility demonstrated by ultrasound. The finding of a monoclonal protein raises the possibility of amyloidosis in association with plasma cell myeloma.

2. The most likely diagnosis is restrictive cardiomyopathy. Although many of the findings in this case are against a diagnosis of chronic ischemic heart disease (IHD), the high prevalence of IHD in developed countries makes it an important consideration in the differential diagnosis.

3. The endomyocardial biopsy shows interstitial deposition of amyloid, which stained positive for Congo red. Myocytes are compressed and have undergone atrophy. Lambda light chains are prone to form amyloid, and patients with multiple myeloma that expresses lambda light chains are at high risk for this complication.

Chapter 4: Krabbe's Disease

1. Krabbe's disease results from homozygous deficiency of an enzyme required to degrade galactolipids produced in the cells that form myelin sheaths about axons in the nervous system (Schwann cells and oligodendroglial cells). Accumulation of galactolipids causes cellular dysfunction resulting in defective myelin deposition and abnormal neuronal function. Examination of the brain by light microscopy would show deficient myelination of the white matter with secondary loss of neurons.

2. Soluble enzyme released by donor leukocytes may be present in serum but is unlikely to cross the blood-brain barrier. Although we do not traditionally think of stem cells as being able to populate the central nervous system, some bone marrow–derived stem cells are capable of populating the brain in young children. Examination of brain tissue from patients with Krabbe's disease treated with bone marrow transplantation has shown that some donor-derived glial cells are present. Infants with Krabbe's disease treated with cord blood stem cells before the onset of symptoms have had a better response than the symptomatic patient described here in whom irreversible neurologic damage had already occurred.

3. Stem cells can be isolated from the small amount of blood remaining in umbilical cords after birth. These cells can be banked and expanded in vitro for therapeutic purposes. Cord blood stem cells are a potentially rich source of therapeutic stem cells.

Chapter 5: Non–Small Cell Lung Cancer with EGFR Mutation

1. Immunohistochemistry allows the detection of specific antigenic epitopes on tissue sections by means of monoclonal or polyclonal antibodies.

2. Pathologic stage determines whether a tumor can be cured by surgery or has advanced beyond the curative ability of a localized therapy. The finding of contralateral metastatic disease in the mediastinum makes this patient AJCC stage IIIB. Stage IIIB tumors are not curable by surgical excision alone.

3. In this case, EGFR gene expression and point mutations are predictive tumor biomarkers because their presence results in an increased likelihood of response to gefitinib, which targets this specific receptor tyrosine kinase.

Chapter 6: Sickle Cell Anemia and Osteomyelitis

1. The bone specimen shows evidence of ongoing acute osteomyelitis. Sections from the central portion of the specimen show a large discrete focus of necrotic bone (sequestrum) with viable bacteria.

2. The antibiotic therapy was ineffective because necrotic tissue is present at the center of the infection. Necrotic tissue provides a nidus for bacterial growth, since penetration of antibiotics into this avascular environment is minimal.

3. Patients with sickle cell anemia have frequent pain crises caused by bone infarcts. Any focus of necrotic tissue is an excellent nidus for the growth of bacteria that are present in the blood (bacteremia). Patients with sickle cell anemia characteristically develop *Salmonella typhi* osteomyelitis although the basis for this tropism is not well understood.

Chapter 7: Hypertrophic Cardiomyopathy

1. All the changes observed in this patient can be explained by heart failure with prominent diastolic dysfunction resulting in backup of pressure to the lungs and venous circulation. The accumulation of edema fluid at multiple sites is typical.

2. The most likely diagnosis is hypertrophic cardiomyopathy. The increased heart size and increased voltage on ECG are both consistent with a large increase in myocardial tissue mass. The patient's family history strongly suggests a genetic cause for his heart disease.

3. The family history is consistent with an autosomal dominant pattern of inheritance, which is typical of hypertrophic cardiomyopathy that results from missense mutations in contractile proteins.

4. The ejection fraction is reduced because this patient has advanced heart failure. The abnormal contractile proteins that cause hypertrophic cardiomyopathy result in defective contraction. The fibrosis associated with hypertrophic cardiomyopathy eventually causes systolic as well as diastolic dysfunction.

Chapter 8: Familial Asthma

1. IL-13 is an important cytokine that tends to reinforce T_H2 immune responses that are significant in many asthma patients.

2. Depending on the extent of his symptoms, corticosteroids and bronchodilators are the traditional drugs of choice. On the basis of recent evidence, you may also select a 5′-lipoxygenase inhibitor to block the formation of leukotrienes, which are important mediators of bronchospasm.

3. Hyperplasia of mucous cells, increased eosinophils, and hypertrophy of bronchial smooth muscle.

Chapter 9: Gastric Malt Lymphoma

1. Based on the morphologic and molecular findings, the tumor is a low-grade B-cell lymphoma of mucosa associated lymphoid tissue (MALT) arising in the setting of chronic *Helicobacter pylori* gastritis.

2. A patient with lymphoma requires clinical staging to assess the extent of disease. In this case, radiographic studies with contrast-enhanced CT of the abdomen and thorax are most appropriate. Bone marrow biopsy could also be performed to assess possible systemic involvement by this low-grade B-cell lymphoma.

3. If this patient has localized disease, a trial of antibiotic therapy to eliminate *H. pylori* is warranted. Some MALT lymphomas completely disappear after antibiotic treatment while other tumors (which have established autocrine growth pathways) persist and require cytotoxic chemotherapy.

Chapter 10: Diabetes Mellitus

1. This patient clearly has type 2 diabetes with insulin resistance documented by increased serum insulin levels in the face of hyperglycemia. The absence of ketosis is also consistent with type 2 diabetes.

2. Central adiposity results in the accumulation of abnormal adipose tissue deposits having high macrophage content. This type of adipose tissue produces more resistin and other substances that interfere with insulin action. Increased numbers of adipocytes also produce leptin, which also interferes with insulin action.

3. Diabetes mellitus is an important risk factor for atherosclerotic cardiovascular disease as well as direct complications of the disease itself.

4. No, leptin gene mutations are very rare causes of obesity that have been described in only a few families. Patients with homozygous leptin mutations become markedly obese very early in life.

Chapter 11: Hodgkin's Disease

1. Multiple cytokines and growth factors, including TGF-β, that are produced by Reed-Sternberg cells stimulate fibrosis. Some of the benign inflammatory cells recruited by Reed-Sternberg cells also produce mediators that stimulate fibrosis.

2. After the diagnosis of Hodgkin's disease is established, the patient's pathologic stage is the most important determinant of therapy. Most patients with stage I disease are cured by localized irradiation while patients with stage III or IV disease can be cured only by systemic chemotherapy.

3. This patient has stage II disease and has a good chance of cure by radiation therapy alone. If disease had been present below the diaphragm or if the diagnosis was mixed cellularity Hodgkin's disease, the patient would be less likely to be cured by irradiation and would have been treated with chemotherapy.

4. The precise role of EBV in Hodgkin's disease is unclear. Epidemiologic studies show a clear association between chronic infection with EBV and increased risk for Hodgkin's disease although tumor development is very rare. Expression of EBV-latent membrane protein (LMP-1) is more common in mixed cellularity Hodgkin's disease than in nodular sclerosis. Specific chromosomal translocations are not known to play an important role in Hodgkin's disease.

Chapter 12: Transitional Cell Carcinoma of the Bladder

1. The patient needs to be staged radiographically to identify possible metastatic spread of transitional cell carcinoma. Transitional cell carcinomas typically metastasize to the lungs and regional lymph nodes.

2. If comorbid disease does not preclude it, radical cystectomy with complete removal of the bladder and associated soft tissue is the preferred therapy for a deeply invasive, high-grade transitional cell carcinoma. An ileal loop ostomy site is created and anastomosed to the ureters to form an artificial bladder.

3. Cigarette smoking is the most important risk factor today. In the past, industrial exposure to aniline dyes and other carcinogens was an important cause of transitional cell carcinoma.

Chapter 13: Breast Cancer

1. HER2/neu gene amplification is a strong predictor of protein overexpression and of response to treatment with a monoclonal antibody directed against HER2/neu (trastuzumab [Herceptin]).

2. HER2/neu is a growth factor receptor, and stimulation of this receptor (by ligand or high receptor density in overexpressing cells) can promote cell cycle progression ($G_0 \rightarrow G_1$) in sensitive cells.

3. The patient has regional metastatic disease, and her other axillary lymph nodes may contain additional tumor deposits.

4. The presence of metastasis in more than three lymph nodes would up-stage this patient to N2 node status and would alter her AJCC tumor stage and her therapy plan. Therefore, evaluation of node status is critical for treatment planning. Axillary dissection can cause permanent lymphedema of the arm, resulting in significant pain and disability.

Chapter 14: New Variant Creutzfeldt-Jakob Disease

1. The patient's young age and rapid clinical course are not consistent with Alzheimer's disease. A diagnosis of Creutzfeldt-Jakob disease (CJD) is a consideration but is

unlikely based on the finding of numerous amyloid plaques throughout the brain. A diagnosis of new variant CJD seems most appropriate in this patient, who resided in England during the peak incidence of bovine spongiform encephalopathy (BSE).

2. In addition to universal precautions, prion-mediated diseases are resistant to most forms of decontamination including autoclaving and formaldehyde. For this reason, great care should be taken to limit contamination during the autopsy to prevent possible spread of disease.

3. The rapid progression of disease does not allow time for removal of damaged neural tissue.

4. The amyloid is composed of prion protein that has assumed a β-pleated sheet conformation.

Index

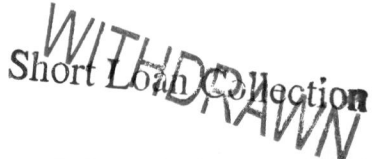